Epidemiology and Control of Hypertension

Epidemiology
and Control
of Hypertension

Editor
OGLESBY PAUL, M.D.

Papers and discussions from the Second International
Symposium on the Epidemiology of Hypertension presen-
ted September 1974 by the Chicago Heart Association; the
Council on Epidemiology and the Council on High Blood
Pressure Research of the American Heart Association; and
the National Heart and Lung Institute.

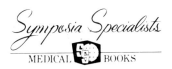

MEDICAL BOOKS

 STRATTON INTERCONTINENTAL MEDICAL BOOK CORPORATION

381 Park Avenue South, New York, New York 10016 and London

Library of Congress Catalog
Card No. 74-27863
ISBN 0-88372-026-4

iv

Contents

viii

Participants

John Abernethy, B. Med. Sc.
Project Director
National Blood Pressure Study
Canberra City, Australia

J. Gordon Barrow, M.D.
Coordinator
Georgia Regional Medical Program
Atlanta, Georgia

Robert Beaglehole, M.D.
Epidemiology Unit
Wellington Hospital
Wellington, New Zealand

Pierre Biron, M.D.
Associate Professor
Department of Pharmacology
University of Montreal
Montreal, Quebec, Canada

Sidney Blumenthal, M.D.
Professor of Pediatric Cardiology
University of Miami
Miami, Florida

Nemat O. Borhani, M.D.
Professor of Medicine
Professor and Chairman
Department of Community Health
School of Medicine
University of California at Davis
Davis, California

John C. Cassel, M.D.
Professor of Epidemiology
Department of Epidemiology
The School of Public Health
The University of North Carolina
Chapel Hill, North Carolina

Theodore Cooper, M.D.
Director
National Heart and Lung Institute
National Institutes of Health
Bethesda, Maryland

Colin T. Dollery, M.B.
Professor of Clinical Pharmacology
Royal Postgraduate Medical School
Hammersmith Hospital
London, England

Manning Feinleib, M.D.
Chief, Epidemiology Branch
Division of Heart and Vascular Diseases
National Heart and Lung Institute
Bethesda, Maryland

Frank A. Finnerty, Jr., M.D.
Professor of Medicine
The Georgetown University
  Medical Division
District of Columbia General Hospital
Washington, D.C.

Edward D. Freis, M.D.
Senior Medical Investigator
Veterans Administration Hospital
Washington, D.C.

S. Hatano, M.D.
Medical Officer
Cardiovascular Diseases
World Health Organization
Geneva, Switzerland

Victor M. Hawthorne, M.D.
Senior Lecturer
Department of Epidemiology &
  Preventive Medicine
University of Glasgow
Ruchill Hospital
Glasgow, Scotland

Walter W. Holland, M.D.
Professor of Clinical Epidemiology
  and Social Medicine
St. Thomas's Hospital and Medical School
London, England

William B. Kannel, M.D.
Medical Director

ix

Framingham Heart Disease and Epidemiology Study
National Heart and Lung Institute
Framingham, Massachusetts

Edward H. Kass, M.D., Ph.D.
William Ellery Channing
Professor of Medicine
Harvard Medical School
Director, Channing Laboratory
Boston, Massachusetts

Walter M. Kirkendall, M.D.
Professor and Director
Program in Internal Medicine
The University of Texas Medical School
  at Houston
Houston, Texas

Herbert G. Langford, M.D.
Professor of Medicine
Chief Endocrinology and
  Hypertension Division
The University of Mississippi
  Medical Center
Jackson, Mississippi

John H. Laragh, M.D.
Master Professor of Medicine
Director, Cardiovascular Center
New York Hospital-Cornell
  Medical Center
New York, New York

Richard Lovell, M.D.
Professor and Chairman
Department of Medicine
University of Melbourne
Royal Melbourne Hospital
Victoria, Australia

Wojciech Nowaczynski, D.Sc.
Director
Steroid Research Department
Clinical Research Institute of Montreal
Montreal, Quebec, Canada

Gaddo Onesti, M.D.
Professor of Medicine
Department of Medicine
Hahnemann Medical College
Philadelphia, Pennsylvania

H. Mitchell Perry, Jr., M.D.
Professor of Medicine

Washington University School of Medicine
Chief of Medical Services
St. Louis V.A. Hospital
St. Louis, Missouri

David L. Sackett, M.D.
Professor of Clinical Epidemiology
  and Biostatistics
Professor of Medicine
McMaster University Medical Centre
Hamilton, Ontario, Canada

James A. Schoenberger, M.D.
Professor and Chairman
Department of Preventive Medicine
Rush-Presbyterian-St. Luke's
  Medical Center
Chicago, Illinois

A. G. Shaper, M.D.
MRC Social Medicine Research Unit
The London School of Hygiene &
  Tropical Medicine
London, England

Norman M. Simon, M.D.
Associate Professor of Medicine
Northwestern University Medical School
Chicago, Illinois

W. McFate Smith, M.D., M.P.H.
Clinical Professor of Medicine and
  Associate Dean
University of California School of Medicine
San Francisco General Hospital
San Francisco, California

Jeremiah Stamler, M.D.
Harry W. Dingman Professor of
  Cardiology
Professor and Chairman
Department of Community Health &
  Preventive Medicine
Northwestern University Medical School
Chicago, Illinois

Louis Tobian, M.D.
Professor of Medicine
Department of Internal Medicine
University of Minnesota Medical School
Minneapolis, Minnesota

Herman A. Tyroler, M.D.
Professor of Epidemiology
Department of Epidemiology
The School of Public Health
The University of North Carolina
Chapel Hill, North Carolina

Gordon Williams, M.D.
Director, Endocrine-Metabolic Unit
Peter Bent Brigham Hospital

Associate Professor of Medicine
Harvard Medical School
Boston, Massachusetts

Warren Winkelstein, Jr., M.D.
Professor of Epidemiology and Dean
School of Public Health
University of California
Berkeley, California

xi

Acknowledgments

The Symposium was made possible by the encouragement and financial
support from
> Chicago Heart Association
> American Heart Association
> Ciba Pharmaceutical Company
> G. D. Searle and Company
> National Heart and Lung Institute,
> National Institutes of Health,
> United States Department of Health, Education
>   and Welfare, Contract No. NO1 HV 52905

Symposium Planning Committees

Chicago Heart Association

Oglesby Paul, M.D., Chairman
Mark Lepper, M.D.
Theodore Pullman, M.D.
James A. Schoenberger, M.D.
Jeremiah Stamler, M.D.
Earl Smith, M.D.
Raymond M. Restivo, Executive Director
Kay R. Westfall, Program Director
Helen Heck, Symposium Secretary
Kathy Kuntzman, Program Assistant

National and International Consultants

Nemat O. Borhani, M.D.
Lewis K. Dahl, M.D.
Colin T. Dollery, M.B.
William Kannel, M.D.
Edward H. Kass, M.D., Ph.D.
Walter M. Kirkendall, M.D.
Herberg G. Langford, M.D.
Richard Lovell, M.D.
Lysle H. Peterson, M.D.
Joseph A. Wilber, M.D.
Robert W. Wissler, Ph.D., M.D.

Foreword

This symposium is one of a series sponsored by the Chicago Heart Association. The Association takes great pride that these symposia have been so well attended and that the documents which have come forth from them have been looked upon as key references in the world medical literature. The subjects of the previous symposia were the pulmonary circulation in 1958 with Dr. Wright R. Adams as editor; the evolution of the atherosclerotic plaque in 1963 with Dr. Richard J. Jones as editor; the first international conference on the epidemiology of hypertension in 1964 with Dr. Theodore N. Pullman, Rose Stamler and Dr. Jeremiah Stamler as editors; the heart and circulation in the newborn and the infant in 1965 with Dr. Donald E. Cassels as editor; and finally the second international symposium on atherosclerosis conducted by our beloved late Louis Katz in 1969. It is our hope that this, our latest undertaking, will prove equally successful and will throw new light on one of the most critically important areas in the whole health field.

James Schoenberger, M.D.

Preface

There is a quotation from T. H. Huxley* appropriate for the start of this symposium: "To a person not instructed in natural history, his country or seaside stroll is a walk through a gallery filled with wonderful works of art, nine tenths of which have their faces turned to the wall." Many of the faces of hypertension are also turned to the wall and it was our hope that during the three days of this symposium some of these faces would be turned around so that they might be recognized with their true identity.

It is gratifying to realize that we have in epidemiology an approach to the problem of hypertension which is relatively new in its application, exciting and already rewarding in new knowledge and complementary to the animal laboratory and to classical clinical investigation. We have a means of studying this frighteningly common and lethal disease as it exists in communities all over the world. We have in this forum a means of exchanging information formally and informally to our great mutual benefit and, what is more important, to the benefit of mankind.

As indicated by Dr. Schoenberger, we organized a meeting in Chicago in 1964 on this same subject. Two years ago, when I had the pleasure of visiting in Australia with Prof. Richard Lovell, he said, "Why don't you in Chicago have another meeting on the epidemiology of hypertension? I think it is time after ten years to have this matter discussed again." I came back home and had a discussion with our local group which responded enthusiastically. We then assessed national and international interest and again were encouraged. We had discussions with Prof. F. Gross regarding his meeting in Milan, and with Dr. Lysle Peterson regarding the World Congress and its meeting in Buenos Aires, and finally arrived at suitable dates. We are deeply grateful to the many individuals who contributed suggestions for topics and speakers, suggestions which resulted in the final program.

We would like particularly to acknowledge the important moral support and financial contributions which have made the meeting possible. The

---

*Huxley, T. H.: *Science and Education.* New York:Appleton, 1894.

National Heart and Lung Institute has been most supportive and helpful and we thank especially Dr. Theodore Cooper for a very sizable and important contribution to this enterprise. Without the help of the Institute, it would have been very difficult to have this meeting proceed. We also wish to thank the American Heart Association and its Councils on Epidemiology and on High Blood Pressure Research which have given us both encouragement and funds. The Chicago Heart Association helped in many indispensable ways, and we should mention especially the importance of staff work done by Ray Restivo, Kay Westfall and Helen Heck. We would like especially to express our gratitude to Dr. Richard Roberts of Ciba, who has assisted in providing a major contribution to make the publication of the proceedings possible. Dr. Scott Smith of G. D. Searle has also been exceedingly helpful. The important work of editing the symposium and including its discussion has been facilitated by the skillful assistance of Joan Wilentz. To all of these and others, our heartfelt thanks.

Oglesby Paul, M.D.

Introduction

The time to control hypertension has come. Basic research and clinical medicine have provided the means of effectively managing most patients with hypertension. Furthermore, the impact and improvement of health and longevity are well acknowledged. Our federal government has demonstrated a growing level of commitment and support. This commitment is shared by members of the scientific community, lay public and Congress, as well. Therefore, a conscious effort will be made to ensure the continuity and stability of productive research and control programs in hypertension.

The evolution of the national effort to combat hypertension rests importantly on the contributions of the epidemiologists. Society is asking us to explain how our therapeutic interventions and our so-called preventive maneuvers will affect the national public health profile. We will be depending, therefore, upon your continuing efforts as we participate in the formulation of public policy and federal programs.

Therefore, this international conference becomes more than a forum for scientists to talk with scientists. It becomes a resource for the physician, public health practitioners and society's leaders.

Theodore Cooper, M.D.

I
Inherited and Environmental Influences

Studies of Hypertension in Twins

M. Feinleib, M.D., R. Garrison, M.S., N. Borhani, M.D.,
R. Rosenman, M.D. and J. Christian, M.D.

Studies of hypertension as a disease and as a genetic trait are beset by problems arising from the variable nature of blood pressure measurements. Clinicians and epidemiologists are aware that the measurements obtained on a patient during an examination are influenced by many environmental and temporal factors. This has led to the development of protocols for standardizing equipment, posture and techniques for recording blood pressure measurements, specification of the time of day and number of measurements and use of adjusted scores and other statistical methods to account for the influence of age, sex and other co-factors. Control of temporal influences may involve multiple measurements over days, weeks, or longer periods. In contrast to the relative stability of other quantitative traits studied by population geneticists, such as height, weight, and even IQ, it is remarkable that any progress at all has been made in elucidating genetic influences on arterial blood pressure.

Yet progress has been made. We think the papers presented give a fairly satisfactory picture of the multifactorial genetic nature of blood pressure and of the importance of environmental factors early in life.

Sir George Pickering has provided adequate arguments at the first symposium on the Epidemiology of Hypertension[1] and elsewhere[2] that essential hypertension is a disease "in which the

M. Feinleib, M.D. *and* R. Garrison, M.S., *Epidemiology Branch, Division of Heart and Vascular Diseases, National Heart and Lung Institute, National Institutes of Health, Bethesda, Md.;* N. Borhani, M.D., *Department of Community Health, University of California, Davis;* R. Rosenman, M.D., *Harold Brunn Institute, Mount Zion Hospital and Medical Center, San Francisco, Calif.;* J. Christian, M.D., *Department of Medical Genetics, Indiana University Medical School, Indianapolis.*

deviation from the norm is quantitative not qualitative." In this respect, essential hypertension is more like anemia than sickle cell disease. The level of blood pressure at which a person is said to be hypertensive is arbitrary. For many years, the tendency was to define hypertension as a percentile of the normal distribution, eg, the top 5%. Recently, the trend has been to use levels above which the rate of anticipated undesirable consequences or risk of disease is sufficient to warrant medical intervention, with due regard for the cost and potential hazard of such intervention. Such arbitrariness necessitates caution in using family studies which posed questions as: "Have you ever been told you had high blood pressure?" or "Do any of your relatives have hypertension?" Yet we cannot rely solely on blood pressure measurements either. Many persons may already be on antihypertensive medication when examined and in large population studies it will be difficult to control for all the environmental and temporal artifacts. However, some of these factors can be analyzed statistically given adequate data for a large number of subjects.

About five years ago the Epidemiology Branch of the Division of Heart and Vascular Diseases, National Heart and Lung Institute, embarked on a program to study the role of familial factors in cardiovascular disease and its antecedent risk factors. This program included family and offspring studies using existing epidemiologic cohorts and a study of twins using the NAS-NRC VA Twin roster. The results of the Twin Study in relation to hypertension are presented.

Methods

Since 1969 the NHLI in collaboration with the NAS-NRC Twin Registry has sponsored the physical examination of 250 monozygous (MZ) and 264 dizygous (DZ) pairs of adult white male twins at five study centers located in New England, Indiana and California, as shown in Table 1. The participants were age 42 to 55 at the time of their examinations. The zygosity of the twins was determined by an extensive series of blood antigen analyses which largely confirmed the twins' opinions of their zygosity. Details of the overall study design and examination protocol have been discussed elsewhere.[3]

TABLE 1. The NHLI Twin Study

Study Center	Dates of Examination	Number of Twin Sets		
		MZ	DZ	Total
Framingham	7/69 - 5/70	55	50	105
Indiana	12/71 - 1/73	68	73	141
San Francisco	7/70 - 1/71	16	38	54
Davis	11/70 - 9/71	33	45	78
	4/73 - 8/73			
Los Angeles	11/71 - 11/72	78	58	136
All	7/69 - 8/73	250	264	514

An effort was made to have both members of each set examined at each center on the same day. All subjects were examined in the morning after an overnight fast. Since the primary purpose of this study was to test for the presence of genetic variance it was important to keep the physicians measuring blood pressures uninformed of twin zygosity. The only practical method was to have different physicians examine co-twins. This minimizes the possibility of recording bias due to facial or anthropometric similarities but at the same time introduces an interobserver component of variability in the within pair differences. Systolic blood pressure (SBP) and fifth phase diastolic pressure (DBP) were measured in a sitting position initially by a nurse and then by the examining physician prior to and immediately following a physical exam. In this report only the first physician reading will be considered.

The analysis of any quantitative character as a threshold trait, that is, considering an individual sick or well according to which side of a cutoff the character falls, can be considered appropriate if one of the following applies: (1) a clearly discontinuous frequency distribution exists and (2) medical treatment is deemed appropriate only above certain levels. Although the definition of hypertension is not universally agreed upon, current practice qualifies blood pressure under criterion (2). This report uses various cutoffs and combinations of SBP and DBP.

Results

The distributions of SBP and DBP for 1026 individual twins that were members of pairs where both co-twins had known values are given in Figures 1 and 2. Despite the pairwise dependence of these observations, the distributions are similar in shape and location to those based on groups of individual males of comparable age.[4,5] As shown in Tables 2 and 3, there were differences in mean blood pressures for the five centers, but no distinct geographic trend could be discerned. The possibility of a difference in blood pressure level for MZ and DZ twins was examined by a two-way analysis of variance. After adjustment for center differences, there was no evidence for different SBP or DBP levels in the two types of twins.

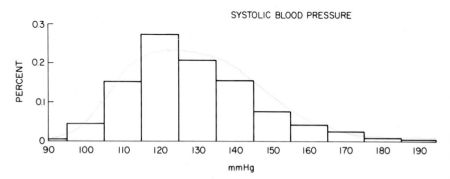

Fig. 1. Distribution of individual SBP measurements for 1026 twins age 42-55.

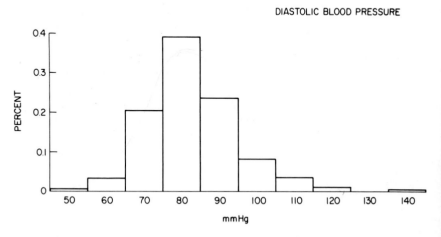

Fig. 2. Distribution of individual DBP measurements for 1026 twins age 42-55.

TABLE 2. Mean Systolic Blood Pressure
by Study Center and Zygosity

	Mean (mm Hg)		
Study Center*	MZ	DZ	Total
Framingham (55,50)	128.8	128.1	128.4
Indiana (68,73)	127.6	124.7	126.1
San Francisco (16,38)	132.9	122.7	125.7
Davis (32,45)	124.8	132.1	129.1
Los Angeles (77,58)	133.2	130.0	131.8
All (248,264)	129.6	127.4	128.5

*(#MZ,#DZ) = Number of pairs.

TABLE 3. Mean Diastolic Blood Pressure

	Mean (mm Hg)		
Study Center*	MZ	DZ	Total
Framingham (55,50)	81.4	81.1	81.3
Indiana (68,73)	80.3	78.8	79.6
San Francisco (16,38)	83.8	77.9	79.7
Davis (32,45)	82.5	85.7	84.4
Los Angeles (77,58)	86.0	82.5	84.5
All (248,264)	82.8	81.1	81.9

*(#MZ,#DZ) = Number of pairs.

The assumptions of the twin model and the estimation and testing of a genetic component of variance when these blood pressure data are considered as a quantitative trait have been presented in detail elsewhere.[6] Tables 4 and 5 summarize the results. The "within pair" estimate of genetic variance has commonly been used to summarize twin data. According to the method of Christian et al[7] this estimate should be used only when there is no evidence of heteroscedasticity, ie, unequal total variances of MZ and DZ twins, whereas the "among component" estimate should be used if there is heteroscedasticity. Thus, for SBP, where there is substantially more variation in MZ twins than DZ (total variances of 346.2 and 268.4, respectively), the unbiased estimate of genetic variance is the "among component" estimate. For both SBP and DBP there is evidence indicating that a substantial portion of the total population variability can be attributed to genetic differences. For SBP it is estimated that as much as 82% of the total variance may be genetic; for DBP as much as 64% may be genetic.

The impact of these genetic parameters can be assessed in several additional ways. One method is to examine the distributions of blood pressures of brothers of individuals having specified levels of blood pressure. Figure 3 shows the distributions of DBP for the brothers of subjects classified at five levels of DBP. Each twin represented in this figure appears as both an "index case" and as a sib of an index case. This double counting avoids the necessity of assigning arbitrary labels to members of the twin pair. The histograms for DBP show similar shapes at all levels with the only notable

TABLE 4. Systolic Blood Pressure

	MZ	DF	DZ	DF
Among pair mean square	538.0	247	336.6	263
Within pair mean square	154.3	248	200.1	264
Total variance	346.2	378.0	268.4	494.5

Estimates of genetic variance	Estimate	F	P
Among pair	402.8	1.60	<.001
Within pair	91.7	1.30	.019
Among component	247.3	1.50	<.001

$$\frac{\text{Genetic variance (A.C.)}}{\text{Total variance (pooled)}} = \frac{247.3}{302.1} = .82$$

TABLE 5. Diastolic Blood Pressure

	MZ	DF	DZ	DF
Among pair mean square	214.0	247	166.7	263
Within pair mean square	57.7	248	95.8	264
Total variance	135.8	371.2	131.2	490.7

Estimates of genetic variance	Estimate	F	P
Among pair	94.6	1.28	.023
Within pair	76.2	1.66	<.001
Among component	85.4	1.38	<.001

$$\frac{\text{Genetic variance (A.C.)}}{\text{Total variance (pooled)}} = \frac{85.4}{133.2} = .64$$

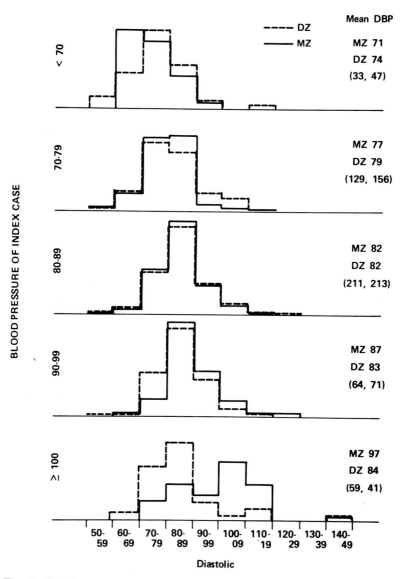

Fig. 3. Distribution of DBP in brothers of individuals having specified levels of DBP, by zygosity.

irregularities occurring among brothers of index cases with DBP 100 mm Hg or greater. The differences in location that are observed between MZ and DZ groups are in every case in the direction expected on the basis of a higher correlation between MZ than between DZ twins: .58 versus .27. For the two classification levels above the median group, the MZ twins show higher levels. For the two lowest groups, the MZ twins show lower levels than DZ. The DZ twins, having the smaller correlation, show greater regression toward the group mean than do the MZ twins. The results for SBP are given in Figure 4 and appear comparable. The skewing of the SBP distribution noted in Figure 1 appears to be present in all seven of these distributions. This suggests that the skewness often observed in SBP distributions is most likely due to measurement properties and not to a genetic mechanism.

The information contained in the high classifications is of practical interest. Two important questions are

1. What is the risk of hypertension in brothers of hypertensives?
2. What is the risk of hypertension in brothers of hypertensives relative to the risk in the general population?

Table 6 gives answers to the first question and Table 7 summarizes the results in terms of relative risks for various levels of SBP and DBP. The probabilities in Table 6 were computed as proband concordance rates where concordance is defined as both members of a pair being within the open ended intervals under consideration.

As expected, the MZ brother of a hypertensive has substantially greater risk of being hypertensive than does a DZ brother. For example, the MZ brother of an individual with DBP$\geq$95 has a .58 chance of having DBP$\geq$95 as opposed to only .19 for a DZ brother. The relative risks were computed by dividing the conditional probabilities by the corresponding unconditional probabilities. The results in Tables 6 and 7 are based on relatively few observations and are therefore subject to considerable sampling variability.

The fact that some subjects in the present study were taking antihypertensive medication complicates the interpretation of the data but also provides additional information. There were six MZ and four DZ pairs where both members were on

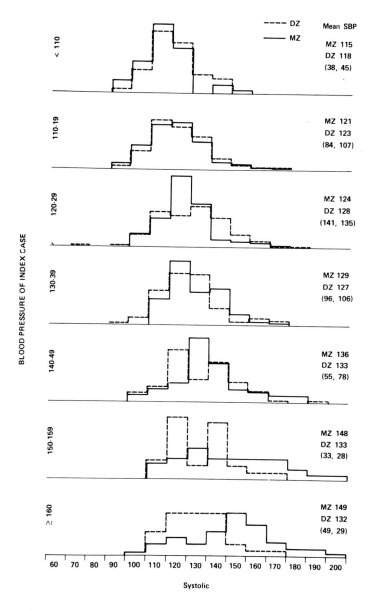

Fig. 4. Distribution of SBP in brothers of individuals having specified levels of SBP, by zygosity.

M. FEINLEIB ET AL

TABLE 6. Probability of Individual Having Blood Pressure Above
Specified Cut Points Conditional on Blood Pressure Level
of his Twin Brother

| | SBP | | | |
| | >140 | | >160 | |
	MZ	DZ	MZ	DZ
Unconditional probability	.28	.26	.10	.06
Given that brother has SBP:				
>140	.58	.43	.27	.08
(137,135)*				
>160	.76	.38	.37	.07
(49,29)				

| | DBP | | | |
| | >95 | | >105 | |
	MZ	DZ	MZ	DZ
Unconditional probability	.15	.12	.06	.04
Given that brother has DBP:				
>95	.58	.19	.32	.15
(72,62)				
>105	.74	.45	.45	.30
(31,20)				

*No. of MZ,DZ twins above specified level.

TABLE 7. Relative Risk of Individual Having Blood Pressure Above
Specified Cut Points Given Brother's Blood Pressure

| | SBP | | | |
| Given That Brother | >140 | | >160 | |
Has SBP:	MZ	DZ	MZ	DZ
>140	2.1	1.7	2.7	1.3
>160	2.7	1.5	3.7	1.2

| | DBP | | | |
| Given That Brother | >95 | | >105 | |
Has DBP:	MZ	DZ	MZ	DZ
>95	3.9	1.6	5.3	3.8
>105	4.9	3.8	7.5	7.5

therapy. In 20 MZ and 28 DZ sets only one member of the pair
was on treatment. In Table 8 the means for the treated and
untreated groups for MZ and DZ twins are listed. All means for
MZ twins are substantially above the population average.
Among DZ twins only the no treatment SBP mean is not

TABLE 8. Mean SBP/DBP for MZ and DZ Pairs
Discordant for Treatment

	No. of Pairs	Treated Brother	Untreated Brother
MZ	20	144.7/91.4	143.2/88.7
DZ	28	145.1/92.4	132.5/86.2

TABLE 9. Relative Risk of Being Classified as Borderline
or Hypertensive Given Brother's Classification

	Relative Risk for Being:			
	Borderline or Hypertensive		Hypertensive	
Given that brother is classified:	MZ	DZ	MZ	DZ
Borderline or hypertensive	1.7	1.4	2.1	1.4
Hypertensive	2.1	1.4	2.9	1.5

markedly elevated. In every case the mean for treated brothers
exceeds that of the untreated sibs with the differences being
larger for DZ twins. Only in one MZ pair and one DZ pair did
treatment appear to contribute to a marked discordance in
blood pressure level, with the treated individual clearly in the
normotensive range and his untreated brother clearly hypertensive.

To account for the potential error introduced by treatment
for hypertension the subjects were classified as hypertensive if
(a) SBP was greater than 159, (b) DBP was greater than 94 or
(c) the individual indicated that he was taking hypotensives or
diuretics prescribed by a physician. Using these criteria 19.9%
of MZ twins and 16.7% of DZ twins were hypertensive. A
category of borderline hypertension was defined as persons with
DBP of 90-94 and/or SBP of 140-159. This group included
15.3% of the MZ and 16.7% of the DZ twins. Table 9 gives the
corresponding relative risks for MZ and DZ brothers of
hypertensives. Brothers of MZ twins with either definite or
borderline hypertension were clearly at increased risks of being
hypertensive. The brothers of DZ hypertensives were also at
greater risk but not as high as for MZ twins.

Discussion

The above data present a clear picture of a major genetic determination of casual arterial blood pressure and of hypertension when defined at a variety of levels. These data are comparable to those reported for previous twin studies of blood pressure[8-10] and hypertension.[11]

Previous studies of the risk of hypertension in relatives of hypertensives vary in design, sample composition and, most important, in criteria for hypertension. Two studies[12,13] report results in terms of mean blood pressures for relatives of hypertensives. For DBP the means range from 82.2 for young relatives of hypertensives to 92.0 for older relatives. Chazan and Winkelstein[13] report a mean DBP of 85.9 for 85 first degree relatives of hypertensives. These findings appear to be comparable to the mean DBP of 84 for the DZ twins in the bottom histogram of Figure 3 and the 86 for untreated DZ brothers in Table 8.

An alternate approach of estimating the proportion of hypertensives in relatives of hypertensives and comparing this with either proportions of hypertensives in relatives of unaffected individuals or the general population has been used in three

TABLE 10. Correlation Between Relatives
for Systolic and Diastolic Blood Pressure

Relatives Compared	No. of Pairs	SBP	R DBP		
MZ twins	248	.55	.58		
DZ twins	264	.25	.27		
Siblings – F'ham	609	.18	.17		
Hayes[17]	545	.20	.17		
Johnson[18]	1464*	.17	.12		
Parents - offspring –					
F'ham	196	.34	.25	.19 (SBP)	.16 (DBP)
Hayes[17]	635	.13	.14		
Siblings and parent - offspring – Miall[19]	623*	.25	.20		
Spouses – F'ham	1644	.07	.07		
Hayes[17]	669	.13	.08		
Johnson[18]	1908	.07	.05		

*No. of families.

additional studies. Sobye,[14] using 160/100 as the criterion for hypertension, found a nearly fourfold excess risk in sibs of hypertensive vs. the general population. Similarly, Perera et al[15] and Ayman[16] found approximately a twofold risk in siblings of hypertensives when slightly less restrictive criteria for hypertension were employed.

The relation of the twin correlations to correlations observed in other relatives is summarized in Table 10. All of the cited studies used age and sex adjusted scores for calculating the correlation coefficients. MZ twins show clearly higher correlations than other relatives. The relatively higher correlations for DZ twins than for ordinary sibs or for parents and offspring are consistent with the hypothesis that shared early environmental factors play a role in determining blood pressure levels.

With all this information it would seem appropriate to ask if we can quantify the relative magnitudes of the environmental and genetic contributions to blood pressure variability. This requires a model relating the various genetic and environmental effects and more information than is currently available. However, we can make some attempt at quantification with a simplified model. Assume that the total population variance of blood pressure, V, is the sum of four additive components: A, additive genetic variance; S, environmental variance shared by members of a sibship, family or household; E, environmental variance that members of a family do not share; and e, random error variance which includes all of the short-term environmental and temporal influences which cause variations in an individual's blood pressure. We assume that there are no genetic effects due to dominance or epistasis and no interaction between the various sources of variability. The error variance can be estimated from the correlation, R_{xx}, between readings in the same individual. At Framingham this ranged from .85 for systolic measurements made during the same exam to .6 for measurements made two years apart. Using these values to indicate an approximate range, the estimates shown in Table 11 are obtained. These estimates are only approximate, but they summarize the order of magnitude of effects as judged from currently available data. The estimates for the shared environmental effects are derived from several alternate sets of assumptions. The overlapping values confirm the consistency of the estimated effect.

TABLE 11. Estimated Relative Contributions
to Blood Pressure Variability

Source	Calculated From	Estimated Relative Contributions
Error	$e/V = 1-R_{xx}$	.15 - .4
Environment		
Nonshared	$E/V = R_{xx}-R_{mz}$	.05 - .3
Shared	$S/V \begin{cases} 2R_{dz}-R_{mz} \\ R_{dz}-R_{Rel} \\ R_{spouses} \end{cases}$	0 .06 - .11 .04 - .13
Genetic	$A/V = 2(R_{mz}-R_{dz})$	.6

The relative contributions of the several sources of variability reflect the situation existing in the populations studied. Population groups with different genetic structures and different ranges of environmental variables might present different relative contributions. However, taking these relative effects at face value we can see why we have been unsuccessful in discovering naturally occurring environmental factors which markedly influence blood pressure levels in the general population. Thus, virtually all hypertension control programs rely on medication to control blood pressure in high-risk patients as opposed, for example, to the alteration of diet used for hyperlipidemia.

It may be pointed out that the polygenic model which appears to underlie the distribution of blood pressures is of relatively little value for purposes of genetic counseling to reduce the population rates of hypertension. However, the high correlations exhibited among relatives could be a powerful motivating factor in recruiting high-risk subjects in community screening programs, and the knowledge that one's blood pressure is, to a large extent, genetically determined may induce hypertensive patients to adhere voluntarily to recommended long-term and even lifelong therapy.

References

1. Pickering, G.: The inheritance of arterial pressure. In Stamler, J., Stamler, R. and Pullman, T. (eds.): *The Epidemiology of Hypertension.* New York:Grune and Stratton, 1967, pp. 18-27.

2. Pickering, G.: *High Blood Pressure*. New York:Grune and Stratton, 1968.
3. Feinleib, M., Christian, J., Borhani, N. et al: The NHLI Twin Study of cardiovascular disease risk factors — organization and methodology. Proceedings of the First International Congress of Twin Studies, Rome, 1974.
4. Winkelstein, W. and Kantor, S.: Some observations on the relationship between age, sex, and blood pressure. In Stamler, J., Stamler, R. and Pullman, T. (eds.): *The Epidemiology of Hypertension*. New York: Grune and Stratton, 1967, pp. 70-81.
5. McDonough, J. R., Garrison, G. E. and Hames, C. G.: Blood pressure and hypertensive disease among negroes and whites — a study in Evans County, Georgia. *Ann. Intern. Med.*, 61:208, 1964.
6. Borhani, N., Feinleib, M., Garrison, R. et al: Detection of genetic variance in blood pressure — the NHLI Twin Study. Proceedings of the First International Congress of Twin Studies, Rome, 1974.
7. Christian, J., Kang, J. and Norton, J.: Choice of an estimate of genetic variance from twin data. *Amer. J. Hum. Genet.*, 26:154, 1974.
8. Lundman, T.: Smoking in relation to coronary heart disease and lung function in twins. A co-twin control study. *Acta. Med. Scand.* 455 (suppl.):1, 1966.
9. Mathers, J., Osborne, R. and DeGeorge, F.: Studies of blood pressure, heart rate and the electrocardiogram in adult twins. *Amer. Heart J.*, 62:634, 1961.
10. Hines, E. A., Jr., McIlhaney, M. and Gage, R.: A study of twins with normal blood pressures and with hypertension. *Trans. Ass. Amer. Physicians*, 70:282, 1957.
11. Vander Molen, R., Brewer, G., Honeyman, M. S. et al: A study of hypertension in twins. *Amer. Heart J.*, 79:454, 1970.
12. Cruz-Coke, R.: The hereditary factor in hypertension. *Acta Genet.*, 9:207, 1959.
13. Chazan, J. and Winkelstein, W.: Household aggregation of hypertension: Report of a preliminary study. *J. Chron. Dis.*, 17:9, 1964.
14. Sobye, P.: Heredity in essential hypertension and nephrosclerosis: A genetic-clinical study of 200 proposite suffering from nephrosclerosis. *Op. dom. Biol. herd. hum. (Kbh)* 16:1-225, 1948.
15. Perera, G., Gearing, F. and Schweitzer, M.: A family study of primary hypertension — final report. *J. Chron. Dis.*, 24:127, 1972.
16. Ayman, D.: Heredity in arteriolar (essential) hypertension — a clinical study of the blood pressure of 1524 members of 277 families. *Arch. Intern. Med.*, 53:792, 1934.
17. Hayes, C., Tyroler, H. and Cassel, J.: Family aggregation of blood pressure in Evans County, Georgia. *Arch. Intern. Med.*, 128:965, 1971.
18. Johnson, B. C., Epstein, F. H. and Kjelsberg, M.: Distribution and familial studies of blood pressure and serum cholesterol levels in a total community, Tecumseh, Michigan. *J. Chron. Dis.*, 18:147, 1965.
19. Miall, W. and Oldham, P.: The hereditary factor in arterial blood-pressure. *Brit. Med. J.*, 1:75, 1963.

Discussion

Dr. Tyroler: I would like to compliment Dr. Feinleib on the reporting of this extremely interesting study. He certainly knows the limitations of the material and stated in qualification of his final remarks that there are alternate explanations of the phenomenon. I would like to identify just three of these which issue both from the material, which he presents, and from related work in other fields which are quite similar. First, in his review of the data there were quoted three instances in which there was evidence of some, though slight, spouse aggregation. This, of course, is a controversial issue in itself and one which we will hear more about later in the program. However, it certainly does speak to the possibility of the effect of shared environment and I suspect also that it influences the interpretations of the similarity among the twins which Dr. Feinleib recorded. Second, he ignored completely the one major associated characteristic which in population studies is clearly associated with blood pressure, that is, weight for height indices. The correlation is not very strong, but is of the same order of magnitude as the correlation between dizygotic twins, namely, approximately 0.2. Similarly, there is clear evidence of aggregation of weight for height in families. I think that as a minimum this variable should be controlled and perhaps it has been already in Dr. Feinleib's studies which he did not report to us. Finally a related problem is the assumption that a monozygotic and dizygotic twin differ only in the amount of sharing of genes. Evidence from behavioral studies and the inheritance of other phenomena show very clearly that there are gross differences in the socialization process, in the sharing of life style, patterns in the personality and other attributes of identical compared with dizygotic twins.

Dr. Feinleib: I think all three questions are extremely important and I think all three of them have anticipated other talks or other studies in progress. I think there is some spouse aggregation. There might be other explanations. The role of obesity is a very important one. We have attempted to adjust for obesity; it does not change the results significantly. The third factor is a perennial one and is an exceedingly difficult subject. Ideally the nearest we can get to it in human populations is to find identical twins that have been separated. It is almost impossible to find such groups.

Dr. Miller, Baltimore: My question relates to sampling. You have excluded some people who were sick, possibly when they were teenagers. You have excluded females, and you have excluded blacks.

Dr. Feinleib: This was not a process of intentional exclusion. These twins were obtained from the rosters of the Veterans Administration starting about ten years ago. All were veterans who had served in World War II or the Korean war. For some reason they decided to use whites only.

Dr. Miller: Suppose the gene has an effect that expresses itself early, before draft age. I want to caution you about generalizing too much.

Dr. Feinleib: We are dealing with adults and any selective factors that may have occurred up to the time they came in for examination would certainly be important, particularly anything that may have contributed to the exclusion of one or the other twin in military service. He would not be eligible for this study. On the other hand, though, a lot of the extraneous conditions like rheumatic fever were weeded out by the early military screening.

Dr. Stamler: I think it is relevant to note that this is a within-population study and if a fundamental, general environmental characteristic is at work permitting the expression of genetic tendency, it would give one pattern. If it is not at work, we would have a very different pattern. For example, if a similar analysis were attempted if there were enough people in the population that Page studied in the Solomon Islands, one might find that an environmental factor is overwhelming and its absence results in virtually no hypertension and no rise in blood pressure with age. In stating that genetic factors account for 60% of variability in a given analysis, it is extremely important that this always be kept in mind. For example, if salt intake is a general conditioner for the development of hypertension in the genetically susceptible and there is a lot of salt intake, we will get the kind of pattern we have. If there is not much salt intake, things will be very different.

Dr. Feinleib: I agree with you completely. I did try to point out that these relations are very approximate and specifically hold only within the range of genetic and environmental variation which exists in the population studied. It is quite evident that if we have diverse populations with different environmental effects, use of medications and maybe diets, we would get quite a different picture.

Dr. Kass: One brief bit of data and then a question simply to reinforce the last two comments. My colleague Frank Sachs, a medical student, studied a large number of vegetarians living in communes. One of the curious findings was that in the 17 communes, there was intracommunal aggregation of just about the same order of magnitude that we usually expect from intrafamilial aggregation. Here it would appear very much as though the common environment and the common dietary constraints were the factors; at least they were the only ones we could think of, since there had been a lot of control of other things such as salt intake and so on. There is a powerful problem here that we are all agreed upon and it is going to be difficult to separate. I do want to ask whether you mean to stress as much as you did the problem of using familial aggregation as a case-finding technique for the high-risk people, given the R is only 0.25 and 0.25 squared gives us a pretty small number.

Dr. Feinleib: I would tend to stress it primarily as a motivating and compliance factor to get people to come in.

Dr. Kass: One final clarification for my benefit and following up Dr. Feinleib's point. You agree with the overwhelming importance of the genetic factor to apply to the environment which you studied. This does not argue that a quite different environment might, for example, abolish hypertension even though the genetic stratum was exactly the same.

Dr. Feinleib: That is correct. If the environment was homogenous, the same for everybody, there would be 100% genetic variability. If the environments were made very disparate, the proportion of elevated blood pressure due to environmental differences would go up. I am sure if we use a black population or non-United States population, we would probably get quite different data.

Studies of Blood Pressure in Spouses

David L. Sackett, M.D.

Family studies of cardiovascular diseases have traditionally focused on genetic rather than environmental issues and have usually confined themselves to the relationships between risk factors and/or disease outcomes among first degree relatives. Concurrent with the gradual ascendancy of a concept of blood pressure as a continuous rather than a discrete variable (Platt and Pickering debate, summarized in Stamler, 1967), there has been a growing interest in family studies which include those members who share the least genetic material. The inclusion of analyses for spouse concordance is now commonplace.

Studies of the magnitude of spouse concordance for risk factors and disease outcomes are important for both basic and applied research. On their own they can contribute to a basic understanding of nature. When coupled with parallel investigations of the first degree relatives, they can help delineate the separate contributions of genetic and environmental forces to the determination of risk factors and disease outcomes. At the same time, these studies may provide the base from which to modify nature. For example, if significant spouse concordance for risk factors and disease outcomes can be demonstrated, programs of intervention and prevention can focus case-finding programs upon the "difficult-to-capture" husbands of the more easily identified hypertensive wives.

Preparation of this paper was supported in part by the following grants: Provincial Research Grant P.R. 32, National Health Grants 606-22-12 and 606-1125-22, Ontario Heart Foundation 14-3, and a Program Grant from the Sun Life Assurance Company of Canada.

David L. Sackett, M.D., M.Sc. Epid., *Professor of Clinical Epidemiology and Biostatistics, Professor of Medicine, McMaster University Medical Centre, Hamilton, Ontario, Canada.*

In reviewing recent studies of blood pressure in spouses, this paper will address two major questions:

1. Does significant spouse concordance for blood pressure exist?

2. If so, does the shared marital environment offer a plausible explanation for the observed concordance?

Before addressing these central questions, two sources of bias in data collection must be confronted. The first arises from the act of *measuring* blood pressure among family members. It is epitomized in the case of the same observer (end-digit preference, hearing acuity, "transference," cuff deflation rate, expectations about spouse concordance, etc.), using the same manometer (mercury level and purity, local irregularities in the internal manometer surface, leaks, etc.), performing the measurement upon multiple family members at the same time of the same day of the same week of the same month. To the extent that each family member is exposed to an identical set of systematic biases, spurious concordance will result. The magnitude of this bias is decreased when a single observer makes all observations upon all subjects (a Herculean — or more properly "Miallean" — task), or when a more "objective" manometer system is introduced, such as the "random-zero" device described by Garrow and now in use (in modified form) in the Hypertension Detection and Follow-Up Trial in the United States.[1] Alternatively, some investigators — particularly when performing retrolective studies — have tested for this source of bias by comparing concordance between true spouse pair members with that observed among spouse pairs generated through the random assignment of wives to other women's husbands who were examined at the same point in calendar time. These "spouse-swapping" analyses have been reported for Buffalo[2] and Framingham[3] and indicate that this first source of bias was not responsible for the spouse concordance for blood pressure observed.

A second source of bias in studies of spouse concordance concerns the *manipulation* of blood pressure data in the subsequent analysis. Because risk factors such as blood pressure show systematic variations with advancing age, the similarity in the age of spouse pair members makes a direct comparison of raw measurements biased; some procedure is required which will remove the age effect from the risk factor under study. In the reports of spouse aggregation summarized here, two general approaches to this problem have been used. Most of these studies use age- and sex-specific scores expressed in standard deviation units. These were developed by fitting simple or complex equations to the changing means and variances of the risk factors which occur with advancing age. If such a standardization technique could remove age effects, and if the resulting scores were normally distributed, the subsequent tests for association could involve the powerful "t-test" family of procedures.

The second general approach to studying risk factor associations treats them as ordinal rather than interval measurements and uses nonparametric tests for association; a good example of this approach is the Ordac method.[2] Although nonparametric testing for ordinal association is less powerful in a statistical sense, it does avoid the introduction of artifacts which may accompany standardization and transformation procedures. It also does not require the assumption of an underlying normal distribution for the risk factor or its derived score.

Both of these approaches have drawbacks. In their original description of the "standardized score" method, Hamilton and Pickering made two relevant points. First, they noted that statistically significant relationships still existed between age and the blood pressure scores they developed, both for systolic ($p = 0.008$) and diastolic ($p = 0.032$) blood pressure. Thus, while the scores may markedly reduce the age effect, they do not totally eliminate its influence on the subsequent analysis. The second point they emphasized is that the resulting blood pressure scores are not normally distributed. This violates (for at least some analysts!) an assumption of the subsequently applied "t-test" family of statistical procedures. Although they pointed out that these departures from normality did not appear to be associated with age, they warned that "such departures are an indication for caution in the use of scores (or for that matter any measurements of arterial pressure)."[4] In analyzing Framingham blood pressures and other risk factors with the Hamilton-Pickering approach, we have found that both points apply. Statistically significant age effects persist, and the resulting standardized scores are not normally distributed.

Although the ordinal association procedures are attractive because they overcome the needs for transformation, standardization and assumptions of normality, they too have drawbacks. First, nonparametric techniques are generally less powerful than the "t-test" family of statistical procedures. As a result, the likelihood of a Type II error is increased, and it may be decided that concordance is absent when, in fact, it is present. Second, the Ordac method proposed by Priore, while ingeniously simple, discards over half of the observations.[2] In summary, the student of familial aggregation of blood pressure or other age-related variables is well advised to assess the strategies and tactics used in the acquisition and manipulation of these data, rather than simply accept a traditional or standard approach.

Does Significant Spouse Concordance for Blood Pressure Exist?

Table 1 summarizes the studies of spouse concordance for blood pressure which have been reported over the past 12 years. Gearing et al studied first degree relatives and 125 spouses of hypertensive and control individuals from the Columbia-Presbyterian Medical Center and the H.I.P.-Yorkville Medical Group in New York.[5] Hypertensives had exhibited repeated diastolic blood pressures of 90 mm Hg or above in the absence of any recognizable secondary cause. Both cases and controls were between the ages of 45 and 65, had spouses and first degree relatives available for examination and were free of diabetes, thyroid, kidney and valvular heart disease, as well as cerebrovascular disease. Although hypertension, as defined, was statistically significantly more frequent among the siblings of hypertensives (45%) than of controls (24%), an identical 17% of the spouses of both hypertensive and control individuals had defined hypertension. These conclusions were confirmed in a subsequent report from this same group.[6]

Chazan and Winkelstein examined everyone living in the households of hypertensive and control patients selected from the outpatient deparment of the E. J. Meyer Memorial Hospital

TABLE 1. Recent Studies of Spouse Concordance for Blood Pressure

Author(s)	Study Sample	Findings (Positive = Statistically Significant)
Gearing et al 1962	125 spouses of defined hypertensives and controls, New York	Negative; frequency of defined hypertension similar for spouses of normotensives and hypertensives
Chazan & Winkelstein 1964	Members of households of 46 hypertensives, controls and first-degree relatives, Buffalo, N.Y.	Positive; unrelated persons in the households of defined hypertensives had higher mean diastolic blood pressure than comparison individuals
Priore 1964	635 spouse pairs in a subset of the sample in Winkelstein et al 1966, Buffalo	Positive; significant Ordac scores for systolic and diastolic blood pressure
Johnson et al 1965	1,908 spouse pairs in a total population sample, Tecumseh, Mich.	Negative; statistically significant correlation coefficients for systolic and diastolic blood pressure in a single age group (wives 50-59)
Winkelstein et al 1966	512 spouse pairs in a random household sample, Buffalo	Positive; significant spouse concordance for couples married more than 15 years, using an empiric ordinal blood pressure classification model
Miall et al	229 spouse pairs in random population samples from two areas in South Wales, U.K.	Negative; regression values of blood pressure scores had negative signs
Tseng 1967	1,652 spouse pairs in total population samples from two areas in Taiwan	Positive; age-sex adjusted scores significant, most marked in the fishing population
Borhani et al 1969	504 spouse pairs in a random household sample, Alameda County, Calif.	Negative; statistically significant Ordac scores for diastolic blood pressure only
Winkelstein et al 1969	(?) same Alameda County sample	Positive; significant spouse concordance for couples married 15 years or more
Hayes et al 1971	669 white and 308 black spouse pairs in a random sample, Evans County, Ga.	Positive; among white spouse pairs, concordance of defined high blood pressure rises (and then falls) with advancing age
Sackett et al 1973	1,259 spouse pairs in the Framingham Heart Epidemiology Study, United States	Positive; cross-sectional analyses showed increasing concordance with longer duration of marriage

in Buffalo, New York, and also studied the household members of the first degree relatives of these patients.[7] Both first degree relatives and unrelated members of the households of hypertensives had higher mean diastolic blood pressures than did the corresponding members of the control households. In concluding that these data suggested an environmental contribution to the determination of hypertension, the authors noted a possible alternative explanation of assortative marriage on the basis of blood pressure.

Priore studied 635 spouse pairs from a random household sample in Buffalo.[2] After suggesting that the traditional age-adjustment techniques for standardizing blood pressure scores were both inadequate and biased, Priore introduced the Ordac, an ordinal method of age correction which classified each subject in an age, sex-specific sextile of the blood pressure range. Comparing the relative locations of members of spouse pairs in this fashion, Priore found statistically significant spouse concordance for both systolic and diastolic blood pressure. Both the Ordac method and the observed result gained additional credibility when it was shown that concordance disappeared when "random marriage" was simulated by a random reassignment of husbands and wives into spouse pairs.

Johnson et al studied blood pressure levels among 1,908 spouse pairs in the total community study in Tecumseh, Michigan,[8] with a standardized score approach. Using the age of the wife as an indicator of the duration of shared environment, they found a statistically significant correlation between spouses for systolic and diastolic blood pressure for only one of the five age groups (wives 50-59). In a subsequent communication from this group, it was concluded that no spouse concordance was present.[9]

Winkelstein et al studied 512 spouse pairs in a random household sample in Buffalo. He used an ordinal classification method which developed empirical interval-estimates of blood pressure on the basis of intra-individual variations over short periods of time.[10] Statistically significant spouse concordance of systolic blood pressure was demonstrated among spouse pairs married for 15 years or more.

Miall et al studied 229 spouse pairs in random population samples from two areas of South Wales, U.K.[11] Age-standardized scores were used and no concordance for blood pressure in these spouse pairs was found; indeed, the regression values had negative signs.

With essentially the same standardization procedures,[4] however, Tseng observed substantial spouse concordance in his study of 1,652 spouse pairs in total population samples from agricultural and fishing populations in Taiwan.[12] It is of particular interest that the correlation coefficients between spouses were of the same general magnitude as those observed between first degree relatives.

Borhani et al, using both a modification of the Ordac method and an interpretation of the method developed by Winkelstein et al, studied 504 spouse pairs in a random household sample of Alameda County, California.[13] Although the Ordac analysis suggested spouse concordance for diastolic blood pressure, the analysis using "Winkelstein's method" was negative. However, Winkelstein et al subsequently suggested that Borhani and co-workers had incorrectly applied the method and, on re-analysis of a data set provided by the Alameda group, demonstrated statistically significant spouse concordance for systolic blood pressure among older spouse pairs.[14]

Haynes et al examined 669 white and 308 black spouse pairs in a random sample of Evans County, Georgia.[15] Positive results were limited to white spouse pairs with the concordance of defined high blood pressure rising sharply with advancing age and then falling beyond age 60. The results were not due to the examination of both members of a spouse pair by the same examiner, and the analysis suggested that the decline in spouse concordance among the elderly could be explained in large part by the high mortality affecting spouse pairs' concordant for high levels of blood pressure.

Finally, Sackett et al examined concordance for blood pressure and a series of other coronary risk factors among 1,259 Framingham spouse pairs who had experienced single, continuous marriages.[3] Using a nonparametric assessment of ordinal age-corrected scores, they demonstrated statistically significant spouse concordance for both systolic and diastolic blood pressure, as well as a number of other coronary risk factors.

Returning now to the central question: *Does significant spouse concordance for blood pressure exist?* I believe that the answer is a qualified "yes." If we limit our consideration to community based study samples, omit the controversial Alameda County study and duplicates such as Priore's[2] analysis of data gathered by Winkelstein,[10] four investigations among 4,092 subjects showed statistically significant spouse concordance for blood pressure, whereas two studies among 2,131 subjects did not. The combined data justify the conclusion that spouse concordance for blood pressure is real.

However: *Is spouse concordance for blood pressure clinically and biologically significant?* Here, the answer is less clear. On the one hand, Tseng found that the degree of blood pressure concordance between spouses may equal that found among first degree relatives,[12] and Winkelstein et al found that parent-child concordance was virtually limited to those families in which spouse concordance existed. In view of these findings it appears warranted to recommend that studies of familial concordance include spouse comparisons.

On the other hand, the magnitude of spouse concordance which has been observed in these investigations does not hold much promise for immediate clinical application. Although hypertensive husbands may have a further increase in their case-fatality rates if their wives are also hypertensive,[15] it does not appear that other potential clinical applications of these findings are likely to be rewarding. For example, case finding among the "difficult-to-capture" husbands of more easily identified wives does not hold much promise. Twenty-six percent of husbands of Framingham wives with diastolic blood pressures $\geqslant 95$ at Exam I also had diastolic hypertension compared with 20% of husbands of wives with diastolic pressures below this level; stated differently, the demonstration of diastolic hypertension ($\geqslant 95$) in a Framingham wife had a sensitivity of only 22% (and a specificity of 86%) in predicting diastolic hypertension in her husband.[3]

In summary, spouse concordance for blood pressure is real and may have biologic importance. The present body of knowledge does not, however, point to immediate clinical application in the detection, evaluation and management of blood pressure disorders. Our efforts in this area must continue to focus upon more urgent issues such as strategies to improve compliance with antihypertensive therapy.[16]

If Spouse Concordance for Blood Pressure Exists, Does the Shared Marital Environment Offer a Plausible Explanation?

On the basis of cross-sectional studies, the answer appears to be "yes," but recent longitudinal analyses have reopened this question, if not answered it in the negative.

Cross-sectional observations of community samples in Buffalo,[10] agricultural areas in Taiwan,[12] Evans County[15] and Framingham[3] all showed increasing spouse concordance for blood pressure with either increasing duration of marriage or simply with advancing age (although declines in concordance among the oldest age groups were noted in Taiwan and in Evans County). In Buffalo, an environmental explanation for this similarity in blood pressure levels received additional support from the demonstration that concordant spouse pairs closely resembled community norms for religion, family size and the congruity of occupation with educational attainment (Winkelstein et al 1965).[10] Thus, cross-sectional studies of the question suggest that the blood pressures of spouse pair members, perhaps in response to the shared marital environment, tended to come together over time, as depicted in Figure 1.

To the extent that these investigations suggest an environmental explanation for spouse concordance, they are vulnerable to an inherent methodologic weakness of the cross-sectional study described by Neyman.[17] Because they are performed at an "instant" in time, cross-sectional studies can make inferences regarding changes over time only by assuming an orderly flow of individuals through succeeding age categories, resulting in the situation depicted in Figure 1.

However, as shown in Figure 2, an alternative series of longitudinal events could result in similar cross-sectional findings. Simplified for purposes of illustration, this explanation involves two different populations of spouse pairs, one of which (pair C-C') was concordant throughout the duration of marriage (and, indeed, was generated through assortative marriage) and the second of which (pairs A-A' and B-B') was discordant

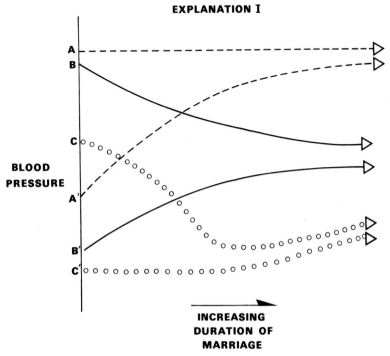

Figure 1.

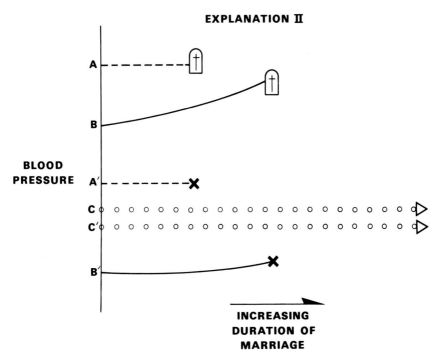

Figure 2.

throughout the marriage. Since discordance necessitates a relatively elevated blood pressure in one member of the spouse pair, one could expect discordant spouse pairs (A-A' and B-B') to be more likely to undergo dissolution through the death of the member with elevated blood pressure. Thus, although cross-sectional data would still suggest increasing spouse concordance as a result of sharing a common environment, this finding would simply have resulted from the uncovering of spouse pairs (C-C') who had been concordant throughout marriage.

A recently reported 12-year longitudinal study of Framingham spouse pairs supports the latter explanation.[3] Using a nonparametric index of ordinal association (Kendall's Tau-A) among age- and sex-specific blood pressure sextiles, Sackett et al made three pertinent observations which are summarized for systolic blood pressure in Figures 3 and 4. First, they found that, among spouse pairs present throughout the 12-year follow-up, concordance for systolic and diastolic blood pressure was high at the start and did not increase over time. Second, successively longer marriage-duration cohorts tended to show greater spouse concordance throughout the 12-year follow-up

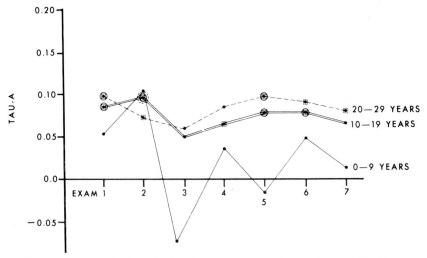

Fig. 3. Longitudinal analysis of spouse concordance for systolic blood pressure.

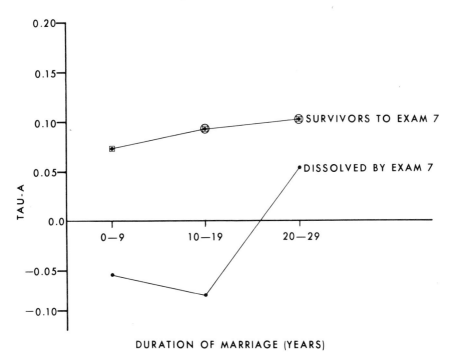

DURATION OF MARRIAGE (YEARS)

Fig. 4. Cross-sectional analysis of spouse concordance for systolic blood pressure — Exam I (Kendall's Tau-A partialled out).

period. Finally (Fig. 4), they repeated a cross-sectional analysis, "partialling out" concordance separately to those spouse pairs who did, and did not, survive the 12-year follow-up. Spouse pairs destined to be dissolved before the end of the follow-up period were either discordant (Tau-A values became negative) or only weakly concordant, and their dissolution uncovered previously and continuously concordant spouse pairs.

Thus, our answer to the question: *If spouse concordance for blood pressure exists, does the shared marital environment offer a plausible explanation?* would have to be a qualified "no" for the present, pending confirmation or refutation of the recent Framingham results. Indeed, the present evidence supports an explanation of spouse concordance on the basis of assortative marriage for similarities in blood pressure, an explanation offered earlier (albeit without enthusiasm) by Winkelstein et al as a potential mechanism for their cross-sectional findings.[10]

In summary, spouse concordance for blood pressure does exist, and it is biologically (but not clinically) important. It does not appear to increase for individual spouse pairs with time, and a plausible explanation for its occurrence is assortative marriage.

On the basis of this review, three recommendations for further studies emerge. First, more work is needed on the development of bias-free, sensitive methods for dealing with blood pressure data. It is important that discussions in this area avoid the obfuscations which biostatisticians and physiologists so often interject in an effort to mask their ignorance of each other's fields. Second, other sources of longitudinal blood pressure data among spouse pairs should be analyzed to confirm or refute the Framingham findings.

Finally, we should carry out studies of the possible mechanisms for this spouse concordance. An attractive hypothesis is assortative marriage, and studies of this distribution and determinants among samples of spouse pairs who do and do not exhibit concordance for blood pressure would be both scientifically rewarding and fun.

References

1. Garrow, J. S.: Zero-muddler for unprejudiced sphygmomanometry. *Lancet*, 2:1205, 1963.
2. Priore, R. L.: The Ordac method of making age-adjustments in data. *J. Chron. Dis.*, 17:241-263, 1964.
3. Sackett, D. L., Anderson, G. D., Milner, R. et al: A longitudinal study of spouse aggregation of coronary risk factors among spouses. Cardiovascular Epidemiology Section, American Heart Association, New Orleans, March 1973.
4. Hamilton, M., Pickering, G. W., Roberts, J. A. F. et al: The aetiology of essential hypertension. II. Scores for arterial blood pressures adjusted for differences in age and sex. *Clin. Sci.*, 13:37-49, 1954.
5. Gearing, F. R., Clark, E. G., Perera, G. A. et al: Hypertension among relatives of hypertensives: Progress report of a family study. *Amer. J. Pub. Health*, 52:2058-2065, 1962.
6. Perera, G. A. Gearing, F. R. and Schweitzer, M. D.: A family study of primary hypertension — final report. *J. Chron. Dis.*, 25:127, 1972.
7. Chazan, J. A. and Winkelstein, W., Jr.: Household aggregation of hypertension: Report of a preliminary study. *J. Chron. Dis.*, 17:9-18, 1964.
8. Johnson, B. C., Epstein, F. H. and Kjelsberg, M. O.: Distributions and familial studies of blood pressure and serum cholesterol levels in a

total community: Tecumseh, Michigan. *J. Chron. Dis.*, 18:147-160, 1965.

9. Deutscher, S., Epstein, F. H. and Kjelsberg, M. O.: Familial aggregation of factors associated with coronary heart disease. *Circulation*, 33:911-924, 1966.

10. Winkelstein, W., Jr., Kantor, S., Ibrahim, M. A. et al: Familial aggregation of blood pressure: A preliminary report. *JAMA*, 195:848-850, 1966.

11. Miall, W. E., Heneage, P., Khosla, T. et al: Factors influencing the degree of resemblance in arterial pressure of close relatives. *Clin. Sci.*, 33:271-283, 1967.

12. Tseng, W.-P.: Blood pressure and hypertension in an agricultural and a fishing population in Taiwan. *Amer. J. Epidem.*, 86:513-525, 1967.

13. Borhani, N. O., Slansky, D., Gaffey, W. et al: Familial aggregation of blood pressure. *Amer. J. Epidem.*, 89:537-546, 1969.

14. Winkelstein, W., Jr., Kantor, S., Ibrahim, M. A. et al: Remarks on the analysis of familial aggregation of blood pressure in the Alameda County Blood Pressure Study. *Amer. J. Epidem.*, 89:615-618, 1969.

15. Hayes, C. G., Tyroler, H. A. and Cassel, J. C.: Family aggregation of blood pressure in Evans County, Georgia. *Arch. Intern. Med.*, 128:965-975, 1971.

16. Sackett, D. L. and Haynes, R. B.: Newsletter on Compliance with Therapeutic Regimens No. 2. McMaster University Medical Centre, Hamilton, Ontario, Canada.

17. Neyman, J.: Statistics: Servant of all sciences. *Science*, 122:401, 1955.

Discussion

Dr. Winkelstein: I think the last two papers were outstanding and I was very impressed with the longitudinal analysis. I have a suspicion though that when this meeting is over we are going to be pretty much in the position we were ten years ago, arguing about the relative importance of genetics and environment. I would suggest that one possible way out of this is that we are going to have to examine the entire family in our attempt to sort out genetic versus environmental factors. Despite what Dr. Sackett has said about assortative marriage, the solution to the problem will still lie in further studies of both the relationship of blood pressure between spouses, between parents and children, and between siblings, but most importantly in the entire constellation in the family situation looking at the environmental influences which are affecting the particular families. I also would like to take slight issue or at least ask him to comment on the possibility of using the phenomenon of familial aggregation as a way of identifying high-risk individuals. This has been attempted in a number of studies and while you pointed out that women were more accessible to diagnosis, it is also true that schoolchildren may offer a very important source for the identification of high-risk individuals.

Dr. Sackett: I think the use of familial aggregation permits more efficient case finding. When one compares, however, the sort of results that Manning reported and the sort of results that I reported, it is much more appropriate to look at it from the point of view of first degree relatives than it is from the point of view of spouses, simply in terms of yield. Your initial comment has been anticipated and hopefully will speed up a logical next phase in the analysis of data which are, in fact, available on families. The issue here is the extent to which one can develop an analogous evaluation of spouses versus first degree relatives which can utilize the analytic progress made in the method-ology developed to assess the difference between monozygous and dizygous twins. I also want to point out that because longitudinal data do not suggest that a shared marital environ-ment is important in determining spouse concordance, this does not mean that environment may not be an important factor in determining blood pressure. These data would be entirely consistent with a major environmental determination of blood pressure acting prior to marriage, simply being markedly reinforced and, indeed, swamped by assortative marriage.

Dr. Lovell: I am not quite clear on what assortative mating means but my question really is in two parts. (1) Ten years ago we spent a good deal of time in this session talking about the relation of blood pressure and body size. Is there any evidence that people marry people of similar somatotypes. Could this be a factor that would tend to render similar blood pressures within marriage? (2) This relates to smoking. Is there evidence that spouses tend to have similar smoking habits? Smokers in general tend to have lower pressures. Could these be factors that might operate?

Dr. Sackett: If one goes into the studies relative to the question of assortative marriages, one would find that they tend to be quite rich in the demonstration of a quite marked influence of physical factors, that is, individuals with similar characteristics being more likely to marry than those without similar characteristics. In Framingham there is substantial spouse concordance for the lipids and for items such as vital capacity. In our analyses of blood pressures, we have looked at the extent to which spouse concordance for blood pressure might simply be a spurious finding based upon similarities or concordance for relative weight, for example. If one looks at spouse pairs who are concordant or discordant for relative weight, one still finds concordance for blood pressure, so that one cannot invoke a relative weight explanation for the observations with regard to blood pressure. A similar situation exists with regard to cigarette smoking which also shows, of course, very pronounced spouse concordance.

Dr. Freis: There is one aspect of these obese studies which bothers me, and that is that the spouses of hypertensive patients might react differently to being approached with the request to measure their blood pressure than the spouses of normal people, with somewhat more alarm and with a temporary rise of blood pressure. Was that controlled in any way?

Dr. Sackett: If one is talking about this in a case-finding technique, of course one has no knowledge of the hypertensive status of the husband. If one talks about the observations on spouses in Framingham, that is a quite different story.

Dr. Feinleib: Dr. Sackett's analysis is based on the assumption that the longer spouses live together the longer they will be sharing the common environment and, therefore, the more similar they should become. An alternate way of looking at this problem is to take people who have been living together and see if after they separate they become less concordant. Figure 1 shows siblings from the Framingham data. The data were analyzed the same way that Dr. Sackett analyzes spouse data, S stands for sister, B for brother. We have sister-brother pairs, sister-sister, brother-brother pairs, and brother-sister pairs. The difference in the sister-brother and the brother-sister is simply which one was older at the time of examination. These were all adults. Remember, the Framingham Study included individuals between the ages of 30 and 60, so this reflects what happened to them during the 16 years after entering the Framingham cohort as adults. The vast majority were no longer living together, although they may have been living together up to

D. L. SACKETT

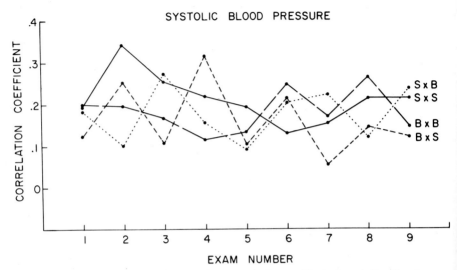

Fig. 1. Correlation coefficients for age- and sex-adjusted systolic blood pressure scores for 609 sibling pairs examined in the Framingham Heart Program over a 16-year period. 5 X 5 = 183 sister-sister pairs, B X B = 141 brother-brother pairs, S X B = 139 sister-brother pairs with sister older than brother, B X S = 146 brother-sister pairs with brother older than sister.

their teen years. We see a remarkable consistency of the correlation coefficient during the 18-year period. Only in the sister-sister set did there seem to be a tendency to fall off, and there only slightly.

The same thing shows up for diastolic pressure (Fig. 2), essentially the same degree of correlation throughout the 16 years of follow-up when they were living apart. Both of these analyses, the sibling and spouse analyses, are based on the assumption that when people live in the same household they share the same environment, and that when they do not live in the same household, they do not share the same environment. I think we have to be a little cautious about this, in that with the freedom of choice that the American population has they have the freedom of choosing to keep their own environment, wherever they go. So even though spouses live in the same household they may have quite dissimilar environments, an environment more similar to the household of origin than to the household into which they marry. It is true also for siblings;

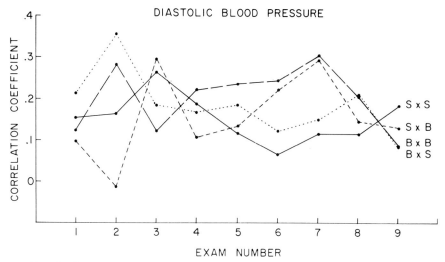

Fig. 2. Correlation coefficients for age- and sex-adjusted diastolic blood pressure scores for 609 sibling pairs examined in the Framingham Heart Program over a 16-year period. S X S = 183 sister-sister pairs, B X B = 141 brother-brother pairs, S X B = 139 sister-brother pairs with sister older than brother, B X S = 146 brother-sister pairs with brother older than sister.

they may be retaining the same environments that they grew up in even though they are now in new family environments. That might explain the consistency of the correlations.

Dr. Sackett: I would agree with your conclusions. It seems to me that assortative marriage suggests, in fact, that there has been a commonality concerning lifestyle and environmental factors which is important in the determination of blood pressure, regardless whether or not there has been geographic commonality; and that this has occurred prior to any association through marriage. Assortative marriage simply says that those with similar environmental background and physical characteristics will tend to aggregate in this phenomenon of marriage.

Studies of Hypertension in Migrants

John Cassel, M.D., M.P.H.

In reviewing the growth of knowledge concerning hypertension, especially essential hypertension, it is sobering and rather depressing to realize how little progress has been made in our understanding of its etiology. Despite spectacular advances in elucidating the pathophysiological mechanisms that control blood pressure levels and concomitant improvements in treatment as well as voluminous and enthusiastic research, we are still powerless to prevent the rise in blood pressure that is so characteristic a feature of aging in developed societies. The situation is aggravated by tantalizing glimpses from across the world of what appear to be almost perfect natural experiments. Had we the skills and wisdom to investigate them appropriately, they might provide invaluable clues, if not explanations, for the apparently inexorable rise of blood pressure with age and the high prevalence of elevated blood pressure and its complications in the modern world.

Beginning in the early 1920s and continuing to the present, there have been reports of populations throughout the world in which blood pressures are low, do not change with age, and in which the major cardiovascular diseases (coronary disease, hypertensive heart disease and stroke) are rare events.[1-2 4] These studies have been conducted on almost every continent and include groups from different parts of Africa, Asia, Australasia, the Americas, the Pacific Islands and Europe. Thus it seems unlikely that there are racial or ethnic groups who are inherently immune to rises in blood pressure. The possibility of some form of genetic immunity is further reduced if, as will be

John Cassel, M.D., M.P.H., *Professor and Chairman, Department of Epidemiology, School of Public Health, University of North Carolina, Chapel Hill.*

shown later, representatives of these groups living under different circumstances are found to have higher blood pressures than the parent group and marked differences in blood pressure levels between the young and the old. Generally, groups with low blood pressures live in small and cohesive societies, relatively insulated from contact with Western and industrialized cultures. A crucial question then is whether a change in these circumstances is associated with changes in blood pressure levels and, if so, the specific nature of the changed circumstances.

The evidence on these points is still somewhat contradictory and has been beset by problems of method and interpretation. Three types of strategies have been used to gather evidence: comparison of ethnically or genetically similar people, studied at the same point in time but living under different degrees of culture contact with modern societies; studies of the same society at different stages of "modernization"; and studies of migrants from low blood pressure societies to more modern societies.

Comparisons of Similar People Living Under Different Degrees of Culture Contact

While no exhaustive review of the literature is intended, examples of some of these studies include comparisons of Polynesians on remote islands with those living on islands more involved in a cash economy[2 5]; Melanesians living in traditional villages and in more European-dominated towns[2 6]; and South African Zulus living in a rural tribal area and in a large city.[2 7] As can be seen from Figure 1, in each of these studies the groups with the greater culture contact had higher blood pressures and a greater tendency for systolic pressures to rise with age (as far as this can be inferred from cross-sectional data). These relationships held for both men and women.

Not all studies have shown such unequivocal results. In another study of Melanesians living in the New Hebrides three groups were compared. One (the culture contact group) lived in the suburbs of the administrative capital and worked in paid employment. The other two lived in areas virtually untouched by civilization. There were almost no differences in the blood

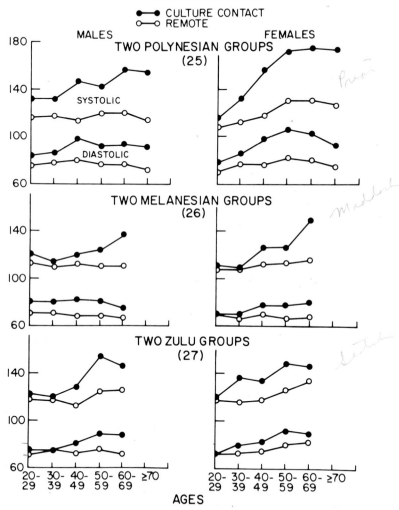

Figure 1.

pressure levels of the three groups at each age level and little difference in the pressures in the old and the young.[2][8]

Interpretation of these studies is difficult. Even when the problems of standardization of blood pressure readings are taken care of (which to a greater or lesser extent was true in each of the studies reported here) there remain sources of potential bias which could have produced spurious differences or disguised real ones. Of these, two of the more important are the assumption of genetic homogeneity of the groups; ie, there may be problems of selection, and the assumption that the "culture contact" group has been exposed to the new culture with sufficient intensity and for sufficient length of time to modify levels of blood pressure.

A few studies have addressed themselves to these problems and have provided reasonably clear-cut answers. Unfortunately they have also created new problems which make interpretation difficult. The problem of selection was investigated by Cruz-Coke[2][9] when he contrasted the blood pressures of two genetically homogeneous populations living in two adjacent but strongly different ecosystems in Chile. The genetic similarity of the two groups was measured by the distribution of blood group allele frequencies and blood pressure recordings were carefully standardized. One group was composed of primitive agriculturists and seminomadic shepherds while the other used more advanced agricultural methods and were subject to urban pressures from the nearby port. The blood pressure in the second group tended to be higher in each succeeding age group, whereas this was not true (beyond age 20) in the first group. Unfortunately, the two groups differed in many respects other than degree of culture contact. The author mentions variations in altitude, temperature, atmospheric pressure, rainfall, humidity, native vegetation, soil, cosmic radiation and oxygen tension — all of which makes it difficult to accept the conclusion that ". . . the present results confirm our previous findings that the rise of blood pressure with age increases significantly when a primitive population emigrates to a civilized region." It does, however, demonstrate that populations with low blood pressures unrelated to age can manifest increased levels of blood pressure with advancing age under changed environmental circumstances. It leaves unclear which circumstances are important and relevant.

The second problem — documenting that the culture contact group is exposed in an important fashion to life styles characteristic of the new culture — has also been addressed in only a few studies. One of these was conducted among the Papago Indians of Arizona by Patrick and Tyroler.[30,31] Using a panel of key informants, 51 Papago Indian communities were scaled according to the degree of their modernization. The ratings were subjected to several reliability tests and validated against conventional criteria of modernization: occupational structure, educational level and kin relatedness. The blood pressures of a stratified random sample of men between the ages of 40 to 49 were measured under carefully standardized conditions. In the villages rated as traditional, 8.3% of the men had systolic pressures over 160 or diastolic over 95. In the modern villages, the comparable figure was 28.3%. Unfortunately these impressive findings are somewhat marred by problems of severe underascertainment in the most traditional villages, but still lend credence to the possibility that where the changes are severe enough (and presumably have acted for sufficient time), patterns of blood pressure do change.

Studies of Societies Undergoing Modernization

Studies in this category share the methodological and interpretative problems of those in the previous category; there are often serious problems of lack of standardization of blood pressure measurements taken at different times by different observers there are difficulties in quantitating the amount and kind of modernization that has occurred and there are the potential problems of selection. Nevertheless, some of the results, both positive and negative, are intriguing. Shaper,[32] for example, quotes three surveys of blood pressures in African men living on the shores of Lake Victoria. In the 1920s blood pressures were moderately low and fell even lower in subjects over 40. Studies in similar groups in the 1930s again showed low pressure patterns but with no fall in level in older age. In the 1960s, however, studies of people living in this same area showed blood pressure patterns with age similar to those seen in developed Western countries. Shaper admits, however, that studies like these can be used only as crude indicators of the possibility that populations can change their blood pressure patterns, primarily because of noncomparability of the samples studied and the methods used.

Somewhat more to the point are two recent studies on islands of the U.S. Trust Territory in the Pacific. These are of special interest because, even though similar in design, the results are divergent. A comparison of the two raises a number of intriguing possibilities. The first study, which so far has produced negative results, is one we conducted on the island of Ponape.[33] Ponape seemed to us to present an almost perfect natural experiment. Despite successive occupations by the Spanish, Germans, and Japanese, three different ethnographic studies at the end of World War II had shown the traditional way of life persisted. Blood pressure studies in 1947 and again in 1950 had shown the by now familiar picture of low blood pressures with little, if any, difference between the young and the old. After World War II, Ponape became part of the U.S. Trust Territory and massive social and cultural change has taken place. These changes are more concentrated in the capital city and diminish with increasing distance from that city. Using a random sample of respondents from the different culture contact zones (with a 95% completion rate) and using the original ethnographic studies as baseline data, we have been able to document rather rigorously the extent of culture change and variations in different parts of the island. The second study, conducted by Labarthe and his colleagues,[34] was on the island of Palau, also now part of the U.S. Trust Territories. Like Ponape, it is inhabited by Micronesians who have a history almost identical to Ponape. As can be seen from Figures 2-4, despite the similarities of the people and their history of culture contact, the blood pressure patterns are very different. On Ponape there is little difference between the 1950 and 1973 blood pressures. Both are low with very modest, if any, difference between the young and the old and no consistent gradient between the culture contact zones. On Palau, on the other hand, there is a much sharper difference between the young and old, and a clear gradient from the remote through the intermediate to the modern zone. Given the similarities of the culture contact, what has protected the Ponapeans? The length of exposure of the two groups is identical and as far as we can tell, using some standard indicators of modernization (one of which is illustrated in Figure 5), the intensity of

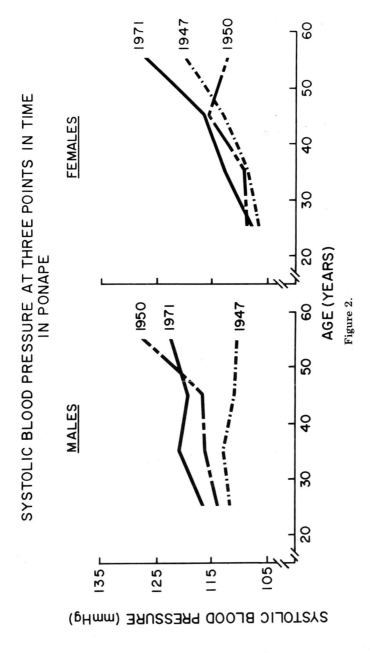

Figure 2.

J. CASSEL

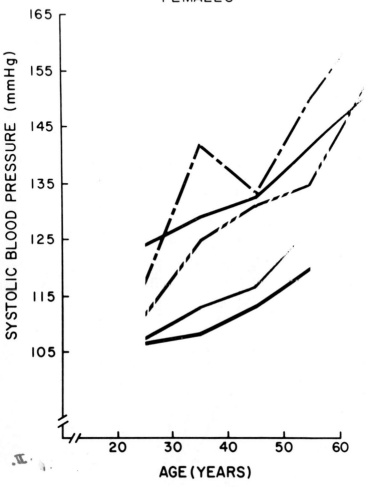

MEAN SYSTOLIC BLOOD PRESSURE (mm Hg) BY AGE
FEMALES

LABARTHE (PALAU, 1968-70)

━━━ PONAPE STUDY (1971)   ⌁⌁⌁ NGERCHELONG (TRADITIONAL)
━━━ MURRILL (PONAPE, 1948) ▬ ▬ ▬ PELELIU (INTERMEDIATE)
            ━━━ KOROR (MODERN)

Figure 3.

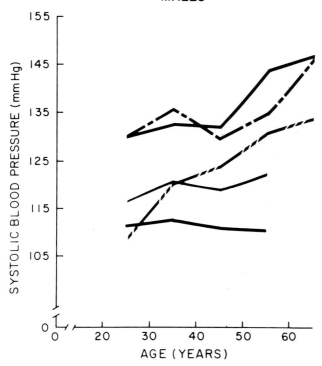

MEAN SYSTOLIC BLOOD PRESSURE (mm Hg) BY AGE: MALES

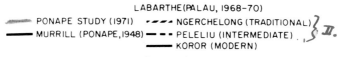

Figure 4.

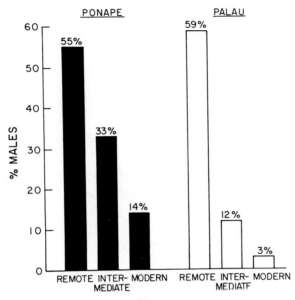

Figure 5.

exposure has not been too different on the two islands. Detailed examination of the relevant elements of the life styles that have changed, and the extent of these changes in the two groups, may provide some important leads. Such comparisons require specification of the relevant aspects of the life style, a task which I address later in this paper.

Studies of Migrants From Low Blood Pressure to Modern Societies

Theoretically, of all the categories of study, investigations of this sort should produce the most clear-cut and unequivocal answers. Ideally, though, to avoid the weaknesses in method common to the previous classes of studies, such investigations should be able to identify migrants before migration, compare them with nonmigrants from the same population (to test for selection factors), follow the migrants over time in their new environment (to ensure that the age relationship of blood pressure is not being produced by selective mortality — a distinct possibility when using cross-sectional data alone), and also follow the nonmigrants over the same period of time (to control for secular changes common to both groups). Furthermore, before and at varying intervals after migration, it will be necessary to quantify those changes in life style and behavior considered relevant in the determination of blood pressure levels. For obvious reasons, few investigators have the opportunity to perform such a complete study (I know of only one, and this is still in its early stages). Most studies have had to content themselves with approximations to the ideal scheme.

Two general approaches have been used: identifying migrant populations at their place of destination and categorizing them on the basis of length of residence, and the more complete approach of identifying populations at their place of origin and comparing them with migrants from these places.

The first approach is exemplified by Stamler's studies[3 5] in which he compared the blood pressure levels of black migrants from the South living in Chicago to Chicago-born blacks (Fig. 6). After 10 to 15 years of city life, the prevalence rate of migrants with diastolic pressures $\geq$ 90 mm equalled those of the Chicago-born; migrants who had been there for less time had a lower rate and those who had been there longer a higher rate, suggesting some form of adaptation by the Chicago-born (albeit imperfect) which has not been achieved by the migrants.

I have chosen four studies to illustrate the second approach. The first is a study by Florey.[3 6] He compared a genetically homogeneous population, part of which lives in the Cape Verde Islands (West Africa) and part of which has migrated over the last 100 years to the East Coast of the United States. As can be seen from Figure 7, the migrants have higher pressures at each age and a sharper difference between the young and the old than do the islanders. (While only systolic pressures are shown in the figure, the same pattern was found for diastolic.) In the second study Shaper[3 2] compared the blood pressures of nomadic Kenyan warriors at different times after their entry into the Kenyan Army with those who did not enter. The recruits showed a significant rise in systolic pressure, not after their first six months in the Army when their weight gain was considerable, but after an average of two years and when their

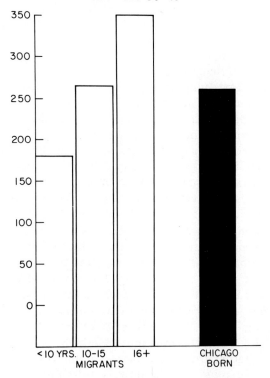

PREVALENCE OF ELEVATED BLOOD PRESSURE
(DIASTOLIC 90mm+) IN CHICAGO BLACKS BY
LENGTH OF RESIDENCE IN CITY (RATE PER 1000)
MEN AGED 30-49

Figure 6.

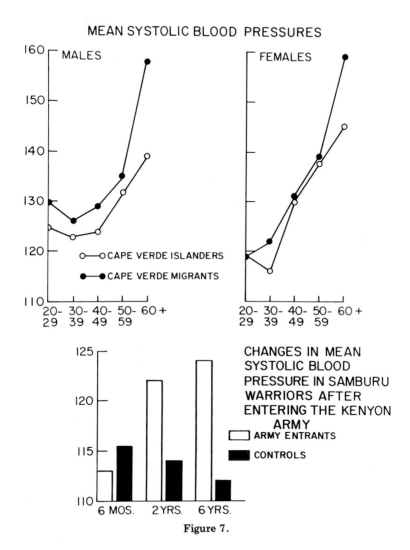

Figure 7.

weight gain was less appreciable than in the earlier period. After six years in the Army, the pressures were still significantly higher than their age-matched controls (Fig. 7). The third study is by Cruz-Coke.[37] He compared Polynesians living on Easter Island with those who migrated to the mainland (Chile). Gene frequencies were measured in the two groups and were found to be similar. The mean diastolic blood pressure of the islanders was 84.2, while those of the migrants was 86.8. (The migrants were on the average 1.6 years older than the islanders.) Furthermore, the regression coefficient of blood pressure on age was only 0.09 for the islanders but 0.34 for the migrants. Finally, Trulson and her colleagues[38] have compared Irish-born Americans (living in the United States) with their brothers living in Ireland. Of the American sample, 32% were classified as hypertensive (systolic blood pressure $\geqslant$ 160 mm or diastolic $\geqslant$ 95 mm) as compared to 21% of the Irish sample.

I feel sure there must have been studies showing no differences in the blood pressure patterns of migrants and nonmigrants but I have not discovered any. I rather suspect that such studies are less likely to be published, which, if true, is a pity. Nevertheless, even if the studies reported here are a selected group, they tend to confirm the findings of the other categories of studies: given certain circumstances, blood pressure patterns do change. This brings us squarely to the question of what these circumstances might be and for how long they operate. Taking the second question first, Scotch's data on the Zulu[39] showed that 36% of those who had spent as little as five to eight years in the city had hypertension (by conventional standards). The effect was particularly notable in women. Stamler, as already reported,[35] found blood pressures in migrants to Chicago were as high as the Chicago-born after 10 to 15 years in the city, and Labarthe[34] found that after 25 years of culture contact on Palau, blood pressures were higher in the old than in the young. It would seem, then, that at the most we are talking of decades, not generational time for these effects to operate, nor does there appear to be a critical age.

Turning now to the nature of the circumstances that might produce such changes in blood pressure patterns, I think it is becoming increasingly unlikely that genetic differences alone will offer a satisfactory explanation. There remains a possibility of genetic differences in susceptibility to environmental factors which needs more study. But even if this is true it leaves unanswered the nature of the environmental factors. Generally speaking, there are two competing sets of hypotheses that have been advanced to identify the relevant environmental factors. One set emphasizes physical factors: caloric intake, physical activity and the associated body build, salt intake and the burden of parasites or diseases such as tuberculosis which produces anemia and wasting in the low blood pressure groups. The alternative set holds that much of the phenomenon can be accounted for by psychosocial factors. Low pressures occur in societies with a coherent value system which remains relatively unchallenged during the lifetime of the oldest inhabitants. Migration to a society with different value systems leads to situations in which previously sanctioned behaviors, especially those the individual acquired during critical learning periods, can no longer be used to express normal behavioral urges. This, in turn, creates repeated autonomic system arousal.

We have no good data to sort out the relative merits of these two sets of hypotheses. We know that there is a modest relationship between weight and blood pressure, for example, and in many studies migrants are heavier than nonmigrants. Some authors have concluded that weight differences are adequate to explain the differences in blood pressure between the groups. If that is universally true, we can stop doing migration studies, as there are easier ways to further our understanding between weight and blood pressure levels than by such relatively complicated and time-consuming approaches. However, a number of studies show that weight differences are not adequate to explain differences in blood pressure.[24] Furthermore, another paper in this series[40] indicates that obesity and weight gain, though obviously important, are by no means complete explanations for the development of elevated blood pressure. The same argument holds for salt intake. While there are reported differences in salt intake in populations with low compared to high blood pressures, we have been relatively unsuccessful in discerning differences within a population between those with low and elevated pressures. I suspect that both sets of hypotheses will be useful, rather than either-or. We will find diet, salt intake and the degree of adaptation to one's niche in society all important in the determination of blood pressure levels.

What we need, then, is a series of prospective studies fulfilling the criteria described above, ones which will eliminate many of the methodological problems which have made interpretation so difficult and which will enable us to quantitate the variables to test both sets of hypotheses. Fortunately, one such study is currently in operation. Preliminary baseline results are now in press in the current issue of the *International Journal of Epidemiology*. This is the study by Prior and his associates on the migration of Tokelau islanders to New Zealand. Planned migration from the Tokelaus to New Zealand was initiated in 1966 and has been continuing since. The only contact between the islands and New Zealand is by ship, which makes the journey once every three or four months. This makes it possible to identify future migrants some months before they leave. Dr. Prior and his colleagues had the foresight to conduct an extensive examination of all the islanders in 1968 (96.4% ascertainment rate). Their data included diet, anthropometry and salt excretion as well as blood pressure levels and cardiovascular status. Two social scientists on the team (Drs. Hooper and Huntsmen) conducted detailed ethnographic studies of the islands for a year or more prior to this date. They have developed scales to measure commitment to Tokelau values and the degree and intensity of social interaction to test some of the more specific psychosocial hypotheses. Furthermore, the migrants are exposed to different sets of circumstances in New Zealand which theoretically should influence their adaptation. Some move to situations where most of their daily contacts are with fellow Tokelau islanders; others are in places where they are relatively isolated from such contact. The Wellington team have set up a surveillance mechanism so that migrants (now numbering some 2,000) can be traced and periodically reexamined. At regular intervals the investigators return to the islands to examine nonmigrants.

Thus we have a most unusual occurrence, an almost perfect "experiment of nature" with investigators on the scene equipped with the imagination and the skill to exploit it fully. Future reports from this group will be awaited with great interest in the hope that some parts of the riddle that has so long puzzled us will now be cleared up.

References

1. Fleming, H. C.: Medical Observations on the Zuni Indians. Contribution to Museum of American Indians, Heye Foundation, 7, No. 2, New York, 1924.
2. Donninson, C. P.: Blood pressure in the African native. *Lancet*, 1:56, 1929.
3. Krakower, A.: Blood pressure of Chinese living in Eastern Canada. *Amer. Heart J.*, 9:376, 1933.
4. Saunders, G. M.: Blood pressure in Yucatans. *Amer. J. Med. Sci*, 185:843, 1933.
5. Kilborn, L. G.: A note on the blood pressure of primitive races with special reference to the Maio of Kiweichaw. *Chin. J. Physiol.* 11:135, 1937.
6. Kean B. H.: Blood pressure studies on West Indians and Panamanians living on Isthmus of Panama. *Arch. Intern. Med.*, 68:466, 1941.
7. Levine, V. E.: The blood pressure of Eskimos. *Fed. Proc.*, 1:121, 1942.
8. Kean, B. H.: Blood pressure of the Cuna Indians. *Amer. J. Trop. Med.*, 24 (suppl.):341, 1944.
9. Alexander, F.: A medical survey of the Aleutian Islands. *New Eng. J. Med.*, 240:1035, 1949.
10. Bibile, S. W. et al: Variation with age and sex of blood pressure and pulse rate for Ceylonese subjects. *Ceylon J. Med. Sci.*, 6:80, 1949.
11. Murrill, R. I.: A blood pressure study of the natives of Ponape Island. *Hum. Biol.*, 21:47, 1949.
12. Murphy, W.: Some observations on blood pressures in the humid tropics. *New Zeal. Med. J.*, 54:64, 1949.
13. Whyte, W. M.: Body fat and blood pressure of natives of New Guinea: Reflections on essential hypertension. *Aust. Ann. Med.*, 7:36, 1958.
14. Padmayati, S. and Gupta, S.: Blood pressure studies in rural and urban groups in Delhi. *Circulation*, 19:393, 1959.
15. Kaminer, B. and Lutz, W. P.: Blood pressure in Bushmen of the Kalahari Desert. *Circulation*, 22:289, 1960.
16. Abrahams, D. G., Able, C. A. and Bernart, G.: Systemic blood pressure in a rural West African community. *W. Afr. Med. J.*, 9:45, 1960.
17. Lowell, R. R. H., Maddocks, I. and Rogerson, G. W.: The casual arterial pressure of Fejians and Indians in Fiji. *Aust. Ann. Med.*, 9:4, 1960.
18. Scotch, N. A.: A preliminary report on the relation of sociocultural factors to hypertension among the Zulu. *Ann. N.Y. Acad. Sci.*, 86:1000, 1960.
19. Maddocks, I.: Possible absence of hypertension in two complete Pacific Island populations. *Lancet*, 2:396, 1961.
20. Scotch, N. A.: Sociocultural factors in the epidemiology of Zulu hypertension. *Amer. J. Pub. Health*, 53:1205, 1963.

21. Fulmer, H. S. and Roberts, R. W.: Coronary heart disease among the Navajo Indians. *Ann. Intern. Med.*, 59:740, 1963.
22. Mann, G. V. et al: Cardiovascular disease in the Masai. *J. Atheroscler. Res.*, 4:289, 1964.
23. Prior, I. A. M.: Population studies in New Zealand and the South Pacific. W.H.O. Report on Cardiovascular Epidemiology in the Pacific. ed. by Fejfar, Z., vol. 28, 1970.
24. Henry, J. P. and Cassel, J. C.: Psychosocial factors in essential hypertension. *Amer. J. Epidem.*, 90:171, 1969.
25. Prior, I. A. M. et al: Sodium intake and blood pressure in two Polynesian populations. *New Eng. J. Med.*, 279:515, 1968.
26. Maddocks, I.: Blood pressures in Melanesians. *Med. J. Aust.*, June: 1123, 1967.
27. Scotch, N. A.: Sociocultural factors in the epidemiology of Zulu hypertension. *Amer. J. Pub. Health*, 53:1205, 1963.
28. Norman-Taylor, W. and Rees, W. H.: Blood pressures in three New Hebrides communities. *Brit. J. Prev. Soc. Med.* 17:141, 1963.
29. Cruz-Coke, R., Donoso, H. and Barrera, R.: Genetic ecology of hypertension. *Clin. Sci. Molec. Med.*, 45:55s, 1973.
30. Patrick, R. C.: Some health consequences of rapid cultural change. Paper presented at Michigan State University, April 25, 1974.
31. Tyroler, H. A.: Blood pressure studies of the Papago Indian. Paper read at the A.H.A. Conference on the Epidemiology of Cardiovascular Diseases, Chicago, Illinois, January 30, 1965.
32. Shaper, A.G.: Cardiovascular disease in the tropics. III. Blood pressure and hypertension. *Brit. Med. J.*, 3:805, 1972.
33. Patrick, R., Cassel, J. C., Tyroler, H. A. et al: The Ponape study of the health effects of cultural change. Paper presented at the annual meeting of the Society for Epidemiological Research at Berkeley, California, June 22, 1974.
34. Labarthe, D. et al: Health effects of modernization in Palau. *Amer. J. Epidem.*, 98:161, 1973.
35. Stamler, J., Berkson, D. M., Lindberg, H. A. et al: Socioeconomic factors in the epidemiology of hypertensive disease. In Stamler, J., Stamler, R. and Pullman, T. N. (eds.): *The Epidemiology of Hypertension.* New York:Grune and Stratton, 1967.
36. Florey, C. du V. and Cuadrado, R. R.: Blood pressure in native Cape Verdeans and in Cape Verdean immigrants and their descendants living in New England. *Hum. Biol.*, 40:189, 1968.
37. Cruz-Coke, R., Etcheverry, R. and Nagel, R.: Influence of migration on blood-pressure of Easter Islanders. *Lancet*, 1:697, 1964.
38. Trulson, M. F., Clancy, R. E., Jessop, W. J. E. et al: Comparisons of siblings in Boston and Ireland. *J. Amer. Diet. Ass.*, 45:225, 1964.
39. Gampel, B., Slome, C., Scotch, N. et al: Urbanization and hypertension among Zulu adults. *J. Chronic Dis.*, 15:67, 1962.
40. Tyroler, H. A., Heyden, S. and Hames, C. G.: Weight and hypertension; Evans County studies of blacks and whites. Paper prepared for presentation at the Epidemiology of Hypertension 2nd International Symposium in Chicago, Illinois, September 18, 1974.

Discussion

Dr. Borhani: I enjoyed Dr. Cassel's excellent presentation. I wonder if he cares to elaborate on the psychosocial aspects influencing differences in blood pressures after migration? Some years ago, as you know, we did report that mortality from coronary heart diseases in California had been dropping between 1950-1960, and then when we analyzed the data by race, we found out that the black population of California did not show the same trend as the white population. The only way we could analyze the problem of migration which we hypothesized was affecting these data was going back to the census data, which provided information on the length of residence in California. We were not able to explain the difference between white and black mortality by migration. The Chicago study by Dr. Stamler and the study that you have just completed perhaps could provide the answer to this question, namely, that migration does influence the blood pressure and that, in turn, affects the coronary heart disease mortality.

Dr. Cassel: The movement of people from a rural type of society into a more urban, industrialized society leads to various phenomena including the loss by some people of rather fragile ties to other important people. It has been argued under those circumstances that this leads, among other things, to constant autonomic nervous system arousal with the possibility of sustained blood pressure which tends to become self-perpetuating. There are animal studies that would tend to confirm this. But to quantitate these factors and prove them human becomes very much more difficult.

Dr. Hoobler, Michigan: I was very much interested in your conclusions which in a much more sophisticated way match some I developed during a sabbatical year in Guatemala. I began with the original premise that possibly the Indian race was immune to the development of hypertension based on early studies of blood pressure in Central America. We did a study* quite carefully on an age-specific population in the rural highlands in Guatemala and found no increase in blood pressure

---

*Hoobler, S., Tejada, C., Guzman, M. et al: Influence of nutrition and "acculturation" on the blood pressure levels and changes with age in the highland Guatemalan Indian, abstracted. *Circulation*, 32 (suppl. II): 1965.

with age and no substantial hypertension. While we were doing this, we contacted a professional colleague practicing near that area and he said there were a lot of Indians in his practice who run several enterprises in the city, and that the frequency of hypertension was just as great as in those of Spanish origin. This led us to do additional studies to examine the blood pressure of large numbers of Indians of the same tribe working in a textile mill. We found that, in fact, they had at all ages the same blood pressure distribution as those of Spanish descent. Then going back and studying the relationship I could only pick out three distinctions: (1) They were slightly heavier in terms of abdominal panniculus, although they were not obese. (2) The textile workers sat all day watching the loom spin while the agricultural workers in the highlands were extremely active all day on their farms. (3) The diet was only slightly modified when the Indians lived in the city. No one had very much meat, but salt intake seemed to be about the same from random urine samples.

Dr. Labarthe, Minnesota: In looking at the results up to the present time, we have tended to focus on the differences among the three areas within the Palau district. Dr. Cassel, referring to earlier surveys, has demonstrated effectively that, in fact, these three areas, while somewhat different among themselves, show in common a striking departure from the pattern shown in Ponape. Two of the hypotheses that have stimulated this sort of investigation have been (1) that it is indeed modernization and contact with the modern culture per se which produces changes in blood pressure, or (2) that blood pressure changes relate more directly to immediate discontinuities or heterogeneity in sociocultural characteristics within groups of individuals at a given time from whatever source of disruption. This suggests the potential interest in looking at these two population studies in Palau and Ponape to see whether there may be differences in the degree of heterogeneity in this respect within the given culture zones in the study. If this hypothesis is correct, we should find greater heterogeneity within each of the three zones in Palau than is the case in Ponape, and this is, perhaps, one of the things we can pursue jointly.

Dr. Cassel: In Ponape, in the capital city, the people are considerably fatter than they are in other areas, but the blood pressures are no higher; in fact, they are a little bit lower than in the more remote areas. So we are dealing with a queer mixture of things.

Dr. Miller, Baltimore: I constantly have a problem when I read the literature about migrant studies. They all seem to indicate that as you move somewhere, your rate of prevalence of hypertension increases. Regarding the people who moved from the southern part of the United States to Chicago, theoretically their blood pressures should have decreased. I am making this point because I think we have not dealt with the subject of who migrates. I am sure that is not a random probability of who migrates.

Dr. Cassel: You are absolutely right; it is not random. Migrants do differ in a number of ways and that is the beauty of the study I mentioned in New Zealand because they do have full and complete information of all people before the act of migration to compare them with those who migrate. In a study we have done, we have positive information. We followed the population for ten years and during that time we know about every person who migrated. We do not know what the health consequences were at the end, but we do know what they were like when they migrated. We and others before us have found that migrants tend to be on the whole somewhat taller, slightly heavier and slightly younger than the nonmigrants. Other studies have showed that they had slightly higher IQs. So there are differences between migrants and nonmigrants. ✓

Hypertension in Japan:
A Review

Shuichi Hatano, M.D.

It has been reported in clinical, pathological and epidemiological studies that cerebrovascular disease is highly prevalent and ischemic heart disease much less prevalent in Japan. Why? Is hypertension more severe or more frequent? A large number of studies and surveys have been carried out to describe the present situation of hypertension in Japan and to elucidate the etiology. The purpose of this paper is to review these studies and present some facts about the Japanese situation, specifically on the following:

1. Is the blood pressure of the Japanese different?
2. Is hypertension evenly distributed among the Japanese?
3. Is the severity of hypertension different in Japan?
4. Is there any change in blood pressure over time?
5. What has been done at the community level to control hypertension and what was the outcome?

Finally, a few hypothetical explanations which fit situations in Japan will be briefly reviewed.

Available Information

An exhaustive review of the Japanese studies is not the purpose of this paper, and a large number of Japanese articles are not introduced. Nevertheless, many references have been made to Japanese literature, and a brief orientation may be worthwhile. Sources of reviewed information in Japan can be classified in three categories. First, a series of surveys conducted by the Japanese government: the national nutrition survey[1] and

Shuichi Hatano, M.D., *Cardiovascular Diseases, World Health Organization, Geneva, Switzerland.*

the adult disease survey[2] which have been conducted on inhabitants in areas selected by probability sampling as representative of Japan and vital statistics for the total population. These surveys cover the whole nation and have been repeated in a standardized way, providing basic information which allows the Japanese situation to be viewed as a whole.

Second, there are the studies that also cover the whole country but on selected populations, such as data from a life insurance company[3] and studies on employees of a big occupation group, such as the Japanese National Railways.[10,36,37] The size of the population is large and the studies include follow-up data that are not included in the government surveys.

Third, more detailed individual studies have been carried out in small areas by universities and institutes. These studies generally provide more accurate information, such as that provided by autopsy on a smaller group of subjects, but are not representative of the whole country.

Most of these studies on hypertension were carried out with the same methods as those recommended by a WHO Expert Committee.[29] However, this does not automatically guarantee comparability of results. Tightly coordinated multicenter epidemiologic studies or studies designed for an international comparison are few. Information on observer bias has seldom been reported to permit critical appraisals. However, an effort has been made in the standardization of cardiovascular survey methods in Japan by the Japanese Association for Cerebro-Cardiovascular Disease Control[44] and others. A single visiting team approach used in some studies[13,23,41,43] would have provided more comparable results. In this retrospective review of already collected data, results are accepted when different investigators of different populations at different times are in agreement.

Blood Pressure in the Japanese

The age-sex specific mean blood pressures of the Japanese population obtained from the national nutrition survey[1] in 1970 and the adult disease survey[2] in 1971, carried out by area sampling, were almost identical. A slightly lower systolic blood pressure was reported in applicants for life insurance in 1953-1954 (Fig. 1).[3] The distribution of blood pressure by age

MEAN BLOOD PRESSURE IN SELECTED POPULATION GROUPS

white

a Bergen, Norway[4] 1950

b Evans County,[5] Ga.,
  USA 1960-62

Japanese

c National nutrition survey[1] 1970

d Life insurance applicants[3] 1953-54

Chinese

e Taipei[6] 1954

f Taipei[7] 1970-71

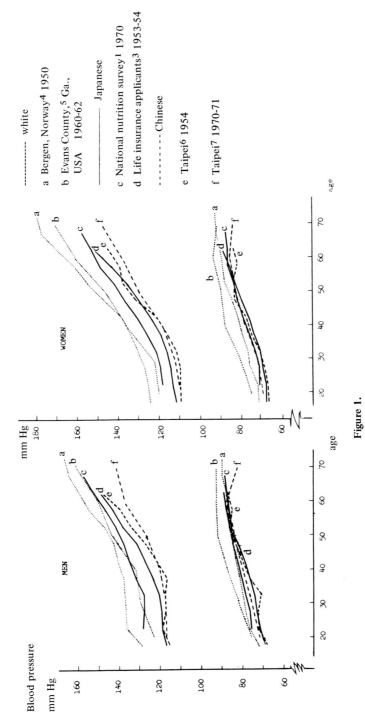

Figure 1.

and sex in the Japanese population is the same as in other countries, though the rise in blood pressure in elderly women is less prominent in the Japanese. Data from Bergen, Norway,[4] and whites in Evans County, Georgia,[5] are referred to for comparison; the mean of both the systolic and the diastolic blood pressure of populations in Bergen and Georgia in both sexes at almost all ages exceeded that of the Japanese.

What about the comparison with the Chinese and Koreans, who are ethnically closer to the Japanese (Table 1)? Two surveys on residents in Taiwan conducted at different times[6,7] showed almost identical results. The Chinese in Taipei had a lower systolic blood pressure than the Japanese, but showed little difference in diastolic blood pressure. A report from Korea[8] showed an equal or only slightly lower blood pressure than the Japanese when young, and the rise in blood pressure with age was not significant, staying even lower than the Chinese in Taiwan after 50 years of age, but the number of old people in this study was small and the methods of recruitment and response rates were not indicated.

Thus, the Japanese as a whole appeared to have a lower blood pressure than white people in Bergen and Georgia and higher blood pressure than populations in Seoul or Taipei. These studies were not coordinated, and further confirmation of results is desirable.

Body build can be a contributing factor to these differences. The average weight-height ratio of obese Japanese (defined as having more than 80% excess of the average ratio) did not even reach the ratio of average Americans.[9] It is not known whether or not the Japanese are hypertensive in a height and weight standardized comparison.

Regional Difference in Blood Pressure

The Japanese are a well-mixed single race living in a small territory which, however, extends over almost the same latitudes as the United States, so that the climate and the life style of the people vary.

The surveys carried out by the government,[1,2] the life insurance study[3] and the results from annual examinations of the Japanese National Railways (JNR)[10] all agree that blood

TABLE 1A. Mean Systolic Blood Pressure in Some Asian Populations

Sex	Age	ALL JAPAN [1] 1970			AKITA *[15] 1963-65			HIROSHIMA & NAGASAKI [14] 1970-72			SEOUL, KOREA [8] ?			TAIPEI, CHINA [6] 1954		
		N	mean	S.D.	N	mean	S.D.	N	mean	S.D.	N	mean	S.D.	N	mean	S.D.
Men	15 - 19	—	—	—	—	—	—	—	—	—	30	115	12	524	115	13
	20 - 24	764	128	14	—	—	—	—	—	—	112	126	12	768	116	14
	25 - 29		127	14	—	—	—	124	115	13	1236	128	14	1169	117	12
	30 - 34	942	127	15	696	137	19	200	117	13	951	125	16	1274	117	14
	35 - 39		131	16				307	122	16				822	121	14
	40 - 44	834	134	19	531	146	26	747	126	19	201	126	16	736	126	14
	45 - 49		137	22				637	126	20				513	133	16
	50 - 54	593	141	23	511	157	30	293	135	25	57	131	20	264	133	21
	55 - 59		146	25				584	135	23				163	139	26
	60 - 64		152	27	333	166	30	594	142	23				64		
	65 - 69	727	157	27				373	146	25	6	136	8			
	70 - 74				29	170	30	302	146	27				82	146	24
	75 - 79		159	27				140	151	27						
	80+							62	153	28					150	30
Women	15 - 19	—	—	—	—	—	—	—	—	—	421	112	10	404	109	11
	20 - 24	1120	116	12	—	—	—	171	112	14	546	117	11	636	109	12
	25 - 29		119	13	—	—	—	247	113	15	459	118	12	616	109	13
	30 - 34	1122	121	13	920	127	17	466	116	16	247	126	18	462	111	15
	35 - 39		125	15				1131	119	17				328	117	21
	40 - 44	1083	130	17	764	137	22	995	123	19	140	126	17	276	120	23
	45 - 49		136	20				682	129	22				197	131	23
	50 - 54	729	141	23	596	148	27	548	133	22	58	131	19	121	137	27
	55 - 59		148	24				572	142	25				91	139	29
	60 - 64		152	26	457	161	31	569	144	26				71	144	34
	65 - 69	894	157	27				463	148	25	11	133	22			
	70 - 74				59	172	32	223	157	16				104	156	29
	75 - 79		163	26				118	157	27						

* Akita, 3 communities age 30-69; 2 communities age 70 & over

TABLE 1B. Mean Diastolic Blood Pressure in Some Asian Populations

Sex	Age	ALL JAPAN 1970			AKITA *15 1963-65			HIROSHIMA & NAGASAKI 14 1970-72			SEOUL, KOREA 8 ?			TAIPEI, CHINA 6 1954		
		N	mean	S.D.	N	mean	S.D.	N	mean	S.D.	N	mean	S.D.	N	mean	S.D.
Men	15 – 19	—	—	—	—	—	—	—	—	—	174	73	11	524	67	13
	20 – 24	764	75	12	—	—	—	124	74	11	247	75	10	766	72	12
	25 – 29		76	12	696	91	14	200	77	11				1169	72	11
	30 – 34	942	78	12	531	102	14	306	81	12	145	78	.10	1274	70	12
	35 – 39		80	13				746	83	13				822	76	11
	40 – 44	834	82	14	511	102	16	237	84	13	108	76	11	735	80	14
	45 – 49		84	14				293	86	14				513	82	14
	50 – 54	593	85	15	334	103	16	384	86	13	209	79	12	534	86	14
	55 – 59		86	15				394	87	14				163	84	14
	60 – 64		87	14				373	85	13	133	79	14			
	65 – 69		88	14				309	83	13						
	70 – 74	727	87	14	29	97	14	146	85	13	61	82	17	82	85	16
	75 – 79							62	82	11						
	80+															
Women	15 – 19	—			—			—			126	72	9	404	66	12
	20 – 24	1120	71	11	—			—			219	75	9	636	67	12
	25 – 29		71	11	920	85	12	170	72	10				616	68	13
	30 – 34	1122	73	12	762	98	13	247	73	11	286	73	14	462	70	13
	35 – 39		76	13				467	76	12				528	75	14
	40 – 44	1083	79	13	596	96	14	1130	77	12	236	74	10	278	78	15
	45 – 49		82	14				995	80	12				197	83	18
	50 – 54	729	83	14	437	100	14	682	82	13	167	75	15	121	83	15
	55 – 59		86	14				548	83	12				91	82	15
	60 – 64		86	14				571	86	13	172	61	16	71	83	15
	65 – 69		87	14				565	86	13						
	70 – 74	894	87	14	59	101	15	462	85	13	146	61	14	164	83	14
	75 – 79							222	84	13						
	80+							117	64	14						

* Akita, 3 communities age 30-69
2 communities age 70 & over

pressure is higher in the northeastern part (Tohoku) of the main island and the northern Japan Sea border and is lower in the southern Pacific border, around the Kyoto and Osaka area and Shikoku Island (the fourth biggest island in the south of Japan). The median values of systolic blood pressure of employees of JNR in its 27 administrative districts is illustrated in Figure 2.[10] Blood pressure was high in Tohoku, a part of Hokkaido (the northernmost island), the western end of the main island and south Kyushu (the westernmost island) and low in the central part of the main island and Shikoku Island. The detailed blood pressure distributions in three representative districts, Osaka (O on the map), Tokyo (T) and Akita (A), are also shown in Figure 8. Employees in the Osaka district showed lower blood pressure at all age groups, those in Akita district higher and those in the Tokyo district a middle level. This regional difference of the blood pressure distribution to some extent corresponds to the death rates from cerebrovascular disease (Fig. 3).[11] The death rate is highest in the northeastern (Tohoku) prefectures, decreases toward the southwest and is lowest in the central part of the main island and Shikoku Island.

However, the blood pressure of populations and the death rate from stroke did not correspond exactly. It is obvious that not all stroke is caused by hypertension and not all hypertensives die from stroke, even in Japan. The comparison among the Japanese in Hiroshima, Honolulu and California clearly indicated this[12]: the prevalence of hypertension was highest in Japanese in California who had lowest mortality and prevalence rates of stroke.

Results from a comparison of individual studies are preliminary, but are more likely to be valid when several other studies indicate the same conclusion. Surveys in a small defined area carried out by individual investigators showed regional differences along the same direction as described above, sometimes revealing bigger differences. Low blood pressure was reported in Osaka,[13] Hiroshima and Nagasaki[14] (Table 1; Fig. 4), which are in the prefectures with a lower death rate from stroke, according to the national mortality statistics (Fig. 3). The population of Hiroshima and Nagasaki showed lower blood pressure than the population in Akita[15] or Bergen[4] in almost all percentiles at all ages, except in the 95th and 75th

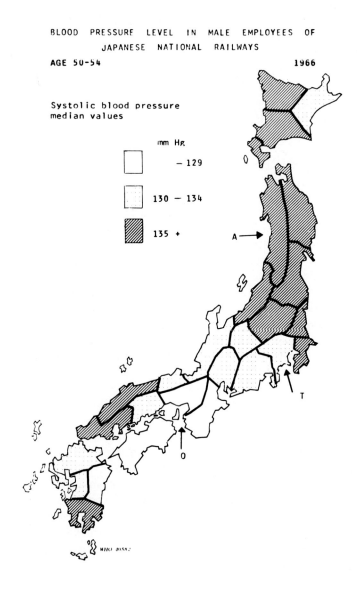

Figure 2.

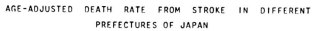

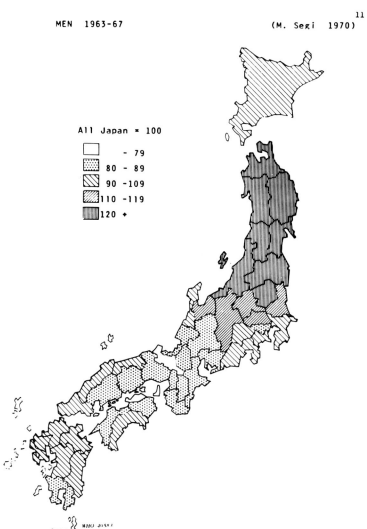

Figure 3.

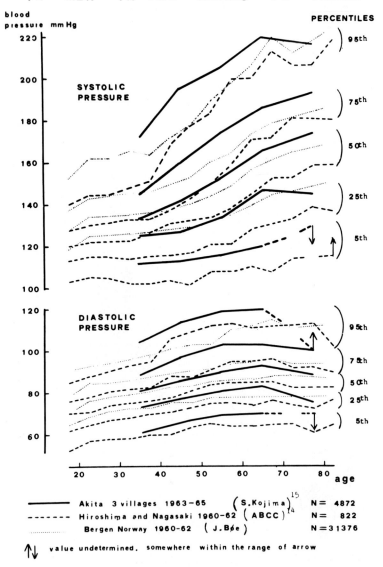

Figure 4.

percentiles, which approached those of the Bergen population in the older age group.

High blood pressure in younger age groups was reported in the population in some communities in the Akita prefecture (Table 1; Fig. 4),[13,15] which is known to have the highest death rate from stroke in all Japan. A very high incidence of stroke in this area was observed in the WHO stroke register project.[16] At the age of 30 to 40 years, the highest 5% of the population in Akita had a higher blood pressure than in Bergen, while the lower three quarters of the population in the two places had nearly the same blood pressure. In older age groups, up to about 70 years, a much larger proportion of the population in Akita was found to have high blood pressure compared to the Bergen population.

The similar upward shift of blood pressure distribution with age was also observed in the JNR employees in the Akita district as compared with the Osaka district, though to a lesser extent (Fig. 8). When these two different groups in Akita were compared, the rural population (Fig. 4) showed a much higher upward trend in blood pressure distribution than JNR employees in the Akita district (Fig. 8). The rural population already had higher blood pressure than JNR employees at 40 to 44 years of age and much higher blood pressure in the 75th and 95th percentiles at 50 to 54 years of age. This exactly reflects the difference between farmers and administrative, managerial, clerical and technical workers, which we shall see in the next section.

Social Differences

Differences in blood pressure appear in other population groups, too. A rise in blood pressure with urbanization or acculturation has been reported from various parts of the world.[17-19] However, inhabitants in probability area samples in agricultural, forestry or fishing areas in Japan revealed higher blood pressures than populations in big cities in men and women in the Japanese national surveys.[1,2]

The blood pressure of men was analyzed in different occupation groups (Fig. 5): agriculture, forestry and fishing; skilled and unskilled laborers and service workers; administra-

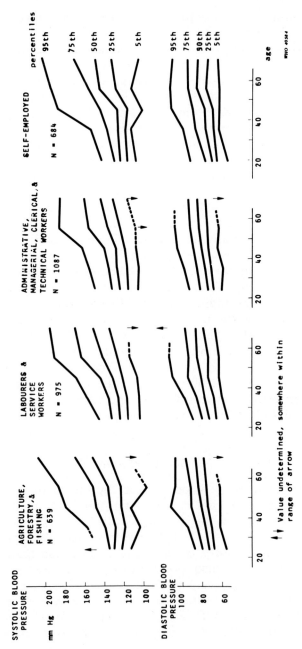

OCCUPATION AND BLOOD PRESSURE DISTRIBUTION IN MEN

5th, 25th 50th, 75th and 95th percentiles

(Japan National Nutrition Survey 1970)[1]

Figure 5.

tive, managerial, clerical and technical workers were combined in this study,[1] composing three large occupation categories. The self-employed were in a separate group. Other, smaller sub-groups are not shown. No remarkable difference was observed in the diastolic blood distribution. The agriculture, forestry and fishing group had a higher systolic blood pressure distribution when young, and the distribution of the systolic blood pressure of 95th percentile was particularly high. All other workers had a lower blood pressure than agricultural workers when young, but their blood pressure scattered in middle age and was almost as high as that of agricultural workers. In administrative, managerial, clerical and technical workers, the trend toward an increase in blood pressure with age was the least marked of all the four occupation groups. However, the difference in the mean blood pressure in middle or old age did not reach a significant level.

Death rates from some selected diseases also revealed a marked difference among occupation groups (Table 2).[20] Administrative and managerial workers have about one half the average death rate from cerebrovascular and hypertensive diseases. Workers in agriculture, forestry and fishing had a 24%-38% higher death rate from these diseases than the average for all workers. This difference is parallel to the blood pressure distribution of the two occupation groups in middle age. The working environment certainly influences the death rate. For example, there is a very high accident rate for miners and masons. Additional contributing factors might be medical knowledge and the health awareness of individuals, economic conditions, the availability of medical services and selection at entry to the occupation. This appears to be so because groups with a lower or higher death rate for cerebrovascular and hypertensive diseases generally had a lower or higher death rate also for malignant neoplasms and accidents, which may not necessarily have the same etiological factors as cardiovascular diseases. What these factors are and to what extent they influence blood pressure are unknown.

Severity of Hypertension in Japan

Is there any difference between hypertensive patients in Japan and those in other countries? Is premature hypertension in Akita severe? Studies were carried out independently and

S. HATANO

TABLE 2. Type of Occupation and Age Standardized Death Rate of Men Aged 15 and Over — Japan 1970

(per 100,000 population)

( ) = relative death rate to all workers (%)

Occupation	All Causes	B26 Ischaemic Heart Disease	B27 Hypertensive Diseases	B30 Cerebrovascular Diseases	B19 Malignant Neoplasm	EB42 EB48 Accident
All workers	482.7 (100.0)	29.6 (100.0)	7.5 (100.0)	110.4 (100.0)	107.4 (100.0)	70.5 (100.0)
Professional & technical workers	424.2 (87.9)	35.3 (119.3)	7.5 (100.0)	90.1 (81.6)	102.5 (95.4)	46.2 (65.5)
Administrative & managerial workers	281.7 (58.4)	24.0 (81.1)	4.2 (56.0)	51.5 (46.6)	84.3 (78.5)	22.2 (31.5)
Clerical & related workers	432.4 (89.6)	31.0 (104.7)	7.0 (93.3)	78.1 (70.7)	123.4 (114.9)	45.1 (64.0)
Sales workers	537.7 (111.4)	39.5 (133.4)	8.9 (118.7)	115.7 (104.8)	131.9 (122.8)	57.6 (61.7)
Service workers	499.9 (103.6)	33.9 (114.5)	8.6 (114.7)	110.4 (100.0)	106.9 (101.4)	59.0 (63.7)
Fishermen, agricultural & forestry workers	621.6 (128.8)	30.9 (104.4)	9.3 (124.0)	152.8 (138.4)	122.4 (114.0)	93.1 (132.1)
Miners & masons	949.9 (196.8)	39.4 (133.1)	5.0 (66.7)	170.0 (154.0)	155.0 (144.3)	329.9 (476.9)
Transport & communication workers	527.6 (109.3)	29.9 (101.0)	7.7 (102.7)	99.3 (89.9)	126.4 (117.7)	120.4 (170.6)
Labourers	400.8 (83.0)	22.3 (75.3)	5.3 (70.7)	84.2 (76.3)	85.2 (76.3)	79.6 (112.9)
Guards, police & defence workers	276.6 (57.3)	22.0 (74.3)	3.8 (50.7)	53.2 (48.2)	72.2 (67.2)	42.8 (60.7)

(Special reports on vital stastistics by occupation & industry 1970) [20]

their comparability is limited.[21],[22] This is just the first step to find out any marked difference, if present.

A comparison within Japan showed that hypertension was more frequent when young, and the frequency of signs of associated organ damage was higher in hypertensive subjects in Akita[23]: the changes in ocular fundi (grade 2 or more of hypertensive or arteriosclerotic changes according to the Scheie classification), proteinuria, glucosuria and the incidence of stroke in middle age were more frequent in the hypertensives in Akita than in hypertensive patients of the same age in farming and mountain villages in Gumma (in the eastern central part of the main island) with also high prevalence of hypertension. This may be attributed to the earlier development and longer duration of hypertension in the population in Akita. The ECG findings did not reveal a significant difference between these villages.

As an indication of the effect of hypertension upon the heart, ECG findings according to the Minnesota code criteria from various population studies in and out of Japan are presented (Table 3). High amplitude R waves were most frequent in Akita.[15] Both the Japanese populations in the two different regions with different prevalence of hypertension[15],[24] revealed less frequent Q waves except Tanushimaru and more frequent high amplitude R waves than white populations.[24],[25] A similar pattern was reported from a Jamaican population, and the racial differences in the prevalence of a high amplitude R wave and its low sensitivity for left ventricular hypertrophy in non-white populations was mentioned.[26] The frequency of high amplitude R waves was also higher in hypertensive subjects than normotensive subjects in other Japanese population studies.[21],[27] When associated with ST segment depression or T wave inversion, a marked increase in future risk of stroke was observed.[22]

Concerning the prevalence of proteinuria as a crude indicator of damage to the kidney, no difference was seen between hypertensive men in Hisayama[21] and white and black American men in Evans County, Georgia.[5]

An important indication of severity of hypertension is prognosis. Available data on cardiovascular disease morbidity or mortality from prospective studies were not presented in such a form as to permit sex and age standardized comparisons

TABLE 3. Frequency of Resting ECG Findings in Men in Selected Communities (Rate per 1,000 Population)

Community year of study	Age	Total No.	Q waves I_1	I_2	I_3	Left axis deviation II_1	High amplitude R-wave III_1	ST-depression IV_1	IV_2	IV_3	T-wave negativity/flattening V_1	V_2	V_3	A-V block VI_1	VI_2	VII_1	Ventricular blocks VII_2	Atrial fibrillation VIII_3	Median blood pressure systolic	diastolic
Japan Akita[15]	40-49	263	0	3.2	7.0		503.9	0	17.7	0	0	10.6	21.2	0	0	0	3.5	0	141	87
Ikawa	50-59	280	3.6	3.6			389.3	14.3	14.3	7.1	3.6	25.0	35.7	0	0	0	17.9	7.1	150	69
1963-65	60-69	198	0	10.1	5.1		363.6	30.3	30.3	0	0	65.7	75.0	0	0	0	35.3	40.4	162	92
Japan Fukuoka[24]	40-49	229	13.1	13.1	0	4.4	83.0	17.5	39.3	39.3	4.4	0	13.1	0	0	0	0	0	124	69
Tanushimaru 1958	50-59	275	0	18.2	0	10.9	69.1	18.2	90.9	50.2	0	7.3	50.9	0	3.6	0	14.5	21.8	135	75
Ushibuka 1960	40-49	234	0	0	0	4.3	145.3	17.1	34.2	29.9	0	4.3	17.1	0	4.3	0	21.4	0	147	70
	50-59	250	4.0	4.0	0	8.0	148.0	4.0	44.0	68.0	4.0	12.0	16.0	0	12.0	0	4.0	0	157	80
USA Railway Switchmen[24] 1957-59	40-49	523	9.6	15.3	11.5	13.4	13.4	0	0	5.7	0	3.8	22.9	0	0	0	3.8	0	131	84
	50-59	312	9.6	25.6	3.2	22.4	19.2	3.2	9.6	9.6	0	9.6	41.7	0	0	6.4	19.2	0	136	67
*Belgium Brussels[25]	40-49	631	3.2	7.9	12.7		15.8	3.2	9.5	0	1.6	9.5	9.5			0				
	50-59	729	8.2	16.5	19.2		19.2	8.2	9.6	20.6	0	19.2	36.9			4.1				
*Jamaica Lawrence Tavern[26] 1962-64	40-49	177	5.6	11.3	5.6	33.9	299.4	5.6	28.2	11.3	5.6	33.9	62.1			0				

between the Japanese and other populations according to blood pressure, except one from JNR. Nevertheless, tentative comparisons of the incidence rate of stroke in the populations in Hiroshima-Nagasaki[22] and Evans County, Georgia[28] and mortality rate from stroke and heart disease in the population in Hisayama[21] and Chicago male workers[30] were attempted, since these studies reported incidence rate or mortality rate according to the blood pressure on entry. The following should be taken as preliminary observations, since the cohorts differed in sex and age structure. It seems that hypertensive Japanese in Hiroshima and Nagasaki had a much higher incidence rate of stroke than hypertensive white and black Americans in Georgia, while the normotensive subjects in both communities showed a similar rate. Hypertensive and borderline hypertensive Japanese in Hisayama had a much higher mortality rate from stroke, and all the normotensive, borderline hypertensive and hypertensive Japanese had a much lower mortality rate from heart disease than the subgroups with comparable blood pressures in the Chicago workers. It should be recalled that the blood pressure among these Japanese populations was lower compared to other places in Japan (Table 2, Fig. 4). Therefore, a very high blood pressure seems to be a significant causative factor, at least in high stroke endemic areas such as Akita, but it cannot be a sufficient explanation for the higher incidence of stroke in these Japanese populations.

This preliminary attempt indicates that the prevalence of proteinuria in hypertensive American and Japanese men was similar. More frequent high amplitude R waves and less frequent Q waves were observed in ECGs among the Japanese. The risk of stroke was higher in the Japanese hypertensive subjects than in the hypertensive white and black Americans, but the risk of ischemic heart disease was much less.

What is the basis for this difference? A comparison of atherosclerosis in the cerebral arteries between Americans in Minnesota and Japanese in Fukuoka showed earlier occurrence, possible higher prevalence and greater severity of atherosclerosis in the small cerebral arteries among the Japanese autopsy population.[31] Coronary atherosclerosis of the Japanese autopsy population was about one-tenth that in the Minnesota cases of the same age.[32]

Are the differences in coronary and cerebral atherosclerosis of ethnic origin? A good answer to this question is given in a study of Japanese inside and outside Japan.[33] A comparison of Japanese in Hiroshima, Honolulu and California revealed a westernization of Japanese in disease pattern as they emigrated toward the Western hemisphere. Japanese in California had about three times the death rate from ischemic heart disease and a quarter the death rate from stroke as compared with the Japanese living in Japan, according to the national mortality statistics in 1950-1954.[34,35] Blood cholesterol level of the Japanese in Japan is low.[13,21-24,44] They are ethnically from the same stock and therefore the way of living must have played a significant role in the difference in death rate from these diseases and presumably in the difference in coronary and cerebral atherosclerosis.

Trends in Blood Pressure

Since 1956 blood pressure measurements have been included in the national nutrition surveys[1] that have been conducted each year in May (with the exception of 1964 and 1966 when the survey was conducted in November only). The mean blood pressure of subjects for different ages and sex in each year is shown (Fig. 6). The blood pressure from life insurance applicants in 1932 and 1953 is also shown as a comparison. The mean blood pressure appeared to be almost the same before and after World War II (a lower blood pressure was reported during and just after the war, probably due to low nutrition). Elevation of the blood pressure then occurred in both men and women, with a plateau around 1960, followed by a gradual decrease. The elevation at the beginning may be partly due to improvement in nutrition and increase in body build. A fluctuation in the initial few years might be attributed to insufficient standardization.

Blood pressure distributions in 1963 and 1970 are compared as an example of how the decrease in mean blood pressure appeared (Fig. 7). The recent reduction was particularly remarkable in middle and old age and in the 95th percentile with higher blood pressure. The decrease was less significant in median values and nonexistent in the fifth percentile. It was

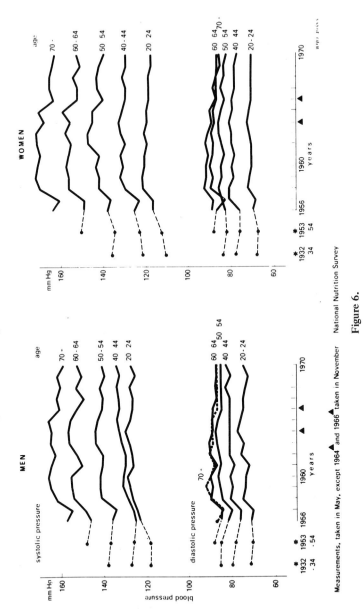

Figure 6.

Measurements, taken in May, except 1964 and 1966 taken in November   National Nutrition Survey

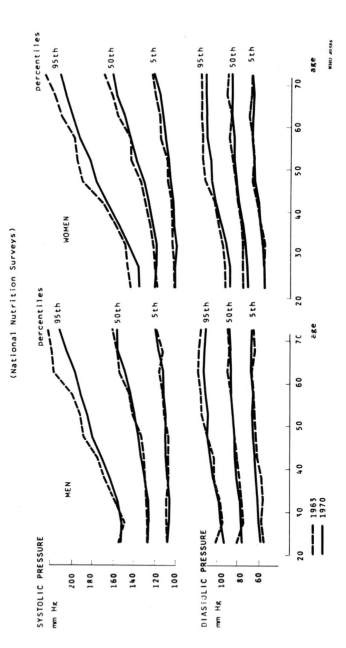

Figure 7.

significant in most age groups in women, but not in men. The same kind of shift was observed in the cohort in Hiroshima and Nagasaki, when blood pressure distributions were compared in a series of follow-ups, in 1960-1962, 1964-1966 and 1970-1972.[14] It also appeared in male employees of the Japanese National Railways[36,37] (Fig. 8).[10] A hypertension control program was begun in 1960 covering all employees aged 40 or over. A blood pressure reduction between 1966 and 1971 was observed in employees aged 50 to 54. They had been under hypertension control for a longer time. The degree of reduction was greater in the 95th percentile. These are populations with high blood pressure which is more likely to be influenced by treatment of hypertension. The reduction was little or non-existent in employees aged 45 to 49, except 95th percentiles. A regional difference appeared in this trend, too. The decrease was more remarkable in the Akita district, where the blood pressure of employees was and still is high, but was not significant in Osaka, where the blood pressure was and still is low.

Employees aged 40-44 who had just entered the age of the target population in the Japan National Railways hypertension control program presented an elevated blood pressure in all three districts. Exceptions were the population with the highest blood pressure, the 95th percentile systolic blood pressure and some diastolic pressure percentiles in Akita, where the early occurrence of hypertension has been known to be more frequent and an intensive hypertension control campaign has been launched. The rising trends of blood pressure in the younger generation may be partly due to change in body build. Employees who reach the age of 40 increase their average body weight by 1 kg every three years.[37] When employees were subdivided by weight index,[38] the prevalence of hypertension at the age of 40 in 1971 increased by roughly 10%-20% from that in 1962 in each subgroup with identical weight indices.[36] Therefore, other, so far unexplained, factors play a significant role.

Trends in Death Rates From Hypertensive Diseases

Similar trends occurred in the reported death rate from cerebrovascular disease and hypertensive disease, which includes hypertensive heart disease and other hypertensive disease, all of

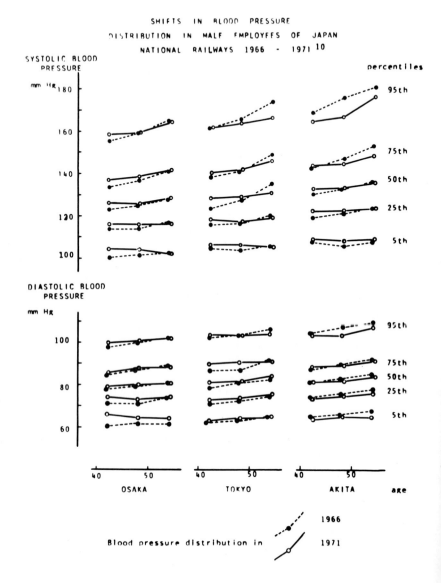

Figure 8.

which can be considered as the outcome of hypertension (Fig. 9).[11,39] The death rates from hypertensive disease rose around 1960 and fell afterward. Death rates from both these diseases have been decreasing more rapidly in younger age groups. These correspond to epidemiological observations in many areas and cannot be merely due to changes in diagnostic habit.

Hypertension Control Programs

Because of the very high death toll from cerebrovascular disease, control of hypertension is of great concern to the government at various levels and also to the public. The Japanese government initiated a hypertension control program in selected areas in 12 prefectures during the period 1969-1972. The program has been extended since 1973 to other areas, in conjunction with a compulsory mass examination for pulmonary tuberculosis.

Local governments are also keen to promote hypertension control. Communities participated actively from the outset of the program, which has been implemented by a medical team from universities, research institutes or central hospitals, together with local general practitioners. Such a program, for example, started in Yachiho Village, Nagano, in 1959[40] and in Yao City, Osaka, in 1964.[41] The center in Fukuoka has been participating since 1971 in an international cooperative hypertension control program coordinated by WHO.[42] Many firms have also developed hypertension control programs of their own, such as the one in the Japanese National Railways, which has covered about 450,000 employees since 1960.[10,36,37] In many of these programs, no reference populations for comparison were set up.

Interim results (Table 4) showed that previously unnoticed hypertension decreased and patients under treatment have increased remarkably ($p < 0.001$) after eight years of intensive program operation on all subjects aged 40 years and more in two communities.[41] A reduction of 27%-44% in the incidence rate of stroke was observed in middle age, the major target population, during the second four-year period as compared with the initial four-year period ($p < 0.05$).[41] However, the incidence rates of cerebral infarction and acute heart attack were also reported to have increased.[36,41] The death rate from

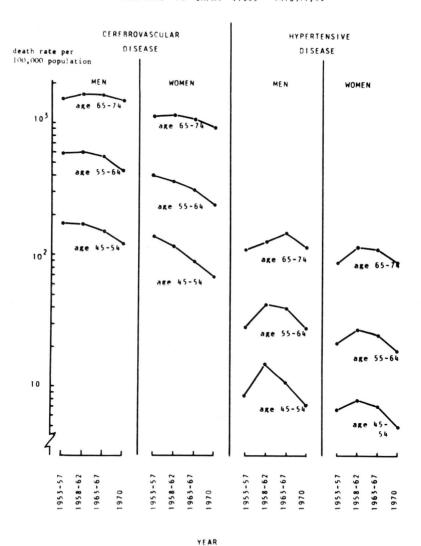

Figure 9.

TABLE 4. Preliminary Results of Hypertension Control During Eight Years in Two Areas in Japan   (Komachi et al 1971)[41]

BASIC DATA	AKITA	OSAKA
No. of Target Population in 1964 (Age: 40 - 69 years)	2741	3713
No. of Hypertensive Patients in 1964 (Prevalence rate in %)	765 (31.5%)	493 (14.9%)

STATUS OF HYPERTENSIVE PATIENTS (%)	AKITA year		OSAKA year	
	1964	1972	1964	1972
Unknown	42.1	7.1	49.5	14.2
Known but untreated	43.0	35.4	37.7	27.4
Known and treated	14.9	57.6	12.8	58.5

CAUSE OF DEATH (per 100,000 per annum)	AKITA year		OSAKA year	
	1964-67	1968-71	1964-67	1968-71
Stroke	538.1	346.6	195.3	114.5
Hypertensive heart disease	27.4	9.1	33.7	26.9
Ischaemic heart disease	36.5	45.6	33.7	40.4
Other & ill-defined heart disease	54.7	27.4	40.4	40.4
Renal diseases	36.5	36.5	20.2	26.9
Other	565.4	647.5	505.0	471.3
All causes	1258.6	1112.6	828.2	720.4
(No. of deaths)	(138)	(122)	(123)	(107)

hypertensive heart disease and stroke decreased greatly. The general declining trends in death rate from stroke all over Japan should also be taken into account in the evaluation of these interventions.

Hypotheses for Differences in Blood Pressure in Populations

Two hypotheses are popular in Japan. One is environmental, related to housing conditions, and the other is biochemical, related to diet.

The observations that blood pressure and death rate from stroke are higher in the colder northern regions and in winter season lead to the hypothesis that cold is one of the causes of hypertension. It was pointed out that room temperature, rather than outdoor temperature, is critical.[43,44] However, the story contradicts the presence of high blood pressure in tropical countries. A small-scale intervention trial on the effect of introducing stoves in a farming village reported failure to reduce the blood pressure.[45]

Many Japanese are fond of a traditional diet of rice, salted pickles, miso and soya sauce, which are produced from fermented beans, cereals and salt. The average daily salt intake of a Japanese adult is 15-20 gm/day[46] and at times as much as 50 gm.[47] A significant correlation has been reported between the death rate from cerebrovascular disease by prefectures[46] or by villages and towns[48] and per capita miso consumption and total salt consumption. In the analysis of the national nutrition survey of Japan,[1] the blood pressure of the upper, middle and lower quintiles for miso consumption followed the same order of size in most age-sex subgroups (Fig. 10). The differences in blood pressure by amount of miso intake were greater and significant in women. High rice intake and high salt consumption are generally associated with a poor and unbalanced diet. Other dietary constituents such as deficiency in animal protein, calcium or vitamins are also considered as a potential contributing factor to hypertension and/or stroke.[23,43,48-50]

The high salt intake hypothesis has certain drawbacks. The Japanese as a whole are high salt consumers, but the national average blood pressure does not appear to be high.[1,2] Blood pressure did not rise in the acute[47] or subacute (one week

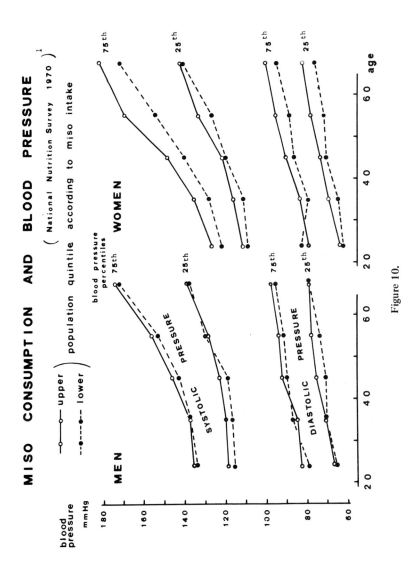

Figure 10.

duration) salt-loading experiment in healthy subjects.[51] However, the author[47] observed a rise in blood pressure in a few subjects whose serum sodium level rose after acute salt ingestion. No correlation could be observed between individual salt consumption estimated by chloride measurement in 24-hour urine and blood pressure in individual subjects.[47] The mechanisms by which chronic salt overload induces high blood pressure in healthy people have not been substantiated. A positive correlation between the cold temperature and the high salt consumption was also suggested.

There are some other diet-related hypotheses to be mentioned, but none have been confirmed. The lower blood pressure in the apple-producing areas in Aomori, near Akita, was ascribed to a high potassium intake from apples, counteracting the hypertensive effect of sodium.[52] A high correlation between acidity, the ratio of sulphuric acid and carbonic acid ion concentration,[53] or the amount of metasilicic acid[54] in river water and the death rate from cerebrovascular disease has been reported, but the correlation between these chemical constituents and blood pressure was not determined. Studies on water hardness in relation to cardiovascular disease developed abroad.[55] The role of cadmium and its accumulation in the kidney and possible hypertensive effect[56] has also been considered. However, no difference in the prevalence of hypertension and proteinuria has been found in Japan when highly cadmium-polluted, slightly polluted and nonpolluted areas were compared.[57]

Conclusion

The available data and reports on hypertension in Japan are reviewed. The following conclusions can be drawn as to the present situation of hypertension in Japan.

The Japanese as a whole are not particularly hypertensive, although the death rate from cerebrovascular disease is high.

The blood pressure distribution of the population differs according to geographical area. It is higher in the northeast and in the northern Japan Sea border and lower in the Osaka and Kyoto districts and surrounding areas. The regional differences in blood pressures parallel the death rates from cerebrovascular disease to some extent, but there are exceptions.

Blood pressure also differs according to social conditions. Rural inhabitants have higher blood pressure than those living in big cities. Men working in agriculture, forestry and fishing have a higher blood pressure than men in some other occupation groups when young.

Hypertensive subjects in Japan appear to have higher incidence and death rates from cerebrovascular disease than hypertensive white and black Americans.

Regional difference was observed inside Japan, too. Hypertensive subjects in some communities in Akita revealed higher frequency of signs of associated organ damage and higher incidence rates of cerebrovascular disease.

The blood pressure of a part of the general population in middle and old age having higher blood pressure (as expressed by the 95th and 75th percentiles in blood pressure distribution) has decreased in recent years. A rise in blood pressure has been observed among younger employees in one occupation group.

Certain hypertension control programs gave rise to improved treatment of hypertension in the community.

Acknowledgments

I would like to express my thanks to all the people who helped to make this review possible, in particular the Japanese Ministry of Health and Welfare, the Bureau of Public Health Affairs (Director-General Dr. T. Saburi), the Nutrition Division (Heads, Drs. S. Anzai and K. Sakaki), the Tuberculosis and Degenerative Disease Control Division (Head, Dr. S. Shimada), the Statistical Information Bureau (Director, Dr. T. Matsuura) and all their staff for special tabulations, and special thanks to Drs. T. Soda and F. Ueda.

In addition, I am indebted to the Atomic Bomb Casualty Commission (Dr. H. Kato), the Akita Prefectural Institute for Hygiene (Dr. S. Kojima), the Japanese National Railways (Dr. Y. Fukuda), the Osaka Center for Adult Diseases (Dr. Y. Komachi), and the Saku Central Hospital (Dr. K. Isomura) for tables on blood pressure distribution of populations.

For all their valuable information, I am grateful to Drs. K. Hamada, K. Itahara, N. Kimura, T. Kobayashi, T. Omae, N. Sasaki and E. Takahashi.

References

1. Japanese Ministry of Health and Welfare: Present status of national nutrition, results of the national nutrition survey 1956-1971. Special tabulations in this report, cited from Koseikyokai: *Kosei no Shihyo*, 20:(9), 1974. (In press.)*
2. Statistical Information Bureau, Japanese Ministry of Health and Welfare: Report of the adult disease survey 1961-62 and 1971-72.*
3. Isshiki, T. and Yoshikawa, T.: Statistical study on blood pressure. Report 1. *Hoken Igaku Zasshi*, 54:29-36, 1956.*
4. Bøe, J., Humerfeld, S. and Wedervang, E. R.: The blood pressure in a population. *Acta Med. Scand.*, suppl. 321, 1957.
5. McDonough, J. R., Garrison, G. E. and Hames, G. C.: Blood pressure and hypertensive disease among negroes and whites. A study in Evans County, Georgia. *Ann. Intern. Med.*, 61:208-228, 1964.
6. Lin, T. Y., Hung, T. P., Chen, C. M. et al: Studies on hypertension among urban Chinese in Taiwan. I. Mean blood pressure readings. *J. Formosa Med. Ass.*, 55:131-138, 1956.
7. Chen, C. M. and Tseng, W. P.: Prevalence of heart disease in Taipei urban population. Presented at the 5th Asian-Pacific Congress of Cardiology, Singapore, October 8-13, 1972.
8. Hong, M. H. and Suh, S. K.: Epidemiological and clinical studies of hypertension in Koreans. *Korea Med. Univ. J.*, 9:55-74, 1974.
9. Tsukamoto, H.: Ijichosa Kenkyu, Medical Department of the Meiji Life Insurance (12) 53-65, 1971.*
10. Fukuda, Y.: Development of cerebral stroke and coronary heart attack. An epidemiological study. Rodo Igaku Kenkyukai, Tokyo, 1970. Special tabulations supplied for this report.*
11. Segi, M., Kurihara, M., Matsuyama, T. et al: Mortality by causes of death and prefectures in Japan (1953-1967) — death rates by age groups and age adjusted death rates. Department of Public Health, Tohoku University School of Medicine, Sendai, 1970.*
12. Marmot, M. G. et al: Epidemiologic studies of coronary heart disease and stroke in Japanese men living in Japan, Hawaii and California: Prevalence of coronary heart disease, hypertension and related abnormalities. (In press.) Cited from Kagan, A.: Epidemiology of hypertension and stroke in Oceania. A background paper for a WHO meeting on the control of hypertension and stroke in the community, Tokyo, March 1974. (Ref. No. CVD/H/74.26.)
13. Komachi, Y., Iida, M., Shimamoto, T. et al: Epidemiological studies on Japanese hypertension and ischaemic heart disease. *Jap. Circ. J.*, 31:563-580, 1967.
14. Atomic Bomb Casualty Commission: Adult health survey, Hiroshima and Nagasaki, Japan. Tabulation No. 2568, 1974.
15. Kojima, S.: Personal communication.*
16. World Health Organization: Community control of stroke and

---

*In Japanese.

hypertension: Report of a WHO meeting. Part I: Stroke. Geneva, December 1973. (Ref. No. CVD/74.3(I).)

17. Henry, J. P. and Cassel, J. C.: Psychosocial factors in essential hypertension. Recent epidemiological and animal experimental evidence. *Amer. J. Epidem.*, 90:171-200, 1969.

18. Shaper, A. G.: Blood pressure studies in East Africa. In Stamler, J., Stamler, R. and Pullman, T. N. (eds.): *The Epidemiology of Hypertension.* Proceedings of an International Symposium. New York and London:Grune and Stratton, 1967, pp. 139-149.

19. Prior, I. A. M., Evans, J. G., Harvey, H. P. B. et al: Sodium intake and blood pressure in two Polynesian populations. *New Eng. J. Med.*, 279:515-520, 1968.

20. Statistical Information Bureau, Japanese Ministry of Health and Welfare: Vital statistics on occupation and industry. A special report of vital statistics, 1970.

21. Katsuki, S., Hirota, Y., Akazome, T. et al: Epidemiological studies on cerebrovascular diseases in Hisayama, Kyushu Island, Japan. Part I. With particular reference to cardiovascular status. *Jap. Heart J.*, 5:12-36, 1964.

22. Johnson, K. G., Yano, K. and Kato, H.: Cerebral vascular disease in Hiroshima. Report of a six-year period of surveillance 1958-64. ABCC Tech. Rep. 23-66, Atomic Bomb Casualty Commission, Hiroshima and Nagasaki, 1966.

23. Kojima, S.: Actual circumstances of adult diseases in agricultural and mountain villages — a survey of cardiovascular diseases in Akita and Gumma prefectures. *Rinsho Eiyo*, 41:681-688, 1972.*

24. Keys, A., Aravanis, C., Blackburn, H. W. et al: Epidemiological studies related to coronary heart disease. Characteristics of men aged 40-59 in seven countries. *Acta Med. Scand.*, suppl. 460, 1966.

25. Rose, G. A., Ahmeteli, L., Checcacci, F. et al: Ischaemic heart disease in middle-aged men. Prevalence comparisons in Europe. *Bull. WHO*, 38:885-895, 1968.

26. Miall, W. E., Del Campo, E., Fodor, J., et al: Longitudinal study of heart disease in a Jamaican rural population. 1. Prevalence, with special reference to ECG findings. *Bull. WHO*, 46:429-442, 1972.

27. Takahashi, N., Kato, K., Suzuki, K. et al: Epidemiologic studies on hypertension and coronary heart disease in a Japanese rural population. III. Electrocardiographic findings in Chiyoda. *Jap. Heart J.*, 5:38-48, 1964.

28. Heyman, A., Karp, H. R., Heyden, S. et al: Cerebrovascular disease in the bi-racial population of Evans County, Georgia. *Stroke*, 2:509-518, 1971.

29. Hypertension and ischaemic heart disease. Preventive aspects. *WHO Techn. Rep. Ser.*, No. 231, Geneva, 1962.

30. Stamler, J., Berkson, D. M. and Lindberg, H. G.: Risk factors: Their role in the etiology and pathogenesis of the atherosclerotic disease. In Geer, J. and Wissler, R. W. (eds.): *The Pathogenesis of Atherosclerosis.* Baltimore:Williams and Wilkins, 1972.

31. Resch, J. A., Okabe, N. and Kimoto, K.: Cerebral atherosclerosis. *Geriatrics*, 24:(11), 111-123, 1969.
32. Kimura, N.: Analysis of 10,000 post mortem examinations in Japan. In *World Trends in Cardiology*. New York:Harper and Brothers, 1956, vol. 1, p. 22. Cited from Ref. 31.
33. Worth, R. M., Kato, H., Rhoads, G. G. et al: Epidemiologic studies of coronary heart disease and stroke in Japanese men living in Japan, Hawaii and California: Mortality. (In preparation.) Cited from Kagan, A.: Epidemiology of hypertension and stroke in Oceania. A background paper for a WHO meeting on the control of hypertension and stroke in the community, Tokyo, March 1974. (Ref. No. CVD/H/74.26.)
34. Gordon, T.: Mortality experience among the Japanese in the United States, Hawaii, and Japan. *Public Health Rep.*, 72:543-553, 1957.
35. World Health Organization: Epid. and vital statist. rep. 15:(2), 1962.
36. Fukuda, Y.: Recent trends and background of cerebrovascular and heart attack. From the standpoint of control in an occupational group. A special report of the 7th annual meeting of the Japanese Association for Cerebro-cardiovascular Disease Control, 1972.*
37. Chiba, Y.: Hypertension and stroke control in a large occupational group. A background paper for a WHO meeting on the control of hypertension and stroke in the community, Tokyo, March 1974. (Ref. No. CVD/H/74.21.)
38. Minowa, S., Takahashi, H., Mayuzumi, N. et al: A study on the standard weight of adults — annex. A graph for calculation of weight index in adults. *Nihon Iji Shinpo.*, No. 1988, 24-29, 1962.*
39. *World Health Statistics Annual, 1970.* Geneva:Wld Hlth Org., 1973, vol. 1.
40. Isomura, K.: The effect of cardiovascular control in an agricultural village with special reference to the hypertension control. *Nihon Rinsho*, 26:860-867, 1968.*
41. Komachi, Y., Iida, M., Shimamoto, T. et al: Evaluation of hypertension control in the community. *Ann. Rep. Centre Adult Dis.* (Osaka), 11:(2), 1-4, 1971.
42. Community control of hypertension: Methodological considerations and protocol of a WHO cooperative project. A background paper for a WHO meeting in Geneva, December 1973. (Ref. No. CVD/S/73.11.)
43. Takahashi, E., Kato, K., Kawakami, Y. et al: Epidemiological studies on hypertension and cerebral haemorrhage in north-east Japan. *Tohoku J. Exp. Med.*, 74:188-210, 1961.
44. Kobayashi, T.: Epidemiological study of cerebral apoplexy and ischaemic heart disease in Japan. *Jap. Circ. J.*, 33:1483-1488, 1969.
45. Wakatsuki, T., Mitsui, Z., Kure, S. et al: Study of coldness and cold injury — continued — Experimental study on how the family life with a stove influences the health of rural in the coldest season. I. *Nihon Noson Igaku Zasshi*, 10:65-76, 1962.*
46. Sasaki, N., Takeda, J., Fukushi, S. et al: Nutritional factors related to the geographical difference in the death rate from apoplexy in Japan. *Nihon Koshueisei Zasshi*, 7:1137-1143, 1960.*

47. Kimura, T.: Excessive salt intake and blood pressure. *Nihon Serigaku Zasshi*, 22:91-95, 1960.*
48. Kojima, S.: Distinctive features of cerebral apoplexy in and around Akita district. *Nihon Koshueisei Zasshi*, 13:907-924, 1966.*
49. Kaneta, S., Ishiguro, K., Kobayashi, S. et al: An epidemiological study on nutrition and cerebrovascular lesions in Tohoku area of Japan. *Tohoku J. Exp. Med.*, 83:398-408, 1964.
50. Takahashi, E.: Geographic distribution of mortality rate from cerebrovascular disease in European countries. *Tohoku J. Exp. Med.*, 92:345-378, 1967.
51. Grant, H. and Reischsmann, F.: The effect of the ingestion of large amount of sodium chloride on the arterial and venous pressure of normal subjects. *Amer. Heart J.*, 32:704, 1946. Cited from Ref. 47.*
52. Sasaki, N., Mitsuhashi, T. and Fukushi, S.: Effects of the ingestion of large amount of apples on blood pressure of farmers in Akita prefecture. *Igaku to Seibutsugaku*, 51:103-105, 1959.*
53. Kobayashi, J.: On geographical relationship between the chemical nature of river water and death rate from apoplexy. *Berichte d. Ohara Inst. f. landwirts. Biol.*, 11:12-21, 1957.
54. Misawa, T., Kitamura, Y., Okada, H. et al: Biological effects of silicic acid in drinking water and foods. First report. The relation between high silicic acid intake and hypertension. *Nihon Iji Shinpo*, (1718) 30 Mon., 3-9, 1957.*
55. Morris, J. N., Crawford, M. D. and Heady, J. A.: Hardness of local water supplies and mortality from cardiovascular disease in the county boroughs of England and Wales. *Lancet*, 1:860-862, 1961.
56. Perry, H. M. Jr., Tipton, I. H., Schroeder, H. A. et al: Variation in the concentration of cadmium in human kidney as a function of age and geographic origin. *J. Chron. Dis.*, 14:259-271, 1961.
57. Tsuchiya, K.: Environmental pollution by cadmium and its health effect on trace elements in relation to cardiovascular diseases. Geneva, Feb. 1971. (Ref. No. CVD/WP/70.14.)

Discussion

Dr. Tobian, Minnesota: I would like to ask one question about the miso. You divided the miso eaters into quintiles. It occurred to me that the highest quintile eats only a small amount more miso soup than the lowest quintile. I would like to know whether they eat very uniformly in the Akita prefecture, or is there really a wide variation in the intake of miso?

Dr. Hatano: This is based on a national nutrition survey, not particularly in Akita.

Dr. Dollery: I think the question was what is the absolute difference in consumption between the different quintiles rather than whether the differences were significant.

Dr. Hatano: The average consumption of miso among the Japanese is about 15 to 20 gm per day. It is remarkably high compared with other nations, but I regret that I have no information about the absolute difference in this survey.

Dr. Mah, Ohio: We have been collecting data on populations with respect to their lipids, their obesity, their blood pressure scores and exercise. We noted that in the cases of spouses, there was quite a close correlation between blood pressure scores and lipids. However, in the case where one of the spouses was doing a considerable amount of exercise, regardless of whether it was the female or the male who was exercising, that person would have a much lower level of lipids and blood pressure. So I suggest exercise may have something to do with it. Again with migrants, lack of exercise is possibly important when a person moves from an active life to an urban center with all the conveniences and few opportunities for the previous high levels of activity. This might, again, offer a reason why blood pressure scores go up. The question I want to direct to Dr. Hatano is the amazing thing about your statistics. Agricultural workers usually score fairly low in blood pressure and yet in your case, the pressures are much higher. In the past decade or so, with mechanization decreasing the amount of physical activity, might this again explain why blood pressure scores have been increasing?

Dr. Hatano: This high blood pressure level among rural populations in Japan has been observed for a long time. I do not think blood pressure has been studied specifically in relation to physical activity.

Dr. Kass: There are a reasonable number of careful studies which have demonstrated that rural populations have higher blood pressures than urban, including the early studies of Comstock. I am so greatly concerned with the sort of fixation that slowly sweeps the field with respect to preformed hypotheses, so that when data do not seem to fit the hypothesis, they are rather commonly disregarded. I think the predominance of high blood pressure in rural populations is rarely taught even by professors of medicine, because we have become so imbued with the idea that urbanization is an important factor in development of high blood pressure. In fact, the evidence for this is almost nonexistent.

Dr. Hatano: I quite agree. These are hypothetical and not confirmed.

Dr. Stamler: I would say a little bit about the U.S. migrant problem in that regard. The fact is that both the data of the National Health Examination Survey in 1960-1962, and the very extensive analyses that Moriyama, Krueger and Stamler did of the mortality data for the period 1959-60-61 indicate that the highest rates tended to be for the South Atlantic and East South Central regions of the United States. The black-white difference was greatest there. When we factored out, as was done with the mortality data, urban versus rural, urbanization was not a key factor. I think it is very important that these facts be kept in mind.

Before we take too seriously the study we did on the migrants, we had better be sure that the data we are looking at were age adjusted. My recollection is that the sample was small and there may not have been age adjustments.

Mrs. Stamler: One interesting aspect about the Chicago data may touch on the very question just raised. It is not necessarily living in the city that is the problem, but it may be the problems of living in the city for certain special groups that accentuate the problem. For example, among the migrants themselves, there was a difference in problems of hypertension among groups answering the following questions in different ways: If they had to choose again, would they migrate? If they would migrate, would they migrate to Chicago again? The people who were worse off were those who said, yes they would migrate but they would not migrate to Chicago again. That means that these were people who found special problems in staying where they were but found even more problems in the place they had chosen to migrate to. So I do not think it is a question of urban versus rural, but a very complicated question of what the social relations were back home and what they found in life here. In regard to age adjustment, our Chicago data were not age adjusted, but the mean ages in various groups were almost identical. So there was that one weakness. Also, the numbers were small, there were no specific prior hypotheses and the study has never been replicated. Therefore, we prefer to be guarded about these findings.

Dr. Lovell: One of the points about the Japanese story is the very striking differences in geographic areas in relation to stroke. I would like to ask Dr. Hatano whether there has been any systematic effort to examine the certification customs in different parts of Japan in validating, in other words, the certification of stroke. In particular, has there been any regional difference in the way in which sudden death has been certified? Is it customary in Japan to certify sudden death as due to cerebrovascular accident or to a myocardial infarction?

Dr. Hatano: I cannot answer the second question. I have not studied sudden death, but in the Hisayama study, in which the autopsy rate was very high, only one out of nine heart disease deaths was diagnosed as "sudden death." Sudden death and ischemic heart disease are still infrequent in Japan, and I do not think one needs to appraise sudden death as a source of falsely exaggerated diagnosis of stroke. In the referred surveys, data on death certificates were corrected with available information from families, attending physicians and hospital data, and a significant difference was still found, for example, between Osaka and Akita.

Dr. Dollery: In other words, you are saying that you think that the death certification is reasonably accurate?

Dr. Hatano: Yes.

Dr. Holland: I think that the Japanese data are very fascinating. Dr. Hatano, you showed a difference in the case-fatality rates for strokes, comparing individuals with similar levels of pressure in Japan and the United States. Can you show the same thing within Japan, in view of the wide variation in pressures and in mortality rates within Japan?

Dr. Hatano: I think this is what we really need to study.

Dr. Tyroler: I would like to expand on the regional variation in mortality. In the southeast United States there are inordinately high prevalence rates of elevated blood pressure and also markedly higher death rates for strokes. What is usually not recognized is that there are microregional variations as well. Within the southeast, there is a clear area of increased cardiovascular disease known for about 20 years or longer and consistent and stable at each mortality analysis, which runs down the coastal plains and covers an area about 1,000 miles, encompassing Evans county. We recently completed a study in North Carolina which shows age specific mortality rates from strokes twice as high, in this zone, as outside this zone within the same state with people of generally similar ethnic background. We have had the opportunity to look at diagnostic customs, certification of deaths and hospital admissions, and we are convinced that this is a real phenomenon and that it is not the southeast per se but it is this high, coastal plain mortality region. In North Carolina, at least, both of these zones, one with the death rate twice that of the other, were rural. So the rural factor alone is not explanatory.

Dr. Miller, Maryland: In reference to the geographical differences in stroke deaths, we are doing a study in Pueblo, Colorado, which has almost no strokes; Savannah, which he just spoke of which has the highest number, and Hagerstown, Maryland, which is intermediate, and I am sorry to say that hypertension does not explain the difference. We have to look somewhere else.

Cooperative Studies of Blood Pressure in Japanese in Japan, Hawaii and the United States

Warren Winkelstein, Jr., M.D.

Introduction

In 1957 Gordon first documented the observation that mortality from stroke and coronary heart disease varied among Japanese migrant populations to Hawaii and California. He found rates highest in Japan, intermediate in Hawaii and lowest in California, while rates for coronary heart disease followed a reverse trend.[1] Since there was no reason to believe that migrant Japanese were genetically different from nonmigrants, these rate variations offered the opportunity to study the effects of changing environment on these major causes of death. Furthermore, the existence of the Atomic Bomb Casualty Commission in Hiroshima and Nagasaki provided the facility to mount epidemiologic studies in an area which had fortuitously been the main source of migrants to Hawaii and California. About 1965, plans were made for a series of comparable collaborative studies in Japan, Hawaii and California to explore the phenomenon.

The data included in this paper have, in large part, already been presented at various meetings in this country and abroad and are scheduled for publication in the *American Journal of Epidemiology*.[2] However, additional analyses of the association of education and occupation with blood pressure level will be presented here.

Warren Winkelstein, Jr., M.D., *Program in Epidemiology, School of Public Health, University of California at Berkeley.*

Methods

Data for men 45-69 years of age were examined in this study. The Japanese sample was selected from the 20,000 people in the Adult Health Study Sample under clinical surveillance by the Atomic Bomb Casualty Commission in Hiroshima and Nagasaki. All males from these two cities between the ages of 45 and 69 and alive on January 1, 1965, were selected for clinical study. About 10% of the 2,989 men satisfying these criteria had emigrated from the cities under study. Of those remaining, approximately 85% underwent examination, yielding a sample of 2,141 men in Japan.

Using selective service registration records in Hawaii, attempts were made to identify all men of Japanese ancestry aged 45-69 and living on Oahu in 1965. Eleven thousand one hundred forty-eight men were located. Of these, 8,006 men (72%) underwent examination between 1965 and 1969.

A special census was used in California to locate Japanese-Americans living in the eight San Francisco Bay Area counties. The 2,733 men 45-69 enumerated were invited to participate in a multiphasic examination in 1969-1970. A total of 1,842 men (67%) were examined.

In each of the three study areas, standardized interviews were used. All subjects completed a self-administered question-naire detailing various demographic and socioeconomic char-acteristics. A medical history questionnaire was then completed. In Japan and Hawaii, the medical history questionnaire was administered by a nurse-interviewer; in California it was self-administered.[3]

In Table 1 the study populations for the three areas are presented according to age and generation. As expected, the Japan-born (Issei) populations of Hawaii and California are considerably older than the second-generation populations (Nisei). The population under study in Japan has an inter-mediate age distribution. Therefore, analyses will be applied to the populations grouped in five-year age intervals from 45 through 69 years.

Blood pressure measurements were obtained in a standard fashion with mercury manometers and regular cuffs applied to the subject's left arm at heart level in the sitting position. Systolic blood pressure was taken at the first phase (appearance

TABLE 1. Study Population According to Age, Area and Generation

| | Japan | | Hawaii | | | | California | | | |
| | | | Issei | | Nisei | | Issei | | Nisei | |
Age	n	%	n	%	n	%	n	%	n	%
45 – 49	302	13.4	19	2.0	1813	25.7	23	8.6	705	44.8
50 – 54	457	20.3	38	4.0	2753	39.0	34	12.6	489	31.0
55 – 59	481	21.4	127	13.5	1465	20.7	34	12.6	238	15.1
60 – 64	543	24.2	501	53.3	836	11.8	55	20.5	111	7.1
65 – 69	466	20.7	256	27.2	195	2.8	123	45.7	32	2.0
Total	2249	100.0	941	100.0	7062	100.0	269	100.0	1575	100.0

of sound) and diastolic blood pressure at the fifth phase (disappearance of sound). The geographic distances between study areas precluded standardization of observers. While this and the use of automated recording devices would have been desirable, it is not unreasonable to assume that this problem did not cause substantial bias in the findings. Of course, we are aware of the extensive data which have led to the distrust of intergroup comparisons of blood pressure levels. However, it is our opinion that intrasubject variability is at least as great a problem and one which has received all too little attention. In this study, the measurements in each of the study areas were made by many separate observers, each of whom had been given explicit training in blood pressure technique in addition to their basic professional preparation. World Health Organization criteria were used to define hypertension, normotension and borderline hypertension.[4]

Relative weights were calculated using a table of "ideal" weights, which is based on the mean weight at each height of men in Hawaii whose back and arm skinfold totaled 10-12 mm.[4] The subject's measured weight was divided by the ideal weight for his height, and this fraction was multiplied by 100 to give the relative weight for each subject.

Since blood pressure distributions, particularly systolic, are generally skewed to the right, it was decided to present the complete percentage distributions and to employ the median and quartiles as descriptive statistics. However, in order that the findings of the study may be compared to those from other populations, the means and standard deviations for the various

104

W. WINKELSTEIN, JR.

age, area and generation groupings are given in an expanded paper.[2] To describe the distributions the blood pressures will be classified into 10 mm intervals bracketing values terminating in zero. This is done to minimize the effect of the expected zero terminal digit preference.

Results

The frequency distributions for systolic and diastolic blood pressure in the Japanese population and in the Honolulu and California Nisei are shown in Figures 1 and 2. The frequency distributions reveal the expected skew for systolic blood pressure and the increasing variability with age. The diastolic distributions do not reveal as much decomposition as systolic with increasing age and show substantial kurtosis at younger ages, ie, excess of values near the mean and far from it.

The medians (50th percentiles) are graphed in Figures 3 and 4. These data show an expected rise in systolic blood pressure with age in each of the five population subgroups. For diastolic blood pressure, only the California Issei show such a pattern.

With respect to blood pressure level, subjects living in Hawaii and Japan have similar levels for both systolic and diastolic pressure, while the California Issei and Nisei are substantially higher in general. However, there are several

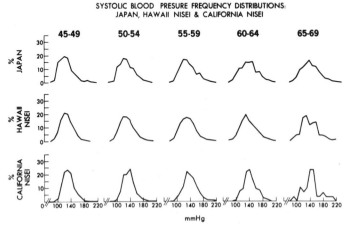

Figure 1.

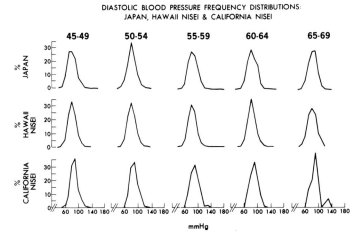

Figure 2.

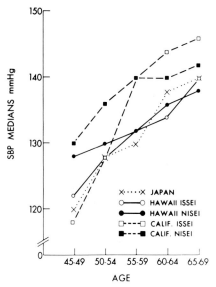

Figure 3.

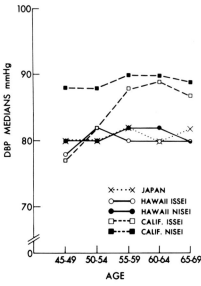

DIASTOLIC BLOOD PRESSURE
MEDIANS BY AGE, AREA AND GENERATION

Figure 4.

exceptions. California Issei have lower median systolic values for the 45-49 year age group than any other subgroup, while Hawaiian Nisei have median systolic values close to the California Nisei. Japanese in the two oldest age groups have higher median systolic blood pressure than the Hawaiian Issei or Nisei. With respect to diastolic blood pressure, the young California Issei again have similarly low median values, although the Hawaiian Nisei are not nearly as high as the California Nisei. In the oldest age group, the Japanese in the home islands have higher median diastolic blood pressure than do the Hawaiian Issei or Nisei.

When the study populations were classified according to qualitative criteria, a similar pattern emerged as shown in Table 2.[3] Definite hypertension was more prevalent in the California cohort than in either the Hawaiian or Japanese cohorts. Exceptions to this occurred in the oldest and youngest age groups where the Japanese cohorts had higher prevalence than the Hawaiian cohort. The pattern of borderline hypertension

TABLE 2. Prevalence of Hypertension for Japanese Males
by Age and Geographical Location

Age	Japan	Hawaii	California	Japan	Hawaii	California
	Definite Hypertension (Prevalence/1000)			Borderline Hypertension (Prevalence/1000)		
45 – 49	139	142	234	163	222	306
50 – 54	194	183	286	203	221	280
55 – 59	255	199	263	199	252	253
60 – 64	280	247	384	239	236	292
65 – 69	318	352	423	278	288	245
Age-Adjusted Rate	223	194	315	215	235	285
No. of men	2127	7998	1795	2127	7998	1795

was slightly different with an upward gradient from Japan to California.

Since body habitus is known to be directly associated with blood pressure level, the data were analyzed to take into account differences in this characteristic among populations. In Table 3 the proportions of each subgroup with relative weight greater than 120% are shown by age. At all ages the Japanese living in the home islands have substantially lower proportions with relative weight greater than 120%. Furthermore, there is no particular age pattern among those in Japan although the oldest age group has the smallest proportion in this relative weight class. The patterns for Hawaii and California are generally similar with the highest proportion of individuals with relative weight greater than 120% in the 45-49 year age group.

TABLE 3. Percent With Relative Weight Greater Than 120
by Age, Area and Generation

Age	Japan	Hawaii		California	
		Issei	Nisei	Issei	Nisei
45 – 49	17.8	63.2	62.0	38.1	69.8
50 – 54	23.9	52.6	56.5	54.5	68.5
55 – 59	24.7	50.4	51.9	57.6	63.4
60 – 64	20.4	39.7	49.8	47.2	53.6
65 – 69	15.2	41.6	46.2	47.0	50.0

W. WINKELSTEIN, JR.

The only deviation from this is the California Issei who have a small proportion of their population in the heavier class. In California there are slightly higher proportions in the heavier groups at all ages for both Issei and Nisei with the exception of the youngest Issei group.

We have adjusted the systolic and diastolic blood pressure medians using a simple method to take account of these differences in relative weight distributions.

Since most relative weight subgroups have substantial numbers of subjects, the observed median can be assumed to be a good estimate of central tendency. Therefore, we have averaged the medians over the various relative weight groupings in order to obtain an adjusted mean for each area and subgroup. This method is analogous to the method of direct age adjustment in which a standard population with equal numbers in each group is used in the adjustment. The adjusted medians along with the unadjusted medians for comparison are shown in Tables 4 and 5.

The systolic and diastolic blood pressure medians for the Japanese in Hiroshima and Nagasaki are essentially unchanged

TABLE 4. Systolic Blood Pressure Medians* Adjusted to
Relative Weight Differences by Age, Area and Generation:
Japan, Hawaii and California
(Unadjusted Medians Shown in Parentheses)

Age	Japan	Hawaii Issei	Hawaii Nisei	California Issei	California Nisei
45 – 49	123 (120)	124** (122)	122 (128)	119** (118)	129 (130)
50 – 54	127 (128)	125 (128)	124 (130)	127 (128)	132 (136)
55 – 59	131 (130)	130 (132)	126 (132)	132 (140)	141 (140)
60 – 64	138 (138)	130 (134)	132 (136)	140 (144)	134 (140)
65 – 69	142 (140)	134 (140)	136 (138)	146 (146)	135 (142)

*Median = mean of medians from the relative weight groups: < 90, 90-100, 100-110, 110-120, 120-130, > 130.
**Values based on n $<$ 30.

TABLE 5. Diastolic Blood Pressure Medians* Adjusted to Relative
Weight Differences by Age, Area and Generation:
Japan, Hawaii and California
(Unadjusted Medians Shown in Parentheses)

Age	Japan	Hawaii		California	
		Issei	Nisei	Issei	Nisei
45 – 49	80	79**	77	76**	85
	(80)	(78)	(80)	(77)	(88)
50 – 54	82	77	78	83	84
	(80)	(82)	(80)	(82)	(88)
55 – 59	84	76	78	84	87
	(82)	(80)	(82)	(88)	(90)
60 – 64	82	78	80	84	85
	(80)	(80)	(82)	(89)	(90)
65 – 69	84	79	79	88	78
	(82)	(80)	(80)	(87)	(89)

*Median = mean of medians from the relative weight groups: < 90, 90-100,
100-110, 110-120, 120-130, > 130.
**Values based on $n < 30$.

by the adjustment procedure. In general, the adjustment results
in lowering median values in both Hawaii and California, thus
decreasing the differences among the three areas. For systolic
blood pressure after adjustment, the California Nisei remain
somewhat higher than other subgroups in the three younger age
groups. For diastolic blood pressure, after adjustment, the
California Nisei have substantially higher pressures only for the
45-49 year age group.

In the search for additional factors associated with blood
pressure level in the three populations, we decided to examine
initially occupation and education. Since occupational status
was defined somewhat differently in each of the three study
areas, we developed a classification based on the educational
achievement of persons classified into the various occupational
groupings. Thus for each area we arrayed the occupations
according to the mean number of years of education reported
by each participant and then arbitrarily divided the distribution
into three homogeneous groupings yielding low, intermediate
and high status occupations. Educational achievement was also

arbitrarily classified into four groups of essentially similar grade completion. The mean systolic blood pressures for each subgroup were then tabulated. In order to obtain sufficient numbers of observations to accomplish the cross-classification, it was necessary to pool age groups 45-59 and 60 and over. For this analysis we have used only systolic blood pressure for the reason reported by our group at the last international symposium on hypertension.[5] We are presenting means rather than medians at this time only because our computer programs are currently being revised and when these tables were prepared, programs to calculate medians were not available. We have tabulated the relative weights according to occupational status and educational achievement and have found that there are no significant trends. This permits the direct examination of the blood pressure values without recourse to further adjustment. The analysis is limited to California and Hawaii Nisei, all Japanese, and the aforementioned age grouping 45-59.

For home island Japanese and for Hawaiian Nisei, there was no apparent association between occupational status or educational achievement and systolic blood pressure. Nor were there any interaction effects. However, for California Nisei there may be an independent association between educational achievement and blood pressure level with occupational status controlled, as well as an interaction effect between the two independent variables. The data are shown in Table 6. In both the intermediate and high occupational status groups there is an inverse association between educational achievement and sys-

TABLE 6. Systolic Blood Pressure Means
According to Occupational Status and
Educational Achievement, California Nisei,
45-59 Years of Age

Educational Achievement (Yrs.)	Occupational Status		
	1 (Low)	2	3 (High)
8	133	140	141
9 – 11	137	138	138
12 – 15	135	136	137
16 & over	138*	133	133

*Values based on less than ten observations.

tolic blood pressure level with an ordered gradient. In the low occupational status group, no such graded response is seen. An examination of the rows in the table confirms the lack of association between occupational status and systolic blood pressure level when education is controlled. The interaction is suggested by examination of the corner cells with the lowest systolic blood pressure readings of the table appearing in the congruent corners and the highest reading occurring in the group representing high occupational status with low educational achievement. Of course, these observations must be viewed cautiously since a full analysis has not yet been accomplished.

Discussion

When the blood pressure distributions were initially examined, it appeared that for most age groups the California Issei and Nisei had substantially higher values than their counterparts in Hawaii and the Japanese in Hiroshima and Nagasaki. Furthermore, the differences between the summary values for the Hawaiian cohorts and the Japanese home island population appeared very small and variable in direction. When the blood pressures were adjusted for relative weight the differences among all three populations became smaller and, for some age groups, disappeared altogether. However, the California cohort remained somewhat higher than the Japanese and Hawaiian cohorts in most comparisons and the home island Japanese had slightly higher adjusted values than the Hawaiian cohort.

It is worth noting that the relative weight distributions of the Hawaiian Japanese were similar to, although somewhat lower than, the California Japanese, while they were substantially higher than the home island cohort. Nevertheless, when adjusted, both the systolic and diastolic blood pressures of the Hawaiian Nisei were in general lower than the Japanese in the home islands. The reason for this paradox is that the relationship between relative weight and blood pressure among the Japanese in the home islands is not as consistent as it is among the Hawaiian Nisei. Consequently, when the blood pressures are adjusted for relative weight, the Hawaiian Nisei, though a heavier subpopulation than the home island Japanese, have generally lower adjusted median blood pressures.

A similar relationship between blood pressure and weight has previously been observed for descendants of Cape Verdeans who migrated to New England in the mid and late 19th century.[6] That is, the migrant population blood pressures were higher than those of their home island counterparts until body weight was taken into account.

Weight is a function of nutrition and energy output. The precise mechanism of its relationship to blood pressure remains unknown. While dietary salt has been suggested as a factor, its role has not been definitively established.[7-10] In the present study, dietary information and physical activity patterns are available for the various subgroups.[11] Thus, in subsequent analyses it may be possible to isolate various components of this complex relationship.

As expected, the pattern of definite hypertension follows the pattern of median blood pressure levels in the three populations. However, as our colleagues have indicated in a separate presentation, hypertensive heart disease was much more common in the home island cohort than in the Japanese-American cohorts. This suggests that there may be additional factors involved in the genesis of hypertensive heart disease.

The analysis of education and occupation is, in a sense, peripheral to the basic issue under consideration here, namely, the comparison of blood pressure levels in the three populations. However, it may shed some light on the problem of intercultural comparisons. There are indications from other sources that the role of occupation and education in Japanese society is quite different than in America. Furthermore, the occupational status of Hawaiian Japanese is much more homogeneous than in the other two populations. The finding of a relationship between blood pressure level and education in the California Nisei and the possible interaction with occupation is of considerable interest, since it has been so difficult to demonstrate any such associations in previous studies of blood pressure.

The underlying assumption which motivated this cross-cultural study was that migrants would experience stresses which would affect their physiologic functions and subsequent disease processes in the course of adjusting to the new culture. Thus, it was expected that blood pressure would follow a gradient from traditional Japanese to acculturated Americans, although the investigators had no prior reason to expect the particular direction of the gradient. Since coronary heart disease and stroke are both associated with high blood pressure, and since the Japan, Hawaii, California gradient for mortality from these diseases was reversed, it is interesting to note that the adjusted medians indicate higher blood pressures in Japan and California than in Hawaii. This, in turn, leads to the conclusion that the differences in stroke and coronary heart disease gradients are most probably due to factors other than blood pressure level.

It has already been suggested that the high stroke rates in Japan are due to high blood pressure and the low rates of coronary disease there to low cholesterol levels.[7] The relatively low stroke rates in California Japanese may be attributable to early elimination of susceptibles with high cholesterol and high blood pressure. The intermediate rates for both stroke and coronary heart disease in Hawaii are consistent with the lower adjusted blood pressure levels and intermediate cholesterol values in that population.

References

1. Gordon, T.: Mortality experience among the Japanese in the United States, Hawaii and Japan. *Public Health Rep.*, 72:543-53, 1957.
2. Winkelstein, W., Kagan, A., Kato, H. et al: Epidemiological studies of coronary heart disease and stroke in Japanese men living in Japan, Hawaii and California: Blood pressure distributions. *Amer. J. Epidem.* (accepted for publication).
3. Marmot, M., Syme, S. L., Kagan, A. et al: Epidemiologic studies of coronary heart disease and stroke in Japanese men living in Japan, Hawaii and California: Prevalence of coronary and hypertensive heart disease and associated risk factors (submitted for publication).
4. Belsky, J. L., Kagan, A. and Syme, S. L.: Epidemiological studies of coronary heart disease and stroke in Japanese men living in Japan, Hawaii and California: Research plan. Atomic Bomb Casualty Commission Technical Report 12-71, 1971.
5. Winkelstein, W. and Kantor, S.: Some observations on the relationships between age, sex and blood pressure. Reprinted from *Epidemiology of Hypertension.* Grune and Stratton, Inc., 1967, pp. 70-81.
6. Florey, C du V and Cuadrado, R. R.: Blood pressure in native Cape Verdeans and in Cape Verdean immigrants and their descendants living in New England. *Hum. Biol.*, 40:189-211, 1968.
7. Switzer, S.: Hypertension and ischemic heart disease in Hiroshima,

Japan. *Circulation*, 28:368-380, 1963.

8. Dahl, L. K. and Love, R. A.: Etiological role of sodium chloride intake in essential hypertension in humans. *JAMA*, 164 (4):397-400, 1957.

9. Chiang, B. N., Perlman, L. V. and Epstein, F. H.: Overweight and hypertension: A review. *Circulation*, 39:403-421, 1969.

10. Sive, P. H., Medalie, J. H., Kahn, H. A. et al: Correlation of weight-height index with diastolic and with systolic blood pressure. *J. Prev. Soc. Med.*, 24:201-204, 1970.

11. Tillotson, J. L., Kato, H., Nichaman, M. Z. et al: Epidemiology of coronary heart disease and stroke in Japanese men living in Japan, Hawaii and California: Methodology for comparison of diet. *Amer. J. Clin. Nutr.*, 26:177-184, 1973.

Discussion

Dr. Sackett: You have found generally higher blood pressures in California than in Japan, suggesting a migration effect. As Dr. Cassel pointed out, one of the problems here is that the data are cross-sectional and one is concerned about blood pressures in these individuals prior to migration. Forgetting about the California Japanese for a moment, it might be desirable to compare blood pressure levels in Japanese in Japan with and without first degree relatives who have migrated to Hawaii or California. If one finds that individuals with migrant relatives have higher blood pressures than those without migrant relatives, one could suggest that people with higher blood pressures migrate. On the other hand, if one finds similar blood pressure levels, it would support the hypothesis that it is the migration which causes the increase in blood pressure rather than migration simply selecting individuals with higher blood pressure.

Dr. Winkelstein: I think your comment is self-contained. We have not done that. The records would be difficult to come by. Most of the migration, I understand, was directly to the two areas. Dr. Kagan might want to comment.

Dr. Kagan, Hawaii: About 85% of people we have been studying in California and Hawaii were born in California or Hawaii of migrant parents, so we cannot really study the effects of such factors.

Dr. Woo-Ming, California: We have done some preliminary work with the Chinese in San Francisco. We have not looked at the migration patterns, but we did come to some interesting conclusions with regard to sex difference, especially in the 35-54 age group. The Chinese women apparently have a prevalence of high blood pressure intermediate between Caucasians and blacks, while the men do not show this finding, at least not in the 35-54 group. Have you noticed any significant sex difference?

Dr. Winkelstein: Our studies do not include women, unfortunately, so we do not have any data on that.

Dr. Roistacher: I suspect that those of us who have been running regressions and analyses of variance by the hundreds would be interested in why you reject parametric analyses.

Dr. Winkelstein: We have rejected them largely because of the intrasubject variability which leads to a very imprecise index of blood pressure level when you use a single value. It is also apparent from the data that have been presented in several papers that the distributions depart markedly from the normal; therefore, they do not meet the usual restrictions of ordinary parametric analysis. When we analyzed familial aggregations, using standard parametric technics, in the Buffalo data, we did not reveal aggregations whereas when we used nonparametric technics, the aggregation was immediately apparent. No one has really, to my knowledge, studied and settled satisfactorily the issue of what the appropriate technics are for the analysis of blood pressure data. They continue to answer always that parametric technics are "robust" and take care of these issues. The data exist in the literature which I think raise serious questions as to the use of the standard parametric analyses.

II
Dietary and Chemical Factors

Electrolytes and Hypertension

Herbert G. Langford, M.D. and Robert L. Watson, D.M.V.

Is electrolyte intake, especially of sodium, a major culprit in the genesis of essential hypertension? And if it is, does it act in a permissive manner, allowing hypertension to occur if sodium intake is above a certain level, or is it a graded phenomenon, with progressively elevated pressure accompanying each increment of sodium intake?

The South Sea Island studies of Maddocks,[1] Prior,[2] Page[3] and Shaper[4] revealed that members of a number of primitive communities have low pressures, that the pressures do not rise with age and that the individuals take very little sodium. Incidentally, they eat food containing a great deal of potassium. We will return to the potassium theme later, but for the moment it seems that a *manner of life* marked by a very low Na and high K ingestion will prevent hypertension.

Granting that a very low Na diet will prevent hypertension may carry us halfway over another hurdle: Are humans rats or rabbits? If rats are given a high salt intake, many will become hypertensive. Rabbits and dogs do not become hypertensive with excess salt consumption unless the renal mass is markedly reduced. The South Seas studies suggest that humans have at least some resemblance to rats and that below a threshold intake of sodium, hypertension does not develop.

Dahl[5] has amplified this view by showing that by selective breeding he can derive salt-sensitive and salt-resistant strains of rats. Of great interest is the fact that his salt-sensitive strain is

Supported in part by a grant from the Hartford Foundation and by NIH-NHLI grant number E-10721.

Herbert G. Langford, M.D., *Professor of Medicine and Physiology; Chief, Endocrine and Hypertension Division, Department of Medicine, and* Robert L. Watson, D.M.V., Ph.D., *Associate Professor, Department of Preventive Medicine; Assistant Professor, Department of Medicine, University of Mississippi School of Medicine, Jackson.*

also more responsive to other hypertensive stimuli such as renal arterial narrowing. A human with a "salt-sensitive" genetic background of the same kind as Dahl's rats would be more likely to become hypertensive if atherosclerosis partially occluded an artery to a kidney than someone from a "salt-resistant" heritage. The genetic propensity to become hypertensive might be expressed in one kin member because of his electrolyte intake, in another member because of his renal atherosclerosis and in still another because of "factors operating through the mind," to use Pickering's happily noncommittal phrase.

To return to the primary theme, let us phrase our question as follows: Is essential hypertension produced by excess Na consumption? Because of the South Sea Island experience we concede that a threshold Na intake or Na/K intake is necessary as a permissive factor.

Several lines of evidence have been offered in support of the Na hypothesis. One cross-cultural argument has been offered which states that the average blood pressure of a population and the average sodium intake are linearly related.[6] We do not believe that the evidence supports this thesis. We would like to know the age, sex, obesity, etc., of the comparison populations and the conditions of measurement. Such data are not available, nor are valid cross-cultural data on salt consumption. In the last decade at least two studies within a single population have failed to find a relationship between Na excretion and blood pressure. Miall in South Wales found that his subjects with higher pressures excreted *less* sodium than those with lower pressures.[7] The Framingham experience, reported by Dawber at the earlier conference, was that there was no relationship between Na excretion and blood pressure.[8]

Our entry into this field was precipitated by observations of Dr. Watson. We did a blood pressure survey of all (95%) high school students of Jackson, Mississippi, and its surrounding county, Hinds. The blood pressures showed socioeconomic and urban-rural gradients: in the city the poorer the family, the higher the child's systolic blood pressure, with the pressures of those living in the rural areas being even higher.[9] All of our studies were done by repeated subsampling of individuals originally identified during the school survey. These study groups are listed below:

1. Forty Negro females randomly allocated from those in the school survey with systolic pressures > 125 mm Hg and 20 Negro females randomly allocated from those with systolic pressures < 105 mm Hg during the school survey. (Overnight urines only were collected.)

2. All Negro female sibling pairs identified in the school survey after exclusions for pregnancy. (N = 194 pairs interviewed.) (ON and 24-hour urines collected for one day.)

3. A proportionate random sample of Negro females drawn from each school in the school survey. (N = 250 drawn = 108 completions.) (ON and 24-hour urines collected for six consecutive days.)

4. A proportionate random sample of white females from each school in the survey. (N = 250 drawn = 105 completed.) (ON and 24-hour urines collected for three days.)

5. A proportionate random sample of white females from each school in the survey. (N = 150 = 77 completed.) (ON urines collected.)

6. All Negro females included in 3 above. (N = 108 = 82 completed.) (ON and 24-hour urines collected for two or three days in winter.)

7. Systematic cluster sample of households after a random start — to identify Negro females ages 35-44 in Jackson only. (N = 40 clusters of 5 = 198 Negro females completed.) (ON and 24-hour urines collected for one day.)

We originally postulated that differing salt intake was the most likely variable to explain the blood pressure gradients that we observed. In our original studies we despaired of a long collection period. A random sample correlated poorly with a 24-hour urine sample, but the correlation of overnight urine with 24-hour urine electrolytes was acceptable. Using this approach, we looked at the urinary electrolyte excretion of girls picked from the "upper" and lower ends of the blood pressure distribution. Though the absolute amount of Na excreted by the "upper" group was greater than that excreted by the lower group, the two groups were not significantly different by the

TABLE 1.

SELECTED MEAN OVERNIGHT URINE VALUES AMONG NEGRO FEMALES WITH ˙HIGH˙ and WITH ˙LOW˙ BLOOD PRESSURES

GROUP	Na/cr	C r. mg./hr.	Na mEq/hr.	K mEq/hr.
"HIGH" (33) PRESSURE 131/69=x̄	0.1297	44.64	5.67	0.85
"LOW" (19) PRESSURE 94/49=x̄	0.1133	39.84	4.45	0.61
F	3.66**	1.11	3.00**	2.83**
t		0.98		

** P < .01

The P values refer to the F test.

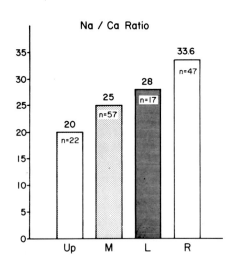

Fig. 1. Na/Ca ratio in urine of black girls aged 19-21, arranged by socioeconomic status. Up = Upper; M = Middle; L = Lower; R = Rural.

"T" test or by nonparametric methods, but they were by the "F" test (Table 1). Perhaps that means that in the group with higher pressures there is a subset where higher pressures are related to their higher salt consumption.

We have now looked at the 24-hour Na excretion and blood pressure of over 600 individuals as listed above, all identified by some appropriate sampling technique from a population base. In no case have we been able to find a significant positive correlation between blood pressure and Na excretion alone. We do find associations that are of interest.

The first is with calcium. M. J. Watson, the nutritionist on our project, first noted the low Ca intake, as measured by dietary recall, of our rural students. We have obtained tantalizing, but not consistent or convincing clues of the relationship between Ca excretion and hypertension. First, the urinary Na/Ca ratio gradient in a subset of black girls resembles that found for their blood pressure (Fig. 1). Second, in two subsets the Na/Ca ratio found in 24-hour urinary samples was significantly higher for individuals from the upper end of the blood pressure distribution curve than for those from the lower end. Third, rats on a low Ca^{++} and given 0.9% NaCl as drinking water took only one half as much saline as those on a normal Ca^{++} diet, but reached the same degree of hypertension (Fig. 2). However, the relationship between Na/Ca ratio and blood pressure has not been consistent in all our studies. A pair-feeding experiment — where one group of rats was fed a low Ca^{++} diet and the other a normal Ca^{++} diet, but both groups given the same high salt intake — failed to disclose any impressive blood pressure differences between the two groups.

Although the calcium story continues to interest us, and because the reputed correlation between hard water and protection from cardiovascular mortality is of possible clinical importance, we must conclude that we have neither clear epidemiologic nor convincing experimental data to link Ca^{++} deficiency and hypertension.

To summarize our conclusions to date, we feel that neither our studies nor other reports establish a causal relation between the intake of sodium and the occurrence of hypertension within the civilized population. The attempt to add calcium to the equation has not been productive.

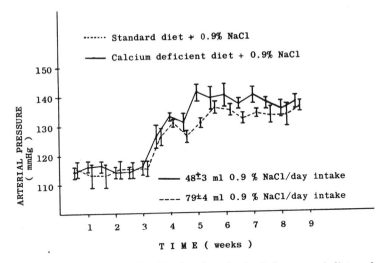

Fig. 2. Blood pressure and saline intake of rats fed a normal diet and a calcium-deficient diet. The blood pressures were not significantly different, but the low calcium rats took in only a little more than half as much saline to reach the same degree of hypertension. (Reprinted from Langford et al.[9])

There are hints in the literature that K may be involved in blood pressure regulation. Two papers in the 1920s reported that treatment with K salts would lower blood pressure in hypertensive patients. Meneely reported that K protected rats from Na produced mortality and produced at certain Na/K ratios a decrease in the Na produced hypertension.[10] Dahl has demonstrated that in his salt-sensitive rats the higher the Na/K ratio of their food, the higher their blood pressure, holding Na constant.[11]

We find that in almost all of our studies the urinary Na/K ratio will be higher in individuals from the upper end of the blood pressure distribution — not always significantly higher, but definitely higher. Figure 3 shows the urinary Na/K ratio in blood pressure in one group of black girls and another of white girls. Both samples were approximately 100 in number and were selected randomly from students we had previously seen in our school surveys. The blood pressure of the black girls is significantly higher, as is the urinary Na/K ratio. We have plotted the blood pressure and Na/K ratio of our two groups of girls and of Dahl's rats at the same Na/K ratios. We cite not as

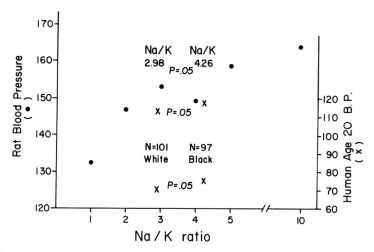

Fig. 3. The basic figure, showing on the left ordinate the blood pressure of Dahl's salt-sensitive strain after prolonged feeding of a defined diet, with the dietary Na/K ratio on the abscissa. If Na is held constant, blood pressure increases as K is decreased. On the same graph are plotted urinary Na/K ratios and blood pressure of a sample of black girls and a sample of white girls. The significantly higher blood pressure of the black girls is accompanied by a significantly higher urinary Na/K ratio.

proof but as parable the comparable slopes of their blood pressures for similar Na/K ratios.

However, none of the studies of overnight or 24-hour urinary excretion of electrolytes versus one or two blood pressure determinations demonstrated a clear and consistent correlation between electrolyte excretion and blood pressure. We next considered the possibility that our failure to find a significant relation between electrolyte excretion and blood pressure might be due to variability of both parameters.

We obtained the cooperation of 108 black girls, age 19-21, whom we had seen in school four years before. They were visited daily for eight days and three blood pressures were determined at each visit. Six 24-hour urine collections were obtained, partitioned into overnight and the rest of the 24-hour specimens.[1][2] Table 2 shows a few of the correlations. An overnight urine predicts the total 24-hour urine excretion well, but not the six-day excretion. Even a 24-hour urine doesn't predict the six-day excretion very well. The same can be said for blood pressure.

TABLE 2.

Electrolyte Excretion

Black Females at Home x̄ 21 years

n=104

Correlation Coefficients (vs. 6 day rates)

Variables	1ST Overnight	1ST 24 hours	1ST 3 days
Na	.420	.664	.900
K	.247	.810	.941
Ca	.552	.741	.948

When we determined correlations between electrolyte excretion measured for the entire collection period and the mean of the 24 blood pressures that had been taken on these individuals, we failed to find a correlation between Na excretion and blood pressure, between Ca excretion and blood pressure, and between Na/Ca ratio and blood pressure. There is one correlation which was reasonably strong and significant: that of the diastolic blood pressure versus the Na/K ratio (Table 3). We suggest that this finding is more than a chance occurrence for the following reasons: (1) In five out of six samples each of about 100 individuals, the Na/K ratio followed the blood pressure, even though the correlation was not significant. In other words, if we divided the individuals by blood pressure, the third with the highest blood pressure would have the highest Na/K ratio and the third with the lowest blood pressure would have the lowest Na/K ratio. (2) The black-white blood pressure difference is accompanied by a significant Na/K ratio difference. (3) An association between Na/K ratio and blood pressure was found in the Evans County study[13] and in the tri-state cardiovascular study of Culler.[14] (4) Two papers in the 1920s, not entirely convincing, describe the successful use of K as an antihypertensive agent.[15,16] (5) When problems of variability were minimized by multiple observations, the correlation of diastolic blood pressure and Na/K ratio was the only significant correlation in the study reported above. (6) Acute infusion of K

TABLE 3. Correlation Between 24 Blood Pressure Determinations
Determined Over Eight Days and Urinary Excretion
of Na, K, Ca and Na/K and Na/Ca Ratios

	S	D	
Na	.119	.026	Negro Females n = 101
K	.012	.050	19.5 yrs.
Ca	.090	.080	8 days BP
Na/K	.121	.372	6 days urine
Na/Ca	.053	.083	p = 0.02

The only significant correlation is between the Na/K ratio and diastolic blood
pressure.

is natriuretic and will lower the blood pressure of hypertensive
patients.[17] (7) Finally, K protects against the blood pressure
raising effect of Na in rats.[10,11]

We conclude with the following hypothesis: In the salt-
sensitive portion of the population, blood pressure will be a
direct function of the sodium intake and an inverse function of
K and perhaps Ca intake.

We believe that the time is now approaching when this
hypothesis should be tested as a means to prevent hypertension.
Modest reduction of sodium intake, plus moderate increase of
potassium intake, could be a dietary modification that the
population could live with and, if it prevents hypertension, live
with their new diet longer than they could with their old.

References

1. Maddocks, I.: Possible absence of essential hypertension in two
   complete Pacific island populations. *Lancet*, 2:396, 1961.
2. Prior, I. A. M., Grimley-Evans, J., Harvey, H. P. B. et al: Sodium
   intake and blood pressure in two Polynesian populations. *New Eng. J.
   Med.*, 279:515, 1968.
3. Page, L. B., Damon, A. and Mollering, R. C.: Antecedents of
   cardiovascular disease in six Solomon Island societies. *Circulation*,
   49:1132-1146, 1974.
4. Shaper, A. G.: Cardiovascular disease in the tropics. III. Blood
   pressure and hypertension. *Brit. Med. J.*, 2:805, 1972.
5. Dahl, L. K., Heine, M. and Tassinari, L.: Effect of chronic excess salt
   ingestion; evidence that genetic factors play an important role in
   susceptibility to experimental hypertension. *J. Exp. Med.*, 115:1173,
   1962.

128   H. G. LANGFORD AND R. L. WATSON

6. Dahl, L. K.: Possible role of salt intake in the development of essential hypertension. In Bock, K. D. and Cuttier, P. T. (eds.): *Essential Hypertension, An International Symposium.* Berlin-Gottingen-Heidelberg:Springer-Verlag, 1960.
7. Miall, W. E. and Oldham, P. D.: Factors influencing blood pressure in the general population. *Clin. Sci.*, 409-444, 1958.
8. Dawber, T. R., Kannel, W. B., Kagan, A. et al: Environmental factors in hypertension. In Stamler, J., Stamler, R., and Pullman, T. N. (eds.): *The Epidemiology of Hypertension.* New York:Grune and Stratton, Inc., 1967, pp. 255-282.
9. Langford, H. G., Watson, R. L. and Douglas, B. H.: Factors affecting blood pressure in population groups. *Trans. Ass. Amer. Physicians,* 81:135-146, 1968.
10. Meneely, G. R., Ball, C. O. T. and Youmans, J. B.: Chronic sodium chloride toxicity: Protective effect of added potassium chloride. *Ann. Intern. Med.*, 47:263, 1957.
11. Dahl, L. K., Leitl, G. and Heine, M.: Influence of dietary potassium, and sodium/potassium molar ratios on the development of salt hypertension. *J. Exp. Med.*, 136:318-328, 1972.
12. Langford, H. G. and Watson, R. L.: Electrolytes, environment and blood pressure. *Clin. Sci. Molec. Med.*, 45:111s-113s, 1973.
13. Grim, C. E., McDonough, J. R., Dahl, L. K. et al: Dietary sodium, potassium and blood pressure. Racial differences in Evans County, Georgia. *Circulation*, 61 and 62, (suppl. 3): 85, 1970.
14. Culler, L.: Personal communication to R. L. Watson.
15. Thompson, W. H. and McQuarrie, I.: Effect of various salts on carbohydrate metabolism and blood pressure in diabetic children. *Proc. Soc. Exp. Biol. Med.*, 31:907, 1933-34.
16. Priddle, W. W.: Observations on the management of hypertension. *Canad. Med. Ass. J.*, 25:5, 1931.
17. Bartorelli, C., Gargano, N. and Leonett, G.: Potassium replacement during long-term diuretic treatment in hypertension. In Gross, F. (ed.): *Antihypertensive Therapy, An International Symposium.* Berlin-Heidelberg-New York:Springer-Verlag, 1966, pp. 422-435.

Discussion

Dr. Miller, Maryland: One of the more important lessons to be learned is the importance of genetic substrates. Why did you not adjust the genetic substrates?

Dr. Langford: I did not adjust for genetic substrates. I think the easiest answer is to say that I do not know how to. I am not sure that there is an innate, in the genes, black-white difference in blood pressure. If we look at the upper socioeconomic blacks in Jackson, Mississippi, versus rural whites, at age 18 the blood pressure difference is abolished for the girls and reversed for the boys. Something more than race is contributing. We are studying the first degree siblings of hypertensives at the moment as sort of an enriched sample in looking for a relationship between electrolyte excretion and blood pressure.

Dr. Cassel: How sure can you be from the studies you have read, including your own, that the sodium potassium ratio precedes the elevation of blood pressure and does not follow it?

Dr. Langford: If the primary variable was sodium I would think this quite tenable, and I do not think our data will reject that. You could make an argument that the hypertensives might have taken more sodium because they are diuresing out more sodium due to pressure diuresis, or the other argument of the much forgotten study from the Harvard physiology department about 1945 that the established renal hypertensive takes in less sodium. I do not think I can permanently reject your hypothesis, but it is not attractive to me on physiological grounds and I guess emotional, too.

Dr. Zinner, Rhode Island: I find these data very interesting and I think you will find in Dr. Kass's presentation some striking resemblances to the data that you have presented. With respect to urinary kallikrein, an enzyme which has been related to hypertension, Dr. Harry Margolius and I have found a strong, positive correlation of urinary potassium concentration and urinary kallikrein, and a negative weak correlation of urinary sodium concentration and urinary kallikrein concentration.

Dr. Beaglehole: I would like to report some negative, longitudinal results which may be relevant here. We have looked at the correlation between the sodium intake in the first year of life in a group of children in New Zealand and related this to blood pressure in the fourth year of life. Controlling for age and race, we found no consistent relationship, certainly no significant relationship.

Dr. Langford: I am interested to hear that. I would like the group to know of a wonderful experiment that is being done by the food manufacturers. You know that the sodium intake of the first six months of life in the United States changed drastically about three or four years ago. It would be fascinating to have the two-year-old blood pressure of the cohorts starting in 1968 with cohorts starting in 1971. If anybody holds captive such a prospective study I hope they will look at it.

Dr. Kass: There is one interesting aspect of this that is not directly related to the electrolyte problem but I think it should be. Many of the studies of black and white children show no racial difference in blood pressure; yours do. It would be very nice to have some sense of what accounts for it. Are your children older? Is there an age when the spread begins to occur? Are the particular circumstances that surround your population more sharply defining the differences at an earlier age? I would greatly welcome some sense to this because many of us have looked at black and white children in an entirely different setting and are impressed that their blood pressures are not dissimilar even though they are destined to become so later.

Dr. Langford: Maybe mine are not children at all, they are adolescents. It may be that socioeconomic and other gradients are fairly marked in Jackson and therefore you might see a difference in blood pressure earlier.

Dr. Simpson, New Zealand: I just wonder whether these surveys, which Dr. Langford and Dr. Beaglehole mentioned, really give the best chance of detecting this relationship of sodium and hypertension. We all know that blood pressure goes up particularly after the age of 35 or 40. Why did Dr. Langford look for this relationship in girls of 19 instead of in women of 39?

Dr. Langford: Dr. Watson and I have had big discussions about whether to study 6-year-olds, 19-year-olds or 40-year-olds. We decided we could not get a timed urine sample in the 6-year-old. We have the 19-year-olds who do not have as many commitments and were cooperative. But we did study many people 35-44 years of age. We could find no correlation in them. I will say that they were not as reliable collectors as the 20-year-olds.

Dr. Blackburn, Minnesota: I do not want to speak if there is someone here representing the Louvain group in Belgium. If there is not, I will make a comment on this problem of the variability of both the sodium excretion and the blood pressure. They found essentially no correlation using ordinary clinic blood pressure measurements. They found a very strong correlation when they used self-recorded home blood pressures.

Current Status of Salt in Hypertension

Louis Tobian, M.D.

Interest in the relationship between salt and hypertension originally centered on the lowering of hypertensive blood pressures with diets very low in sodium chloride. Ambard and Beaujard first proclaimed this principle, and F. M. Allen vigorously urged low salt diets 25 years later. Then, William Kempner[1] introduced the rice diet which had its antihypertensive effect as a low salt diet. Perera noted that even a week on a high salt intake would slightly raise the blood pressure of subjects with established hypertension. McQuarrie showed definitively that a high salt intake would produce hypertension in a 13-year-old boy, whereas normal salt intake would bring the blood pressure back to normal.

Provocative animal experiments were also performed in these early days. Lenel, Katz and Rodbard made chickens hypertensive by offering only 1% saline solution for drinking water. Sapirstein made rats hypertensive by allowing them to drink only a 2% saline solution. In Meneely's classic experiment,[2] various diets containing salt in very small or very large amounts and with various intermediate levels were fed to rats over a nine month period. It was seen that each increment in salt intake brought a concomitant increase in blood pressure. The rats eating the 10% salt in the dry diet developed frank hypertension. At 2% to 5% salt in the diet, borderline or mild hypertension was observed. At the higher levels of blood pressure, obvious nephrosclerosis was encountered. In these early days, it was also clear that the full expression of deoxycorticosterone hypertension in the rat could best be

Louis Tobian, M.D., *Division of Hypertension-Nephrology, Department of Internal Medicine, University of Minnesota Hospital and School of Medicine, Minneapolis.*

obtained if a high NaCl intake were given along with the deoxycorticosterone. Conversely, a very low sodium intake completely prevented a rise in blood pressure after deoxycorticosterone. Potassium feeding reduces the hypertension resulting from concomitant NaCl feeding.

Such reports prompted epidemiologic studies concerning salt and hypertension. Maddocks and Prior[3] noted that natives in small villages in New Guinea had virtually no hypertension and that the blood pressures in old men were no higher than those in young men. This demonstrated that blood pressure is not necessarily compelled to rise with advancing age, but genetically similar natives nearly always developed their share of hypertension when they moved to modern coastal cities. The salt in the citified diet was suspected as a cause of this emergence of hypertension.

Lot Page recently extended these observations in Solomon Island natives. In a primitive inland village there was no hypertension at all and no rise of average pressure with advancing age. In another primitive village located on an offshore island, there was a significant amount of hypertension and the average blood pressure tended to rise with advancing age. The main difference between the two villages was that the natives living by the ocean cooked their fish in salty sea water. Cooked fish acquired about 3% salt in the meat and hence provided this population with significantly more dietary sodium.

Dr. Shaper reported that Samburu farmers greatly increase their salt intake to 18 gm a day when they are drafted into the army and begin to eat army rations. Their blood pressure does not rise during the first army year, but does begin to show a rise starting with the second year of high salt rations.

At the other end of the salt spectrum, Japanese farmers in the northern prefecture of Akita eat a huge amount of salt daily as part of their dietary custom, which is related to the preservation of food. They may eat as much as 20 to 35 gm of salt per day. Eighty-four percent of the farm villagers in this area have a systolic blood pressure over 140 mm Hg.[4] The most prevalent cause of death there is stroke.

To summarize these population studies, areas with very high salt intakes have a high incidence of hypertension. Areas with a low salt intake, less than 4 gm of NaCl daily, have a very low incidence of hypertension and blood pressure does not rise with advancing years. Such a low intake of salt, 4 gm daily, is compatible with very vigorous health. Chimpanzees in the jungle are on low salt diets and possess great athletic prowess.

In the United States, Dahl found that the employees of Brookhaven National Laboratory who did not salt their food had approximately a 1% incidence of hypertension, while 12.7% of those who salted heavily had hypertension. Gifford could not find a relationship of salt to the incidence of hypertension in the Cleveland area. However, he did note that heavy salt users had significantly more complications from their hypertension than did light users.

In rats, one can induce hypertension with high sodium feedings. The hypertension persists indefinitely even after a normal diet is resumed.[5] It is as if the salt and the hypertension have somehow produced a permanent change, especially in the kidney, so that hypertension becomes a permanent adaptation. The same mechanism may be involved in the permanent hypertension after deoxycorticosterone therapy.

Dahl advanced an intriguing concept with regard to salt intake and hypertension. Everyone knows that some individuals can eat huge amounts of salt but still have a normal blood pressure and live a fine octogenarian life. It is clear that essential hypertension has a strong hereditary aspect. Such individuals are highly resistant to hypertension and a reasonable salt intake is not going to affect them. To document the principle, Dahl started with a single strain of rats and bred from them a race very susceptible to salt hypertension and a second race highly resistant to salt hypertension. The resistant rats are also relatively resistant to all other forms of experimental hypertension except one-kidney Goldblatt hypertension.[6] When these two strains of rats are fed a fairly low sodium intake (0.3% NaCl in the diet), their blood pressures are quite similar while young; with adulthood, the hypertension-prone strain has a pressure about 15 mm Hg higher than the hypertension-resistant strain. Thus, this is a form of high normal or borderline "essential" hypertension which develops in sensitive rats maintained on a low salt diet.

In my view, it is very reasonable to suppose that human beings resemble Dahl rats. If a human subject is truly resistant to hypertension, reasonable amounts of salt in the diet will not change this. If another human subject is hereditarily susceptible to essential hypertension, he may be able to avoid hypertension by remaining on a low salt intake throughout life. However, if he eats 10 gm of salt daily, his hereditary predisposition will become apparent as his blood pressure gradually begins to rise into the hypertensive range.

Early prehistoric man is thought to have been a sodium deficient herbivore, desperate for dietary sodium in order to survive and multiply. The taste receptors for salt in the human tongue are of interest in this connection. Evolution has equipped humans to cope with sodium deficiency rather than sodium excess. It is no wonder, then, that certain specific human beings become hypertensive when they eat excessive amounts of salt.

It is particularly easy to produce salt hypertension in young rats and more difficult in adult rats. This is troubling because in the recent past most items of commercial baby food had a very high salt content. Dahl was able to induce hypertension in his susceptible rats by feeding them the commercial baby food sold in grocery stores. Such salt-laden baby food is probably harmful to an infant who is susceptible to subsequent hypertension. Along this same line, cow's milk has four times more sodium per cubic centimeter than human milk.

By what mechanism does salt feeding produce hypertension in susceptible rats or men? In susceptible rats, it is easy to produce hypertension by feeding 8% NaCl in the diet,[2] a situation reminiscent of Japanese farmers. Such rats readily come into sodium balance, and it had been theorized that the hypertension results from damage to the kidney caused by the large amount of NaCl which is excreted every day.

To test this proposition, we fed the 8% NaCl diet to two groups of rats. One group (130 rats) drank tap water *ad libitum*, another group (111 rats) had 0.01% of the thiazide diuretic Enduron in their drinking water and a control group (35 rats) ate a normal diet with 0.3% NaCl. These diet regimens were continued for 4¼ months. As can be seen in Table 1, final blood pressure for the group on a normal salt intake averaged 121 mm Hg. The group with the 8% salt diet had an average pressure of 148 mm Hg. The group on the 8% salt diet plus thiazide had an average pressure of 122. Thus, the high NaCl intake produced a significant degree of hypertension. The average rise of 27 mm Hg amounted to a 22% increase in pressure. When a thiazide diuretic was combined with this same high sodium intake, the hypertension was completely prevented. If we consider all pressures above 140 as hypertensive, both the group on a normal salt intake and the group on 8% NaCl plus thiazide had a zero incidence of hypertension. The group on the 8% NaCl diet without thiazide had a 48% incidence of hypertension.

In a separate group of rats, we determined the inulin space as an index of extracellular fluid volume after eight days on the three regimens. The rats on the 8% NaCl diet without thiazide had an inulin space of 29.8 ml/100 gm of body weight (Table 1). The rats on the 8% salt diet plus thiazide had an inulin space of 28.5. Thus, the addition of thiazide brought about a 4.6% difference in ECF volume, a significant drop with a p value of 0.03. The rats on the 8% salt diet plus thiazide had an ECF volume fairly close to that of the control rats on the normal sodium intake. This study would indicate that the mere passage of NaCl through the renal tubular system does not necessarily cause hypertension. A high NaCl intake may produce hypertension if it increases extracellular fluid volume. The same high NaCl intake produces no hypertension if extracellular fluid expansion is prevented.

This brings us to question how a chronically high extracellular fluid volume, such as that produced by salt feeding, can bring on hypertension.

TABLE 1. Effect of Thiazide on NaCl Induced Hypertension

	Final BP (mm Hg)	% Above 140 (mm Hg)	Inulin Space (ml/100 gm)
8% NaCl (130 rats)	148 ↑ $p < .0001$ ↓	48% ↑ $p < 0.0001$ ↓	29.8 ↑ 4.6% diff. $p < 0.03$ ↓
8% NaCl + thiazide (111 rats)	122	0%	28.5
0.3% NaCl (35 rats)	121	0%	28.0

There are several situations in which an inappropriately high extracellular fluid volume in the body is associated with a large "effective" blood volume. I am not referring here to the edema states of congestive heart failure, cirrhosis, or nephrosis, in which the total ECF volume is high but the "effective" blood volume is actually low. In the states with a high ECF volume and a high "effective" blood volume, we often find a high incidence of hypertension. One example would be mineralo-corticoid hypertension. If too much deoxycorticosterone is given to a rat, or if too much aldosterone emerges from a human adrenal adenoma, this induces the kidney to retain sodium and water until "escape" begins to occur. At this point, no further sodium will be retained, but the general level of body sodium and water is slightly elevated. Over a long period of time this can produce hypertension in a susceptible animal. Another example would be giving a large sodium load to a mammal with deficient renal function. The dog studies of Coleman and Guyton exemplify this.[7] A dog with only one third of its normal renal mass is given 2 liters of saline a day to drink. There is an initial tendency to retain sodium and water, and these dogs develop hypertension. We see this in human subjects with advanced renal parenchymal disease who eat a fairly large amount of salt. They commonly have high blood volumes and considerable hypertension. We also see it in uremic human subjects whose kidneys are almost totally destroyed by disease. They usually have hypertension when their ECF volume is elevated from dietary salt and water, but the hypertension usually disappears when the ECF volume is brought back to low normal levels with the dialysis machine. This reversible change in arterial pressure may be repeated two times a week coinciding with the dialysis cycle.

Moreover, some patients with acute glomerulonephritis and marked sodium and water retention have a high blood and ECF volume and a high arterial pressure. In all these instances the veins could easily accommodate the modest elevation of blood volume. However, the extra volume will often increase venous filling pressure, which in turn will increase cardiac output. The higher cardiac output, of course, tends to increase arterial pressure. Furthermore, a rise in cardiac output produced in this way induces tissue blood flows which are inappropriately high for metabolic needs. This situation would stimulate an auto-regulation of blood flow in many tissue beds, certainly in brain, muscle, gut and kidney. As an autoregulatory response, most tissue beds would undergo arteriolar vasoconstriction, raising the general peripheral resistance. The combination of the higher cardiac output and increased vasoconstriction would tend to raise the blood pressure even higher; and as the arterial pressure increases, the cardiac output would gradually come back to normal levels. After a time the cardiac output would be about normal while the peripheral resistance and blood pressure remained elevated. Thus, the underlying tendency to a higher cardiac output can be completely masked. The higher arterial pressure, through the medium of pressure diuresis, would enhance the sodium and water output by the kidney in those situations where renal function was fairly well preserved. This would tend to bring ECF volume somewhat closer to normal. However, the original renal abnormality would tend to preserve a slight ECF expansion.

Most of the partially nephrectomized dogs of Coleman and Guyton undergo just these changes.[7] It is a very reasonable way to explain how a high ECF volume can bring about an arterial hypertension with peripheral vasoconstriction. Ultimately, the systemic peripheral arterioles will undergo a "waterlogging"[8] and thickening of their walls[9] just as we see in all hypertension. This arteriolar waterlogging and thickening will also occur in the renal afferent arteries and arterioles. Moreover, this process of thickening will itself make a major contribution to the increased peripheral resistance, even though it was not the original cause of it.[8,9] This general mechanism is probably operative in the hypertension of many azotemic and uremic patients.

Though this formulation is reasonable as it stands, addition-al elements are necessary for the hypertension brought on by excessive ECF volume. Bartter has given 20 mg of deoxycortico-sterone daily for three weeks to human volunteers and has produced no hypertension. The ECF volume must have risen maximally at the end of one week, but no hypertension subsequently occurred. These people were simply not suscep-tible to hypertension in spite of the effect of mineralocorticoid on ECF volume. Similarly, Dahl injected deoxycorticosterone into his two strains of rats, one sensitive and one resistant to salt hypertension. The sensitive strain promptly became hypertensive, but the resistant strain did not.[6] Even though the DOCA exerted its mineralocorticoid effect on the rats of the resistant strain and raised ECF volume a bit, hypertension did not ensue. In both instances, some genetic susceptibility is required before the high ECF volume will produce hypertension. Muirhead also gave large saline loads to bilaterally nephrectomized rabbits and produced a sizable rise in blood pressure; but if these same nephrectomized rabbits had fragments of renal medulla implanted subcutaneously, the same saline load would produce only a very small rise in blood pressure. Evidently, the fragments of renal medulla were releasing humoral agents which prevented the volume-induced hypertension.

Moreover, there are some uremic human subjects who have a normal arterial pressure. Onesti found that ECF expansion in some of these people does not produce a significant rise in blood pressure and peripheral resistance. Thus, increased ECF volume seems to bring about hypertension only in a susceptible subject. Part of this susceptibility may be related to thickened arterioles. However, the explanation of susceptibility is still mainly an enigma.

When thiazide drugs or spironolactone are given to patients, the arterial blood pressure is usually lowered and the hypertensive process can be reversed. These diuretics produce a slight decrease in ECF volume, which would decrease venous filling pressure and cardiac output. The autoregulatory response to this would bring about systemic arteriolar dilatation. The lower cardiac output and the vasodilatation should lower arterial blood pressure. This would amount to antihypertensive whole-body autoregulation or reverse autoregulation. Such reverse autoregulation could also be a mechanism that partially accounts for the antihypertensive action of both propranolol and guanethidine. Both agents lower cardiac output, which could eventually induce a lowered peripheral resistance by reverse autoregulation. Thus, adaptation to a rise or a drop in ECF volume can ultimately influence the peripheral arteriole to enhance or reduce hypertension. One of the main antihypertensive actions of the kidneys is to excrete the daily sodium load without any tendency to a rise in ECF volume. Failure to do this encourages hypertension.

Considering body fluid volumes, Dustan and Tarazi noted in the treatment of clinical hypertension that when blood pressure was successfully lowered, plasma volume was also lowered. A low sodium intake is particularly effective in the treatment of the hypertension associated with renal parenchymal disease. This would be expected since the diseased kidney usually exhibits an impairment of sodium excretion. With a normal salt intake in this situation extracellular volume builds up before sodium balance is attained. Curtailing salt consumption would reduce the excretory load on the diseased kidney and thereby reduce somewhat ECF volume. As mentioned above, this should reduce hypertensive pressure levels.

We can feed rats 8% salt for four months and then regular chow for three months. Some rats show permanent hypertension in the "post-salt" period and some have normal pressure levels in the same interval. The kidneys from these two types of rats were isolated and perfused with blood from donor rats at varying inflow pressures. With each increase in the inflow pressure in the isolated kidneys, the urinary output of sodium and water also increased. Figure 1 shows the sodium output per minute per kilogram of rat weight for three levels of inflow pressure. The top line represents kidneys from 15 "post-salt" normotensive rats. As the inflow pressure goes from 100 to 130

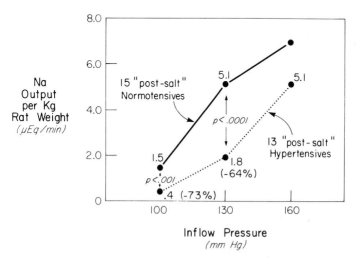

Figure 1.

to 160, the sodium output increases with each rise in pressure. The lower line represents kidneys from 14 rats of the "post-salt" hypertensive group and they follow the same general principle, more sodium output with each rise in inflow pressure. The weight of the kidneys per 100 gm of body weight and the weight of the rats were about the same in the two groups. The noteworthy feature here is that the curve representing kidneys from hypertensive rats is significantly shifted to the right. At 130 mm Hg inflow pressure, the kidneys from the hypertensive rats put out 1.8μEq of Na/Kg body weight/min, which is 64% less sodium than the 5.1μEq output of kidneys from the normotensive rats. This is a highly significant difference with a p value of .0001. At 100 mm Hg inflow pressure, the kidneys from hypertensive rats had a 73% lower Na excretion compared to kidneys of "post-salt" normotensive rats. Thus, if the hypertensive kidneys are perfused at normal inflow pressures, they put out grossly subnormal amounts of sodium. However, the hypertensive kidney can catch up on its sodium output if it is perfused at an elevated pressure. Figure 1 indicates a hypertensive kidney perfused at 160 mm Hg will put out about the same amount of sodium as a normotensive kidney perfused at 130 mm Hg.

Figure 2 shows the urine volume at the various inflow pressures. Again, at normal inflow pressures of 130 mm Hg as well as at 100 mm Hg, the hypertensive kidneys put out about 58% to 67% less urine volume per minute than the normotensive kidneys, a significant difference with a p value of .001. However, when the hypertensive kidneys are perfused at 160, the urine volume increases briskly and exceeds the volume put out by normotensive kidneys perfused at 130.

Thus, if hypertensive kidneys are perfused at a normal pressure, they will excrete subnormal amounts of both sodium and water. If this occurred in the body, it would lead to sodium and water retention. Such sodium and water retention tends to produce and maintain the hypertensive state. Once a hypertensive level of inflow pressure is reached, the hypertensive kidneys can then excrete a normal amount of sodium and water. This shift in the pressure natriuresis curve suggests that the hypertensive kidney needs a high arterial pressure for adequate sodium excretion. Any trend toward a normal blood pressure

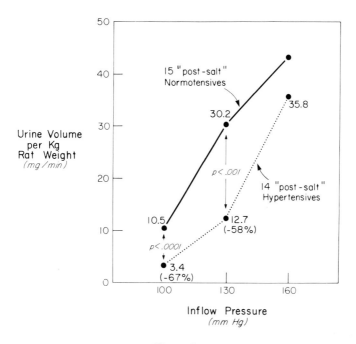

Figure 2.

would be thwarted by sodium retention. Thus, hypertension tends to be maintained.

Salt feeding for three days in 130 gm rats can raise cardiac output by 13.4%.[10] After seven days of salt feeding the cardiac output of these young rats has returned to normal. This sequence of a temporary rise in cardiac output is reminiscent of the Coleman-Guyton dog. Apparently, salt feeding can some-times activate the same mechanism.

I say "sometimes" because of certain salt feeding experiments at the University of Iowa. When young normotensive subjects are fed 400 mEq of salt for four weeks, their forearm flow goes up, their forearm vascular resistance goes down and the blood pressure stays the same. When the same procedure is applied to young subjects with borderline hypertension, the forearm vascular resistance goes up instead of down and arterial pressure rises. These very mild hypertensives respond complete-ly differently to a dietary salt load. Extracellular fluid volume increases in both groups, but only the borderline hypertensives show a rise in blood pressure and peripheral resistance.

We conclude with some other aspects of the relation between salt and hypertension. Hypertensive arteries have an increased Na content per unit of dry weight.[8] This may add to the thickening of the artery wall with a resulting increase in vascular resistance. It may also be related to enhanced vasoconstriction.

In rats with three types of experimental hypertension, the sodium concentration in the renal papilla is markedly reduced.[5,11,12] The lipid granules in the cytoplasm of the papillary interstitial cells are reduced concomitantly.[5,11,12] The sodium and the lipid granules go up and down together.

In normotensive Kyoto Wistar rats, a low salt intake significantly increases urinary kallikrein while a high salt intake does not change urinary kallikrein.[13] In direct contrast, in Kyoto Wistar spontaneously hypertensive rats, urinary kallikrein does not change with a low Na diet but increases briskly with a high Na intake. The presence of hypertension reverses the usual kallikrein response to Na feeding.[13] Moreover, human hypertensive subjects excrete a sodium load much more rapidly than their normotensive counterparts.

In one-kidney Goldblatt hypertension[14] or in mild two-kidney Goldblatt hypertension, definite sodium retention accounts partially for the rise in arterial pressure. However, if the sodium retention is prevented by a very low Na diet and diuretics, the animal will become hypertensive anyhow, by means of the renin-angiotensin system.

I have tried to survey the current status of both dietary and extracellular salt in hypertension. It is apparent that we are still groping for the answer to the key question: Why does salt increase peripheral resistance in people susceptible to hypertension and does not in those resistant to hypertension?

References

1. Kempner, W.: Treatment of kidney disease and hypertensive vascular disease with rice diet. *N. Carolina Med. J.*, 5:125, 1944.
2. Meneely, G. R., Tucker, R. G., Darby, W. J. et al: Chronic sodium chloride toxicity in the albino rat. II. Occurrence of hypertension and of a syndrome of edema and renal failure. *J. Exp. Med.*, 98:71, 1953.

3. Prior, I. A. M. and Evans, J. G.: Sodium intake and blood pressure in Pacific populations. *Israel J. Med. Sci.*, 5:608, 1969.
4. Takahashi, E., Sasaki, N., Takeda, J. et al: The geographic distribution of cerebral hemorrhage and hypertension in Japan. *Hum. Biol.*, 29:139, 1957.
5. Tobian, L., Ishii, M., and Duke, M.: Relationship of cytoplasmic granules in renal papillary interstitial cells to "post-salt" hypertension. *J. Lab. Clin. Med.*, 73:309, 1969.
6. Dahl, L. K., Heine, M., and Tassinari, L.: Effects of chronic excess salt ingestion: Role of genetic factors in both DOCA-salt and renal hypertension. *J. Exp. Med.*, 118:605, 1963.
7. Coleman, T. G. and Guyton, A. C.: Hypertension caused by salt loading in the dog. III. Onset transients of cardiac ouput and other variables. *Circ. Res.*, 25:153, 1969.
8. Tobian, L. and Binion, J. T.: Tissue cations and water in arterial hypertension. *Circulation*, 5:754, 1952.
9. Folkow, D.: The haemodynamic consequences of adaptive structural changes of the resistance vessels in hypertension. *Clin. Sci.*, 41:1, 1971.
10. Tobian, L. and Ganguli, M.: Rise in cardiac output after a high NaCl diet in young rats. *Fed. Proc.*, 33:337, 1974.
11. Ishii, M. and Tobian, L.: Interstitial cell granules in renal papilla and the solute composition of renal tissue in rats with Goldblatt hypertension. *J. Lab. Clin. Med.*, 74:47, 1969.
12. Tobian, L. and Ishii, M.: Interstitial cell granules and solutes in renal papilla in post-Goldblatt hypertension. *Amer. J. Physiol.*, 217:1699, 1969.
13. Geller, R. G., Margolius, H. S. and Pisano, J. J.: Effect of dietary sodium content on kallikrein excretion in spontaneously hypertensive rats. *Fed. Proc.*, 33:642, 1974.
14. Tobian, L., Coffee, K. and McCrea, P.: Contrasting exchangeable sodium in rats with different types of Goldblatt hypertension. *Amer. J. Physiol.*, 217:458, 1969.

Discussion

Dr. Meneely, Louisiana: I would like to comment on the papers of both Dr. Langford and Dr. Tobian. First, I would like to thank them for what they call my work. I was indeed a participant but there were a number of other people in the group and they certainly were heavy contributors to it. A lot of people overlook the fact that the Kempner diet is not only a low sodium diet but it is also a high potassium diet. I too have always worried about Dahl's study of ". . .salt before tasting, salt after tasting, never salt. . . ." You are not alone in being the only ones who could not repeat it. We could not, either. We thought the reason we failed with the questions of salt before eating and so on was that we did it on 3,000 potential draftees back in World War II, too young a group. We got zilch as a result. We decided our problem was that we had too narrow an age spread in our population. Further, when elevated blood pressure was found, we were usually able to elicit a history of kidney trouble. Besides that, it was abundantly obvious in spot-checking 24-hour urine outputs that the subjects had no idea how heavily they were salting their food. Also, I think there is an overlooked point about Dahl's Brookhaven population — it was a recently assembled population. They were all brought to Brookhaven from different parts of the country and they had not yet settled down to the local salt intake depending upon what is for sale in the stores and what people in the neighborhood are accustomed to eating. Therefore, we thought there was a wider spread of salt intake than in a more settled local population.

We described a group of rats which ate 2.5% or 5.6% sodium chloride. They got hypertension, moderate hypertension, and their lifespan was greatly shortened. They got all the tissue changes that are seen in human hypertension. They did not have increased sodium spaces. When extra potassium was given to those animals, they did not have changes in the sodium space either; the sodium space stayed the same. They did not get reductions in blood pressure, but they outlived the controls, the median duration of life being increased by eight months.

Dr. Tobian: One fascinating set of studies was done at the University of Iowa Medical Center and Dr. Kirkendall was in on that first paper. The first study was on normal students. They had various levels of salt intake for about a month. When they were given about 400 mEq of sodium a day, the blood pressures of these individuals did not rise. The forearm blood flow rose. If the blood pressure stayed the same and the forearm blood flow rose, we have to assume that their vascular resistance went down. They also had an increased glomerular filtration so we presume some vascular resistance in the kidney might have gone down. They have subsequently done another study on young people with borderline hypertension. I think it had more or less the same format with a greatly different effect. They gave them a 400 mEg salt intake also. They did not get an increase in forearm blood flow. In fact, they got a decrease in blood flow and presumably an increase in vascular resistance. Instead of having no effect on blood pressure, they had a rise in blood pressure. This is a little reminiscent of the old study of Perera 30 years ago.

It is a matter of to whom you feed salt. If you are an R-rat or an R-person or dog, you can get this extra salt. It might raise your cardiac output a little bit, it might decrease your peripheral resistance, but your blood pressure stays level But give the same kind of treatment to an S-individual and something totally different happens. Their peripheral resistance goes up, the blood pressure goes up, and you just do not get the same response.

Dr. Langford: I agree that this is true for rats and may be true for men.

Dr. Kirkendall: I wanted to set you straight on one thing. The first group of individuals we studied may have been students but they came from the state penitentiary.

Dr. Langford: That I did not know. What about the second group?

Dr. Kirkendall. The second group consisted of volunteers from the community.

It is of great interest to me in those studies that enormous hemodynamic changes occurred. Not only, as Dr. Tobian pointed out, was there a sharp increase in forearm blood flow and a dramatic increase in filtration rate but also, as you would expect, an increase in the right atrial pressure. We did not do cardiac output, but I assumed the cardiac output was up at this time. We did not change potassium intake at any time during these studies so our subjects received 100 mEq in all three of the experiments. I think one of the more fascinating things was that there was a reduction in potassium excretion as sodium intake decreased as though there was a retention of potassium to compensate for less sodium. Although there was no significant change, there were suggestions that total body potassium increased as well. I agree with Dr. Langford that this subject is not closed, for one must not look simply at sodium, as most investigators have.

Dr. Holland: As an epidemiologist I would like to ask a question of the last two speakers. Why is it that their findings have never really been reconciled with carefully done epidemiologic studies? I am at a loss to understand why none of the epidemiologic studies on populations which have measured differences in salt intake and salt excretion — in either total population groups or on random samples in which there has been a careful description of the population and with response rates of more than 90 or 95% — none have been able to confirm the pathophysiologic mechanisms that you have proposed.

Dr. Tobian: My own guess about this with regard to the United States is that the people in the United States are fantastically homogeneous and they all tend to do the same thing. I think they all eat a lot of salt. There is hardly anyone in the whole country that is on a low salt diet.

Dr. Langford: I think none of it has been done very well. We cannot really reject or accept the null hypotheses, and accuracy of measurement has not been gone into well. Actually, Dr. Holland, there has been very little measurement at all. We don't propose correlation with sodium alone, but with the ratio of sodium to potassium.

Metals and Human Hypertension

H. Mitchell Perry, Jr., M.D. and Elizabeth F. Perry, A.B.

Introduction

Excluding the alkali metals (sodium and potassium) and the alkaline earths (calcium and magnesium) three metals have been seriously suggested as possible contributors to human hypertension: lead, mercury and cadmium. Although one could mention lead (in deference to the older literature) and mercury (because of its chemical similarity to cadmium), only cadmium seems to be a serious candidate, and this paper will be limited to the evidence that cadmium may affect human blood pressure. No tight logical argument for the involvement of cadmium can be made; however, I have tried to collect the relevant material, realizing that some vital data are missing and others are diffuse or equivocal. My purpose is not to persuade you of a role for cadmium, the data are not that conclusive. Rather I am trying to convince you that the field warrants further work.

A very brief outline of the facts that suggest a relationship between cadmium and hypertension follows. At present, cadmium has no known biologic effects in man except for its well-recognized toxic effects which are associated with extensive and easily demonstrable exposure. Nonetheless, all adult human beings have had significant long-term, low-level cadmium exposure which has resulted in a considerable, but *apparently* inert accumulation of cadmium in the body. This cadmium is concentrated in the kidney where it is bound to a specific protein, metallothionein. Zinc and other metals are also bound to metallothionein, which has no known function. Cadmium is

Supported by the Veterans Administration Research Service.

H. Mitchell Perry, Jr., M.D. *and* Elizabeth F. Perry, A.B., *Medical Service, Veterans Administration Hospital, and the Hypertension Division, Department of Medicine, Washington University School of Medicine, St. Louis, Mo.*

bound more tightly than zinc and can displace it. Hypertensive human beings have been reported to have more renal cadmium than normotensive subjects. Long-term and relatively low-level cadmium feeding in animals has produced hypertension. Although the mechanism of the cadmium-induced hypertension in animals is not known, cadmium has been shown to influence cardiac output, circulating renin and salt and water metabolism. Perhaps the slow accumulation of cadmium in man during the first three or four decades of life has a previously unrecognized chronic effect which raises the blood pressure and is responsible for part of human essential hypertension. It seems likely, however, that no convincing case for cadmium involvement will be made until a reasonable mechanism by which it might raise blood pressure is proposed and can be supported by adequate data. It is obviously very difficult to prove that a common and initially asymptomatic disease is a late manifestation of long-term, low-level exposure to an ever present environmental contaminant.

Cadmium-Induced Hypertension in Animals

Probably the strongest evidence for the involvement of cadmium in the control of blood pressure is that hypertension can be induced in rats by feeding them low doses of cadmium. Since this topic has been recently reviewed in some detail,[1] it will be treated very briefly. Small amounts of parenteral cadmium can produce a prompt and marked increase in blood pressure.[2] More applicable to the human situation, chronic feeding of relatively small amounts of cadmium (1 to 5 parts per million in drinking water) can induce hypertension over a period of months. Schroeder, who first reported this, observed very marked hypertension.[3] Our animals and those of Sorenson and his co-workers, on the other hand, have had definite but much less marked increases in pressure, the average increase in systolic pressure being 15-20 mg Hg.[4,5] The kidneys of "cadmium-hypertensive" rats had cadmium concentrations comparable to the kidneys of the average American adult with no known exposure to cadmium.[6] Finally, cadmium-induced hypertension can be modified by other substances, particularly by zinc and selenium, and also by giving cadmium in hard water.[7-9]

Water Hardness and Cardiovascular Mortality

There is an entirely statistical but nonetheless impressive correlation between water hardness and total cardiovascular death rate. The correlation is negative so that the softer the water the higher the death rate. This intriguing and self-contained set of data initially seemed far removed from cadmium and the possibility of cadmium-induced hypertension, but it is briefly summarized here because a possible connection has recently been suggested. In 1957, Kobayashi made the original observation that the stroke rate was related to the acidity of local river water.[10] This induced Schroeder to seek and find a correlation between cardiovascular death rates and hardness of the drinking water.[11] Morris and co-workers found similar relationships in Great Britain,[12] and other groups of investigators have generally been able to confirm these findings in whole or in part,[13-18] although a few investigations in restricted geographical areas with relatively narrow ranges of water hardness have failed to find a relationship.[19-21] In the positive studies, ischemic heart disease was usually the most strongly correlated component of cardiovascular disease; cerebrovascular disease, which of course accounts for far fewer deaths, was less often correlated; and hypertension, which is rarely a direct and recognizable cause of death, could be shown to be correlated in only two studies. Crawford and Crawford tried to elucidate these relationships by comparing the coronary arteries of subjects from regions with soft and hard water. Those "soft water" subjects who died of myocardial infarction had less arteriosclerosis than "hard water" subjects, whereas "soft water" subjects dying of other causes had more arteriosclerosis. The coronary arteries of all "soft water" subjects had less calcium and magnesium.[22] In addition, preliminary results suggest differences in the tissue concentrations of several trace metals, particularly cadmium but also lead and chromium. The "soft water" subjects had an average of twice as much bone cadmium at autopsy as the "hard water" subjects.[23]

Renal Cadmium and Blood Pressure

Cadmium has no known biologic function, and there is very little of it in the human body at birth.[24] During the fourth decade, however, most of the considerable adult body burden (about 15 mg in the average American) has been accumulated.[25] By far the highest concentration occurs in the kidney.[26] Moreover, based on limited data, there seem to be considerable geographic differences in renal cadmium concentration. Figure 1 shows cumulative frequency graphs for renal cadmium concentration in autopsy material from nine countries. In brief, African Negroids had an average of about 1,200μg of cadmium per gram of kidney ash; Caucasoids from America, Europe and Asia had 2,200; and Asiatic Mongoloids

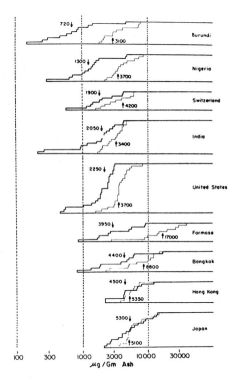

Fig. 1. Cumulative frequency graphs of the renal concentrations of cadmium and zinc for each of the nine national groups comprising 119 adult subjects. The distribution of the individual concentrations is shown for cadmium by heavy lines and for zinc by fine lines. Figures cite and arrows point to median values. The vertical scale indicates the number of patients. For instance, in the top graph each of the 11 subjects from Burundi is represented by one of the steps. The horizontal scale is logarithmic.[24]

had 5,200. Statistically these three groups were significantly different.[24]

With the variability in the human body burden of cadmium clearly in mind, several studies can be mentioned which suggest that hypertensive subjects have significantly more renal cadmium than otherwise similar but normotensive subjects. These data have been summarized in Table 1. Schroeder compared 117 normotensive Americans who died sudden accidental deaths with 17 hypertensive Americans who died similarly. The normotensive group had an average of $2,940\mu g$ of cadmium per gram kidney ash; whereas the hypertensive group had $4,220\mu g$. The difference was highly significant ($p < 0.005$).[27] Despite a wider range of renal cadmium concentrations, a similar trend was observed in a heterogeneous group of subjects from various parts of the world.[27] In Czechoslovakia, Lener and Bibr found a similar difference with very small numbers of patients.[28] Morgan, in contrast, did not find any difference in the mean renal cadmium concentrations of hypertensive versus normal subjects, although she did observe that the hypertensive group had a higher median concentration than the normotensive group.[29] Thus her data were not inconsistent with hypertension being associated with an elevated renal cadmium.

The limited autopsy data just cited, suggesting a relationship between renal cadmium concentration and human hyperten-

TABLE 1. Renal Cadmium as a Function of Blood Pressure*

	Patients	$\mu g/g$ Tissue Mean	$\mu g/10$ mg Ash Median	Mean	Significance and Author
Hypertensive	17		37	42	$p < 0.005$
Normotensive	117		29	29	Schroeder – U.S.
Hypertensive	17		49	51	$p < 0.025$
Normotensive	23		27	32	Schroeder – foreign
Hypertensive	12		27	25	Not significant
Normotensive	25		22	25	Morgan – Alabama
Hypertensive	12	36			Significant
Normotensive	10	27			Lener

*Values for renal cadmium in hypertensive and normotensive subjects. Note: To make the values for ash and wet weight roughly comparable, the values for the latter are expressed in the unusual units of μg Cd/10 mg ash. (Tipton's figures indicate that mean renal ash weight is 1.1% of wet weight.[47])

sion, should logically be extended by studying renal cadmium in much larger numbers of hypertensive and normotensive subjects. It is difficult, however, to measure either the renal or the total body burden of cadmium in living patients because of its very long biologic half life resulting from essentially permanent trapping by metallothionein. Moreover, the absolute renal burden of cadmium may not be the critical factor. Rather, the cadmium burden relative to that of substances like zinc or selenium may be important.

Blood Cadmium and Blood Pressure

There is little to suggest that the body burden of cadmium is reflected by the cadmium concentration, either in whole blood or in any circulating compartment. Perhaps, with appropriate standardization, the body burden will be found to bear some relation to cadmium concentration in erythrocytes, since in animals that compartment is correlated with long-term exposure.[30] Circulating extracellular cadmium, on the other hand, seems to be more closely related to recent absorption.[31,32] It should be both simple and important to determine whether there is a correlation between levels of circulating cadmium and human blood pressure; however, only the most preliminary data are available. Thind observed a higher mean level of plasma cadmium in ten patients with essential hypertension $(0.30\pm0.28\mu g/100$ ml$)$ than in 15 normal subjects $(0.20\pm0.06\mu g/100$ ml$)$; however, his groups were not only very small but they also differed in other things besides blood pressure.[33] In contrast, Mertz et al, while studying renal excretion of cadmium, found no significant difference in the serum cadmium levels of six normal subjects and 12 hypertensive patients, most of whom had renal disease.[34] Wester also found no significant difference in the serum cadmium levels of 16 hypertensive patients when he compared them to eight normotensive subjects.[35]

Urine Cadmium and Blood Pressure

With respect to a possible relationship between urinary cadmium and body burden, Friberg's early experiments with rabbits suggested that very little cadmium appeared in the urine

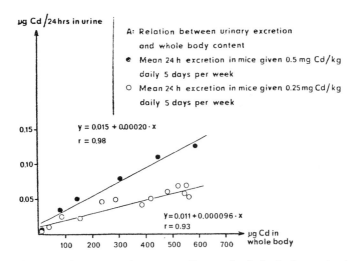

Fig. 2. Relation between urinary excretion and whole body content of cadmium in mice given daily injections of radio cadmium at one of two dosage levels: 0.25 or 0.5 mg Cd/kg. (From Nordberg.[36])

until a toxic level had accumulated in the kidney. Then both protein and cadmium suddenly appeared in relatively large amounts.[30] Recently, however, working with mice and apparently more sensitive techniques, the same group reported that urinary cadmium did reflect body burden before any evidence of renal failure occurred. Their data show a good correlation between the daily excretion of cadmium in urine and the body burden of cadmium for animals receiving a constant daily dose (Fig. 2); however, the level of excretion depended upon daily dose as well as body burden.[36]

Until recently the low levels of urinary cadmium in man (about $2\mu g/day$)[37] were thought to be unrelated to body burden.[38] Recent data, however, suggest that in Japan urinary excretion of cadmium follows a definite pattern increasing with age to a maximum at about 35 years and then decreasing slightly (Fig. 3).[39] Although nothing is known about the actual body burden of these subjects, the curve of Figure 3 is reminiscent of Schroeder's curve for renal cadmium concentration in Americans as a function of age.[25] Despite these Japanese data which raise the question of a relationship between excretion and body burden, no evidence has been

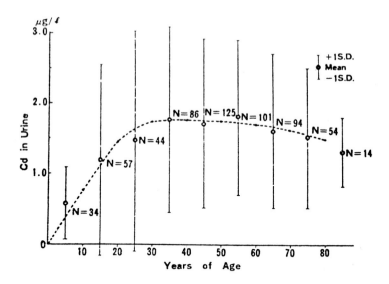

Fig. 3. Average cadmium concentration in urine within different age groups in Tokyo. (From Tsuchiya, Seki and Sugita.[39])

advanced for a relationship between body burden and urinary cadmium in exposed workers without proteinuria.[40]

There are no convincing data clearly demonstrating a relationship between urinary cadmium and human essential hypertension, or one of the recognized secondary types of hypertension; however, some interesting observations have been made, both in the mid-50s and more recently. A comparison of the trace metal content in the urines of 15 patients with severe hypertension (most had malignant stages) and 15 normotensive subjects revealed generally similar concentrations of ten trace metals and markedly different concentrations of the 11th, cadmium. For the "hypertensives," the cadmium concentration averaged 50 parts per billion (ppb) versus less than 1 ppb for the "normals." Moreover, when therapy had controlled the blood pressure and halted the rapidly progressive renal dysfunction, eight of the hypertensive patients were retested, and the average urinary cadmium had diminished from 50 to 5 ppb.[41] These data are difficult to interpret in view of the rapid renal destruction that accompanies severe and particularly "malignant" hypertension, but it seems likely that in conjunction with the marked proteinuria and rapidly decreasing renal mass, the hypertensive patients were also rapidly losing a lifetime's accumulation of renal cadmium, hence the very high urinary cadmium levels.

In 1969, Szadkowski and co-workers failed to find a significant relationship between urinary cadmium and blood pressure in 105 men and 64 women. These investigators studied a relatively large group of subjects, including some with high blood pressure. Unfortunately, no data are given except the mean and standard deviation for blood pressure (137 ± 30/83 ± 16 mm Hg) and for urinary cadmium (1.25 ± 1.02μg of cadmium/gm of creatinine).[42] It is difficult to know how many subjects had meaningful and persistent hypertension.

In contrast, in 1972 Mertz and co-workers reported that hypertensive subjects tended to excrete more urinary cadmium than normotensive individuals. Of 29 subjects examined, six were normotensive and two had essential hypertension, while the remainder had hypertension associated with renal disease of varying severity. Individual serum and urinary cadmium concentrations are tabulated along with data defining renal function, but no blood pressure data are cited.[34] Since the large majority of the subjects of this study had obvious renal disease, most of the data are not relevant to the thesis suggested here, ie, that excess cadmium in an apparently normal kidney may produce hypertension.

A recent study reveals higher concentrations of cadmium, but not zinc, in the urine of 90 hypertensive women from New Zealand when compared with 106 normotensive but otherwise similar women. The mean values were 32μg and 23μg of cadmium per liter of urine for hypertensive and normotensive subjects, respectively. The difference was significant, with $p < 0.02$[43]; however, the results are difficult to interpret because of the abnormally high cadmium excretion in both groups. Another recent study by Wester failed to show any significant differences in the concentrations of 17 trace elements, including cadmium, in the urines of 16 hypertensive and eight normotensive subjects. However, there was a significant increase in the urinary concentrations of five elements, including both cadmium and zinc, following therapy with oral diuretics.[35]

Hypertension in Populations With High Cadmium Exposure

If cadmium is involved in human hypertension, an excess of hypertension might be expected in those with high occupational exposure. Any such excess would, however, be extremely difficult to document. Hypertension has certainly been noted in industrially exposed populations, but available data do not permit a conclusion as to whether the incidence differs from an unexposed but otherwise similar population. As an example of the problem involved, Friberg observed that one third (14 of 43) of the workers exposed to cadmium for more than nine years had systolic pressures of 160 mm Hg or more and that one fifth (9 of 43) had diastolic pressures of 100 mm Hg or more.[44] In an earlier publication apparently involving the same 43 workers, he compared them to 15 somewhat younger patients with cadmium exposures of four years or less. None of the 15 had systolic pressures as high as 150 or diastolic pressures as high as 100 mm Hg.[45] However, this difference in blood pressure is very difficult to interpret because of the small numbers involved and because of the difference in the ages of the two groups. (Their mean ages were 44 and 35 years.) In more general terms, the limiting factor in drawing any conclusions from the blood pressures of exposed workers is the lack of data for comparable subjects without overt exposure.

The absence of hypertension in subjects with chronic cadmium poisoning and associated renal failure or in Japanese with advanced "itai-itai" disease is cited as strong evidence against cadmium being involved in human hypertension. This argument is not entirely convincing. Exposure of animals to excessive cadmium produces toxicity, but not hypertension; however, there is a critical intermediate range of exposure which is associated with elevated blood pressure, but no other recognizable effect.[4] Moreover, at the time of death chronic cadmium poisoning of man, including "itai-itai" disease, is characterized by markedly shrunken, "end stage" kidneys with abnormally low rather than high cadmium concentrations. It is not really surprising that shrunken kidneys, composed largely of scar tissue, should have lost most of whatever parenchymatous cadmium they once contained. Likewise, any hypertension associated with an earlier heavy burden of cadmium might be expected to have "burned out."

However, if cadmium is involved in human hypertension, one might reasonably expect that subjects *without* clinical cadmium toxicity, but living in cadmium-polluted areas and hence having unusually high cadmium exposures, should show an excess of hypertension. The critical blood pressure data for such populations are not readily available, but very preliminary observations of areas around alkaline accumulator factories in Scandinavia or of areas adjacent to the "itai-itai" regions of Japan do not suggest any great increase in hypertension.

Treatment of Hypertension by Removing Cadmium

If human essential hypertension is related to an absolute excess of renal cadmium or to an excess of renal cadmium with respect to zinc or some other substances, it might be theoretically possible to lower blood pressure by removing cadmium. Few available chelating agents, however, have a significantly greater affinity for cadmium than for zinc; hence they could not be expected to remove cadmium differentially. Na_2 ZnCDTA (the zinc chelate of disodium 1,2-cyclohexylene-dinitrilotetraacetate hydrous) which has been available on an experimental basis (Cooper Laboratories), has 100 times the affinity for cadmium that it has for zinc. Schroeder reported that this compound lowered cadmium-induced hypertension in rats.[7]

We have given the chelate to nine hypertensive patients and observed some possible antihypertensive effect; but the results are far too meager and equivocal to provide evidence for cadmium involvement in hypertension; at best they can be thought of as consistent with the possibility. In these very preliminary studies, the subjects were kept on a hospital research ward for 5 to 15 days until their diastolic pressures were relatively stable. (The mean pretreatment diastolic pressure was 122 with a standard deviation of 7.8 mm Hg.) During the next 5 to 15 days, parenteral chelate was administered, and the mean diastolic pressure fell 3 to 17 mm Hg. (The average fall for the nine patients was 11 mm Hg.) The total chelate administered per subject ranged from 2.88 gm to 19.44 gm each gram of which has the potential to bind 0.24 gm of cadmium. The apparent change in pressure persisted relatively briefly. The effect began to disappear a few days after the last dose of chelate and within two to four weeks, the pressures had reverted to approximately their preinjection values.

Summary

There are data which raise the question of whether cadmium might be involved in human hypertension. It must be emphasized that they are far from conclusive. They can be summarized as follows:

1. Chronic low-level cadmium ingestion can induce hypertension in rats without any other obvious effects. Moreover, the renal cadmium levels of such chronically cadmium-fed rats are comparable to those of the average adult American without any unusual cadmium exposure.
2. A considerable series of reports has indicated that soft water is statistically associated with an increase in the total cardiovascular death rate. Preliminary observations suggest that one population exposed to soft water had an average of twice as much bone cadmium as its matched "hard water" population, raising the possibility that cadmium-induced hypertension could explain some or all of the excess mortality associated with soft water.
3. Limited studies suggest that hypertensive subjects have higher renal cadmium concentrations than do normotensive subjects dying sudden accidental deaths. An element of uncertainty is introduced by the wide variability of renal cadmium concentrations in apparently unexposed populations from different geographic areas.
4. There are some data suggesting that hypertensive patients have higher levels of urinary cadmium than do normotensives; however, there are no adequate data for patients without malignant hypertension and rapidly progressing renal dysfunction. Moreover, even a clearcut finding of abnormally high urinary cadmium levels in hypertensive patients would be difficult to interpret.
5. Very limited data involving clinically normal subjects from areas of high cadmium pollution adjacent to accumulator factories in Sweden or to the "itai-itai"

regions in Japan show little evidence of excess hypertension. Even more limited preliminary data suggest that a cadmium-binding chelate may lower elevated human blood pressure. The same compound has been reported to control cadmium-induced hypertension in rats.

References

1. Perry, H. M., Jr.: A Review of Hypertension Induced in Animals by Chronic Ingestion of Cadmium. Nutrition Foundation. (In press.)
2. Perry, H. M., Jr. and Yunice, A.: Acute pressor effects of intra-arterial cadmium and mercuric ions in anesthetized rats. *Proc. Soc. Exp. Biol. Med.*, 120:805, 1965.
3. Schroeder, H. A. and Vinton, W. H., Jr.: Hypertension induced in rats by small doses of cadmium. *Amer. J. Physiol.*, 202:515, 1962.
4. Perry, H. M., Jr. and Erlanger, M. W.: Metal-induced hypertension following chronic feeding of low doses of cadmium and mercury. *J. Lab. Clin. Med.*, 83:541, 1974.
5. Sorenson, J. R. J., Sastry, S., Kober, T. E. et al: Cadmium-induced hypertension in male Sprague-Dawley rats. Ann. Report of Center for Study of Human Environment March 31, 1973, Department of Environmental Health, College of Medicine, University of Cincinnati, Ohio, (preliminary report), pp 93-96.
6. Schroeder, H. A., Kroll, B. A., Little, J. W. et al: Hypertension in rats from injection of cadmium. *Arch. Environ. Health*, 13:788, 1966.
7. Schroeder, H. A. and Buckman, J. B.: Cadmium hypertension: Its reversal in rats by a zinc chelate. *Arch. Environ. Health*, 14:693, 1967.
8. Perry, H. M., Jr. and Erlanger, M. W.: Prevention of cadmium-induced hypertension by selenium. *Fed. Proc.*, 33:357, 1974.
9. Perry, H. M., Jr., Erlanger, M. W. and Perry, E. F.: Reversal of cadmium-induced hypertension by selenium or hard water. 8th Annual Conference on Trace Substances in Environmental Health, Columbia, Missouri, 1974.
10. Kobayashi, J.: Geographical relationship between chemical nature of river water and death rate from apoplexy. *Benchte Ohara Inst. Landivertsch Biologie*, 11:12, 1957.
11. Schroeder, H. A.: Relation between mortality from cardiovascular disease and treated water supplies. *JAMA*, 172:1902, 1960.
12. Morris, J. N., Crawford, M. D. and Heady, J. R.: Hardness of local water supplies and mortality from cardiovascular disease. *Lancet*, 1:860, 1961.
13. Biersteker, K.: Hardness of drinking water and mortality. *T. Soc. Geneesk.*, 45:658, 1967.
14. Bjorck, G., Bostrom, H. and Eistron, A.: On the relationship between water hardness and death rate in cardiovascular diseases. *Acta Med. Scand.*, 178:239, 1965.

15. Bostrom, H. and Wester, P. O.: Trace elements in drinking water and death rate in cardiovascular disease. *Acta Med. Scand.*, 181:465, 1967.
16. Masironi, R.: Cardiovascular mortality in relation to radioactivity and hardness of local water supplies in the USA. *Bull. WHO*, 43:687, 1970.
17. Muss, D. L.: Relationship between water quality and deaths from cardiovascular disease. *J. Amer. Water Works Ass.*, 54:1371, 1962.
18. Robertson, J. S.: Mortality and hardness of water. *Lancet*, 2:348, 1968.
19. Lindeman, R. D. and Assenzo, J. R.: Correlations between water hardness and cardiovascular deaths in Oklahoma Counties. *Amer. J. Public Health*, 54:1071, 1964.
20. Mulcahy, R.: The influence of water hardness and rainfall on the incidence of cardiovascular and cerebrovascular mortality in Ireland. *J. Irish Med. Ass.*, 55:17, 1964.
21. Osancova, K. and Hejda, S. in Hartog, D. et al (eds.): *Dietary Studies and Epidemiology of Heart Diseases.* Stichting tot Wetenschappelijka Voorlichting op Voedingsbied. The Hague, 1968.
22. Crawford, T. and Crawford, M. D.: Prevalence and pathological changes of ischemic heart-disease in a hard-water and in a soft-water area. *Lancet*, 1:229, 1967.
23. Crawford, M. D.: Personal communication.
24. Perry, H. M., Jr., Tipton, I. H., Schroeder, H. A. et al: Variation in the concentration of cadmium in human kidney as a function of age and geographic origin. *J. Chronic Dis.*, 14:259, 1961.
25. Schroeder, H. A. and Balassa, J. J.: Abnormal trace metals in man: Cadmium. *J. Chronic Dis.*, 14:236, 1961.
26. Perry, H. M., Jr., Tipton, I. H., Schroeder, H. A. et al: Variability in the metal content of human organs. *J. Lab. Clin. Med.*, 60:245, 1962.
27. Schroeder, H. A.: Cadmium as a factor in hypertension. *J. Chronic Dis.*, 18:647, 1965.
28. Lener, J. and Bibr, B.: Cadmium and hypertension. *Lancet*, 1:970, 1971.
29. Morgan, J. M.: Tissue cadmium concentration in man. *Arch. Intern. Med.*, 123:405, 1969.
30. Friberg, L.: Further investigations on chronic cadmium poisoning. A study on rabbits with radioactive cadmium. *Arch. Ind. Hyg. Occup. Med.*, 5:30, 1952.
31. Eybl, V., Sykora, J. and Mertl, F.: Wirkung von Ca ADTA und Ca DTPA bei der Kadmiumvergiftung. *Acta Biol. Med. German*, 17:178, 1966.
32. Lucis, O. J., Lynk, M. E. and Lucis, R.: Turnover of cadmium 109 in rats. *Arch. Environ. Health*, 18:307, 1969.
33. Thind, G. S.: Role of cadmium in human and experimental hypertension. *J. Air Pollut. Contr. Ass.*, 22:267, 1972.
34. Mertz, D. P., Koschnik, R. and Wilk, G.: Renal Aussheidungsbedingunge von Cadmium beim normotensiven und hypertensiven Menschen. *Z. Klin. Chem. u Khn Biochem.*, 10:21, 1972.

35. Wester, P. O.: Trace elements in serum and urine from hypertensive patients before and after treatment with chlorthalidone. *Acta Med. Scand.*, 194:505, 1973.
36. Nordberg, G. F.: Cadmium metabolism and toxicity. *Environ. Physiol. Biochem.*, 2:7, 1972.
37. Friberg, L., Piscator, M., Nordberg, G. F. et al: *Cadmium in the Environment*, ed. 2. CRC Press, Inc., 1974, pp. 66 and 67.
38. Piscator, M.: Cadmium Toxicity — Industrial and Environmental Experience. In Proceedings of the 17th International Congress on Occupational Health, to be published, 1974.
39. Tsuchiya, K., Seki, Y. and Sugita, M.: Biologic Threshold Limits of Lead and Cadmium, Proceedings of the 17th International Congress on Occupational Health, to be published, 1974.
40. Friberg, L., Piscator, M., Nordberg, G. F. et al: *Cadmium in the Environment*, ed 2. CRC Press, Inc., 1974, pp. 65-72.
41. Schroeder, H. A. and Perry, H. M., Jr.: Essential and abnormal trace metals in cardiovascular diseases. *Proceedings of the Annual Meeting, Council for High Blood Pressure Res.*, 4:71, 1956.
42. Szadkowski, D., Schaller, K. H. and Lehnert, G.: Renal Cadmiumaus Sheiduno, Lebensalter und Arterieller Blutdruck. *Arch. Klin. Chem.*, 7:551, 1969.
43. McKenzie, J. M. and Kay, D. L.: Urinary excretion of cadmium, zinc and copper in normotensive and hypertensive women. World Health Organization, April 1973.
44. Friberg, L. and Mystrom, A.: Synpunkter pa den kroniska kadmium forgettningens prognos. *Svensk. Lakartidn.*, 49:43, 1952.
45. Friberg, L.: Health hazards in the manufacture of alkaline accumulators with special reference to chronic cadmium poisoning. *Acta Med. Scand.*, 138: (suppl. 240): 124, 1950.
46. Tipton, I. H.: In Seven, M. D. (ed.): *The Distribution of Trace Metals in the Human Body, Metal-Binding in Medicine*. Philadelphia, Pa.: Lippincott, 1960, p. 27.
47. Perry, H. M., Jr.: Minerals in cardiovascular disease. *J. Amer. Diet. Ass.*, 62:631-636, 1973.

Discussion

Dr. Quintanilla, Illinois: The acute administration of cadmium enhances sodium reabsorption in the kidney. I wonder if this has been explored as a possible mechanism for cadmium-induced hypertension?

Dr. Perry: There are some data which suggest that cadmium chronically fed and inducing hypertension also does cause a retention of sodium, and if I were guessing, I would think this was the most likely mechanism of the hypertension that is induced by cadmium feeding. However, the two speakers who preceded me make me wonder if I can use this as a mechanism.

Dr. Stanley, England: We did get some differences in chromium, the soft-water towns having lower bone chromiums than the hard-water towns. This, perhaps, ties in with Dr. Mertz's work and Dr. Schroeder's speculations on chromium deficiency perhaps being involved in atherosclerotic heart disease. I do not know much about chromium in hypertension. We have done some very preliminary analyses of tissue levels of trace elements, and I think that one must just say that it points out the tremendous difficulties in such analyses. We know so little of trace element metabolism that if we actually look at trace element levels in organs, we do not really know what they mean. There is evidence of heterogeneity within renal tissue. Stein's work has shown that if you take the renal cortex and then the renal medulla, there is a gradient from outer cortex to inner cortex and from outer medulla to inner medulla. If you just take samples from the cortex or medulla, you would not pick up this heterogeneity. Also, the form of the trace element is important as to what actually is active and what exactly in the kidney you might be looking at. It might not be kidney cadmium that is important at all, although it might be coming out in population studies. I cannot sit down without talking about interactions with other trace elements. You mentioned selenium and mercury. I think you cannot look at cadmium without also looking at selenium and mercury because their interactions may lead to a relative deficiency or a relative excess of metal within the body. I do not think you can just talk about total cadmium excess.

Dr. Dollery: I appreciate that when you were presenting the human data about the chelate, you did so with caution. I would reinforce that caution because it seems to me that the blood pressure change could very well be a placebo effect.

Dr. Lawton, Iowa: Dr. Perry, I would like to ask you regarding your current concepts about a possible protective function of zinc and what your current considerations are regarding the use of the cadmium-zinc ratio with relation to hypertension.

Dr. Perry: I cannot answer that question easily. There is no doubt that zinc can influence the hypertension induced by feeding cadmium. In general, one can counteract the effect of cadmium by adding zinc. The two are usually competitive, but the relationship is complex and currently available data are inadequate to make any further definitive statement.

Water Hardness and Hypertension

A. G. Shaper, M.D., D. G. Clayton, M. A.
and Fiona Stanley, M.D.

There is a general, but not universal acceptance that a strong statistical association exists between cardiovascular mortality and the mineral content of drinking water; the softer the drinking water, the higher the death rate.[1-5] This inverse relationship between the hardness of drinking water and cardiovascular death rates has been found in many countries since the initial report from Japan in 1957. There have been studies in which no such relationship has been found, but these have tended to involve small population groups and to cover areas without strong contrasts in the hardness of drinking water. There have also been studies which suggest that soft water increases the risk of death in general, rather than death from cardiovascular causes in particular. It is important to emphasize that between the various countries reporting an association between cardiovascular mortality and water hardness, there have been differences in the specific components of cardiovascular mortality implicated. The purpose of this paper is not to claim that the Water Story is fundamentally a problem of hypertension, but merely to explore the possibility that hypertension may in some way be involved in the problem.

It is of some interest to start at the beginning with the report from Japan by Kobayashi in 1957, in which he examined the geographic relationship between the chemical nature of river water and the death rate from apoplexy.[6] At that time, stroke was the major cause of death in Japan and there were considerable differences in death rates in different parts of

A. G. Shaper, M.D., D. G. Clayton, M.A. *and* Fiona Stanley, M.D., *MRC Social Medicine Unit, London School of Hygiene & Tropical Medicine, London, England.*

Japan. Kobayashi reported that Japanese rivers were characterized by a low level of calcium carbonate, and in some
districts there were rivers containing larger quantities of
sulphate than carbonate, ie, with a high SO_4/CO_3 ratio. The
geographic distribution of death rates from apoplexy was
compared with the distribution of the SO_4/CO_3 ratios and this
suggested a close correlation even within individual prefectures.
He suggested that for some reason, the excess of inorganic acid
induced apoplexy and that calcium carbonate prevented
apoplexy.

Schroeder reexamined Kobayashi's data and found higher
correlations with "all heart disease" than with stroke.[7]
Schroeder went on to examine data from the United States and
found considerable differences in cardiovascular death rates
between the soft-water and hard-water areas. When he subdivided cardiovascular disease into its component parts, the
strongest correlation was for "hypertension with heart disease."
There was also a strong correlation with ischemic heart disease
in white persons aged 55 to 64 years. Hypertension per se and
stroke showed fewer striking relationships to the hardness of
drinking water.[8,9]

More recent work from the United States has compared the
death rate for inhabitants of the basins of two hard-water and
two soft-water rivers, involving some 7.5 million people along
the Ohio and Columbia rivers (soft) and the Missouri and
Colorado rivers (hard). The noncardiovascular death rates were
virtually the same in all four river basins, but death rates from
arteriosclerotic heart disease and hypertensive heart disease
were lower in the hard-water regions.[10]

Studies from England and Wales have reported similar
negative correlations between total cardiovascular death rates
and the hardness of drinking water.[11] The correlations were
greatest with water calcium and with the carbonate fraction
(reflecting temporary hardness); correlations with sodium were
much lower and were negligible with magnesium. Among the
groupings within cardiovascular disease, the correlations were
substantial and highly significant for cerebrovascular deaths and
for those certified (at that time) to "myocardial degeneration."
In coronary heart disease, the correlation was large only in
middle-aged (45-64 years) men, and correlations with death

from hypertensive heart disease or hypertension without heart disease were not significant.[11] However, the rates for hypertensive heart disease and for hypertension without heart disease are much lower than those for the major cardiovascular groupings and, therefore, are not as reliable. In later United Kingdom studies, correlations were significant for cerebrovascular, coronary and "other" heart disease, and no specific comments were made regarding hypertension.[12,13]

It is clear from the American and British studies, as well as from reports from other countries, that there is no clear universal relationship with one particular form of cardiovascular disease. Whatever mechanism is involved must be common to deaths from ischemic heart disease, cerebrovascular disease, hypertensive heart disease and those conditions labeled as "myocardial degeneration." Any one of the major processes in cardiovascular disease could be involved — hypertension, myocardial function, intravascular thrombosis or mural atheroma.

The MRC Social Medicine Unit set up a series of exploratory studies in 12 towns in England and Wales, six with hard water and low cardiovascular death rates and six with soft water and high cardiovascular death rates. They were chosen from the two extremes of the water-calcium and death rate distribution and were matched as far as possible for size and latitude. Several types of studies were mounted in the 12 towns.

1. A study of all *death certificates* for the year 1970, together with additional information from the certifying doctor regarding the terminal episode, previous medical history and length of residence in the towns. This study was concerned with sudden death and its possible contribution to the excess mortality in soft-water towns and also with the possible role of hypertension.

2. *Necropsy material* was obtained from the above cases dying naturally or from accidents for a morbid anatomic study of the myocardium and coronary arteries. We were looking for differences in coronary atherosclerosis and for evidence of hypertension or previous myocardial injury.

3. *Clinical* and biochemical measurements were made in some 500 middle-aged sedentary workers resident in these towns to assess whether there might be differences in blood

pressure levels or other risk factors for cardiovascular disease between hard- and soft-water areas.[14]

The study of all *death certificates* for 1970 for the 12 towns showed that a significantly higher proportion of deaths in the soft towns took place within one hour of the onset of acute symptoms. In male subjects with no previous history of coronary disease, the length of terminal episode was less than one hour in 54% of IHD deaths in soft-water towns compared with 38% in hard-water towns. In those with some history of coronary disease, deaths within one hour comprised 43% of IHD deaths in soft-water towns and 33% in hard-water towns. These differences were significant and when both groups were combined, the percentages of sudden deaths in the six soft-water towns were consistently higher than those obtained in the six hard-water towns (Table 1, Fig. 1).

Prospective studies have shown that a raised blood pressure is one of the risk factors associated with sudden death from ischemic heart disease.[15] We have examined the data for a diagnosis of hypertension either as a cause of death, as contributing to death or as mentioned by the general practitioner or other doctor. Since the number of cases is limited and the reporting of hypertension on death certificates and on the questionnaires completed by the doctors is probably inadequate, not too much reliance should be placed on these findings, but they are of some interest. In both males and females over 55, the proportion of IHD deaths in which hypertension is mentioned, either in the death certificates or in subsequent inquiries, is substantially higher in the soft-water towns (Table 2).

TABLE 1. 12 Towns Death Certification Study.
Percentage of IHD Deaths Under One Hour
in Males 30-59 Years (1970)

| | 6 Soft-Water Towns | | 6 Hard-Water Towns | |
	IHD Deaths*	% Sudden	IHD Deaths	% Sudden
No history of IHD	205	54	144	38
Some history of IHD	170	43	141	33

*Excluding a few deaths where no information concerning terminal episode was available.

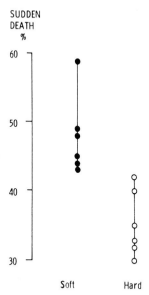

Fig. 1. Sudden death (< 1 hour) as a percentage of IHD deaths in males 30-59 in six soft-water and six hard-water towns.

In the study of *necropsy material* obtained from cases dying naturally or from accidents, the findings in the two groups of towns were very similar as regards coronary artery disease and hypertension as determined by heart weight, ventricular thickness and renal vascular pathology.

Clinical study. There were no significant differences between the soft-water and hard-water town men in age distribution, in mean height or weight; the mean subscapular skinfold thickness was greater in the soft-water towns, but no

TABLE 2. 12 Towns Study. Diagnosis of Hypertension as
a Cause of Death, Contributing to Death or Mentioned
by Doctor on Subsequent Inquiry

| | 6 Soft-Water Towns | | 6 Hard-Water Towns | |
	IHD Deaths	% Hypertension	IHD Deaths	% Hypertension
Males > 55 years	170	38	139	27
Females > 55 years	51	83	25	56

TABLE 3. 12 Towns Study. Clinical Findings
in Men Aged 40-65 Years

	6 Soft-Water Towns		6 Hard-Water Towns
No. of men examined	245		244
Heart rate (per min)	77.8	$p < 0.01$	74.0
Plasma-cholesterol (mg/100 ml)	245.0	$p < 0.05$	237.0
Systolic BP (mm Hg)	139.0		136.9
Diastolic BP (mm Hg)	87.5	$p < 0.01$	84.7
Systolic BP > 180 mm Hg	4.9%		2.1%
> 160 mm Hg	13.9%		10.9%
Diastolic BP > 110 mm Hg	4.1%		1.7%
> 100 mm Hg	11.9%		7.9%

difference was observed for the triceps or suprailiac measurements. Smoking habits were similar in the two groups of towns. There was a significant difference in the *heart rate* as calculated from the ECG records, with a higher heart rate in soft-water groups. This was surprisingly consistent between the towns, the one exception being the town with the smallest number of men in the study. Plasma cholesterol concentrations were higher in the soft-water group, but this finding was not very consistent between the groups (Table 3).

Mean blood pressures were higher in the soft-water group, the most significant difference being in casual diastolic pressure. The findings were again surprisingly consistent between the two groups of towns; the one soft-water town with the lower blood pressure than the other soft-water towns happened to be one with a high cigarette smoking rate, and this may be of some significance. The distributions of casual diastolic blood pressure showed differences at all levels between hard- and soft-water towns. Differences in systolic pressure were predominantly limited to the upper extremes of the distributions. There was an interesting difference between the hard- and soft-water towns in the relation between age and blood pressure. There was little or no difference between the two groups at ages 40-50, but quite pronounced differences at ages 55-64. The increase in mean blood pressure with age was less pronounced in the hard-water group; indeed, the mean diastolic blood pressure did not increase with age in this group (Fig. 2).

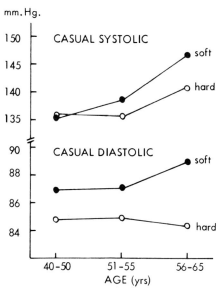

Fig. 2. 12 Towns Study. Mean blood pressure by age in men 40-65 in soft-water and hard-water towns.

In both hard- and soft-water towns there was a fair degree of correlation between systolic blood pressure and heart rate in men less than 50 years of age ($r \cong 0.4$). In older men, the correlation was less marked in the hard-water towns and completely disappeared in the soft-water towns (Table 4).

The difference of 2.8 mm Hg in mean casual diastolic pressure between hard- and soft-water towns, although statistically significant at the 1% level, may seem irrelevant to the clinically orientated. We would remind you that even small

TABLE 4. 12 Towns Study. Correlations between
Systolic Blood Pressure and Heart Rate.
(Number of Men in Brackets)

	6 Soft-Water Towns	6 Hard-Water Towns
Men < 50 years	0.38	0.43
	(103)	(97)
Men > 50 years	0.05	0.29
	(116)	(124)

differences in mean levels may reflect quite large differences in the percentage of the population at the extremes of the distribution. The percentage of subjects with casual systolic pressure over 180 mm Hg may appear small and not worthy of attention: 2% in the hard-water towns and 5% in the soft-water towns in men aged 40-65. If one applies these percentages to the male population of England and Wales, it means the difference between dealing with 140,000 hypertensive subjects or 360,000 hypertensive subjects. For diastolic blood pressure >110 mm Hg, the figures would be 140,000 and 290,000.

It must be emphasized that this was an exploratory pilot study involving small numbers and that confirmation of these findings must be sought in larger and different studies.

No significant differences were found in 12-hour urine samples between residents of the two groups of towns in terms of their bulk biochemical constituents. The variance of these measurements was very large and a study of this size could have detected only very marked differences. It is of interest that another urinary excretion study, based on single specimens of urine, has shown different results.[16] This study covered a hard-water town (London) and four soft-water towns (including single urine specimens provided by our subjects in three of our six soft-water towns). The amounts of calcium, magnesium and potassium excreted in the hard- and soft-water areas were not significantly different, but the sodium excretion was significantly higher in the soft-water areas. As the main source of sodium is dietary salt, the authors suggest that this is the source of the higher sodium excreted in the soft-water towns. Commenting on this study, Langford and Watson[17] emphasize that random urine samples do not truly reflect the usual excretion of electrolytes. Based on their own studies, they suggest that the combination of a low calcium intake and a high sodium intake may represent a hypertensinogenic situation.[18] It would be of considerable interest to determine whether higher sodium intakes are characteristic of soft-water areas.

In the serum, there were no significant differences in concentration of the major electrolytes (sodium, potassium, calcium and magnesium). There was, however, a significant difference in albumin concentration, the men in the hard-water towns having more albumin in their serum ($p < 0.01$). This difference was very small, amounting to only about a 2% increase, but was extremely consistent. There was a less consistent difference in phosphate concentrations, again higher in the hard-water towns (p < 0.05).

We can venture no explanation for these findings. In an attempt to determine whether there was a relationship between the serum biochemistry differences and the blood pressure differences, a multiple regression analysis was carried out. Serum albumin and serum phosphate concentrations were both associated with blood pressure, particularly with systolic blood pressure. The association of blood pressure with albumin was *positive*, the association with phosphate was *negative* and both achieved a high level of statistical significance (p < 0.01 in each group of towns). However, it does not seem likely that the biochemical differences explain the difference in blood pressure. In fact, if anything, these relationships would predict a difference in blood pressure in the reverse direction, ie, higher blood pressures in the hard-water towns.

Conclusion

There would appear to be some circumstantial evidence to suggest that hypertension plays a role in the regional variation in cardiovascular mortality in the United Kingdom. There is certainly enough evidence to warrant the further examination of the relationship between water hardness and hypertension in the United Kingdom, with an emphasis on longitudinal and prospective community studies.

References

1. Masironi, R.: Trace elements in cardiovascular disease. *Bull. WHO*, 40:305-312, 1969.
2. Crawford, M. D., Gardner, M. J. and Morris, J. N.: Cardiovascular disease and the mineral content of drinking water. *Brit. Med. Bull.*, 27:21-24, 1971.
3. Crawford, M. D.: Hardness of drinking water and cardiovascular disease. *Proc. Nutr. Soc.*, 31:347-353, 1972.
4. Masironi, R., Miesch, A. T., Crawford, M. D. et al: Geochemical environments, trace elements and cardiovascular disease. *Bull. WHO*, 47:139-150, 1972.
5. Neri, L. C., Hewitt, D. and Schreiber, G. B.: Can epidemiology elucidate the water story? *Amer. Epidem.*, 99:75-88, 1974.

6. Kobayashi, J.: On geographic relationship between the chemical nature of river water and death rate from apoplexy (preliminary report). *Berichte des Ohara Instituts fur Landwirtschaftliche Biologie*, 11:12-21, 1957.

7. Schroeder, H. A.: Degenerative cardiovascular disease in the Orient. II. Hypertension. *J. Chronic Dis.*, 8:312-333, 1958.

8. Schroeder, H. A.: Relationship between mortality from cardiovascular disease and treated water supplies: Variations in states and 163 largest municipalities of the United States. *JAMA*, 172:1902-1908, 1960.

9. Schroeder, H. A.: Relations between hardness of water and death rates from certain chronic and degenerative diseases in the United States. *J. Chronic Dis.*, 12:586-591, 1960.

10. Masironi, R.: Cardiovascular mortality in relation to radioactivity and hardness of local water supplies in the U.S.A. *Bull. WHO*, 43:687-697, 1970.

11. Morris, J. N., Crawford, M. D. and Heady, J. A.: Hardness of local water supplies and mortality from cardiovascular disease in the county boroughs of England and Wales. *Lancet*, 1:860-862, 1961.

12. Crawford, M. D., Gardner, M. J. and Morris, J. N.: Mortality and hardness of local water supplies. *Lancet*, 1:827-831, 1968.

13. Gardner, M. J. Crawford, M. D. and Morris, J. N.: Patterns of mortality in middle age and early old age in the county boroughs of England and Wales. *Brit. J. Prev. Soc. Med.*, 23:133-140, 1969.

14. Stitt, F. W., Clayton, D. G., Crawford, M. D. et al: Clinical and biochemical indicators of cardiovascular disease among men living in hard and soft water areas. *Lancet*, 1:122-126, 1973.

15. Kannel, W. B., Dawber, T. R., Kogan, A. et al: Factors of risk in the development of coronary heart disease. Six years follow-up experience. The Framingham Study. *Ann. Intern. Med.* 55:33-50, 1961.

16. Dauncey, M. J. and Widdowson, E. M.: Urinary excretions of calcium, magnesium, sodium and potassium in hard and soft water areas. *Lancet*, 1:711-715, 1972.

17. Langford, H. G. and Watson, R. W.: Urinary excretion of calcium and sodium in hard and soft water areas (correspondence). *Lancet*, 1:1293-1294, 1972.

18. Langford, H. G., Watson, R. L. and Douglas, B. H.: Factors affecting blood pressure in population groups. *Trans. Ass. Amer. Physicians*, 81:135-146, 1968.

Discussion

Dr. Cassel: Let me ask you two questions. In your mind do you think the relationships you are showing between hard water and various risk factors indicate that soft water is somehow responsible for the elevation of risk factors or do you think given the risk factors the softness of the water leads to the excess of CHD? Second, how do you reconcile your findings with George Comstock's when he found in a case control study in Hagerstown no difference between cases and non-cases in terms of the tapwater analysis?

Dr. Shaper: I think that there is very little direct relation between water hardness and the other risk factors. What is of importance now is to find out, let us say using the United Kingdom, whether risk factors function differently in areas differing in water hardness resulting in different morbidity and mortality patterns. Only a prospective study of this kind can really give an answer to that question and this is the hypothesis that we will be exploring. As to Comstock and the case control studies in tapwater, I doubt whether anybody will get an answer out of the water hardness story from that type of an approach. I do not think it can pay off unless it is on a prospective basis and involving fairly large numbers.

Dr. Kagan, Hawaii: I would like a clarification on what you said on how you chose these towns. Did you say that you had chosen these towns simply because they were soft water towns, or because they were soft water towns which had high cardiovascular mortality rates?

Dr. Shaper: This is a frequent criticism of the 12-town study. The statement is made: "So you chose six towns with soft water and high cardiovascular mortality and six towns with hard water and low cardiovascular mortality; what else did you expect to find?" — the supposition being that if you look at areas which differ in their cardiovascular mortality that, ipso facto, they will also differ in every cardiovascular aspect that you can possibly measure. There is no evidence for this. If you have, I will be glad to hear it. I would emphasize that when these 12 towns were originally chosen, they were quite deliberately chosen on the basis that if these 12 towns did not show any differences between hard and soft water in risk factors, then that kind of an approach was not worth pursuing on a larger scale.

Dr. Kass: The question that one might raise is whether hard water and soft water effects might not be limited to those who had had the exposure in the very early stages of life. If, for example, the Comstock population was like most American populations and subject to a great deal of movement, then one would be more concerned with where these people lived for the first year or two of life rather than where they are living now and where their water came from. I wondered along these lines whether your two outlying towns were characterized by a great deal of migrant population change in contrast to the towns that were not so different from the others.

Dr. Shaper: That is an important and interesting question. We have been very concerned with the residence problem and in all the studies that we carried out, we have noted how long people have lived in the area and where they have lived before. The two groups of towns are in areas of very low population mobility. This is true of most of England compared with the United States. In the studies that we are proposing in the next 25 towns, family studies will be included. In terms of duration, how long does a person have to be in a hard or soft water area? There are two or three interesting suggestions. Margaret Crawford and others from our Unit published a paper on changes in cardiovascular mortality following changes in water supply. While she could not put a time period on it, it did seem that in England and Wales, in the very few areas in which the water had become softer the cardiovascular mortality had increased, and in those where it had become harder, mortality had decreased. I believe there is one study in the United States from Florida which suggests that a similar thing can happen over a period of four years with a change in water supply.

Dr. Lovell: I do not know if you skated over this deliberately, but I rather took the point that at the beginning of your statement you said that total mortality was involved here. Is it specifically cardiovascular mortality or changes in other forms of mortality? Could you tell us a little more about the age and sex pattern that is affected by this?

Dr. Shaper: I did skate over it! There are some very good papers that suggest that we are dealing with a general mortality problem and not a specific cardiovascular one. The major burden of the evidence, on the other hand, seems to suggest that there is something that is predominantly cardiovascular. However, in England and Wales correlations for bronchitis are also very high. I think one must not forget this. Although we try to explain them away on socioeconomic and industrialization differences, I am not sure that we can explain them away so easily. There is also a relationship with neonatal abnormalities and stillbirths.

Dr. Sackett: I think perhaps these outlying towns may salvage what might be in the eyes of some of us an unfortunate design of selecting towns that are both soft and deadly. Because you do have some soft water towns with relatively low levels of coronary risk factors, I will be quite interested in how the mortality rates there compare with the other soft water towns with high coronary risk factors. Your sample is not going to be very large, but that may tell you a lot more than looking at the other ten of the 12 communities.

Dr. Shaper: I think this is absolutely key to the future of this kind of work. That there are soft water towns with a low cardiovascular mortality is quite clear. And there are hard water towns with moderate cardiovascular mortality, certainly not low. I think that these particular kinds of towns are almost certainly more important to this kind of study than the others. We have taken this to heart and in the next 25 towns will be particularly examining this problem.

Dr. Miller, Maryland: I do not think it is fair that you should discourage retrospective studies in the area of water hardness. For example, it is quite reasonable that a study could be completed in people who have used hard water for years and now have died. Have you adjusted for fatality rates in your towns?

Dr. Shaper: I think that retrospective studies can make a contribution but nobody is suggesting that the water factor, if it is a cardiovascular risk factor, is the only cardiovascular risk factor or the most important one. It has been suggested that at best it might make a 15% difference in the mortality rates. There is nothing wrong with doing retrospective studies of this kind; I just do not think that they are going to give us an answer to whether there really is a water factor or the nature of that water factor. In terms of adjusting for mortality, the answer is no.

Dr. Tuomilehto, Finland: I gather from your figures that hard water because of high calcium concentration is a big problem in cardiovascular disease. Is there any difference in how people take in calcium?

Dr. Shaper: I do not know that this is a calcium story and the amount of calcium that you get in your drinking water is relatively limited, which makes the possibility that this is strictly a calcium story fairly unlikely. There may be differences in the way you take your calcium. There is no doubt that cooking in hard or soft water can have considerable effects on calcium content of foods. However, I do not think that adding or subtracting calcium, in a simple way, is going to make differences in the cardiovascular mortality rate.

Weight and Hypertension: Evans County Studies of Blacks and Whites

Herman A. Tyroler, M.D., Siegfried Heyden, M.D.
and Curtis G. Hames, M.D.

"That there is a definite correlation between blood pressure and the relation of body weight to height has been found so often as to leave room for no doubt." With these words, Pickering[1] introduced the topic of our presentation. He then cited studies, some of which are now more than 50 years old, confirming the correlation obtained both in the observational mode and following clinical maneuvers designed to lower weight. Since the last international symposium on hypertension ten years ago, there has been an additional large number of confirmations of these findings in community as well as clinical settings and in observational as well as experimental investigations.[2]

Longitudinal observation of cohorts sampled from total, geographically defined residential populations have documented the association of weight with blood pressure in the Framingham,[3,4] Tecumseh,[5] and Rhonda Fach and Vale of Glamorgan[6] studies. Similar conclusions have resulted from the longitudinal studies of male cohorts ascertained and sampled from such institutionally and occupationally defined and diverse populations as steel mill workers,[7] college students,[8] aviators[9] and Israeli civil servants.[10]

Given this plethora of information, it is not our purpose here to test once more, in another population, for the

The work reported here was supported in part by USPHS Grant No. HL 03391 and the NHLI Hypertension Detection and Follow-Up Program.

Herman A. Tyroler, M.D., *Professor, Department of Epidemiology, The School of Public Health, University of North Carolina, Chapel Hill;* Siegfried Heyden, M.D., *Professor, Department of Community Health Sciences, Duke University Medical School, Durham, N.C.;* and Curtis G. Hames, M.D., *General Practitioner — Chairman, Evans County Health Department, Claxton, Ga.*

177

correlation of blood pressure with weight. Rather we shall report on an integrated series of studies performed within one biracial community setting and derive the implications of these studies for blood pressure control programs. The studies were performed in Evans County and include cross-sectional and longitudinal naturalistic observation of a total community, plus a randomized, open trial of the effects of experimental modification of the weight of a representative sample of overweight individuals with high blood pressure drawn from the same population. Finally, the information derived from these studies will be used to estimate the potential for community control of high blood pressure by weight control in a total geographically defined population. The estimation of the potential for community intervention will be undertaken from an epidemiologic perspective, consistent with contemporaneous international interest in screening, detection and management programs for the control of elevated blood pressure in populations.

Methods

The Evans County Cardiovascular Disease Study was initiated with a prevalence survey of all adult residents of this biracial, predominantly rural county, located in the Coastal Plains of Georgia, in the period 1960-1962. Following a private census, 92% of those eligible were examined.[11] Follow-up reexaminations began in 1967, with completion rates of 91% of the survivors of the original cohort.[12] The average period of time between the first and second examination was 87 months. For convenience, this is referred to as a seven-year incidence study.

All studies of the change in a characteristic of a cohort measured at two or more points in time, of logical necessity, are restricted to the subset of individuals who survive and are ascertained for reexamination. The weight and blood pressure of reexamined Evans County residents would be different from the original total cohort if weight and blood pressure were associated with the probability of dying, migrating or not participating in the repeat examination. We have studied this relationship and have found no statistically significant evidence of blood pressure or of weight adjusted for height differences, between migrants out of Evans County and those remaining.[13] The same study, not surprisingly, did disclose consistent and statistically significant higher mean baseline examination blood pressure values within each race/sex group for those who died prior to their scheduled reexamination.

The blood pressure of each subject was measured by one of two examining physicians at the time of the original and repeat surveys. Three readings were taken with the use of mercury sphygmomanometers with cuff widths of 14 cm. First and fifth phase (disappearance) of Korotkoff sounds were employed to designate systolic and diastolic pressures. The first reading was performed at the first examination after completion of a standardized history; at the follow-up survey examination, the first reading was taken at time of arrival at clinic. In each instance, the left arm was used with the subject sitting and the first of the three readings taken was used for the present analyses. Efforts to maximize interobserver comparability and to adjust for noted instrument differences are reported elsewhere.[14]

All subjects had height and weight measured without shoes and with light clothing on. The Quetelet Index was calculated as weight (pounds)/height^2 (inches) $\times$ 100. The Quetelet Index was chosen as a body mass index from a large series including weight/height and the Ponderal Index, based on a review of population weight for height indices[15] as being least correlated with height and most correlated with independent measures of obesity, although others have argued that the most valid index of obesity should be sex, population specific in its use of power functions of height and weight, and that all are far from highly correlated with obesity.[16] Sex specific, age standardized scores were constructed by subtracting the mean for the appropriate five year age/sex specific value from each subject's observed Quetelet Index and dividing by the standard deviation for that group .

$$z = \frac{\text{Observed}_{QI} - \text{Age Sex Specific Mean}_{QI}}{\text{Age Sex Specific SD}_{QI}}$$

The association between weight characteristics as risk factors and the incidence of elevated blood pressure was measured by calculating the percentage of the disease (in the entire population) attributable to exposure to the risk factor.[17] This association is equivalent to the percent reduction in cases which would have occurred if groups of individuals in Evans County, who were either overweight or gained weight, had had the incidence rate of those who were not overweight or had not gained weight. As discussed and derived by Leviton,[17] this statistic has been variously referred to as attributable risk. Others have termed it population attributable risk proportion. It is a function of (1) the ratio of the incidence of high blood pressure in individuals with and without the weight characteristics (eg, being overweight) — ie, the relative risk — and (2) the prevalence of the weight characteristic in the population.

$$\text{Pop AR \%} = \frac{b\ (R-1)}{b\ (R-1) + 1} \times 100$$

where Pop AR % = population attributable risk percent

b = proportion of population with weight characteristic (eg, overweight)

R = relative risk (eg, incidence of DBP $\geq$ 95 in initially normotensives with DBP $<$ 90 who were overweight at intake/the incidence of DBP $\geq$ 95 in initially normotensives with DBP $<$ 90 who were not overweight at intake)

The population attributable risk percent is treated as a statistical population measure of association and as equivalent to the potential for percent reduction in new cases of high diastolic blood pressure. It was computed in relation to weight at intake and weight gain for the two race groups and for all residents age 35-59 in Evans County in 1960.

Results and Discussion

Correlation and Regression Analyses

Despite earlier controversy, there is no longer doubt that blood pressure is continuously distributed in populations, without any natural breakpoints and without evidence of any clear critical levels below which individuals are protected from, and above which they are at risk of, vascular sequelae of elevated blood pressure. Similar statements can be made for the distribution and consequences of weight measures adjusted for height. Given these properties, the association between the two is most appropriately represented by correlation analysis. The correlation coefficient between diastolic blood pressure and Quetelet Index in Evans County residents age 35-59 in 1960 was 0.26, a value not dissimilar to that reported in other population-based studies, such as Tecumseh.[18] It is also possible to represent this relationship as though fixed weight for height levels had been assigned and the blood pressure observed. In this regression mode of analysis, there is, in the Evans County data, evidence of differences between the white and black population (Table 1 and Fig. 1). The change in blood pressure per unit change of the age standardized Quetelet Index (ie, the regression coefficient) is greater for white than it is for black examinees. The average blood pressure is considerably higher in the black than in the white population at all weight levels; however, because of the stronger association of blood pressure with weight in whites, the difference in blood pressure between the two races is decreased among the more overweight individuals and, conversely, is exaggerated among individuals who are leaner. We shall return later to the implications of these findings for community intervention studies. At this point we note only that a weaker relationship between blood pressure and weight in the black (particularly in black males) than in the white population was also observed in the Charleston cardio-vascular disease survey.[19]

The relationship between change of weight and change of diastolic blood pressure in the period from 1960 to 1967 is set out in Table 1 and in Figure 2. Change in blood pressure over time is associated with change in weight. The correlation coefficient for change of diastolic blood pressure with change of weight for all race/sex groups combined was 0.22 and there was no clear evidence of major differences among the race/sex groups. The average change of blood pressure per pound change of weight was of relatively small magnitude (0.2 mm), indicating an average increment or decrement of only 4 mm Hg for a concomitant weight change of 20 pounds.

TABLE 1. Regression and Correlation Analysis of Diastolic Blood Pressure
and Weight Relationships by Race and Sex
Evans County Residents Age 35-59

Cross Sectional Study, 1960. Diastolic Blood Pressure 1960.
As a Function of Age Standardized Sex Specific Quetelet Index, 1960

	WM	WF	BM	BF	All
Regression Coefficient	4.48	5.38	2.01	3.02	4.34
Constant Term	89.12	89.90	100.40	99.60	93.13
Correlation Coefficient	0.32	0.35	0.11	0.18	0.26

Longitudinal Study, 1960-1967
Change in Diastolic Blood Pressure As a Function of Weight Change

	WM	WF	BM	BF	All
Regression Coefficient	0.15	0.25	0.20	0.17	0.20
Constant Term	0.25	1.16	-2.41	-0.86	-0.07
Correlation Coefficient	0.16	0.29	0.19	0.20	0.22

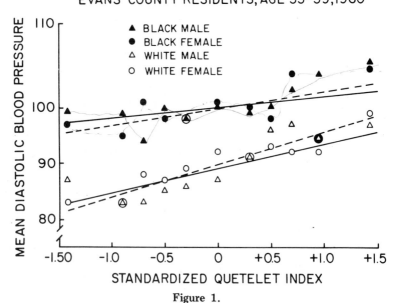

Figure 1.

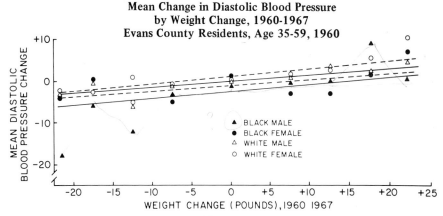

Mean Change in Diastolic Blood Pressure
by Weight Change, 1960-1967
Evans County Residents, Age 35-59, 1960

▲ BLACK MALE
● BLACK FEMALE
△ WHITE MALE
○ WHITE FEMALE

Figure 2.

In principle, it is possible to regard all individuals of a population as target subjects for an intervention effort. With this population perspective, one can attempt to manipulate the total distribution of weight at a point in time and also modify the distribution of weight change over time. Assuming both the feasibility of this effort and a causal relation between weight and blood pressure change, we could simulate weight change and then estimate the potential change in the total population distribution of blood pressure. Epidemiologically attractive as this approach is in principle, focusing as it does on a total population approach, it is beyond the realm of most current applications of our intervention technology. Although there are several innovative approaches under test at present directed toward total communities utilizing the mass media and techniques such as information diffusion and group educational processes, most current intervention programs involve a categorical approach to hypertension as a disease entity and a limited identification of either high-risk persons for preventive purposes or the identification of patients for therapeutic maneuvers. Accordingly, the remainder of our analyses and our estimations of potential community impact are based upon this categorical approach.

Remission Rates of High Blood Pressure

The relationship between blood pressure and weight changes from 1960 to 1967 among all Evans County examinees of both sexes with high diastolic pressure in 1960 is set out in Table 2

TABLE 2. Percent Remission Rate of High Diastolic Blood
Pressure (≥ 95 mm Hg) to Normal (< 90 mm Hg) in Relation to
Weight Change from 1960 to 1967 by Race and Level of 1960
Diastolic Blood Pressure

			White		
			1960-1967 Weight Change		
			Loss < 9		
	No. of	Gain	Through	Loss	All Weight
1960 DBP	Examinees	≥ 10 lbs.	Gain < 9	≤ 10 lbs.	Change
95-99	74	19.0	37.8	43.8	33.8
100-104	73	5.0	17.1	22.2	15.1
≥ 105	103	5.3	8.2	11.4	8.7
≥ 95	250	10.0	19.8	21.7	18.0

TABLE 3. Percent Remission Rate of High Diastolic Blood
Pressure (≥ 95 mm Hg) to Normal (< 90 mm Hg) in Relation to
Weight Change from 1960 to 1967 by Race and Level of 1960
Diastolic Blood Pressure

			Black		
			1960-1967 Weight Change		
			Loss < 9		
	No. of	Gain	Through	Loss	All Weight
1960 DBP	Examinees	≥ 10 lbs.	Gain < 9	≥ 10 lbs.	Change
95-99	58	20.0	25.8	17.6	22.4
100-104	72	0.0	22.2	7.7	13.9
≥ 105	166	4.7	8.0	12.5	8.4
≥ 95	296	6.3	15.5	12.1	12.5

for whites and Table 3 for blacks. Eighteen percent of the white
and 12.5% of the black population examinees with diastolic
blood pressure equal to or greater than 95 mm Hg in 1960
reverted to pressures below 90 mm in 1967. There was a strong
relationship of this remission rate to weight change for both
whites and blacks. The remission rate was twice as large for
subjects losing ten or more pounds than it was for subjects
gaining ten or more pounds, and for whites this relationship
obtained at all levels of initial diastolic blood pressure. The
Evans County data indicate that in the absence of weight
change, the probability of remission of high diastolic blood
pressure was lower as the initial blood pressure was higher, but
that for whites at all initial diastolic blood pressure levels equal

to or greater than 95 mm Hg, there was a strong relationship of weight change to remission rates. The remission rates were lower for blacks than for whites, and a clear relation to weight change was present only for blacks with initial diastolic blood pressure of 105 mm Hg or higher. The differences between black and white remission rates were minimal among those examinees with highest initial diastolic blood pressure levels (ie, $\geq$ 105 mm Hg).

A Community-Based Diet Experiment

A community-based experiment of the effect of diet and weight loss on high blood pressure was undertaken, sampling overweight subjects with elevated blood pressure from the total Evans County Cardiovascular Survey population.[20] Eligibility criteria required subjects to have had diastolic blood pressure equal to or greater than 90 mm Hg upon examination both in the 1960 and 1967 surveys as well as one or more readings over 95 mm Hg.

Eligible study subjects were reexamined in June 1971, at which time they had to be under age 65 and free of either history or clinical evidence of coronary heart disease or stroke. They were then randomly allocated into either a dietary management treatment group or comparison group. Subjects randomly allocated to the control comparison group were told of their elevated pressure and advised to seek treatment from their usual medical care sources. This was an open, community-based trial, with blinding of the observer of blood pressure measurements at the completion of the experiment.

The dietary experiment, under the direction of S.H., consisted of a low calorie, low salt diet providing 700 calories per day, from approximately 50 gm of carbohydrate, 60 gm of protein, 30 gm of fat with a goal intake of about 1 gm of sodium chloride daily. Potassium containing salt supplements were prescribed and distributed free of charge.

For a very obese, physically inactive individual, this is essentially a maintenance rather than a weight reduction diet; therefore, according to the initial degree of obesity and physical activity, between one and three days of intermittent fasting per week was recommended, allowing ad libitum intake of non-caloric liquids. Instruction was provided, both in group and individual sessions, by S.H. and a local resident trained as a

TABLE 4. Evans County Weight Reduction Experiment
Comparison of Treatment and Control Groups
Pre-intervention Measurements (July 1971)

		Treatment Group No. of Subjects		Control Group No. of Subjects
Total Subjects		63		64
H_x Drug R_x: Yes		28		27
		Mean		*Mean*
Age (years)		53.9		53.9
SBP (mm Hg)		166.8		167.8
DBP (mm Hg)		103.2		101.2
Weight (pounds) Total		195.0		197.2
All Males		201.8		201.2
All Females		192.9		195.1
Height (inches) Total		65.0		65.4
All Males		69.4		69.1
All Females		63.3		63.5
Relative Weight (% "ideal")	*Mean*	*No. of Subjects*	*Mean*	*No. of Subjects*
Total	156	63	154	64
WM	134	11	135	15
WF	159	18	152	17
BM	135	6	135	7
BF	168	28	174	25

nurse auxiliary. Weekly visits were scheduled for blood pressure measurements and review of weight and diet status for the first two to four months of the program. These were then spaced once a month and finally every two months when casual blood pressure was below 90 mm Hg.

The characteristics of the treatment and control group at intake are set out in Table 4. The total sample of eligibles, numbering 143, was randomized into 72 subjects in the treatment and 71 in the control group. Early removal of nine subjects from the treatment group and seven from the control group, primarily due to noncompliance, produced follow-up study subjects numbering 63 in the treatment and 64 in the control group. The two groups were most similar with respect to their age, blood pressure, weight indices and history of drug therapy at intake. The average age of the population was 54 years, average systolic blood pressure 167 mm Hg and the average diastolic blood pressure was 102. The relative weight of the population was 156%, ie, as a group they averaged 56%

EVANS COUNTY
WEIGHT REDUCTION EXPERIMENT
AVERAGE WEIGHT, NUMBER OF SUBJECTS WITH
ELEVATED BLOOD PRESSURE AND NUMBER USING
ANTIHYPERTENSIVE DRUGS DURING FIRST
YEAR OF PROGRAM

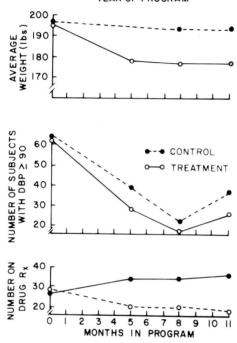

Figure 3.

above the "ideal" weight based on Metropolitan Life Insurance standards. Subjects in both the treatment and control group were of approximately the same race/sex composition, with black females most numerous, followed by white females, white males and black males. This distribution is not equivalent to the relative prevalence of high blood pressure in the target community and reflects the lower initial participation rate of black males. The mean relative weight was highest in black females, who averaged 71% above the ideal weight for their height. White females were 56% and white and black males approximately 35% above ideal weight.

The progress of these two groups of subjects during a one year follow-up is summarized in Figure 3. It will be noted that there was a sizable reduction in weight in the treatment group from an average of 195 pounds to a final weight of 177 pounds, representing an average loss of 18 pounds per subject. There was much less evidence of weight reduction in the control group, a decline from 197 to 193 pounds. Parallel decreases in blood pressure occurred in these two groups. It should be noted, however, that there was a divergence over time in the number of subjects on hypotensive drug therapy in the two groups. At intake, 28 subjects in the treatment group were on hypotensive drug therapy in comparison with 27 in the control group. The number in the control group on drug therapy increased during the year of follow-up to 36, while the number in the diet treatment group on drug therapy declined to 18, while its blood pressure decrease was taking place.

At one year follow-up, an independent observer, not knowing whether subjects were in the treatment or control group, reexamined each subject and produced blood pressure measurements indicating a decline of 18 mm systolic pressure in the treatment group and 12 mm in the control group (a statistically significant difference) and an average diastolic decrease of 13 mm Hg in the treatment group and 8 mm Hg in the control group, a difference not statistically significant. The number of subjects with diastolic pressure less than 90 mm Hg was 32 in the diet treatment group and 25 in the control group.

Some of the decline in blood pressure for both the treatment and control groups can probably be attributed to psychological effects of intensive follow-up including familiarization with blood pressure measurement procedures. Some of the decrease in the control group is probably attributable to increase in the number of subjects using hypotensive medication. The fact that statistically significant differences in the systolic blood pressure and modest differences in diastolic pressure in the treatment and control group were achieved at one year follow-up despite decreasing drug utilization in the diet treatment group lends credence to attributing some impact of the dietary program in achieving blood pressure reduction.

Additional evidence for the effect of weight reduction on decrease in blood pressure comes from inspection of the relationship between weight change and blood pressure change as set out in Figure 4. There is a correlation coefficient of

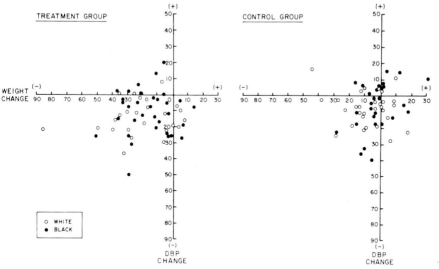

Figure 4.

approximately 0.25 between weight change and diastolic blood pressure change for both the treatment and the control group. It is of interest that this correlation is of the same magnitude for the experiment as observed in the naturalistic community study between 1960 and 1967. It is important, however, to point out that although there is a statistically significant association, the correlation coefficient is small. Therefore, weight reduction per se, during the experiment, statistically explains only a small proportion of all the blood pressure change. Alternative explanations, in addition to regression to the mean, the psychotherapeutic benefits of the instructional program and the procedural familiarization effect previously alluded to, include the benefits of salt restriction and the possible hypotensive effect of the use of potassium supplements.

This experiment has demonstrated that subjects in a free living community who are both overweight and have elevated blood pressure but are otherwise healthy can be screened and recruited into a weight reduction program. Of 72 subjects randomized into the dietary program, 58 remained in the program for one year and 62 of 71 in the control group were followed for the same period of time.

Obviously, longer periods of observation are necessary to determine the long-term effectiveness of a program of this type as measured by compliance and successful maintenance of diet and weight loss and ultimately the impact, if any, on morbidity and mortality. It does seem apparent, however, that satisfactory participation, compliance, reduced hypotensive drug use and successful, measurable blood pressure reduction has been achieved for a one year period in obese hypertensives identified from a population screening given the regimen described here.

The Potential for Primary Prevention
of Elevated Blood Pressure by Weight Control

In contrast to the treatment of overweight patients with elevated blood pressure, the approach of primary prevention is prophylactic reduction of the weight of normotensives to prevent the emergence of elevated blood pressure. We do not have the experience of an experimental primary prevention trial; however, the potential for such an effort can be estimated by observation of the incidence of high blood pressure in relation to weight characteristics. There were 582 Evans County residents age 35-59 with diastolic pressure below 90 mm Hg in 1960 who were reexamined in 1967. The seven year percent incidence of high diastolic blood pressure (ie, increase to pressure 95 or higher) was 16.8% for this cohort (Table 5). That is, an average of slightly more than 2% of these subjects, screened and found to be normotensive in 1960, had elevations of blood pressure per year of follow-up. The magnitude of this incidence has important consequences for community intervention programs. Periodic screening will be mandatory for community high blood pressure detection and control.

It is also clear that there is a strong relationship of incidence of high blood pressure to weight change. The incidence rate was twice as great for subjects whose weight increased ten or more pounds than it was for those who did not gain ten pounds in the seven year follow-up. The association was even stronger in relationship to baseline overweight status, independently of weight change. Overweight in this context was arbitrarily defined as a Quetelet Index value in the upper 12.5% of Evans County examinees' five year age/sex specific distributions in

TABLE 5. The Seven-year Percent Incidence of Diastolic Blood
Pressure ⩾ 95 in Individuals With Diastolic Blood Pressure < 90 in 1960
in Relation to Baseline Weight and Weight Gain
Evans County Residents, Age 35-59, 1960

| | | Weight Status, 1960 | | All Weight |
		Normal	Overweight*	Levels
	Change ⩽ + 9 lbs.	9.9	36.7	13.1
Weight Change	Change ⩾ + 10 lbs.	20.9	58.3	26.1
	All Weight Change Levels	12.9	43.9	16.8

*Overweight = Subjects with weight-height (Quetelet) index in the upper 12.5%
of their five year age/sex specific distribution in 1960.

1960. The seven year incidence of diastolic pressure equal to or
greater than 95 mm Hg was 44% for those overweight,
contrasted with 13% for those of normal weight, a relative risk
of 3.4. As is evident from Table 5, there is an association of
both baseline weight and weight gain with the incidence of
elevated blood pressure. Controlling for either baseline weight
or weight gain, the association of the other weight characteristic
with incidence of high blood pressure remains.

The relationships are set out in the form of incidence and
relative risk of incidence of high diastolic pressure by various
combinations of weight characteristics in Tables 6 and 7. It will
be noted that subjects who were both overweight at intake and
gained more than ten pounds had an almost six times greater
risk of developing elevated blood pressure than those who were
of normal weight and did not gain as much as ten pounds. The
respective incidence figures were 58.3% contrasted with 9.9%. An
additional finding disclosed in these tables is that excess
baseline weight and weight gain are each associated with the
incidence of elevated diastolic blood pressure to all observed
levels greater than 95 mm Hg. That is, the importance, as
measured by relative risk, of weight characteristics was the same
in predicting the incidence of blood pressure to a level of 95 to
99 mm Hg as it was for subjects increasing pressure to levels of
100 to 104, and approximately the same for individuals
increasing to a level of 105 mm Hg or greater. The relationship
(to weight), however, was not present for subjects with

TABLE 6. The Seven-year Percent Incidence of Different Levels of
High Diastolic Blood Pressure by Weight Characteristics
Evans County Residents With Diastolic Blood Pressure < 90 in 1960

No. of Examinees	Weight Characteristics		Percent Incidence from DBP < 90 in 1960 to the Following Diastolic Blood Pressure Levels in 1967				
	Overweight in 1960	Weight Gain ≥ 10 lbs. 1960-1967					
			90-94	95-99	100-104	≥ 105	≥ 95
365	–	–	15.1	2.5	4.4	3.0	9.9
144	–	+	24.3	6.3	9.7	4.9	20.9
49	+	–	24.5	2.0	24.5	10.2	36.7
24	+	+	12.5	12.5	25.0	20.8	58.3
582							
414		–	16.2	2.4	6.8	3.9	13.1
168		+	22.6	7.1	11.9	7.1	26.1
582							
509	–		17.7	3.5	5.9	3.5	12.9
73	+		20.5	5.5	24.7	13.7	43.9
582							
365	–	–	15.1	2.5	4.4	3.0	9.9
217	Either + or +		23.0	6.0	14.7	7.8	28.5
582	Total Population with DBP < 90 in 1960		18.0	3.8	8.2	4.8	16.8

transition from pressures below 90 to borderline values of 90 to
94 mm Hg. The observational data thus indicate that baseline
weight and weight gain are strongly associated with the risk of
developing elevated blood pressure, other than to readings in
the borderline range.

Some of these associations can be explained as spurious and
related to the inaccurate, nonvalid approximation to intra-
arterial pressure obtained by the indirect auscultatory method
in obese subjects[21] plus the effects of wide diameter arms and
relatively small blood pressure cuffs. Others[22] have argued that
the correlation of arm circumference with blood pressure in
population studies is an indirect one attributable to obesity,
because of the high correlation of arm circumference with body
weight. Some of our findings, however, cannot be explained by
invoking the argument of "cuff" hypertension. In particular,
subjects who were overweight in 1960 and did not gain ten or
more pounds had an almost four times greater risk of

TABLE 7. The Seven-year Relative Risk of Incidence of High Diastolic
Blood Pressure by Weight Characteristics
Evans County Residents with Diastolic Blood Pressure < 90 in 1960

Weight Characteristics						
Overweight in 1960	*Weight Gain ⩾ 10 lbs. 1960-1967*	*Relative Risk of Transition from Diastolic Blood Pressure < 90 in 1960 to the Following Diastolic Blood Pressure Levels in 1967*				
		90-94	95-99	100-104	⩾105	⩾95
–	–	1.00	1.00	1.00	1.00	1.00
–	+	1.61	2.52	2.20	1.63	2.11
+	–	1.62	0.80	5.57	3.40	3.71
+	+	0.83	5.00	5.68	6.93	5.89
	–	1.00	1.00	1.00	1.00	1.00
	+	1.40	2.96	1.75	1.82	1.99
–		1.00	1.00	1.00	1.00	1.00
+		1.16	1.57	4.19	3.91	3.40
–	–	1.00	1.00	1.00	1.00	1.00
Either + or	+	1.52	2.40	3.34	2.60	2.88

developing high blood pressure (ie, greater than 95 mm Hg)
than did subjects who were both free of weight gain and were
not overweight in 1960. The importance of weight characteristics, per se, is also emphasized in their equal relationship to
the incidence of successively higher levels of blood pressure.
Clearly, overweight individuals whose pressure increased
between the baseline and follow-up reading without weight gain
could not have the second elevated reading explained by
spuriously elevated readings, attributed to a wide arm circumference and a proportionately smaller blood pressure cuff, in
the absence of major changes in weight and arm circumference
between the two blood pressure readings. The inadequacy of
"cuff hypertension" as an explanation for the increased
incidence of high blood pressure in overweight normotensives
who did not gain weight does not rule out its possible
importance in explaining other findings, such as the association
between being overweight and having elevated pressure at a
point in time, or gaining weight and developing elevated
pressure.

The potential for primary prevention of high diastolic blood
pressure in the Evans County cohort was estimated from these
observational findings by computing the population attributable

risk percent (Table 8). Assuming causal relationships between weight and blood pressure and assuming our capability to modify weight, the potential for reduction of new cases, that is, the primary prevention of high diastolic blood pressure, is 22% by preventing weight gain in the Evans County cohort and there is the potential for a 23% reduction in incidence by controlling the weight of those who were overweight in 1960. Were both of these attributes to be controlled, there is a potential for reduction in incidence of high blood pressure cases of 41% in the Evans County cohort. These are sizable potential reductions. Each would involve target intervention populations of different sizes. It would require intervention in more than a third of the population (37.3%) to achieve the 41% reduction in all cases by achieving weight loss among those overweight in 1960 and preventing weight gain between 1960 and 1967. Almost as large a group (28.9% of the population) would have to be ascertained in advance and prevented from weight gain to achieve the 22% reduction in cases attributed to weight gain and that, of course, assumes that the individuals who were subse-

TABLE 8. The Potential for Primary Prevention of High Diastolic Blood Pressure (DBP ⩾ 95) by Control of Weight and Weight Gain Evans County 1960-1967

| Weight Characteristics | | | | | |
Overweight in 1960	Weight Gain ⩾ 10 lbs. 1960-1967	PAR	% of Pop.	R.R.	Pop. AR %
−	−	365	62.7	1.00	−
−	+	144	24.7	2.11	−
+	−	49	8.4	3.71	−
+	+	24	4.1	5.89	−
	−	414	71.1	1.00	−
	+	168	28.9	1.99	22.2
−		509	87.5	1.00	−
+		73	12.5	3.40	23.1
−	−	365	62.7	1.00	−
Either + or	+	217	37.3	2.88	41.2
Total Population with DBP < 90 in 1960		582	100	−	−

quently to gain weight could be identified prior to the event, a technical capability we do not possess at present. Therefore, in point of fact, all subjects in the cohort would have to be "treated" to achieve this goal. In sharp contrast, it was possible and feasible to identify only 12.5% of the population classified as overweight in 1960. Assuming that their weight could be reduced to the level of the remainder of the population, and assuming further that this carried with it a reduction in incidence rate to the level of the remaining population, an almost one quarter reduction (23.1%) in the total population incidence of elevated blood pressure potentially could have been achieved in the Evans County cohort. This clearly is both a sizable proportion of all cases and also one which quantitatively would be worthy of achievement, if it were possible to do so by the detection and intervention of only one in eight of the population at risk in the total community.

The potential for primary prevention of elevated blood pressure in the community is considerable as estimated in Evans County. It is, as was discussed earlier, a function both of the relative risk of incidence of high blood pressure in relationship to weight characteristics, and also of the prevalence of the various weight characteristics in the community. One associated characteristic which potentially could secondarily influence each of these parameters is the race composition of the community. It is well known that the prevalence of elevated blood pressure is markedly higher in the black than in the white population. Few data are available on the incidence of high blood pressure in community-based black populations. Therefore, it was of interest to compare the incidence of high blood pressure and its relation to weight characteristics in the blacks and whites of Evans County. The overall incidence of high blood pressure was two times higher in blacks than in whites (Table 9 and Fig. 5). The total incidence was 16.8%; for blacks it was 28%, for whites 13.8%. The difference between black and white incidence figures is highly related to weight characteristics. For those not overweight and without weight gain, the black incidence rate is almost three times higher than the white (20.3% contrasted with 7.2%). In sharp contrast, among individuals who were both overweight in 1960 and had a weight gain of ten or more pounds, the incidence rate was extremely high for both blacks and whites and there was very little

TABLE 9. The Seven-year Incidence of Diastolic Blood Pressure
≥ 95 in Individuals with Diastolic Blood Pressure < 90 in 1960
in Relation to Weight Characteristics by Race
Evans County Residents, Age 35-59 in 1960

Weight Characteristics				
Overweight in 1960	Weight Gain ≥ 10 lbs 1960-1967	All White	All Black	Total
−	−	7.2	20.3	9.9
−	+	17.1	33.3	20.9
+	−	35.1	41.6	36.7
+	+	55.6	66.6	58.3
	−	10.3	23.3	13.1
	+	22.6	38.5	26.1
−		9.9	24.3	12.9
+		41.8	50.0	43.9
Either +　　or　　+		25.3	39.2	28.5
Total Population with DBP < 90 in 1960		13.8	28.0	16.8

difference between them (66.6% for blacks and 55.6% for whites). The different relation of weight to incidence of high blood pressure for blacks and whites is quite similar to the cross-sectional regression analyses (Fig. 1). The influences these relationships have on the potential for reduction in incidence of elevated diastolic blood pressure is set out in Table 10. It will be noted that the distribution of weight characteristics is quite similar for whites and blacks. This, however, disguises a race/sex difference. The white male population had a much higher prevalence of overweight individuals in 1960 than did black males, and conversely the black female population had a much higher proportion of overweight subjects than did the white females. Race/sex specific estimates are not presented because of the relatively small number of normotensives at risk in the higher cardiovascular disease region within which Evans County is located. In contrast to the similarity in distribution of weight characteristics, the relative risk of developing elevated diastolic blood pressure is dissimilar in the two races. The relative risk is consistently and considerably higher for whites than it is for

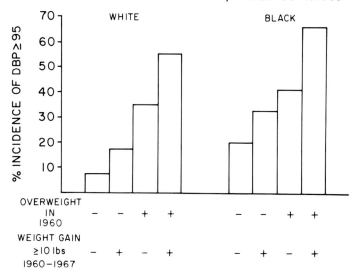

THE SEVEN YEAR INCIDENCE OF DIASTOLIC BLOOD
PRESSURE ≥ 95 IN INDIVIDUALS WITH DIASTOLIC BLOOD
PRESSURE < 90 IN 1960 IN RELATION TO BASELINE
WEIGHT AND WEIGHT GAIN BY RACE
EVANS COUNTY RESIDENTS, AGE 35–59 IN 1960

Figure 5.

blacks and is similar for the two sexes in each race group. The potential for reduction in incidence of high blood pressure by control of weight characteristics, therefore, is different in the two races and reflects the higher relative risk in whites. By controlling both baseline weight and weight gain, there is a potential for prevention of 27.5% of the new cases of high blood pressure in blacks and a potential prevention of almost one half of the incidence in white cases (47.7%). Of more practical import, there is a potential for a 27.9% reduction in incidence in whites and 16.9% in blacks by weight control of 12% of whites and 14% of blacks who are overweight. The data clearly indicate the existence and operation of factors in addition to weight characteristics which must be identified to account for the excess incidence of elevated pressure in the black. The data, nevertheless, highlight the strong potential for primary prevention on a community basis, for reduction in

TABLE 10. Comparison of Potential for Primary Prevention of High Diastolic Blood Pressure (DBP ⩾ 95) by Control of Weight Characteristics in Evans County Whites and Blacks

| Weight Characteristics | | % of Pop. with Weight Characteristics | | Relative Risk of DBP < 90 → DBP ⩾ 95 | | Potential % Reduction in Incidence of DBP ⩾ 95 | |
Overweight in 1960	Weight Gain ⩾ 10 lbs. 1960-1967	W	B	W	B	W	B
–	–	63.7	59.2	1.00	1.00	–	–
–	+	24.3	26.4	2.38	1.64	–	–
+	–	8.1	9.6	4.88	2.05	–	–
+	+	3.9	4.8	7.72	3.28	–	–
		100.0	100.0				
	–	71.8	68.8	1.00	1.00		
	+	28.2	31.2	2.19	1.65	25.1	16.9
		100.0	100.0				
–		88.0	85.6	1.00	1.00		
+		12.0	14.4	4.22	2.06	27.9	13.2
		100.0	100.0				
–	–	63.7	59.2	1.00	1.00		
Either + or	+	36.3	40.8	3.51	1.93	47.7	27.5
		100.0	100.0				
Total Population with DBP < 90 in 1960		457	125				

incidence of elevated blood pressure, particularly in the white population.

Summary and Conclusions

The seven-year experience of the Evans County cohort reported here confirms the cross-sectional association of weight and blood pressure. Being overweight is associated with both increased prevalence and incidence of high blood pressure and weight change is associated with blood pressure change. Weight increase is associated with increased incidence of high blood pressure in normotensives and a decreased remission rate in those with high blood pressure. Weight decrease is associated with increased rates of remission of those with high blood pressure and decreased incidence rates of high blood pressure in normotensives. In addition, an open, community-based trial indicated that a significant number of overweight individuals with high blood pressure could be brought to and maintained in blood pressure remission for one year by dietary management. These associations are stronger for whites than blacks.

The limitations of the experience and data presented should be obvious. In the observational surveys, single, casual blood pressure determinations were used for the analyses and they were obtained initially more than 14 years ago under less than the optimally rigorous conditions of objective measurement, free of observer bias, which would be incorporated in a contemporaneous population survey. The blood pressure measurements used, however, have had both concurrent and predictive validation, ie, the Evans County high blood pressure cohorts, identified as they have been for these weight studies, do have predictively higher prevalence[1 4] and incidence rates of cardiovascular disease[2 3] than the "normotensive" cohort.

There are considerations other than the reliability and validity of the measurements reported, which limit their usefulness for primary prevention estimates. The attributable and relative risk estimates of elevated blood pressure, given various combinations of weight characteristics, are but measures of association permitting approximations of the potential for the control of high blood pressure. They were derived in Evans County, located in a region with high prevalence and incidence of high blood pressure and may not be applicable elsewhere.

Of greater practical importance are current limitations in our ability to achieve weight control in a normotensive population and the paucity of knowledge we have of the potential this has for reduction of morbidity and mortality. The cumulative, long-term experience of many investigators in this field has been so discouraging that it has prompted comments such as, "Obesity is a relatively incurable disease. This situation makes proper clinical trials impossible."[2 4] Without arguing with this summation and evaluation of experience to date, we would suggest that the strengths of the association of weight with incidence of high blood pressure, the commonness of over-weight individuals, the short-term modest, but apparently useful, success of our community-based experiment of the dietary management of high blood pressure, and the absence of any other currently known approaches with any potential for a major primary prevention impact, all argue for the need for community-based experimental trials of primary prevention of high blood pressure by diet and weight control.

References

1. Pickering, G.: *High Blood Pressure*, ed. 2. New York:Grune & Stratton, Inc., 1968, p. 215.
2. Chiang, B. W., Perlman, L. V. and Epstein, F. H.: Overweight and hypertension: A review. *Circulation*, 39:403, 1969.
3. Kannel, W. B., Brand, N., Skinner, J. J. et al: The relation of adiposity to blood pressure and development of hypertension: The Framingham Study. *Ann. Intern. Med.*, 67:48, 1967.
4. Ashley, F. W. and Kannel, W. B.: Relation of weight change to changes in atherogenic traits: The Framingham Study. *J. Chronic Dis.*, 27:103, 1974.
5. Johnson, B. C., Karunas, T. M. and Epstein, F. H.: Longitudinal change in blood pressure in individuals, families, and social groups. *Clin. Sci. Molec. Med.*, 45:35s, 1973.
6. Miall, W. E., Bell, R. A. and Lovell, B. A.: Relation between change in blood pressure and weight. *Brit. J. Prev. Soc. Med.*, 22:73, 1968.
7. Ulrych, M., Tauber, J. and Shapiro, A. P.: Long term study of the relationship between blood pressure, age, and body weight in steelmill workers. *Clin. Sci. Molec. Med.*, 45:107s, 1973.
8. Paffenbarger, R. S., Thorne, M. C. and Wing, A. L.: Chronic disease in former college students. VIII. Characteristics in youth predisposing to hypertension in later years. *Amer. J. Epidem.*, 88:25, 1968.
9. Oberman, A., Lane, W. D., Harlan, W. R. et al: Trends in systolic blood pressure in the thousand aviator cohort over a twenty-four year period. *Circulation*, 36:812, 1967.
10. Kahn, H., Medalie, J. H., Neufeld, H. M. et al: The incidence of hypertension and associated factors: The Israel Ischemic Heart Disease Study. *Amer. Heart J.*, 84:171, 1972.
11. McDonough, J. R., Hames, C. G. and Stulb, S. C.: Cardiovascular Disease Field Study in Evans County, Ga. *Public Health Rep.*, 78:1051, 1963.
12. Cornoni, J. C., Waller, L. E., Cassel, J. C. et al: Evans County Cardiovascular and Cerebrovascular Epidemiologic Study: The incidence study — study design and methods. *Arch. Intern. Med.*, 128:896, 1971.
13. Wetherbee, H. and Tyroler, H. A.: The relation of migration to coronary heart disease risk factors. *Arch. Intern. Med.*, 128:976, 1971.
14. McDonough, J. R., Garrison, G. E. and Hames, C. G.: Blood pressure and hypertensive disease among Negroes and Whites: A study in Evans County, Georgia. *Ann. Intern. Med.*, 61:208, 1964.
15. Khosla, T. and Lowe, C. R.: Indices of obesity derived from body weight and height. *Brit. J. Prev. Soc. Med.*, 21:121, 1967.

16. Florey, C du V.: The use and interpretation of Ponderal Index and other weight-height ratios in epidemiologic studies. *J. Chronic Dis.*, 23:93, 1970.
17. Leviton, A.: Definitions of attributable risk. Letter to the editor. *Amer. J. Epidem.*, 98:231, 1973.
18. Epstein, F. H., Francis, T., Hayner, W. D. et al: Prevalence of chronic diseases and distribution of selected physiologic variables in a total community, Tecumseh, Michigan. *Amer. J. Epidem.*, 81:307, 1965.
19. Klein, B. E. K., Cornoni, J. C., Jones, F. et al: Overweight indices as correlates of coronary heart diseases and blood pressure. *Hum. Biol.*, 45:329, 1973.
20. Heyden, S., Tyroler, H. A., Hames, C. G. et al: Diet treatment of obese hypertensives. *Clin. Sci. Molec. Med.*, 45:209s, 1973.
21. Neilsen, P. O. and Jauniche, H.: The accuracy of auscultatory measurement of arm blood pressure in very obese subjects. *Acta Med. Scand.*, 195:403, 1974.
22. Khosla, T. and Lowe, C. R.: Arterial pressure and arm circumference. *Brit. J. Prev. Soc. Med.*, 19:159, 1965.
23. Tyroler, H. A., Heyden, S., Bartel, A. et al: Blood pressure and cholesterol as coronary heart disease risk factors. *Arch. Intern. Med.*, 128:907, 1971.
24. Mann, G. V.: The influence of obesity on health. *New Eng. J. Med.*, 291:187, 1974.

Discussion

Dr. Borhani: First, I would like to congratulate you on this beautiful work. I have two questions: (1) I notice that after the eighth month in the diet study the blood pressures of both controls and cases start rising. I wonder if that trend is going to continue and what your thoughts would be on this. (2) Do you have any explanation why the relative risk is so much higher among the whites? Is it because they gain more weight and more rapidly, or do you have another explanation?

Dr. Tyroler: I would agree with you on the extraordinary importance of the incidence figures in blacks. To the best of my knowledge, this is the first in a population base setting. In a place like Evans County the cumulative incidence figures suggest that community control is going to require much more than one-time screening to ascertain cases for intervention. Also, the incidence for blacks approaches 4% per year. Those screened and found to be normal have an extraordinarily high risk of subsequent development of elevated pressure and continuous monitoring would be necessary. As far as your second question is concerned, the relative risk of elevation of diastolic blood pressure is higher among whites. I am going beyond the data now, but I suggest there is almost a saturation phenomenon. Almost all the expression of elevated blood pressure has taken place in the blacks, and there is not much more room for further expression. When you get to 50% or 60% of the population manifesting this on prevalence, 4% per year as showing it on incidence, I do not think there is much room for more expression. As to your final question, Dr. Heyden had his groups of counselors work intensively with his population for one year. I think it is an extraordinary achievement. I think it is important to point out that this was not a clinic for overweight individuals who said they wanted help. These were individuals who were sampled from the total community and he was able, by his intensive methods, to achieve the weight reduction over the time that you observed in one year. In the ensuing two years there was slippage. We have preliminary data, which I am not prepared to discuss in detail, to show that at the end of the three-year follow-up there was some slippage, but a weight difference persisted over the three-year period.

Dr. Labarthe, Minnesota: One of the things that is always perplexing, in blood pressure measurements, particularly over extended intervals, is the problem of intra-individual variability in blood pressure. Recently, we have been looking into this problem in a cohort within the Chicago Gas Company. A rather interesting finding is that the amount of variability within individuals in this cohort over a five-year period was not very different than has been reported in only a few months in some other population-based studies. This raises some concern. For example, a shift from one blood pressure class to another, on remeasurement, may be nearly as much a result of remeasurement itself as it is a result of the time interval between observations. The implications for "incidence of hypertension" are quite important. It may be that the seven-year incidence observed here, which would have to be divided by seven to give an average annual incidence, might in fact be the same amount of change that would be observed if the remeasurement were done within a year or two years rather than seven. It may not differ very much from a remeasurement over ten years. Thus, the absolute value of *average annual* incidence seems quite sensitive to the time interval between observations. We may wonder whether, in fact, incidence in its usual sense has the usual applicability to so variable a characteristic as blood pressure. One reason why this is a crucial question here is that blood pressure fluctuates more than weight. Thus, the relationship between conversion to the arbitrary class "hypertension" and concurrent change in weight is very closely dependent upon the particular time interval over which you have remeasured the blood pressure and allowed weight to change.

Dr. Tyroler: I think that is a point well taken. In partial confirmation of that is the finding in the Framingham Study that elevated blood pressure among normally weighted individuals is a strong risk factor for the incidence of obesity on sequential examinations. Another point almost unnecessary to mention before this audience is the fact that we are talking about incidence of an arbitrary phenomenon. The relationships are continuous. Clearly different estimates of impact and attributable risk would be obtained with different cut points, and I chose the arbitrary cut points I did simply because they are the ones that have some clinical justification and are the guide rules for an intervention program.

Dr. Meneely, Louisiana: I would like to inquire about the follow-up of Dahl's observations on that group of obese subjects in whom he reduced salt and maintained calories. The blood pressure went down, whereas, when he reduced calories and kept salt up the blood pressure stayed up and the weight went down. What has become of further studies in that line?

Dr. Tyroler: This particular experiment does not speak to that point. From the research design point of view, one can only call it a diet modification study and there was both salt restriction and weight loss operative here.

Question: I also would like to compliment your report. Have you looked at, or do you intend to look at those who regained weight?

Dr. Tyroler: It is going to be extraordinarily complex to disentangle effects of the type that you ask about. Those who did not lose weight and in whom the blood pressure remained high were put on antihypertensive medication, and those who lost and then gained weight and whose blood pressure rose would then be put on medication also.

Dr. James, Ohio: Did you categorize your patient data in terms of activity status, ie, comparing the nonsedentary patient to sedentary patients?

Dr. Tyroler: We do not have the rigorous data that would be appropriate to answer your question, but in a certain sense a natural experiment was going on in Evans County. The black population in the 1960s, when this study was underway, was predominantly occupied with hard, manual labor. The black male was exquisitely lean, the Quetelet Index was markedly lower, the weight for height indices were markedly less and skin folds were markedly lower for the black than white. The caloric intake was much higher, the body weight was lower and they had much higher blood pressures than the whites in the community.

III
Endocrine and Hormonal Factors

Problems of the Radioimmunoassay of Renin Activity

Walter M. Kirkendall, M.D., Merrill Overturf, Ph.D.,
Robert E. Druilhet, Ph.D. and Patricia Arnold, B.S.

Introduction

Recent interest in the identification of a subgroup of low-renin hypertensives by the use of plasma renin activity (PRA) assay has brought into sharp focus the need for results which are accurate, reproducible and comparable among investigators. The most widely used methods for the determination of renin activity are those based on the indirect method of measuring by radioimmunoassay the angiotensin I (AI) generated during a controlled incubation of plasma.[1]

The abundant literature concerning the methodologies involved with the radioimmunoassay of plasma renin activity (PRA) indicates that there are many problems associated with it. The numerous procedural modifications alone indicate dissatisfaction among the proponents of the various methods. The various methods which have been proposed, and the conflicting data obtained, are apparently the result of an inability to recognize, much less control, all of the variables inherent in the system. The following is a list of some of the various controllable and noncontrollable variables.

Supported in part by the National Institutes of Health Grant HL-1517 from the National Heart and Lung Institute and by a Grant-In-Aid from E.R. Squibb and Sons.

Walter M. Kirkendall, M.D., *Professor and Director, Program in Internal Medicine;* Merrill Overturf, Ph.D., *Assistant Professor of Internal Medicine;* Robert E. Druilhet, Ph.D., *Senior Research Associate in Internal Medicine;* and Patricia Arnold, B.S., *Laboratory Technician in Internal Medicine, The University of Texas Medical School at Houston.*

Controllable Variables

1. *Chemically and radio-pure standard angiotensin I can be obtained* and stored for a period of time with minimal difficulty.
2. *Theoretically, specific angiotensin I antibodies can be obtained.* However, there is reason to believe that many peptides are present in plasma which may react with the angiotensin I antibodies. Heptapeptides (Arg^2....Phe^8) and hexapeptides (Val^3....Phe^8) are known to occur in human plasma and have been shown to react with "specific" angiotensin I antibodies.[2] An important question to be answered is "What is the concentration in plasma, at any specific time or physiological state, of these peptides and other peptides which may cross-react with AI antibodies and compete for binding sites?"
3. *Incubation conditions can be controlled.* However, it is not clearly resolved what the optimal conditions are. The literature is controversial as to whether a low or a more neutral pH should be utilized and whether the incubation period should be long or short. Differences of opinion arise, not only from considerations regarding a preference for a physiological pH or maximum angiotensin I generation which is obtained at a low pH, but also regarding the linearity of the angiotensin I generation. Some authors assert that the generation of AI is linear for as long as 40 hours,[3] while others indicate that it is necessary to anticipate nonlinearity from samples even when incubated for 60 minutes.[4]

Noncontrollable Variables

1. *Antibody specificity.* Since there are no data which indicate all the possible peptides occurring in human plasma at any one time, it is currently impossible to rule out completely the occurrence of all cross-reactive polypeptides in terms of AI antibodies. Cross-reactivity studies must be performed with these peptides that are known to occur in human plasma such as angiotensin II, the hepta- and hexapeptide angiotensin metabolites, bradykinin and vasopressin. However, it must be real-

ized that a large number of unidentified short-chain peptides occur in plasma which compete, either alone or in combination, for antibody binding sites thus modifying and falsely indicating a variously high or low "renin activity."

2. *Substrate concentration.* Angiotensin I generation rate depends upon the concentration of the substrate and the renin concentration of plasma. With low concentrations of substrate it is predictable that the reaction rate would be proportional to the substrate concentration. Conversely, high substrate concentrations lead to an increase in angiotensin I generation rate. At high substrate concentrations renin would be saturated with substrate and the reaction would follow zero order kinetics. Thus, the initial velocity at high substrate concentrations (Vmax) would depend only on the enzyme concentration. As the reaction proceeds, there would be a decrease in substrate concentration, due to enzymatic consumption of the substrate, resulting in a decrease in the reaction rate. Therefore, the effect of decreasing substrate concentration can be lessened by decreasing the reaction time (short incubation time). It is held by some investigators,[5,6] though not by all,[7,8] that plasma substrate concentration is seldom great enough to provide zero order kinetics. If substrate concentration is rate-limiting, the velocity at which a certain plasma sample forms angiotensin I (PRA) would be a variable determined not only by the concentration of renin but also by the substrate concentration. To control the level of substrate concentration is of prime importance in the kinetics of all enzyme reactions. Considering existing RIA procedures for determining PRA, the use of endogenous substrates precludes this requisite.

3. *Renin.* A further complication in RIA assays is the evidence that renin is not an enzyme entity, but rather a large family of enzymes with differing configurations but similar reaction rates.[9] Recent studies have shown that several molecular weight forms of human kidney "renin" are differentially inhibited by various acid protease inhibitors.[10,11] By inference, it would appear

that "renin activity" has historically expressed the sum
total of the angiotensin I formed by the actions of these
systems.

4. *Naturally occurring renin inhibitors and activators.*
Little is known regarding the various substances which
have been found that either inhibit or activate renin.
Changes in the renin-substrate reaction velocities have
provided some evidence for the loss of plasma renin
inhibitors or the presence of activators.[7] Direct evidence
for the occurrence of a lyso-phospholipid in human
plasma which inhibits PRA has been obtained.[12,13] It
has recently been shown that some phospholipids from
human kidneys can substantially accelerate the renin-
substrate reaction in vitro.[14] The qualitative and quantitative occurrence of these substances and their possible
synergistic relationships might conceivably have significant effects on the amount of angiotensin I generated
by a given plasma sample. Where these substances are
synthesized, what pathways are involved and what
controls their syntheses are significant questions for
future research.

Assay Conditions

Standard methods for the collection and storage of samples
for PRA determination are well documented and should be
adhered to in order to provide the laboratory with proper
material. Interestingly, it has been found that plasma pH
increases upon storage ($-20°C$) up to a practically constant value
of 8.3 ± 0.2 after 15-20 days.[15] This could have significant
effects upon PRA results when unaltered incubations are
performed. Whether prolonged storage will result in loss or
change in PRA is not yet certain. Recently, we completed a
year-long drug study during which many PRA samples were
drawn, frozen and assayed as a batch at the completion of the
study. Our results strongly indicated that there had been a
considerable loss of PRA with time.

From a practical viewpoint, reliable PRA measurements can
be obtained by using antibodies with high specificity, as far as
this can reasonably be determined, a mono-iodinated chemically
pure labeled antigen, and careful technical manipulation with

suitable controls. Whether these reagent requirements can be met by the components of commercial kits is doubtful.

Studies Using Commercial Kits*

A study concerning the performance of three commonly used commercially available PRA assay kits has recently been conducted by us. Our purpose was to evaluate the kits with regard to reproducibility, sensitivity, ease of performance and effects of kit age. Although several similar studies have been reported,[4,16,17] changes in kit reagents and protocol with the intention of improving overall performance made a more recent evaluation necessary. In addition, the effects of the pH of the incubation medium upon PRA results were determined by using split samples assayed by two independent laboratories.

Reproducibility

Plasma was collected from normal individuals and immediately aliquoted into 2.3 ml portions, a sufficient quantity for duplicate assay, and frozen. On a test day (TD) one aliquot of each sample was thawed at $5°C$ and assayed. Unless otherwise stated, the manufacturer's directions were followed as nearly as possible. The values obtained from repetitive assays on aliquoted samples with the components of a particular kit varied. For example, one NEN kit over a period of one month (six test days) with plasma samples of n=8 resulted in means of 1.37 ± 0.97 S.D. (TD-1) to 1.16 ± 0.56 S.D. (TD-6). Another NEN kit gave $\bar{x}$=3.78 ± 2.55 (TD-1) and $\bar{x}$=1.48 ± 0.93 (TD-6). Similar results were also obtained for kits supplied by SQ and S-M.

Sensitivity

When the standard curves obtained with various kits from the same manufacturer were examined, it was found that great differences in sensitivity were obtained, ie, sensitivity is decreased greatly when the slope of a plot of B/F or "b" vs. angiotensin I is decreased; the sharper the slope the higher the

---

*The kits which were evaluated were obtained from Schwarz-Mann, Orangeburg, N. Y. (S-M); New England Nuclear Corp., Boston, Mass. (NEN); and E.R. Squibb and Sons, New Brunswick, N.J. (SQ).

sensitivity. The degree of the slope is dictated not only by the sensitivity of the antibody but the purity of the labeled and unlabeled AI. Our experience has been that in many instances where the slope of B/F is relatively flat, the labeled AI solution contained several contaminating radio-labeled compounds and/or possessed AI of low specific activity. On other occasions it was found that the antibody lacked sensitivity. While there is no known procedure to stimulate the production of highly specific antisera, such antisera can be selected by demonstrable high sensitivity, ie, on the basis of the slope of the response curve. Similarly, radio and chemically pure AI with high specific activity can be obtained with known methods. Strict quality control can insure a high level of purity. In practical terms, when sensitivity is low it becomes impossible to distinguish between low and normal levels of renin activity. Accordingly, "low renin hypertension" cannot be diagnosed. A standard curve with a very sharp slope is usually not as important a requisite for distinguishing between normal and high renin activity states since the normal PRA values nearly always fall somewhere on the upper part of the curve and high values will be far below, perhaps locating on the horizontal plane. In other words, the discrimination (sensitivity) needed to distinguish between low and normal PRA is several times greater than that needed to distinguish between normal and elevated PRA. Our experience with commercial kits has revealed that several of them have been so insensitive that low renin activity levels were unmeasurable. On a statistical basis, because the mean of normal plasmas was very low and the standard deviation great, a low renin activity would be indicated by a result of near zero, with a standard deviation encompassing values of zero.

An assay curve which has a sharp slope does not necessarily herald satisfactory results for there are other problems. Some problems are well recognized and some are not. Many of them may evolve from the fact that the standard curves are obtained from a simple aqueous buffer solution and samples which are read from the curves contain plasma. Indeed, it has been shown that some samples contain "nonspecific" proteins which interfere with PRA assays.[18,19] The formation of large cryoprecipitates by certain plasmas may also affect the results of PRA assays; however, no relevant data are available.

Effect of Age

PRA data obtained from kits sold by S-M and NEN also indicated that either the antibody and/or the labeled or unlabeled antigen were undergoing degradations over a period of one month. This was shown by (1) the gradual decrease in the slope of the standard curve and (2) the gradual lowering of the calculated PRA levels of split repetitive samples. In general, SQ kits did not demonstrate these phenomena.

As would be expected from the foregoing discussion, when PRA determinations were performed on split samples with kits from various manufacturers, the results were similar (Figs. 1 and 2). From these two figures which compare the results of S-M with SQ and NEN with SQ, only a moderately strong correlation coefficient of r = 0.75 (P <0.05) was obtained.

Effect of pH

Studies designed to examine the effects of the pH of the plasma incubation medium and the age of the kit were

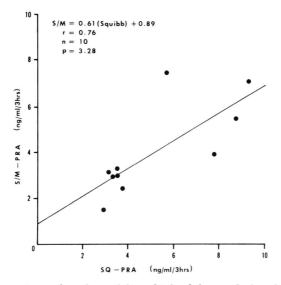

Fig. 1. Ten values of renin activity obtained by analysis with SQ kit reagents are plotted against corresponding S-M values.

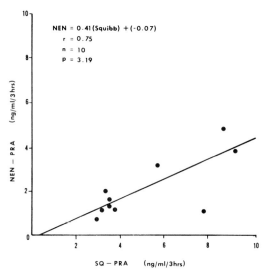

Fig. 2. Ten values of renin activity obtained by analysis with SQ kit reagents are plotted against corresponding NEN values.

performed with a kit supplied by SQ. A quantity of blood was drawn from 15 normal individuals, aliquoted into 2.3 ml plasma portions and immediately frozen. One half of the plasma aliquots from each individual were shipped to another laboratory. Three test days (TD) were chosen. The first TD was designed to conform to the day that both groups had the "fresh" kit materials. TD-2 and TD-3 represented 15 and 30 days subsequent to TD-1. The plasma samples were drawn seven days prior to TD-1. Three incubation protocols were performed in duplicate by each laboratory on each of the 15 samples. One incubation was performed on unaltered plasma (physiological pH), a second incubation was done at pH 7.4 using 2M tris-maleate buffer and a third incubation was done at pH 5.7 by adjusting the plasma with maleic acid.

Table 1 presents a summary of the data. Several observations are immediately apparent. The amount of angiotensin I formed (PRA) at either pH 7.4 or pH 5.7 was more than twofold greater than that generated by unaltered plasma. This conclusion holds for both laboratories over the 30-day test period. These results present a confounding situation since the literature indicates that more angiotensin I (AI) is generated in a

TABLE 1. Renin RIA Results of the UTMSH/Squibb Study*

Test Day		Physiological (unaltered) pH		pH 7.4 (Tris-maleate Buffer)		pH 5.7 (Maleic Acid Solution)	
		U.T.	Squibb	U.T.	Squibb	U.T.	Squibb
I	n	5	5	5	5	5	5
	X̄	0.47	0.59	1.27	1.66	1.32	1.19
	S.D.	0.20	0.24	0.58	0.79	0.37	0.61
	Range	0.26-0.70	0.37-0.91	0.60-1.99	0.80-2.46	0.89-1.62	0.51-1.77
	Calculated Range	0.44	0.54	1.39	1.66	0.73	1.26
II	n	5	5	5	5	5	5
	X̄	0.51	0.90	1.71	1.93	1.80	2.21
	S.D.	0.24	0.47	0.76	0.74	0.75	0.99
	Range	0.29-0.87	0.44-1.40	0.93-2.63	1.02-2.77	1.06-2.84	1.10-3.42
	Calculated Range	0.58	0.96	1.70	1.75	1.78	2.32
III	n	5	5	5	5	5	5
	X̄	0.40	0.67	1.01	1.73	2.00	1.54
	S.D.	0.23	0.32	0.44	0.75	1.06	0.77
	Range	0.21-0.78	0.33-1.03	0.52-1.48	0.87-2.43	0.93-2.46	0.72-2.58
	Calculated Range	0.57	0.70	0.96	1.56	1.53	1.86

*Includes only those results which were never too high to calculate accurately.

more acid medium. It would be anticipated that the pH 5.7 incubation would generate more AI than the unaltered incubation which is known to become even more alkaline as the incubation proceeds.[4,20] However, no explanation is apparent regarding the similar results obtained from incubations buffered at pH 7.4 and the incubations at the adjusted pH 5.7.

It is also evident that although 15 plasma samples were assayed for each of the three incubation conditions some data could not be used (Table 1). For example, because some values were obtained which were indicative of PRA which were too high to calculate accurately (% bound values were too low to read from standard curve), the "n" values dropped from 15 to 5 in terms of the overall data. In this regard, it was those incubations at pH 5.7 and 7.4 which gave the "off-curve" PRA values.

Inter-Laboratory Comparison

Table 2 presents a comparison of the data obtained from the two laboratories. A series of nine test groups revealed a significant difference (p <0.05) in four of the groups. Because no other explanation was tenable, such as type of incubation or age of reagents, we concluded that even when split samples were assayed with essentially identical antibodies, antigens, and so forth, results from one laboratory to another are very difficult to compare. Considering this, it is not surprising that the

TABLE 2. Test of Significant Difference of PRA Results
Obtained From Split Samples

Test Day	Incubation Condition	n	LAB I vs. LAB II
I	Unaltered	14	NSD[1]
	pH 7.4	9	NSD
	pH 5.7	10	<0.05
II	Unaltered	12	<0.01
	pH 7.4	6	NSD
	pH 5.7	6	<0.05
III	Unaltered	14	<0.01
	pH 7.4	10	<0.01
	pH 5.7	6	NSD

[1]NSD = No significant difference, otherwise statistically significant difference at level indicated.

TABLE 3. Test of Significant Difference of PRA Results Obtained from Split Samples for Each Laboratory and Test Day

Test Day	Incubation Condition	n	UTMSH Results	n	Squibb Results
I vs. II	Unaltered	14	NSD[1]	12	<0.01
I vs. II	pH 7.4	6	<0.05	8	<0.01
I vs. II	pH 5.7	8	<0.05	8	<0.01
I vs. III	Unaltered	14	<0.01	14	<0.05
I vs III	pH 7.4	10	<0.01	9	NSD
I vs. III	pH 5.7	10	NSD	6	<0.05
II vs. III	Unaltered	14	<0.01	14	<0.01
II vs. III	pH 7.4	6	<0.01	6	<0.01
II vs. III	pH 5.7	9	<0.05	9	<0.05

[1]NSD = No significant difference, otherwise statistically significant difference at level indicated.

literature is replete with PRA methodologies as well as conflicting and controversial results.

In an evaluation of differences of PRA results obtained from one test day to another (Table 3), it was found that statistically significant ($p < 0.05$) differences were present in all but three groups (Lab I = 2 groups and Lab II = 1 group). An explanation for these differences is not apparent in that no particular trend was demonstrated. Similar results were obtained when the data were compared on an "incubation condition" basis (Table 4). These results were expected as it is

TABLE 4. Test of Significance of PRA Results Obtained from Split Samples Comparing Incubation Conditions by Each Laboratory

Test Day	Incubation Condition	n	UTMSH	n	Squibb
I	Unaltered - pH 7.4	10	<0.01	10	<0.01
I	Unaltered - pH 5.7	10	<0.01	14	<0.01
I	pH 7.4 - pH 5.7	10	<0.05	10	<0.01
II	Unaltered - pH 7.4	6	<0.01	7	<0.01
II	Unaltered - pH 5.7	9	<0.01	6	<0.01
II	pH 7.4 - pH 5.7	5	NSD[1]	7	NSD
III	Unaltered - pH 7.4	14	<0.01	10	<0.01
III	Unaltered - pH 5.7	12	<0.01	6	<0.01
III	pH 7.4 - pH 5.7	12	<0.01	6	NSD

[1]NSD = No significant difference, otherwise statistically significant difference at level indicated.

well established that the incubation condition is a very important parameter of AI generation. In this respect, however, it is interesting but probably coincidental that neither laboratory demonstrated a difference in PRA incubation of pH 7.4 and 5.7 on the TD-2.

Summary

A simple, accurate summary statement regarding the RIA for the assay of PRA is not possible; the assay is not simple, but quite demanding. The manipulative procedures are deceptively easy, and the biological and chemical-radiochemical components require exacting standardization. The great need is for an international reservoir of highly specific angiotensin I antibody and well-standardized pure angiotensin I which could be distributed to those involved with conducting RIA. Until such a source is available it must remain the responsibility of commercial sources and laboratory personnel to establish and adhere to their individual criteria of antibody specificity and AI purity. Correspondingly, RIA results from one laboratory to another will remain essentially incomparable until a common source of reagents is available and standardized techniques are utilized.

References

1. Haber, E., Koerner, T., Page, L. B. et al: Application of a radio-immunoassay for angiotensin I to the physiologic measurements of plasma renin activity in normal human subjects. *J. Clin. Endocr.*, 29:1349, 1969.
2. Cain, M. D., Catt, K. J. and Coghlan, J. P.: Effect of circulating fragments of angiotensin II on radioimmunoassay in arterial and venous blood. *J. Clin. Endocr.* 29:1639, 1969.
3. Lash, B. and Fleischer, N.: Radioimmunoassay of angiotensin I for estimation of plasma renin activity. *Clin. Chem.*, 20:620, 1974.
4. Osmond, D. H., McFadzean, P. A. and Scaiff, K. D.: Renin activity by radioimmunoassay: The plasma incubation step. *Clin. Biochem.*, 7:52, 1974.
5. Skinner, S. L., Lumbers, E. R. and Symonds, E. M.: Alteration by oral contraceptives of normal menstrual changes in plasma renin activity, concentration, and substrate. *Clin. Sci.*, 36:67, 1969.
6. Weinberger, M. H., Collins, R. D., Dowy, A. J. et al: Hypertension induced by oral contraceptives containing estrogen and gestagen. *Ann. Intern. Med.*, 71:891, 1969.

7. Rieger, D., Romero, J. C., Lazar, J. et al: Definition and use of renin reaction velocity in the study of human hypertension. *J. Lab. Clin. Med.*, 80:342, 1972.

8. Haas, E. and Goldblatt, H.: Kinetic constants of the human renin and human angiotensinogen reaction. *Circ. Res.*, 20:45, 1967.

9. Skeggs, L. T., Lentz, K.E., Kahn, J. R. et al: Multiple forms of human kidney renin. In Genest, J. and Koiw, E. (eds.): *Hypertension.* New York:Springer-Verlag, 1972.

10. Overturf, M., Leonard, M. and Kirkendall, W. M.: Inhibition of human renin activity by pepstatin. *Biochem. Pharmacol.*, 23:671, 1974.

11. Druilhet, R., Overturf, M. and Kirkendall, W. M.: The effects of streptomyces protease inhibitors on human kidney renin. *The Pharmacologist*, 16:600, 1974.

12. Osmond, D. H., Smeby, R. R. and Bumpus, F. M.: Quantitative studies of renin preinhibitor and total phospholipids in organs and in plasma and erythrocytes of control, nephrectomized and very old rats. *J. Lab. Clin. Med.*, 73:795, 1969.

13. Baggio, B., Favaro, S., Antonello, A. et al: A procedure for the determination of a renin inhibitor in human plasma. *Clin. Chim. Acta*, 45:67, 1973.

14. Overturf, M., Druilhet, R. and Kirkendall, W. M.: Effects of human kidney lipids on human kidney renin activity. *The Pharmacologist*, 16:710, 1974.

15. Malvano, R., Zucchelli, G. C., Rosa, U. et al: Measurement of plasma renin activity by angiotensin I radioimmunoassay: (1) an assessment of some methodological aspects. *J. Nucl. Biol. Med.*, 16:24,1972.

16. Goldberg, S. D. and Spierto, F. W.: Plasma renin activity: A method for rapid screening by radioimmunoassay and a comparison of two commercially available kits. *Clin. Chem.*, 19:1396, 1973.

17. Sealey, J. E. and Laragh, J. H.: Searching out low renin patients: Limitations of some commonly used methods. *Amer. J. Med.*, 55:303, 1973.

18. Menard, J. and Catt, K. J.: Measurement of renin activity, concentration and substrate in rat plasma by radioimmunoassay of angiotensin I. *Endocrinology*, 90:422, 1972.

19. Viol, G. W., Keane, P. M., Speed, J. F. et al: Assay of plasma renin activity using commercially available reagents. *Clin. Biochem.*, 5:251, 1972.

The Renin-Angiotensin-Aldosterone System in Relation to Type of Hypertension

John H. Laragh, M.D.

I would like to discuss an approach we have found workable for analyzing the whole population of essential hypertension on a physiological basis. Surely, such an approach should yield information about the mechanisms and natural history of essential hypertension which will result in more specific therapy.

This analysis is based on our studies of the endocrine mechanisms involved in high blood pressure. Every physician knows that the kidney plays a key role in all high blood pressure and that dietary salt is also critical. A third factor in high blood pressure is the activity of the adrenocortical hormone aldosterone and some of its analogues which act on the kidney to retain sodium and cause kaluresis. Although there are many other theories, I would like to focus on these endocrine systems and how they explain the mechanisms of hypertension. I do not propose that the renin-angiotensin-aldosterone system causes all hypertension, but I do propose it as a cybernetic basis for blood pressure regulation that can be expected to be askew in every hypertensive patient, even if only reactively. Deviations in the system or one of its substrates can tell you where you are.

When aldosterone was discovered in 1955 we, like many others, set about to learn how to measure it. It is a difficult measurement even today. We finally learned how to do it by double isotope secretion rate methodology, but each measure-

John H. Laragh, M.D., *Master Professor of Medicine and Director, Cardiovascular Center, New York Hospital-Cornell Medical Center, New York, N.Y.*

ment took four to six weeks to complete. We asked a pedestrian question, but one still relevant: What would you find about the sodium-retaining hormone aldosterone in a whole population of high blood pressure patients if you could measure it? We found that there are two conditions in which the hormone is increased. The first is primary aldosteronism, producing values from 5μg to 1,500μg per day. The other is malignant hypertension, in which enormous amounts of aldosterone are produced with values soaring to 10,000μg/day. However, essential hypertension and most other forms did not show much abnormality in the salt-retaining hormone.

We believed the finding of such massive quantities of aldosterone in the blood of patients with malignant hypertension provided an important clue toward understanding this lethal disease. As an experiment, we infused the renal substance angiotensin II into volunteers and demonstrated a subsequent 50%-250% increase in the adrenocortical secretion of aldosterone. Of course, this pointed to the existence of a renal interaction which seemed intimately involved in malignant hypertension and, even more broadly, in sodium balance just as it is in lower forms of life, as in fish, where the adrenals are wrapped within the kidneys.

Figure 1 depicts the workings of the system as we found it in malignant hypertension. It also provides the basis for analysis of all hypertension. In malignant hypertension the kidneys sustain a critical degree of damage for reasons which are not always clear. When that happens, an inappropriate excess of the enzyme renin is dumped into the bloodstream. Renin has no physiologic actions of its own except to generate angiotensin II from a plasma substrate. Angiotensin II, the most powerful pressor substance known, acts on the arterioles to constrict and raise blood pressure. At the same time it elicits secretion of aldosterone by the adrenal glands. Aldosterone, in turn, acts on the normal kidney to cause salt retention and hydremia, an action that in normal subjects restores sodium balance, turns off the initial signal for renin release and brings the system back to the null point in what is called a perfect, closed, negative feedback loop. But in malignant hypertension the kidneys are damaged beyond function and cannot respond to the command of aldosterone. A vicious circle develops — more renin, more

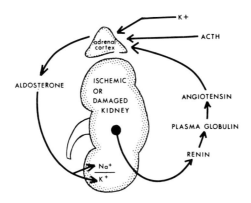

RENAL–ADRENAL INTERACTION
INVOLVING ANGIOTENSIN, ALDOSTERONE
AND Na⁺K⁺ METABOLISM

Fig. 1. The renal-adrenal axis involving renin, angiotensin and aldosterone in regulation of sodium and potassium balance and blood pressure. The interaction is depicted as first identified in patients with malignant hypertension in whom, because of defective feedback, it becomes involved in pathogenesis. From Laragh et al (*Amer. J. Med.*, 52:633-652, 1972).

angiotensin and more hypertension, more aldosterone, rupture of the arterioles, necrotizing arteritis and death.

This pathogenic sequence for malignant hypertension is now widely supported by evidence. For example, renin and aldosterone injected together will produce vasculitis and death in rats in 24 hours. When the hormones are injected separately, nothing happens. The complete syndrome can also be duplicated in dogs by clamping the renal arteries tightly. An enormous literature indicates that massive excesses of aldosterone and renin are vasculotoxic to animals.

The next question is whether subtler, milder increases in these hormones over a longer period of time could have something to do with the cardiovascular damage of the more indolent benign essential hypertension. At any rate, with a knowledge of the workings of this system one can analyze and identify all hypertensive patients in its terms. For example, a patient with a high aldosterone secretion (almost always reflected by a low plasma potassium) and an elevated renin most probably has a kidney disorder causing the derangement. If the renin is subnormal, it points to an adrenocortical form of hypertension with excess primary secretion of steroid. As a start, this approach allows clearly the differentiation of renal and adrenal forms of high blood pressure.

Renin, an enzyme made in the kidney, interacts on a first order basis with a substrate produced by the liver to make angiotensin I, which is converted in the lungs to the active vasoconstricting octapeptide. The system is accelerated in the presence of large quantities of substrate and depressed by small substrate quantities. A rare entity of great epidemiologic significance illustrates this: oral contraceptive hypertension. The first recognized case of this phenomenon involved a 33-year-old woman who came to us in 1966 with an unexplained high blood pressure of 220/130. All tests, including a renal angiogram, were negative. As she was leaving she mentioned that she had been on the Pill for five years. We told her to stop. She returned normotensive in three months. She did not believe the relationship and was disenchanted with withdrawal from the Pill, so we put her back on the medication. Severe hypertension again developed and again was controlled by withdrawing the Pill. This kind of contraceptive hypertension is characterized by a high substrate for renin induced by the estrogen in the medication. There are only a few hundred such cases in the world literature so far, a rare frequency considering that about 10 million women take oral contraceptives. It is a real phenomenon, however, and when it occurs it can produce severe strokes or malignant hypertension. This finding is of great interest in terms of the mechanisms involved and it is relevant to other medical uses of estrogen. Here it illustrates the collision of two coexisting epidemiologic phenomena.

Returning now to the mechanisms, we observe that the renin-angiotensin-aldosterone system is a cybernetic control complex whose "push-pull" features permit a wide range of options in the maintenance of normal blood pressure. That is to say, a low aspect of one control factor is automatically compensated (if the system is working well) by a high aspect of another. Regulation of salt balance is the nominal intent of the process, and a significant measure of its efficiency is supplied by its end product — the sodium discharged in the urine, as measured over a 24-hour period. Such a measurement is meaningful, however, only if we also know how much sodium was supplied in the diet. We still cannot make a fair assessment unless we also know what all this sodium traffic is doing to the hormonal controls and whether or not the hormonal response is appropriate to blood pressure requirements. To draw an analogy: You will not find most diabetic patients if you measure only insulin and not glucose.

The field in which all these factors normally interact cuts a rather broad swath across the statistical landscape, as can be seen in Figure 2, which is a nomogram obtained from a study of normotensive medical students. It depicts the relationships, within the confines of clinically normal blood pressure, of 24-hour sodium excretion, plasma renin and aldosterone. Hypertensive patients in whom the findings are related to this nomogram can then be classified according to the level of plasma hormone — renin, most practically — and the appropriateness of this state of affairs to their level of sodium balance. Thus, there are hypertensives with high, normal and low renin — these designations being made not on absolute but on physiologic terms.

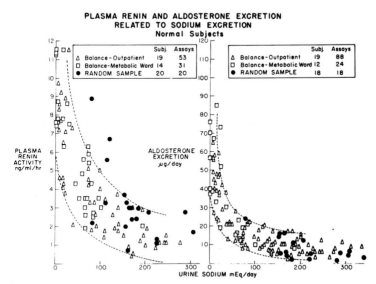

Fig. 2. Plasma renin and aldosterone excretion related to sodium excretion in normal subjects. From Laragh et al (*Amer. J. Med.*, 52:633-652, 1972).

The concept provides epidemiologists with a classification. What are the practical implications and use of it? Figure 3 illustrates one answer. It represents a population of 219 patients with essential hypertension, studied by Brunner of our group. He found 27% to be in the low, 57% in the normal and 16% in the high renin category. The significant clinical evaluation was that patients with low and normal renin were equally hypertensive, but those with high renin were markedly more hypertensive. Moreover, the group with low renin was significantly older, suggesting that they enjoyed a far more favorable mortality rate than their less physiologically compensated counterparts.

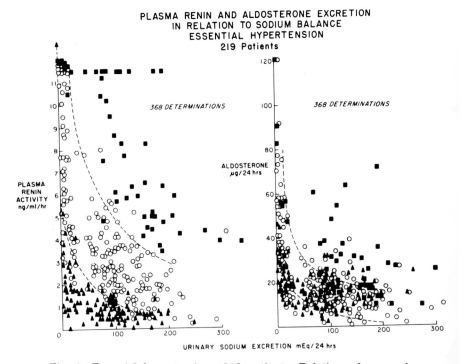

Fig. 3. Essential hypertension: 219 patients. Relation of noon plasma renin activity and of the corresponding daily aldosterone excretion to the concurrent daily rate of sodium excretion. Triangles=low renin, open circles=normal renin, squares=high renin essential hypertension. From Brunner et al (*New Eng. J. Med.*, 286:441, 1972).

Tables 1 and 2 depict a longitudinal study by Brunner covering ten years of experience with hypertensive patients. He analyzed three major events in hypertensive patients: cardiac enlargement, stroke and heart attack. He found, first of all, that low, normal or high renin patients had a fairly equal distribution of left ventricular hypertrophy, indicating a fairly equal degree or duration of high blood pressure. But the surprising finding was that in the first 59 consecutive patients with low renin essential hypertension neither a stroke nor a heart attack had occurred, whereas in the normal or high renin group, a combined incidence of 11% to 14% was experienced.

According to our statisticians, this is highly significant. It does not indicate, as some of our friendly colleagues have misinterpreted us to say, that low renin patients are utterly immortal. It just says that they are at much less risk of developing a stroke or heart attack than are the high or normal renin patients. This observation may provide an explanation for the phenomenon that those who treat high blood pressure patients have observed: the natural history of essential hypertension is not uniform. We all have seen patients with systolic blood pressures of even 300 mm Hg who have disdained all

TABLE 1. Incidence of Cardiovascular Complications

	Left Ventricular Enlargement	Strokes or Heart Attacks* total	strokes	heart attacks
LOW RENIN	12 20%	0%	0%	0%
NORMAL RENIN	18 15%	14 11%	8 6%	6 5%
HIGH RENIN	8 22%	5 14%	4 11%	2 6%
TOTAL	38 17%	19 9%	12 5%	8 4%

*One patient in high renin group had both stroke and heart attack

Modified from Brunner et al (*New Eng. J. Med.*, 286:441, 1972).

TABLE 2. Epidemiologic
and Clinical Characteristics
in Essential Hypertension

	Number of Patients	Mean Diastolic Blood Pressure mmHg	Mean Age years	Known Duration of Hypertension years	Percent Black
LOW RENIN	**59** 27%	**104.9** ±14.2	**46.5** ±11.3	**8.5** ±6.8	**42**
NORMAL RENIN	**124** 57%	**103.5** ±16.9	**37.5** ±12.0	**7.2** ±6.9	**24**
HIGH RENIN	**36** 16%	**124.0** ±19.9	**43.1** ±9.8	**6.8** ±6.2	**11**
TOTAL	**219** 100%				**27**

mean
standard deviation

Modified from Brunner et al (*New Eng. J. Med.*, 286:441, 1972).

therapy and gone on to live a long and merry life. Our studies suggest that those who beat the rap are in the low renin category. It has been well demonstrated that massive excesses of renin and aldosterone have produced vascular injury and cardiovascular damage, strokes and kidney failure in malignant hypertension. Here, we suggest that subtle excesses of renin, relative or absolute, over a protracted period of time may also be a factor in inducing vascular injury.

Another dimension for epidemiologic and clinical consideration is that when patients are profiled according to these physiologic indices, one can move beyond empiric therapy, while recognizing its proven value. In some cases it is a shotgun approach using two or three drugs. But when the endocrine profile of the hypertensive patient is known, the right and specific drug for the particular biochemical lesion can be selected.

All hypertensive drugs currently available can be simply divided into two categories — those which inhibit renin secretion and those which stimulate it. Of the renin inhibitors, the most powerful is propranolol, a beta receptor blocking drug with a checkered history as an antihypertensive agent. It is followed in diminishing order of potency by clonidine, methyldopa, reserpine and the ganglionic blockers. The renin stimulators are of two types. First are the diuretics and aldosterone blockers; they produce enormous rises in renin in all patients who take them. The reaction is a homeostatic defense response to sodium depletion. Second are the vasodilator drugs which produce reactive reninemia, too, by the baroreceptor system. Now, how can this information be put together usefully?

Figure 4 shows the findings in a patient with malignant hypertension, which is a renin-caused, renin-dependent vasculitis. The proof of that has come in recent years by observations that total nephrectomy will relieve malignant hypertension and cure the high blood pressure and the vascular lesion. This malignant hypertensive patient, with encephalopathy, weakness

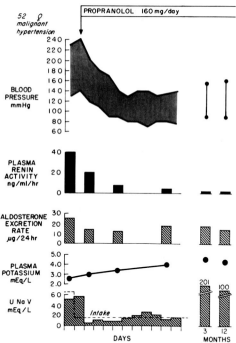

Fig. 4. Propranolol treatment alone in one patient with malignant hypertension resulting in normalization of blood pressure, plasma renin activity, plasma potassium levels and aldosterone excretion rates. These responses were well sustained over a period of 12 months on continuing propranolol therapy. The correction of blood pressure occurred without any change in sodium balance. From Bühler et al (*Amer. J. Cardiol.*, 32:511-522, 1973).

in one arm and one leg, and difficulty in speaking was treated with propranolol alone, because we knew this drug lowered renin. The treatment brought her blood pressure from 240/140 to 130/65. She has now been on propranolol alone ever since for several years and has remained normotensive. The high plasma aldosterone also came down to normal; plasma potassium (which was low because plasma aldosterone was high) came up to normal with no particular repletion; and the sodium balance shows no net change.

The approach also works on essential hypertensives who have been profiled. Figure 5 shows that propranolol alone normalizes and greatly improves the pressure in all the high

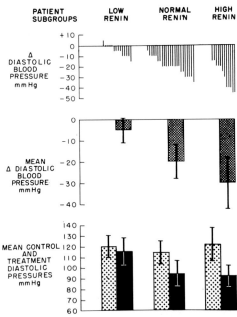

Fig. 5. Propranolol-induced changes in diastolic blood pressure in 74 patients. Absolute changes in diastolic pressure in each individual patient are depicted in the upper section. Other results are expressed as mean±SEM for the low, normal and high renin subgroups. In the lower section, the dotted bars represent control blood pressures and the solid bars pressures after propranolol administration. From Bühler et al (*Amer. J. Cardiol.*, 32:511-522, 1973).

renin patients, has an intermediate but potent effect in the normal renin patient, but fitting the theory beautifully, fails to work at all in low renin hypertension. The latter fact perhaps explains the disenchantment with results in many studies that used the drug without renin profiling.

This experience shows that an endocrine profile analysis, about ready for massive application, can point to causal mechanisms, provide information about prognosis and, more importantly, can allow the physician to predict with a high order of accuracy which drug will work in which patient.

A little exaggeration may serve to simplify and illustrate a physiologic classification of the hypertensions. Table 3 tabulates the physiologic profiles observed in the extremes of high and low renin states. It also cites the hazards and suggests appropriate treatment. The vasoconstricted high renin and the vasodilated low renin patient alike have high peripheral resistance, but the former with low plasma volume and low cardiac

TABLE 3. High Blood Pressure Mechanisms

Relatively Predominant Features

High Renin (vasoconstricted)		Low Renin (vasodilated)
High	Peripheral resistance	High
High	Aldosterone	Low to high
Low	Plasma volume	High
Low	Cardiac output	High
High	Hematocrit	Low
High	Blood urea	Low
High	Blood viscosity	Low
Low	Tissue perfusion	High
Yes	Postural hypotension	No

Clinical Examples

High renin essential	Low renin essential
Renovascular and malignant	Primary aldosteronism

Vascular Sequellae

(+)	Stroke	(−)
(+)	Heart attack	(−)
(+)	Renal damage	(−)
(+)	Retinopathy-encephalopathy	(−)

Treatments

No	Diuretics	Yes
Yes	Antirenin drugs	No
Yes	Direct vasodilators	±
Yes	Adrenergic blockers	±

From Laragh (*Amer. J. Med.*, 55:261-274, 1973).

output, and the latter with high values in these respects. Other physiologic parameters are also proposed. The high renin patient, whose aldosterone is also high, will have a richer, more viscous blood and a higher blood urea with low tissue perfusion from a constricted microcirculation and he will tend toward postural hypotension. Such a patient is the high renin essential hypertensive or the one with renovascular or malignant disease, and he is at risk of cardiovascular and cerebrovascular complications. For him, antirenin and vasodilator drugs are obviously indicated; his constricted circulation must be corrected. On the other hand, the low renin patient, who may be an essential hypertensive or one suffering from primary aldosteronism, is doing comparatively well on the physiologic indices except for his hypertension and a possibly high aldosterone level. Hemodynamically, his chief problem is his excessive volume expansion. The effective way to correct this is to dry him out with diuretics.

Obviously, not all patients fall into such neatly opposed ranks. The concept illustrated here must be understood to be a simplification, but a useful one. Like most rules it is nearly always proved by its exceptions. My hope is that the system it is based on can provide the epidemiologist with a working basis for classification in the further investigation into the nature and distribution of hypertensive disease states.

Bibliography

Brunner, H. R., Laragh, J. H., Baer, L. et al: Essential hypertension, renin and aldosterone, heart attack and stroke. *New Eng. J. Med.*, 286:441, 1972.

Brunner, H. R., Sealey, J. E. and Laragh, J. H.: Renin as a risk factor in essential hypertension: More evidence. In Laragh, J. H. (ed.): *Hypertension Manual.* New York:Dun-Donnelley Publishing Corp., 1974, pp. 71-86.

Bühler, F. R., Laragh, J. H., Vaughan, E. D., Jr. et al: The antihypertensive action of propranolol: Specific anti-renin responses in high and normal renin forms of essential, renal, renovascular and malignant hypertension. *Amer. J. Cardiol.*, 32:511-522, 1973.

Laragh, J. H.: Evaluation and care of the hypertensive patient. *Amer. J. Med.*, 52:565-569, 1972.

Laragh, J. H.: Vasoconstriction-volume analysis for understanding and treating hypertension: The use of renin and aldosterone profiles. *Amer. J. Med.*, 55:261-274, 1973.

Laragh, J. H., Baer, L., Brunner, H. R. et al: Renin, angiotensin and aldosterone system in pathogenesis and management of hypertensive vascular disease. *Amer. J. Med.*, 52:633-652, 1972.
Vaughan, E. D., Jr., Laragh, J. H., Gavras, I. et al: The volume factor in low and normal renin essential hypertension: Its treatment with either spironolactone or chlorthalidone. *Amer. J. Cardiol.*, 32:523-532, 1973.

Discussion

Dr. Langford: Some years ago, Dr. Irvine Page referred to serotonin as providing tenure for the pharmacologist. Dr. Laragh's approach is tenure for a lot of people. Let me ask the following questions: First, do you have any data on the reproducibility of typing of a person? Second, where are your low renin hypertensives coming from? Are the normal or high renin cases converting into low renin ones, or the low renin ones being recruited from people who are previously normotensive? Third, to put up a postulate, granted the correctness of your protection mechanism of low renin, some of these patients are uniquely responsive to the thiazide diuretics. You may have picked out those who were responsive to therapy and treated them before and after typing. The lower blood pressure produced by therapy then protected these individuals from cardiovascular events.

Dr. Laragh: At my age I think I have the license to take the last question first because right now it is the only one I remember. I do not believe we have tended to treat the more responsive low renin patients. Indeed, we have had treatment failures in low renin patients who do not respond to anything, just as many as we do in the other two groups. Second, they are equally hypertensive in individual cases, sometimes very impressively so. We believe diuretics work in all hypertension. Our data show no particular skewing except that about two thirds of low renin patients will respond to diuretics compared with only a third of normal renin patients. That is because there is a renin factor, we would say, in the normal renin and high renin group. But you do get an effect. The other question, does the leopard change his spots? Everybody who does renin profiling is worried about that, and only a large number of longitudinal and prospective analyses will tell us. I can only say that our patients, who are increasing in numbers, and who have been restudied and withdrawn from drugs two to six years later, nearly always have the same profile. I cannot even anecdotally tell you about someone who was normal or high who became low. I think that sequence would be a very disturbing phenomenon to any of us. Everyone agrees renin goes down with age, but the age-related trend is trivial in the data that I have seen when it is compared with the differences that we discriminate among our patients.

Dr. Miller, Maryland: You had a slide that showed that low renin had the best cardiovascular outcome, high renin had the worst, and normal renin was intermediate. I think we need to talk about relative risk in an area like this as opposed to saying that something is normal or had the worst outcome. What makes a renin normal? If we are going to do epidemiological studies on a biochemical parameter, we ought to use numbers, and later as one starts to philosophize maybe employ these nice terms. The other comment is to caution that if your people all came from hospitals, they were there because they were sick. One should not jump to the conclusion too fast about what normal renin really represents in the population. How sensitive is your method, and could Dr. Kirkendall repeat it?

Dr. Laragh: I think your points are well taken. First of all, I would only stand behind the data for the population that we studied. I would ask anybody here to study any other populations; they might find something different. I would not say for a minute that what we found in these 400+ patients applies to everybody, but that is all we can handle. I think we need to go on to see what ambulant patients and normal subjects do in the free-ranging situation. However, if history is any guide, the results will probably not differ dramatically from a sample this size. I also agree with you that the terminology is troublesome. The reproducibility of methods becomes a tactical problem. In our own studies the pattern never varies. I should not use the word "never," but I could test somebody 50 times — if he was high renin and he would remain high. The translation of that into mass study always has a lag time and always an error. These tests, even though they have problems, as Dr. Kirkendall indicated, are not that tough. For example, it was the same with such measurements as blood cholesterol or glucose, which for many years were epidemiologically unreliable. We are involved now with this, transferring it from the research laboratory to the commercial laboratories. I do not think that is beyond solution and I think we have a tactical problem which probably merits a symposium of its own, but I think it is near solution.

Dr. Kirkendall: I think if we pay as much attention to the plasma renin activity measurements as we have to the measurement of the blood pressure by indirect methods, we will be fine.

Dr. Tuomilehto, Finland: I noticed in your material that the low renin group had a higher average age than the normal renin group. Do you feel that it is due to some different symptomatology so that the low renin group is asymptomatic and seeking medical help later?

Dr. Laragh: The fact that the low renin group, as a group, is a little older has several interesting implications. From our own prejudice, it means that they have less vascular damage even though they are older. From your point of view we do not recognize them until older. Maybe they do not get it until they are older, but maybe they get it just as early as everybody else but have a much longer latent period before anything sends them to the physician. There are a number of things here about that which would need some special analysis.

Dr. Sackett: There is a third explanation for your low renin group being older. They could represent a group of survivors, the susceptibles from which have been wiped out in an earlier point in time. Second, could you describe the increase in plasma renin activity which occurs with the administration of thiazide drugs? These drugs have a good record in terms of lowering the occurrence of hypertensive complications. Is it your suggestion that these benefits would have even been greater had drugs like propranolol been used in some of these high renin, essential hypertensives?

Dr. Laragh: Your point is well taken. On diuretic therapy, renin is often very high, five- to sixfold or more than in the control period, and it stays high. Now, I would like to say — and I do not have the proof for it — that high blood pressure, the level of the pressure per se, is a risk factor. Instead, we just say that if you have high blood pressure and a high renin, you are more vasoconstricted and that you are much worse off than if you were not vasoconstricted. When you give a thiazide diuretic and the renin goes up, it rises only because the pressure goes down. It is a reaction to depletion of body volume and sodium stores. I believe there is a lot of evidence from various circumstances to indicate that reactive hyperreninemia is not a risk factor. For instance, the cirrhotic patient has enormous renins with no vascular damage, and he is trying to keep his blood volume normal. The hypertensive on a thiazide, who develops a reactive or compensatory high renin, is trying to keep his blood volume in bounds and maintain his pressure. His pressure has dropped down and he is making renin reactively. That is different than making it inappropriately as an untreated hypertensive does.

Dr. Simpson, New Zealand: I think when this work is extrapolated into the field of therapy, particularly with beta blockers, that it is a little oversimplified. To say that a patient with a high cardiac output should not be treated preferentially with a beta blocker is looking at it purely from the point of view of renin. Obviously, these drugs do many other things and certainly I believe beta blockers are very satisfactory in many cases of hypertension, not, I think, only those with high renins. There is also difficulty in the fact that some beta blockers are less efficient at lowering renin than others. Finally from the purely practical point of view, I am a bit uncertain about the advisability of using purely beta blockers in cases of very severe, accelerated hypertension. I certainly lost one patient in trying to use beta blockers in an acute stage.

Dr. Laragh: I think your points are pertinent. While we predict a high cardiac output in low renin patients, we have not proven that. Nevertheless, I believe it has to be something close to that if they are volume-expanded. I think you have a cause and effect presumption in your mind because propranolol and beta blockers certainly lower cardiac output; but in my opinion, there is very fragile or no evidence to show that is how they lower high blood pressure. Blood pressure does not go down at all on intravenous propranolol, but the cardiac output often goes down 30%-40%. The published world literature has had a great deal of trouble with this, with many groups saying one thing and then changing in subsequent studies. I think the best explanation for the major blood pressure lowering effect of beta blockers is the effect on peripheral resistance. This can be clearly related to renin. Some people say the new beta blockers do not lower renin, but we have rechecked some of our data and we get a massive lowering of renin with every beta blocker we have ever tested. I think some of the studies in question were done in the recumbent position where we would agree the effect of beta blockers is apt to be minimal. I think the idea that cardiac output is the main factor in the antihypertensive effect is certainly a respectable idea, but it is one without any data to prove it so far. Finally, when you lower blood pressure in a malignant hypertensive, cardiac work is so enormously relieved and the risk of failure is eased. That is the best thing that you can do for the myocardium. Much more benefit derives from that than from any inotropic effect that you would get from digitalis, let us say. We do believe that heart failure is a major risk of propranolol in low renin patients, because there it fails to lower blood pressure but lowers cardiac power, and then failure is a real problem. I think in that framework I would also agree with you. One has to be very careful with a negative inotropic drug in a very sick patient on the brink of heart failure. We did this study to show the relevance of renin to the malignant syndrome. We didn't mean to suppose that you would obliterate all other reasonable approaches to a sick patient in whom this negative inotropic effect could be adverse.

Mrs. Stamler, Illinois: Dr. Laragh, your data indicate a higher percentage of persons with low renin among your black patients as compared to your white patients. How does that fit in with the general epidemiologic data in the United States, both morbidity and mortality, showing that hypertension is more severe in blacks, causes hypertensive heart disease at an earlier age, et cetera?

Dr. Laragh: Right. There is no question that blacks have much more hypertension of all types than whites and, as you indicate, that young blacks under the age of 40 have a very severe form of hypertension, replete with malignant hypertension, kidney failure, strokes, and death, much more than whites. Now, there is also no question that there are a lot of older blacks with mild hypertension living a long life. Our data suggest that there are at least two populations among the blacks. Whenever we get a hypertensive black between the age of 20 and 40 and do our renin typing, it is nearly always normal, and sometimes high — we have only seen one black under the age of 40 who had the low renin pattern. This young group as you know is the one so prone to vascular injury. On the other hand, among the older blacks over the age of 50, low renin hypertension is the predominant form, and those blacks are not prone to the vascular damage found in the young blacks. At least, such is our experience, and I think we can cite studies, including one here from Chicago, which suggest that, too. So we explain it by two populations of different risk: young blacks with bad hypertension who rarely exhibit low renin, older blacks with indolent hypertension, with low renin common in the latter group.

Dr. Meneely, Louisiana: There seems to be a growing body of evidence from animal experimental data which suggests that there are break points in the hypertensive pattern. If you are following an animal which appears to have benign essential hypertension, suddenly the blood pressure may start to rise steeply. The syndrome turns into another disease, with quite a different clinical pattern. I would be interested to hear whether you have seen this abrupt onset of a "malignant" phase?

Dr. Laragh: No, but I think the break point, as you call it, is something that we would all like to be able to anticipate, obviously. Perhaps others in the group can speak with more involvement with animals than I can, but I was impressed with the fact that the stroke-prone strain of Okimoto rats was significantly more hypertensive than the stroke-resistant animals. I don't think that there is any question that a rising pressure is a factor inducing what you call the break point of a stroke or a heart attack or kidney failure. What our data suggest — and I certainly have no specific evidence for it — is that if in addition to a rising pressure the patient also has renin-associated increased vasoconstriction, he is at the maximum risk. So the extrapolation of our data, which need to be proved or tested further, is that plasma renin is an indicator of risk, too. We believe that we have high renin patients who are essential who then go on and have the so-called break point developing malignant hypertension or renal failure or a stroke. I should tell you that of that 17% with high renin in our group many of them have fallen into trouble with strokes and heart attacks and

that continues to be so. In fact, I think the world experience
indicates that high renin essential hypertension is the worst kind
to have. The only dispute that remains is that some people hang
tenaciously to the view that normal renin is no worse than low.
I think that everyone thinks high renin is bad, or, at least, if
they don't, I would be surprised.

Dr. Berglund, Sweden: I would like to throw some new
wood onto the fire of the discussion by reporting on the
relation of plasma renin activity (PRA) to blood pressure and
hypertensive organ manifestations in an epidemiological study.

Figure 1 shows the criteria for selection of the material.
From among all the 50-year-old men in Göteborg (n=1122) 863
came to a screening examination which was a part of a primary
preventive trial. A random 10% subsample was drawn and after
exclusion of ten subjects with hypertension, the reference group

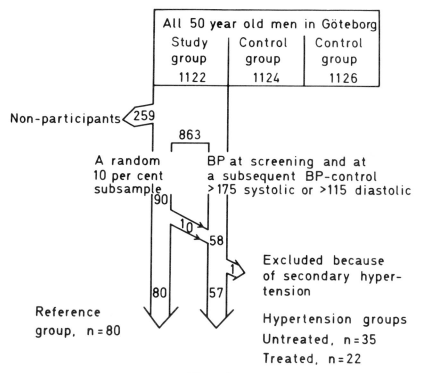

Figure 1.

(n=80) was created. All subjects who at screening and a subsequent blood pressure measurement had blood pressure above 175 systolic or above 115 diastolic and were not on antihypertensive treatment created the untreated hypertension group (n=35). In the reference group the distribution was roughly normal and slightly skewed to the right. In the hypertension group the mode seemed to be somewhat displaced to the left and the positive skewness was more pronounced.

In order to study how low, normal and high PRA with regard to sodium excretion were related to blood pressure and hypertensive organ manifestations, an analysis adapting the technique of the Laragh group was used. Figure 2 shows the relationship between PRA and urinary sodium excretion in the reference group. Arbitrarily drawn borders for the normal relationship between these two variables are shown in the figure. Ninety percent of the subjects had values within these borders.

Figure 3 shows the same relationship between PRA and urinary sodium excretion in the untreated hypertension group. The borders for the normal relationship divide the group into those with low (n=10), normal (n=16) and high PRA (n=8) with regard to sodium excretion.

From the low to the normal to the high PRA group, there was a *decrease* in resting blood pressure and an increase in GFR. That is the opposite of what Dr. Laragh and his group have previously found. Furthermore, with regard to sodium excretion, those with low renin had a reversed diurnal rhythm of urine excretion with small volume and high concentration during the day and a low urinary sodium excretion. Although not statistically significant, those with high PRA tended to have a lower frequency of signs of left ventricular hypertrophy on x-ray, of electrophysiological signs of heart involvement, and of signs of decreased left ventricular distensibility, ie, a more benign hypertension. Finally, a question.

Dr. Laragh, I wonder whether the better response to propranolol treatment in the high renin group which you showed us could be due to the fact that the high renin group in your material had a significantly higher initial diastolic blood pressure than the normal and low renin groups?

PRA (ng/ml/h)

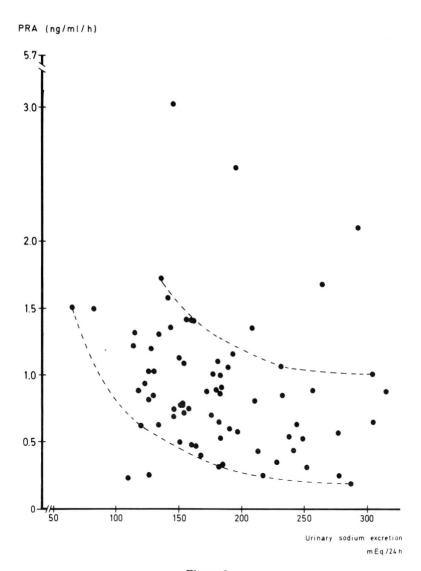

Figure 2.

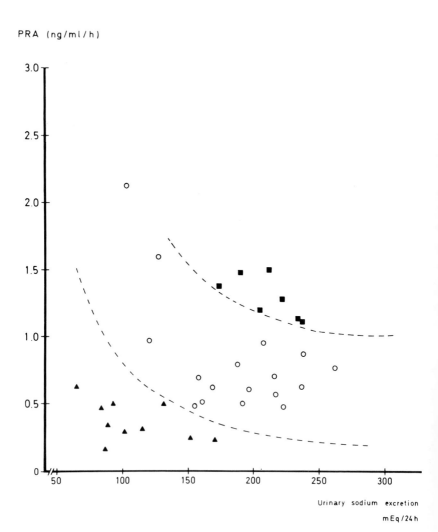

Figure 3.

Dr. Laragh: You just said that your low renin men had higher blood pressures.

Dr. Berglund: Yes, they had.

Dr. Laragh: You asked me the question, maybe propranolol works because they have higher pressure?

Dr. Berglund: I wonder whether they have higher blood pressure from the beginning.

Dr. Laragh: Well, the problem with that is that there is no evidence as far as I know that the degree of prior elevated pressure has anything to do with the antihypertensive action of a drug; in fact, it is usually the reverse. So, I don't understand your suggestion that the drug works in high renin cases because they have more hypertension. That is not known to be a relationship with any other drug, isn't that right? You are saying that the bigger they are, the harder they fall. I don't believe that is true of blood pressure. The higher it is, usually, the harder it is to get it down. Even so, that would have to be proven. I don't think that is the explanation for why propranolol works in high renin. I think that is making it hard. Rather, I think that when we virtually eliminate renin and the blood pressure goes down, the coincidence is certainly so striking that one has to deal with that as the best bet until you find a better one. But there could be other bets. You say that the low renin cases have a reduced GFR.

Dr. Berglund: Yes, the low renin group had a reduced GFR compared to the normal and the high renin groups. They also had a tendency, although not statistically significant, toward lower urinary epinephrine excretion and toward a higher prevalence of heart involvement.

Dr. Laragh: Yes, well, there are several questions. I am aware of some of your data. It is surprising to me that your low renins are more hypertensive than any other groups. I can't explain that. But what really has my head scratching — and actually we are doing some studies because you did — is that you say that the low renin group has the highest renal resistance. We haven't done a study yet, but we are willing to bet our shirt that the high renin group is the most vasoconstricted and has the highest renal resistance. As for the low, I don't know. I only know some studies, such as Dr. Hollenberg's in Boston, and I believe that he thinks as we do that the low renin group has relative renal hyperemia. I cannot understand the low renin group having the most vasoconstriction within the kidney, which is what you are saying. Now, I accept your data, but I can tell you that we are going to look into it.

Dr. Tobian: Did the study from Göteborg, Sweden, really show that the low renin patients had a higher blood pressure than the high renin patients? Did I understand that correctly?

Dr. Berglund: Yes, that is right. When the patients had rested for one hour in a soundproof room, there was a statistically significant difference. The low renin group had a blood pressure of 173/108 and the high renin group had a blood pressure of only 136/88, so there was a very big difference after one hour's rest.

Dr. Dollery: Surely, much of the difference between Dr. Laragh's and Dr. Berglund's group is, essentially, in selection. The Swedish group is dealing with a population sample, whereas Dr. Laragh is dealing with a clinic sample, heavily biased toward malignant hypertension and accelerated hypertension coming into the hospital, and that is a high renin group. It is also a group with a bad prognosis and high complication incidence, so I don't think that there is really any difference between what the two are saying. My personal bias would be to look at the Swedish group's data as being the more reliable, as to what use one can make of renin data in the population at large, although Dr. Laragh's data may be more applicable to a clinic population.

I strongly resist this categorization into low, normal and high renin. What is the statistical justification for this division? On what statistical basis is the division made? I have never heard a clear explanation of that. Clearly it is a reasonably even distribution curve, with somewhat of a skew toward high values in the hypertensives. Where does one draw the cutting points? I am not in the renin field, but I have heard many papers at meetings where other groups do not seem exactly to be able to reproduce, for example, the responsiveness of particular categories of renin hypertensives to beta blockers. We have done two trials since this work came out: one with propranolol and the other with ICI-66082, and in neither trial is there a strong relationship between either the initial renin or the change in renin and the blood pressure response to the beta blocking drug.

My feeling would be that one has to be rather cautious in translating these data into action in the population and community.

Dr. Laragh: I think that those points are certainly worth raising. We all need more data but you must realize that the Göteborg data are based upon a handful of patients, as compared to our data, which are based upon many times the number. All assembled, it is extremely unlikely that low renin patients have the highest renal resistance and the highest blood pressures. I don't think that anybody else but the Göteborg group has found the low renin to have the highest pressures, so I think that what we would have to do is take their data, do the renins blind and exchange them, and we would be most pleased to do that. Also, if you look at their data, the analysis is not done to the advantage of discrimination. There is nobody on a low salt diet, and very few numbers; there is no discriminatory power. I don't think that he is in a position, when he does it out on that side of the curve, to do the thing properly. All I ask you to do is to look at the numbers because we have to work with numbers. So I don't think that that can be translated epidemiologically on such a pitifully small number measured at the high part of the salt curve when the implications of what he has said, interesting as they may be, have not been found by anybody else. Much of what we have done has been found by other people. Our classification has been reproduced in many laboratories. Dr. Williams has a similar approach. I don't say that it is identical, but I think that he will say that he finds low, normal and high, and that we can repeatedly identify them and so can most of the workers in this country. You have to look at it that way. To say that the clinic population is altogether different from a handful of 30 or 40 people who walked in the door in Göteborg is a very daring and interesting statement. I think that the renal resistance data will have to come into play. As far as the beta blockers in renin are concerned, there are two or three reports in the world literature — and we can only deal with the published data — in which the renin seems to go up rather than down. In data reported in the *British Medical Journal*, patients were measured in the recumbent position; I don't think that a renin in the recumbent position is relevant to the study of propranolol. We have checked some of those very blockers and we have found them to nearly obliterate renin. Now, that doesn't mean that an alternate explanation is not in the cards. I think that a study has to be done in which the physiological test and the renin test can stand a double-blind exchange.

Dynamic Studies of Aldosterone Secretion in Patients With Essential Hypertension

Gordon H. Williams, M.D. and Robert G. Dluhy, M.D.

Introduction

Previous studies of the renin-angiotensin-aldosterone axis in patients with essential hypertension have occasionally revealed abnormalities in aldosterone secretion[1,2] or more commonly hyporesponsive plasma renin activity following volume depletion.[3-9] However, most studies have assessed these responses at a single point in time before and after achievement of sodium balance. The present study was performed in patients with essential hypertension who had a normal renin response to sodium restriction and upright posture in order to determine if there were abnormalities in the acute regulation of renin, angiotensin, or aldosterone. The acute responses of these parameters were assessed in sodium-restricted subjects following intravenous volume expansion with isotonic saline or following assumption of the upright posture.

Materials and Methods

Twenty-eight patients with essential hypertension who were previously documented to have normal renin responses to

These investigations were supported in part by the Smith Kline & French Foundation and the John A. Hartford Foundation, Grant 9893. The clinical studies were carried out on The Clinical Research Center of the Peter Bent Brigham Hospital supported by Grant 8-MO1-FR-31-06.

Gordon H. Williams, M.D., *Associate Professor of Medicine, Harvard Medical School; Director, Department of Endocrinology, Peter Bent Brigham Hospital, Boston, Mass.* and Robert G. Dluhy, M.D., *Assistant Professor of Medicine, Harvard Medical School; Associate Director, Department of Endocrinology, Peter Bent Brigham Hospital, Boston, Mass.*

sodium restriction and upright posture[10,11] were studied at the Clinical Research Center of the Peter Bent Brigham Hospital and their responses compared with 18 normal controls.[12,13] Secondary causes of hypertension were excluded by a rapid sequence intravenous pyelogram, urinalysis, serum creatinine, serum electrolytes and 24-hour urinary VMA, metanephrine and 17-hydroxycorticoid determinations which were required to be normal in all patients.

Protocols

All antihypertensive medications were discontinued at least two weeks prior to admission. All patients were maintained on a constant activity pattern simulating normal daily activity and were fed an isocaloric 10 mEq sodium/100 mEq potassium diet. Twenty-four-hour urines were collected daily and analyzed for sodium, potassium and creatinine. The following determinations were performed on each blood sample by methods previously described[14,15]: plasma renin activity (PRA), angiotensin II (AII), plasma aldosterone (PA), plasma cortisol and serum sodium and potassium. All studies were performed when subjects achieved metabolic balance after an overnight fast and supine for at least 12 hours.

Ten normotensive and 14 hypertensive subjects received an infusion of 0.9% sodium chloride at a constant rate of 500 ml/hr for six hours beginning at 8 a.m. During the infusion study, blood samples were obtained every 10 minutes for 30 minutes and then at one, two, four, six and eight hours. In 14 hypertensive and eight normotensive subjects, blood samples were obtained supine and then 3, 5, 10, 20, 30, 60, 90, 120 and 240 minutes after assuming the upright posture. Upright activity was maintained by walking at a constant rate (3-4 ft/sec) for four hours on a 300 foot course. The upright posture study was repeated in the same subjects in balance on a 200 mEq sodium/100 mEq potassium diet.

Results

Saline Infusion

Normal controls. Figure 1 summarizes the mean results in the previously reported normal control subjects.[12] Mean PRA levels declined rapidly after the start of the saline infusion with a significant fall by 10 minutes and a 50% decline by 60 minutes. The pattern of response for plasma angiotensin II and aldosterone was almost identical to the PRA response except that aldosterone did not significantly decline until 20 to 30 minutes. The mean 24-hour urine sodium and potassium excretions on the day of saline infusion were 180 ± 16 and 72 ± 3 mEq/24 hr, respectively, while the mean weight gain was 1.2 ± 0.2 kg.

Hypertensive subjects. Figure 2 shows the changes of the various parameters in response to the saline infusion in all 14 essential hypertensive patients.[10] Mean PRA levels did not significantly decline until 60 minutes and did not fall to 50% of control until 120-240 minutes after the start of the saline

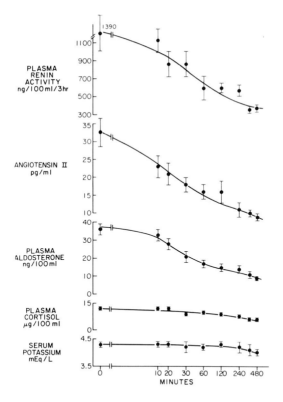

Fig. 1. Mean response of PRA, AII, and aldosterone to the infusion of normal saline at a rate of 500 cm³/hr for 6 hours. Responses are plotted against time on a log scale.

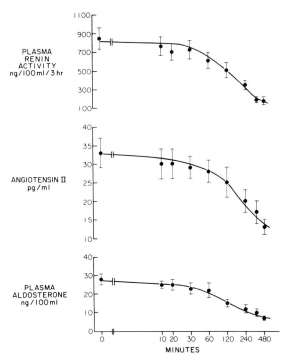

Fig. 2. The mean ± SEM of plasma renin activity, angiotensin II and aldosterone in 14 hypertensive subjects following infusion of 0.9% sodium chloride (500 ml/hr for six hours). Subjects were in balance on a 10 mEq Na/100 mEq K diet.

infusion. Thereafter, the rate of decline of PRA was similar to the control subjects and by 360-480 minutes all hypertensive subjects demonstrated normal suppression of PRA. Plasma AII responded similarly except a significant fall from baseline did not occur until 120 minutes. Likewise, PA levels did not significantly decline below control until 120 minutes, compared to the normal response where a significant decline occurred at 20-30 minutes. Throughout all saline infusion studies, changes in PRA, AII and PA were significantly correlated with each other. There were no significant changes in serum sodium or potassium, and plasma cortisol levels exhibited only the expected diurnal fall during the infusion studies.

Five of the 14 hypertensive subjects demonstrated a response to saline infusion identical to the normotensive

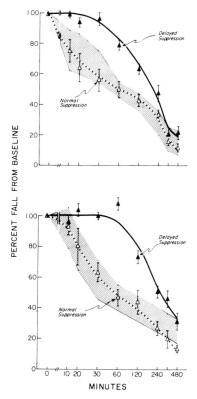

Fig. 3. The mean ± SEM percent change from control of plasma renin activity and plasma aldosterone following infusion of 0.9% sodium chloride (500 ml/hr for six hours) in 14 hypertensive patients with a normal renin response to sodium restriction. The response of normal subjects (mean ± S.D.) is shaded. The renin responsive patients were divided into those with normal suppression (5) and those with a delayed suppression (9).

controls (Fig. 3). Mean PRA levels fell significantly by 20 minutes and had fallen 45% below baseline by 60 minutes. Likewise, AII and aldosterone levels both significantly declined by 30 minutes and fell approximately 50% below baseline by 60 minutes. As a reflection of intravascular volume expansion, the mean hematocrit levels declined to 97% of control at 30 minutes and 87% of control at 360 minutes, similar to the response in normotensive subjects.[10] Nine hypertensive patients demonstrated a significantly delayed response of the renin-aldosterone system to saline infusion (Fig. 3). The mean PRA levels did not fall significantly from control until 120 minutes and a 50% decline did not occur until after 240 minutes. Plasma AII levels and PA also did not decline below control until 120 minutes and did not show a 50% reduction until 240-360 minutes. Mean hematocrit levels declined to 94% of control at 30 minutes and 82% of control at 360 minutes.

Urinary sodium excretion on the saline infusion day in the hypertensive patients as a whole (124 ± 21 mEq/24 hr) was significantly less (p < 0.05) than that seen in normotensive controls. In addition, the nine hypertensive patients with delayed renin-aldosterone suppression following saline infusion excreted significantly less sodium (92 ± 17 mEq/24 hr) and gained significantly more weight (p < 0.05) than those with normal suppression (178 ± 38 mEq/24 hr) or normal controls (180 ± 16 mEq/24 hr). In addition, potassium excretion was greater (p < 0.05) in the hypertensive delayed responders (88 ± 6 mEq/24 hr) than the normal responders (73 ± 3 mEq/24 hr) or normotensive subjects (72 ± 3 mEq/24 hr).

There were no significant differences between the two groups of hypertensive patients with regard to age; duration or level of blood pressure; renal function (ie, creatinine clearance and IVP); or admission serum or urine sodium and potassium.

Upright Posture Study

Normal controls. In eight normal subjects on a 10 mEq sodium/100 mEq potassium diet, the mean 24-hour urine sodium excretion was 6 ± 1 and potassium 71 ± 2 mEq.[1][3] Basal PRA (4.5 ± 0.8 ng/ml/hr) and AII levels (42 ± 9 pg/ml) increased at the earliest (1 min) sampling period but a significant rise did not occur until after five minutes of assuming the upright posture (Fig. 4). A significant increase above basal aldosterone levels (33 ± 6 ng/100 ml) did not occur until 20 minutes after assuming the upright position. There was a twofold increase in all parameters by 20-60 minutes with a peak three- to fourfold increase occurring between 90 and 150 minutes. The levels then plateaued for an additional 60-90 minutes and at the final sampling period, there was a slight decline. There were no significant differences in the serum sodium or potassium levels throughout the study and plasma cortisol showed the expected diurnal fall.

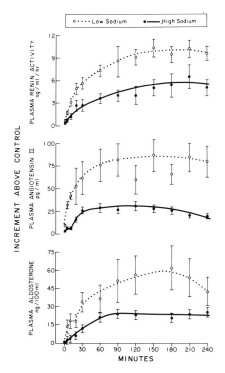

Fig. 4. Increments (mean ± SEM) above control of plasma renin activity, angiotensin II and plasma aldosterone following the assumption of upright posture in normal subjects on low (10 mEq) or high (200 mEq) sodium intakes.

In the same eight normal subjects on a 200 mEq sodium/100 mEq potassium intake, mean 24-hour urine sodium excretion was 203 ± 12 and potassium 78 ± 3 mEq. As expected, all supine control values were significantly lower on the high sodium than on the low sodium intake. In contrast to the sodium-restricted study, significant increments above the basal renin (1.6 ± 0.4 ng/ml/hr) and AII levels (19 ± 4 pg/ml) did not occur until 20-30 minutes after assuming the upright posture (Fig. 4). Plasma aldosterone levels similarly demonstrated a delay in response to upright posture. Peak levels were again reached by 90-120 minutes, plateaued for another 90-120 minutes, but did not decline toward the end of the study. Plasma sodium and potassium did not change, while plasma cortisol showed only the expected diurnal fall.

In both sodium-restricted and sodium-loaded subjects, there were significant positive correlations between the plasma renin and plasma aldosterone responses to postural change. However, the slopes of the regression relationships were significantly different ($p < 0.0001$) on the two dietary intakes (Fig. 5). Thus, a given increment in plasma renin activity was associated with a greater increment in aldosterone levels on the sodium-restricted compared to the sodium-loaded diet.

Hypertensive subjects. Figure 6 correlates the plasma renin activity and aldosterone responses to upright posture in 14 essential hypertensive patients on a sodium-restricted diet.[11] Nine responded normally while five had altered response patterns with decreased plasma aldosterone levels for given levels of PRA. While the abnormal responders achieved normal plasma aldosterone levels in response to upright posture, their mean levels of upright PRA were significantly greater than normal (18 ± 20 ng/ml/hr vs 38 ± 3 ng/ml/hr). Thus, the ratio of the increment of aldosterone to the increment of renin

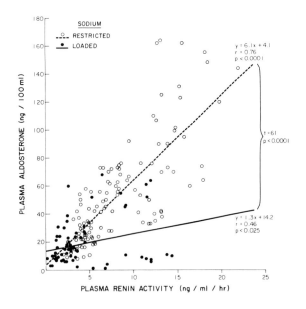

Fig. 5. Regression relationships between posture-induced changes in plasma renin activity and plasma aldosterone in sodium-restricted and sodium-loaded subjects.

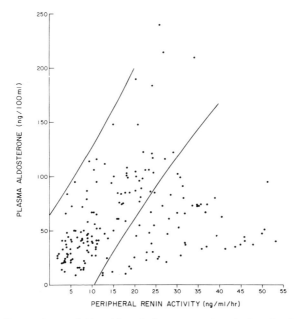

Fig. 6. Regression relationships between posture-induced changes in plasma renin activity and plasma aldosterone in 14 sodium-restricted hypertensive patients. The 99% confidence intervals of the responses of normal subjects are given by the solid lines.

activity was less in the abnormal response group (all less than 2.3), while all normal responders were greater (Fig. 7). There were no significant differences between the normal and abnormal hypertensive subjects with regard to age; duration or level of hypertension; renal function; or admission or study day sodium and potassium levels.

The mean response patterns were similar when the same subjects had upright posture studies repeated on a 200 mEq sodium diet. Although separation into the same two groups was more difficult, the abnormal responders had higher basal and upright levels of PRA, normal PA levels and a lowered aldosterone to renin increment ratio compared to the normal responders (Fig. 8). Thus, on high and low sodium intakes, a group of patients with essential hypertension with normal plasma renin activity following sodium restriction and upright posture had an altered renin-aldosterone relationship which was more readily appreciated on a sodium restricted diet.

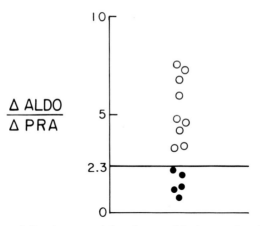

Fig. 7. Ratio of the increment in plasma aldosterone to plasma renin activity induced by upright posture in 14 hypertensive subjects. Open circles represent the normal and closed circles the abnormal responders with a clear separation of the two groups at a ratio of 2.3.

Discussion

There have been few investigations of the acute responsiveness of the renin-angiotensin-aldosterone axis. Assumption of the upright posture or acute volume depletion after furosemide administration has been reported to produce significant increments in PA levels within 30-60 minutes.[16-18] Return to the supine position led to a 50% fall in PRA within 5-10 minutes.[17] Studies of acute volume expansion have been limited but suggest a rapid suppression of renin and aldosterone secretion. Pickens and Enoch reported that PRA fell 37% from control four hours after volume expansion with 500 ml dextran infusion.[19] Kem, Weinberger, Mayes and Nugent described that plasma aldosterone levels fell to less than 50% of control after a four-hour saline infusion (2 liters) and assumption of the supine position.[20] The present study extends these observations during the early time period (0-60 min) and demonstrates that in the sodium-depleted state, the renin-angiotensin-aldosterone axis can be rapidly suppressed by small volumes of sodium chloride or rapidly activated by assuming the upright posture in normal subjects. Furthermore, the relationship between postural-induced changes in PRA and PA was significantly altered by the state of sodium balance with increased glomerulosa cell sensitivity induced by dietary sodium restriction. This enhanced

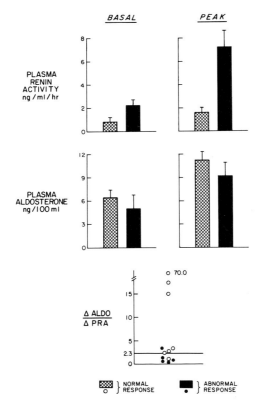

Fig. 8. Mean ± SEM of plasma aldosterone and renin activity responses to upright posture in 14 hypertensive subjects on a 200 mEq Na/100 mEq K diet. The patients were divided into normal and abnormal groups according to their renin-aldosterone posture responses during sodium restriction.

adrenal sensitivity associated with dietary sodium restriction is not only seen with postural changes, since previous studies in normal subjects have demonstrated a similar enhancement with ACTH[21,22] and angiotensin infusions.[23,24] Finally, this important influence of dietary sodium on adrenal sensitivity indicates that random upright hormone measurements on unspecified sodium intakes would not be usful in assessing the renin-angiotensin-aldosterone axis in normal or hypertensive subjects.

The present data suggest that patients with essential hypertension who have normal renin responsiveness to sodium restriction and upright posture can be divided into two subgroups, either on the basis of their renin-aldosterone responses to upright posture or to saline infusion. Sixty-five percent of the hypertensive patients studied had a delayed suppression of PRA, AII, and PA following isotonic saline infusion. Further evidence that there were two distinct populations of patients was the significant difference between the time necessary to produce a significant (40%) fall in PRA in the slowest responder (60 min) in comparison with the fastest delayed responder (180 min).

There have been relatively few studies of patients with essential hypertension assessing the acute response of the renin-angiotensin-aldosterone axis following volume expansion. Kem and co-workers[20] reported that the plasma renin and aldosterone responses of 18 patients with essential hypertension on an ad lib diet before and after a four hour infusion of saline were normal. Since the present study demonstrates that subjects in all hypertensive subgroups achieved comparable suppression after four hours of saline infusion, it is not surprising that similar abnormalities were not observed in the patients of Kem et al. Krakoff et al reported the plasma renin response in subjects with essential hypertension on a 95 mEq sodium intake following infusion of isotonic saline over a 60-minute period.[25] The authors concluded that plasma renin fell to a variable degree following infusion of isotonic saline in subjects with essential hypertension. However, examination of their data indicates that their renin-responsive hypertensive group can also be subdivided into two groups. Only three of their nine subjects showed a significant (40%-50%) 60-minute postsaline infusion decline in plasma renin activity, a proportion similar to the 35% reported in the present study. These three subjects also had a mean sodium excretion of 90 mEq/3 hr in contrast to 46 mEq/3 hr in the individuals who had a less significant fall in renin activity.

The reasons for the different response patterns of the renin-responsive essential hypertensive patients following saline infusion are not clear. Subjects with normal and delayed suppression did not appear different with regard to baseline parameters. Mean age, distribution of female to male and white to black, duration and severity of hypertension, and urine sodium and potassium on admission and on the day prior to saline infusion were the same in the two groups. The two groups also seemed to be in the same volume state prior to saline infusion. While the delayed suppression group did lose more weight and had slightly higher hematocrits after achieving sodium balance, their sodium-restricted upright plasma renin levels and aldosterone secretion rates on the day prior to the study tended to be lower. Further, since the decline in hematocrits following saline infusion was comparable or greater in the delayed suppression group, it is unlikely that these subjects were more volume depleted prior to the infusion or that their abnormal response pattern represents a difference in the magnitude of intravascular volume expansion. Thus, one possibility is that the delayed suppression group is simply less sensitive to a comparable degree of volume expansion. This could occur if there was a higher receptor threshold or a sluggish response system. If this were so, a similar sluggish response to sodium restriction in these subjects might he anticipated. Because none was found, either the response system is not altered or the chronicity of the stimulus from sodium restriction is able to overcome the deficiency. Alternatively, the data could be explained by an altered response to the infusion of sodium per se. Recent studies in normal men have provided evidence for a sodium-dependent mechanism that can suppress renin and aldosterone secretion independent of changes in intravascular volume.[12,25] (Fig. 9). While these studies do not distinguish between renin regulation by a sodium-dependent intrarenal mechanism versus a change in extrarenal-extracellular fluid, they strongly suggest that sodium has a role independent of its ability to expand intravascular volume in regulating renin release. Thus, it is possible that the delayed suppression seen in some hypertensive subjects in the present study reflects a loss of sensitivity of this sodium-sensing mechanism.

An abnormal renin-aldosterone relationship was also seen in patients with essential hypertension following assumption of the upright posture. Sixty-five percent had normal postural responses while 35% had increased levels of PRA for the level of aldosterone achieved. The difference between the normal and abnormal response groups was not related to age; duration or level of blood pressure; renal function; or sodium-potassium balance. The greater than normal renin postural increment in the abnormal response group could be related to the greater

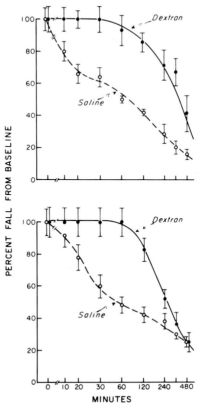

Fig. 9. Comparison of the rate of response of PRA and aldosterone to saline and dextran infusions. Results are expressed as the mean ± SEM percent fall from the baseline plotted against time on a log scale.

volume deficit recorded in these subjects as they achieved low sodium balance (3.4 ± 0.5 vs. 1.6 ± 0.3 kg). The inappropriately normal plasma aldosterone levels recorded in the presence of elevated levels of PRA did not appear to be related to a change in aldosterone metabolism or potassium balance, since the secretion rate of aldosterone and plasma potassium levels were comparable in the two groups. Furthermore, since the abnormal interrelationship was seen in the same patients under conditions of sodium loading or sodium restriction, it is unlikely that volume contraction per se can explain the altered renin-aldosterone relationship. Thus, it is possible that hypertensive patients with an abnormal renin-aldosterone response demonstrate decreased glomerulosa cell sensitivity to levels of AII. In fact, the renin-aldosterone regression relationship in the sodium-restricted state in the abnormal responder subgroup is similar to that observed in normal subjects on a high sodium intake.[13]

The role of these abnormalities in the pathogenesis of essential hypertension is speculative. The renin-responsive group with delayed suppression had a subnormal natriuresis following saline loading. The present study does not characterize the pattern of natriuresis, since excretion measurements were only obtained over the entire 24-hour period encompassing the day of saline infusion. Thus, it is impossible to temporally relate changes in the renin-angiotensin-aldosterone axis with changes in sodium excretion. However, if we speculate that the renin-angiotensin-aldosterone axis mediates this subnormal natriuresis, it is likely that the delayed suppression of AII is more important because AII has a major role in modifying the renal excretion of sodium and water, presumably through its effect on renal blood flow.[26-32] Moreover, the sodium-retentive tendency and failure to normally suppress AII levels in this subgroup could combine to elevate arterial pressure since sodium enhances the pressor effect of AII. Finally, hypertensive subjects with abnormal renin-aldosterone postural responses appear to require higher than normal levels of PRA and AII to achieve normal levels of aldosterone. Thus, it is speculated that increased levels of AII are required in order to modulate the renin-angiotensin-aldosterone volume feedback loop with increased levels of arterial blood pressure as a potential secondary side effect.

References

1. Collins, R. D., Weinberger, M. H., Dowdy, A. J. et al: Abnormally sustained aldosterone secretion during salt loading in patients with various forms of benign hypertension: Relation to plasma renin activity. *J. Clin. Invest.*, 49:1415, 1970.
2. Nowaczynski, W., Kuchel, O. and Genest, J.: A decreased metabolic clearance rate of aldosterone in benign essential hypertension. *J. Clin. Invest.*, 50:2184, 1971.
3. Weinberger, M. H., Dowdy, A. J., Nokes, G. W. et al: Plasma renin activity and aldosterone secretion in hypertensive patients during high and low sodium intake and administration of diuretic. *J. Clin. Endocr.*, 28:359, 1968.

4. Williams, G. H., Rose, L. I., Dluhy, R. G. et al: Abnormal responsiveness of the renin aldosterone system to acute stimulation in patients with essential hypertension. *Ann. Intern. Med.,* 72:317, 1970.

5. Jose, A. and Kaplan, N. M.: Plasma renin activity in the diagnosis of primary aldosteronism. *Arch. Intern. Med.,* 123:141, 1969.

6. Espiner, E. A., Christlieb, A. R., Amsterdam, E. A. et al: The pattern of plasma renin activity and aldosterone secretion in normal and hypertensive subjects before and after saline infusion. *Amer. J. Cardiol.,* 27:585, 1971.

7. Brunner, H. R., Laragh, J. H., Baer, L. et al: Essential hypertension: Renin and aldosterone, heart attack and stroke. *New Eng. J. Med.,* 286:441, 1972.

8. Tuck, M. L., Williams, G. H., Cain, J. P. et al: Relation of age, diastolic pressure and known duration of hypertension to presence of low renin essential hypertension. *Amer. J. Cardiol.,* 32:637, 1973.

9. Crane, M. G., Harris, J. J. and Varner, J. J. Jr.: Hyporeninemic hypertension. *Amer. J. Med.,* 52:457, 1972.

10. Tuck, M. L., Dluhy, R. G. and Williams, G. H.: A delayed suppression of plasma aldosterone during saline infusion in patients with essential hypertension. Abstracts of The Endocrine Society 55th Annual Meeting, June 1973, p. 52.

11. Himathongkam, T., Dluhy, R. G., Tuck, M. L. et al: Abnormal renin-angiotensin-aldosterone dynamics in the "normal renin" hypertensive patient. Abstracts of The Endocrine Society 56th Annual Meeting, June 1974, p. 58.

12. Tuck, M. L., Dluhy, R. G. and Williams, G. H.: A specific role for saline or the sodium ion in the regulation of renin and aldosterone secretion. *J. Clin. Invest.,* 53:988, 1974.

13. Tuck, M. L., Dluhy, R. G. and Williams, G. H.: Sequential responses of the renin-angiotensin-aldosterone axis to acute postural change: Effect of dietary sodium. *J. Lab. Clin. Med.* (In press, 1975.)

14. Underwood, R. H. and Williams, G. H.: The simultaneous measurement of aldosterone, cortisol, and corticosterone in human peripheral plasma by displacement analysis. *J. Lab. Clin. Med.,* 79:848, 1972.

15. Emanuel, R. L., Cain, J. P. and Williams, G. H.: Double antibody radioimmunoassay of renin activity and angiotensin II in human peripheral plasma. *J. Lab. Clin. Med.,* 81:632, 1973.

16. Rosenthal, J., Boucher, R., Nowaczynski, W. et al: Acute changes in plasma volume, renin activity, and free aldosterone levels in healthy subjects following furosemide administration. *Canad. J. Physiol. Pharmacol.,* 46:85, 1968.

17. Oparil, S., Vassaux, C., Sanders, C. A. et al: Role of renin in acute postural homeostasis. *Circulation,* 41:89, 1970.

18. Bayard, F., Alicandri, C. L., Beitins, I. Z. et al: A dynamic study of plasma renin activity and aldosterone concentration in normal and hypertensive patients. *Metabolism,* 20:513, 1971.

19. Pickens, P. T. and Enoch, B. A.: Changes in plasma renin activity produced by infusions of dextran and dextrose. *Cardiov. Res. Cent.*

Bull., 2:157, 1968.

20. Kem, D. C., Weinberger, M. H., Mayes, D. M. et al: Saline suppression of plasma aldosterone in hypertension. *Arch. Intern. Med.*, 128:380, 1971.
21. Venning, E. H., Dyrenfurth, I., Dossetor, J. B et al: Influence of alterations in sodium intake on urinary aldosterone response to corticotropin in normal individuals and patients with essential hypertension. *Metabolism*, 11:254, 1962.
22. Tucci, J. R., Espiner, E. A., Jagger, P. I. et al: ACTH stimulation of aldosterone secretion in normal subjects and in patients with chronic adrenocortical insufficiency. *J. Clin. Endocr.*, 27:568, 1967.
23. Oelkers, W., Brown, J. J., Fraser, R. et al: Sensitization of the adrenal cortex to angiotensin II in sodium-depleted man. *Circ. Res.*, 34:69, 1974.
24. Hollenberg, N. K., Chenitz, W. R., Adams, D. F. et al: Reciprocal influence of salt intake on adrenal glomerulosa and renal vascular responses to angiotensin II in normal man. *J. Clin. Invest.*, 54:34, 1974.
25. Krakoff, L. R., Goodwin, F. J., Baer, L. et al: The role of renin in the exaggerated natriuresis of hypertension. *Circulation*, 42:335, 1970.
26. Brown, J. J. and Peart, W. S.: The effect of angiotension on urine flow and electrolyte excretion in hypertensive subjects. *Clin. Sci.*, 22:1, 1962.
27. Bentzel, C. J. and Meltzer, J. I.: Angiotensin II, norepinephrine and renal transport of electrolytes and water in normal man and in cirrhosis with ascites. *J. Clin. Invest.*, 42:1179, 1963.
28. Leyssac, P. P.: The *in vivo* effect of angiotensin on the proximal tubular reabsorption of salt in rat kidneys. *Acta Physiol. Scand.* 62:436, 1964.
29. Page, I. H. and Bumpus, F. M.: Angiotensin. *Physiol. Rev.*, 41:331, 1961.
30. Tobian, L., Coffee, K., Ferreira, D. et al: The effect of renal perfusion pressure on the net transport of sodium out of distal tubular urine as studied with the stop-flow technique. *J. Clin. Invest.*, 43:118, 1964.
31. Vagnucci, A. I., Lauler, D. P., Hickler, R. G. et al: Acute infusion of synthetic angiotensin II in patients with essential hypertension. *Circulation*, 29:523, 1964.
32. Hollenberg, N. K., Solomon, H. S., Adams, D. F. et al: Renal vascular responses to angiotensin and norepinephrine in normal man. *Circ. Res.*, 31:750, 1972.

Discussion

Dr. Kirkendall, Moderator: Have you found any dichotomy in any of your normal or hypertensive studies between plasma renin activity and angio-II levels?

Dr. Williams: No, we have not found any dichotomy in any subject. We have looked very carefully, because that is an obvious thing to look for. The only additional comment in connection with the study is that maybe if we can perfect the AII assay, we may end up with a better way of assessing the system than using renin activity, but that is probably much further away than trying to standardize the renin activity.

Dr. Kirkendall: That is right. I think right now the AII assay is tougher than the plasma renin assay.

Dr. Williams: Much more difficult.

Dr. Quintanilla, Illinois: I have a question about the last part of your study, when you compared the effect of saline with dextran. Saline and dextran produce quite different expansion of the vascular volume. Did you measure the actual blood volume?

Dr. Williams: We didn't actually measure the volume. We used the hematocrit, which is a poor man's volume measurer, and with it, the dextran produced a little greater intravascular volume expansion than did the saline.

Aldosterone, Deoxycorticosterone, 18-Hydroxydeoxycorticosterone and Progesterone in Benign Essential Hypertension

W. Nowaczynski, D.Sc., O. Kuchel, M.D., Sc.D.
and J. Genest, C.C., M.D.

Introduction

Disturbances of sodium regulation have long been recognized to be associated with experimental and clinical hypertension. Restriction of sodium intake reduces the blood pressure in both the experimental animal and man,[1,2] while the administration of large doses of salt accelerates the development of hypertension in animals.[2,3] Sodium content is increased in the arteries of patients with essential hypertension as well as in animals experimentally made hypertensive, and natriuretics or antagonists of mineralocorticoids lower the blood pressure[2] or prevent the development of experimental hypertension.

We shall review aldosterone metabolism in hypertension first, since aldosterone is the major physiological factor controlling sodium conservation and excretion of potassium, since hyperaldosteronism in Conn's syndrome[4] is a well-documented cause of curable hypertension and since aldosterone production

This study was generously supported through grants from the Medical Research Council of Canada (Grant Nos. MA-1549, MT-2915, MR-3708 and the Group Grant on Hypertension), the Quebec Heart Foundation and the Searle Co., Chicago.

W. Nowaczynski, D.Sc., *Professor of Medicine, University of Montreal and McGill University, Director, Steroid Research Department;* O. Kuchel, M.D., Sc.D., F.R.C.P.(C), *Professor of Medicine, University of Montreal and McGill University, Senior Investigator; and* J. Genest, C.C., M.D., F.R.C.P.(C), F.A.C.P., *Professor of Medicine, University of Montreal and McGill University, Scientific Director, Steroid Research Department, Clinical Research Institute of Montreal and Hôtel-Dieu Hospital of Montreal, Canada.*

can be markedly elevated in the malignant phase of hypertension.[5]

In essential hypertension, a slightly higher than normal excretion of the urinary oxo-conjugate of aldosterone has been reported by some investigators, whereas others have found normal or even low secretion rates.[6] In addition, it was found that aldosterone may not be normally suppressible during high sodium intake in most patients with essential hypertension.[7,8]

The aim of our studies has been to determine whether the abnormal handling of electrolytes in essential hypertension could be related to certain changes in the metabolism of aldosterone. Some aspects of this metabolism have been investigated in detail and are reported here. Some other mineralocorticoids may be involved as well; these are dealt with later.

Methods and Materials

Plasma Aldosterone Concentration

Many observations in this study rely on estimation of the plasma concentration of aldosterone. Because this concentration is normally low, double-isotope procedures or radioimmunoassays were necessary for accurate estimations. It must be emphasized that because the plasma concentration of aldosterone is sensitive to a wide variety of changes in normal physiological conditions, one must be exceptionally careful to define the conditions under which it is studied in order to obtain a true indication of circulating concentrations.

The secretion rate and plasma concentration of aldosterone in normal subjects are influenced markedly by several factors such as dietary sodium and potassium content, postural adaptation,[6,9-15] circadian periodicity[14] and the course of the normal menstrual cycle.[10,14,16,17]

A rapid, specific, precise and reproducible radioimmunoassay for plasma and urinary aldosterone has been developed which uses a sheep antibody preparation.[10] Aldosterone is purified by a blank-free column chromatography on washed wet Sephadex LH-20.

Normal ranges for plasma aldosterone established under various physiological conditions by this procedure[10] are com-

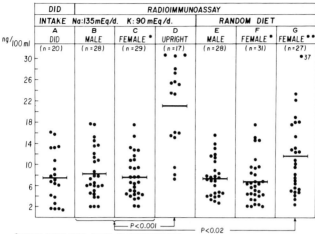

Fig. 1. Plasma aldosterone (ng/100 ml) in control subjects in recumbent posture at 0800h: A, in 20 men and women (7.5 ± 4.8 SD) by double-isotope derivative assay (DID) on a diet containing 135 mEq Na and 90 mEq K; B, and C, as for A, by radioimmunoassay in men (8.3 ± 4.6) and women (7.7 ± 4.0); D, as for B, and C, (17 subjects) but in upright posture (21.2 ± 8.3 SD). E, and F, as for B, and C, respectively, but on random diet (7.4 ± 3.6, 6.8 ± 4.1); G, as for C, and F, with blood samples obtained later than the sixth day from the onset of the menstruation (13.4 ± 7.8). C vs. G p < 0.02; B+C vs. D, p < 0.001.

pared in Figure 1 with those obtained by our double-isotope assay.[1][8] The two assays evidently give similar values.

Figure 1 indicates that the recumbent plasma concentration of aldosterone is much the same in male and female subjects (provided that the blood sampling is done at the beginning of the follicular phase of the menstrual cycle) on both controlled and random diet. Higher recumbent values are obtained in female subjects studied later in the course of the menstrual cycle or in subjects in the upright posture. It should be added that because this plasma concentration depends upon a very labile equilibrium between the secretion rate (SR) and the metabolic clearance rate (MCR) — clearance mainly by the liver[9] but also by the kidney[8] — and because the MCR is very sensitive to changes in hepatic blood flow, which is considerably lower in the upright than in the recumbent posture,[9] the true baseline recumbent value can be obtained only after the subject has been recumbent for several hours. Some discrepancies between results reported by different laboratories may be explained by the failure to recognize the importance of these factors.

Other Methods

The metabolic clearance rates (MCR) of aldosterone, deoxy-corticosterone (DOC), and 18-hydroxydeoxycorticosterone (18-OH DOC) were determined by continuous infusion[19] and the urinary excretion of the oxo- and tetra-hydrometabolites of aldosterone by double-isotope dilution procedures.[18,20] Tritiated tetrahydroglucuronide and 18-oxo-conjugate markers[20] were used for correction of procedural losses.[6] Plasma progesterone,[21] cortisol and corticosterone[22] were determined by a modification of the procedure of Murphy. Double-isotope dilution assays were used to determine the secretion rates (SR) of aldosterone,[18] 18-OH DOC,[23,24] DOC[25] and corticosterone.[25] Plasma renin activity was determined by the method of Boucher et al.[26]

Patients and Control Subjects

All patients were thoroughly investigated[27,28] by all the tests currently available to be sure they were free of secondary types of hypertension.

Ages ranged between 25 and 55 years. The diagnosis of benign essential hypertension (BEH) was made on the basis of a thorough physical examination and the results of numerous determinations including normal serum electrolytes (sodium, potassium, bicarbonates), normal urinalysis, vanillylmandelic acid excretion, rapid sequence intravenous pyelography and renal angiography, absence of retinopathy, normal renal function evaluated by blood urea and creatinine and the excretion of phenolsulfonaphthalein and creatinine clearance, normal electrocardiogram without evidence of left ventricular hypertrophy, normal renal arteriogram and the absence of evident signs of arterio-atherosclerosis of the large vessels.

These patients were divided into two groups. The first one consisted of patients labeled as stable BEH, with blood pressure reading always above 140/90 mm Hg, before and at the time of the study. The second group, categorized as labile BEH, had blood pressure often higher than 140/90 mm Hg, but returning to normal levels under conditions of rest and emotional reassurance. The majority of patients with labile BEH have never been treated. The medication of the other patients was discontinued at least five days prior to the study.

Normotensive controls were healthy laboratory personnel (men and women) and medical students with an age range of 20 to 52.

Unless otherwise stated, all normal subjects and patients had steroid determinations between 0830h and 0900h after having remained in the recumbent position since the night before. This was on the fourth day of a controlled diet containing 135 mEq of sodium and 90 mEq of potassium per day or a sodium-restricted diet of 10 mEq of sodium and 90 mEq of potassium per day.

In addition, patients with low-renin BEH have also been studied. Every patient had at least two renin determinations, one recumbent with a normal sodium and potassium intake (135 mEq of sodium and 90 mEq of potassium daily) and another after stimulation either by upright posture or low-salt diet and/or furosemide. Patients showing plasma renin activities of less than 0.5 ng/ml/hr during stimulation by upright posture and/or less than 1.5 ng/ml/hr after stimulation by salt-poor diet or furosemide and upright posture were considered to have low-renin BEH.

Aldosterone in BEH

The involvement of aldosterone in the pathogenesis of benign essential hypertension remained controversial for many years. Previous observations of our group, subsequently confirmed by other investigators, indicated a significant mean increase in the excretion of the aldosterone oxo-conjugate in patients with BEH,[29-33] while other investigators reported a usually normal or even decreased secretion rate of aldosterone in several similar series of patients.[34-38]

In a more recent study in this laboratory, aldosterone metabolism was investigated in 16 patients with normal plasma renin activity by a concomitant measurement of plasma concentration, SR and MCR of aldosterone. The mean MCR of aldosterone was found to be significantly ($p < 0.001$) lower in patients with BEH than in normal controls, while the plasma

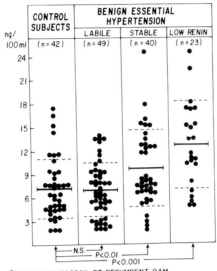

Fig. 2. Mean recumbent (0900h) plasma aldosterone concentrations were 7.1 ng/100 ml ± 3.5 SD in 49 patients with labile BEH, 9.7 ng/100 ml in 40 patients with stable BEH (p < 0.01) and 12.8 ng/100 ml ± 5.7 SD in 23 patients with BEH and low plasma renin activity (p < 0.001), versus 7.2 ng/100 ml ± 3.8 SD in 42 control subjects.

concentration (double-isotope determination) tended to be high and the SR tended to be low.[6,11,19]

A subsequent study on larger groups of subjects showed the mean plasma aldosterone concentrations (by radioimmuno-assay) to be significantly higher than normal in patients with stable BEH and low-renin BEH, while they were not different from controls in labile BEH[12,14,18,39,40] (Fig. 2). The aldosterone MCR was significantly lower[11,12,14,39,40] in patients with stable BEH and labile BEH (p < 0.001 in the two groups) than in control subjects (Fig. 3). In a single patient with BEH and low plasma renin activity, a decreased MCR of 614 1/24 h/m² was found.

The MCR of aldosterone and its plasma concentration, determined in six control subjects and 29 patients with BEH, were negatively correlated (Fig. 4).

Since aldosterone is metabolized mainly by the liver, the findings of a decreased MCR of aldosterone suggested that

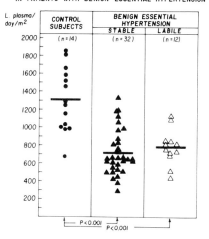

ALDOSTERONE METABOLIC CLEARANCE RATE
IN PATIENTS WITH BENIGN ESSENTIAL HYPERTENSION

Figure 3.

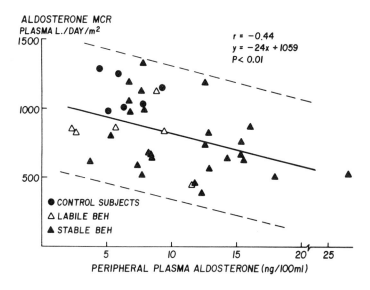

Figure 4.

either the hepatic blood flow was lower in patients with BEH or that the removal of this hormone by the liver cells was impaired.[12,14] However, for steroids having normally high hepatic extractions (most of the corticosteroids), the hepatic blood flow would have to be considerably reduced to result in measurable differences of the hepatic clearance rates. The hepatic blood flow in BEH was found to be normal by Wilkins[41] or reduced by 20% first by Wollheim[42] and recently in our laboratory.[43] The major finding of our study was that patients with BEH present a significantly (about 12%) lower splanchnic blood flow than controls.[43] A negative correlation between the mean arterial blood pressure and the splanchnic blood flow was also shown. This implies that the hepatic blood flow and arterial blood pressure could be influenced by the same pathologic factors. A large enough decrease in hepatic blood flow may diminish or contribute to a decrease in the inactivation of physiologic or pharmacologic agents that are metabolized by the liver. Because tetrahydroaldosterone-glucuronide derives mainly from liver metabolism, in contrast to the 18-oxo-conjugate which is mainly of renal origin, the excretion of these two main metabolites of aldosterone was measured in controls and patients with BEH.[11,12,14,18,40] The urines were collected from 0800h to 1200h in subjects recumbent since the night before, in order to eliminate postural and circadian variations.

In control subjects, the four-hour excretion of the aldosterone oxo-conjugate was about four times lower than that of the tetrahydroglucuronide (Fig. 5). The excretion of the same two metabolites in patients with labile BEH was higher for the oxo-conjugate and lower for the tetrahydroglucuronide. In patients with stable BEH, the mean excretion of the same metabolites was modified similarly, although to a lesser extent than in patients with labile BEH.

In other studies, the protein binding of aldosterone, a potential factor that can affect the metabolism of steroids, was investigated in patients with labile or stable BEH.[12,14,40] The mean percentage of aldosterone bound to a transcortin-like plasma fraction (TLPF) was found to be significantly ($p < 0.001$) higher, as expected,[12,19] in patients with labile and stable BEH, as well as in low-renin BEH than in healthy subjects[14] (Fig. 6).

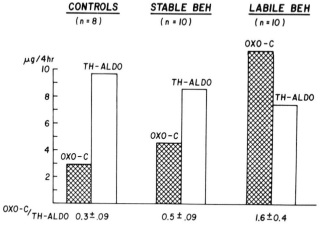

Fig. 5. In eight control subjects, the four hour excretion (from 0800h to 1200h) of the oxo-conjugate of aldosterone was 4.87μg ± 4.6 SD versus 13.5 ± 12.6 SD for the tetrahydroglucuronide, with a mean ratio of 4.0. The excretion of the same metabolites in patients with labile BEH was 7.2μg ± 4.6 SD and 6.7 ± 3.7 SD and in patients with stable BEH 10.1 ± 9.0 SD versus 10.6 ± 5.9 SD, respectively.

Using a dynamic approach we have also found that in response to the stimulation of assuming the upright posture, patients with labile BEH have a significant decrease in the urinary 18-oxo-conjugate of aldosterone, in contrast to the increase in normal subjects (Fig. 7). In patients with stable BEH, this increase is less pronounced.[11,12,14,40] Many of these patients had a greater than normal response of plasma aldosterone to the upright posture[11,12,14,40] (Fig. 7).

In another series of experiments, it was shown that the MCR of aldosterone did not change in response to severe sodium restriction or loading (Fig. 8) or to upright posture[12,14,40] in patients with BEH (Fig. 9).

Modified circadian rhythms of plasma concentration and the TLPF binding of aldosterone, indicating a small excess of circulating aldosterone between 2000h and 0000h, have been found in recumbent patients with BEH[12] (Fig. 10). This circadian rhythm, determined again in two of the control subjects after dexamethasone administration, showed much

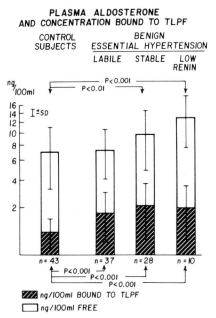

PLASMA ALDOSTERONE
AND CONCENTRATION BOUND TO TLPF

Fig. 6. Recumbent plasma concentration (0800h-0900h) of aldosterone and percentage bound to transcortin-like plasma fraction (TLPF) was 7.1 ng/100 ml ± 3.9 SD in 43 control subjects, 7.3 ng/100 ml ± 3.3 SD in 37 patients with labile, 9.7 ng/100 ml ± 4.9 SD in 28 patients with stable and 13.0 ng/100 ml ± 5.5 SD in 10 patients with low plasma renin activity BEH. The mean concentration of TLPF bound aldosterone was 0.8 ng/100 ml ± 0.6 SD in control subjects, 1.7 ng/100 ml ± 1.3 SD in patients with labile, 2.1 ng/100 ml ± 1.6 SD in patients with stable and 2.0 ng/100 ml ± 1.5 SD in patients with low plasma renin activity BEH, respectively.

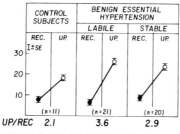

Figure 7.

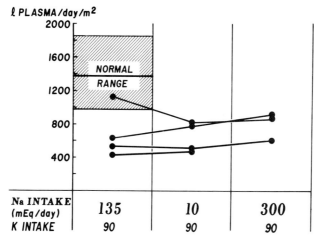

Figure 8.

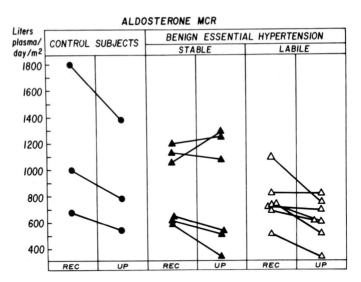

Figure 9.

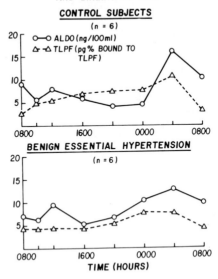

Figure 10.

lower values for plasma aldosterone at all times except for the peak at 0400h which was only slightly lower. This last experiment suggests that the elevation of plasma aldosterone observed between 0800h and noon may be ACTH-dependent while the early morning peak (0400h) is not.

In addition, the mean excretion of aldosterone 21-sulfate was found to be slightly higher in patients with BEH (2.8µg/day) than in normal controls (2.1µg/day)[20] (Fig. 11). Because of the small number of subjects studied, this difference must be considered as suggestive only. However, the increased excretion of some steroid sulfates in patients with BEH may be related to a compensated shift of liver enzymes, reflected by an increase in the hepatic sulfokinase activity and the impaired ability of the liver to reduce ring A of the steroids.[20]

In one case of surgically confirmed primary hyperaldosteronism, an overproduction of aldosterone was indicated by excessive excretion of the oxo-conjugate and a six-times-normal excretion of aldosterone 21-sulfate[20] (Fig. 11).

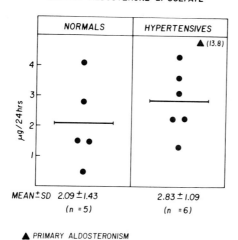

Fig. 11. Urinary excretion of aldosterone 21-sulfate in control subjects, patients with BEH and one case with primary hyperaldosteronism.

Comments on Aldosterone

The above studies explain in part the conflicting earlier results on the metabolism of aldosterone in BEH.[2,6,19] Some researchers confirmed our earlier findings derived from spot determinations of increased excretion of the 18-oxo-conjugate of aldosterone in most patients with BEH, while other groups found no difference with normotensive controls.[2,6,19] In most of these studies in BEH, either urinary excretion or SR of aldosterone determined over hours has been related to single or multiple but instantaneous determinations of plasma concentrations.

The data on Figure 3, obtained with the most accurate double-isotope dilution procedure, confirm a significant increase in the excretion of the oxo-conjugate in recumbent patients with BEH. This is probably due to an impaired hepatic metabolism of aldosterone and not to an increase of its secretion which tends to be low-normal or, even occasionally, subnormal. The latter observation has already been made, though not recognized, by Cope et al[44] who found that the SR of aldosterone was subnormal in three, and between the lower limit and the normal mean in six, out of a total of 13 patients with essential hypertension — then later by Katsushima et al.[36] In addition, the above experiments indicate that lying down increases and standing decreases the concentration of the urinary oxo-conjugate to a greater extent in BEH than in normal controls. Therefore, the 24-hour excretion in patients will greatly depend upon the number of hours the patient was ambulatory or recumbent in bed. These observations certainly account for some of the conflicting data in the literature on the excretion of the urinary 18-oxo-conjugate, since at this time the importance of posture was not fully recognized. They probably also explain the excessive day-to-day fluctuations recorded in this measurement, especially in patients with early asymptomatic BEH.[45,46]

Our studies also suggest that the hepatic metabolism of aldosterone in BEH is modified (a) because of a relatively small decrease in the hepatic blood flow[42,43] and (b) because of an increased binding of aldosterone to TLPF,[14,40] both probably contributing to a significant decrease in the MCR of aldosterone.[6,11,12,14,19,40] The low MCR probably contributes to the significantly higher mean recumbent plasma aldosterone concentration in patients with stable and especially with low-renin BEH (studied for the first time). The significant negative correlation between the MCR and the plasma concentration of aldosterone (Fig. 4) with progressively decreasing ratio from groups of control subjects, patients with labile, and finally patients with stable BEH is compatible with this reasoning.[14,40]

Because of the higher degree of binding of aldosterone to TLPF the amount of this hormone not cleared by the liver and presented to the kidneys will be higher in BEH. However, since globulin-bound aldosterone is not filtrable by the kidney,[47] and consequently is inactive at the tubular level, it will have to re-enter the renal extracellular space where it will be metabolized to the oxo-conjugate, which will then be actively secreted.[48] All this implies an impaired tubular activity of aldosterone under baseline conditions in recumbent patients with BEH and possibly a higher tissue activity of aldosterone in some area of the outer distribution pool.[14,40]

In conclusion, the greater degree of binding of aldosterone to TLPF in BEH may partly explain the lower metabolic clearance rate of aldosterone, the relative increase in the excretion of the aldosterone oxo-conjugate and the relative decrease in urinary tetrahydroaldosterone. Certain subtle changes in the metabolism of aldosterone in BEH become more evident when the system is not only examined under steady conditions, but also investigated dynamically. When patients with BEH assume upright posture, and at certain times during the day, increased binding of aldosterone to TLPF and a small decrease in hepatic blood flow in BEH could bring about or contribute to a retarded response of circulating aldosterone to suppression or stimulation of its production, the consequence being transient excessive levels of circulating aldosterone.

Serious difficulties in research on hypertension stem from the heterogeneity and progressive character of this disorder as well as of most of its biochemical and hemodynamic parameters. This is especially obvious for aldosterone metabolism, which is affected differently at various stages of this disease. Certain parameters under investigation were more modified in labile BEH, where the majority of patients had not been treated previously. It remains to be established whether any differences between the labile and stable forms of BEH are due to the evolution of the disease or could partially be the effect of treatment in patients with stable BEH prior to the study period.

Recent evidence[48, 49] suggests that as much as 98% of the sodium filtered off into the glomerular filtrate is normally reabsorbed in the tubule even in the absence of aldosterone. Aldosterone seems to exert its action in maintaining normal homeostasis, especially in regard to sodium concentration and probably also extracellular fluid volume, within the narrow limit of the remaining 2%. It is therefore quite likely that the abnormal handling of sodium, which may be a primary cause of essential hypertension, may be related to very subtle changes in concentrations of the physiologically active, free portion of aldosterone remaining after binding to circulating proteins. In addition, this latter parameter could affect aldosterone activity in some compartments out of the extracellular volume of distribution.

Our studies indicate that in BEH, because of the modified metabolism of aldosterone, neither urinary excretion nor

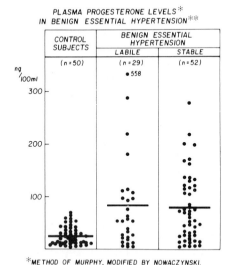

Fig. 12. Mean plasma progesterone was 25.7 ng/100 ml ± 2.5 SE in 50 control subjects versus 84 ± 21 in 29 patients with labile (p < 0.001) and 79.4 ± 8.9 in 52 with stable (p < 0.001) BEH.

aldosterone SR or plasma concentration, in isolated determinations, will give any reliable indication of the adrenal contribution to a clinical situation. In order to obtain the true basal concentration of free plasma aldosterone active at the receptor sites, it is necessary to fractionally measure its plasma concentration and protein binding and consider the posture and diurnal variation as well as variations during the course of the menstrual cycle. Some of the abnormalities in aldosterone metabolism in BEH can be revealed only by dynamic approaches. Many discrepancies in the literature concerning the metabolism of aldosterone in BEH may perhaps now be explained by the nonrecognition of these factors and also — since metabolism of aldosterone seems to be modified differently in various forms or phases of essential hypertension — by selection of populations with different types and severity of hypertension. Over the years, there has been a gradual improvement in criteria for the diagnosis and classification of patients; some abnormalities can be revealed only by the highly sophisticated methods now available.

Progesterone

Plasma progesterone levels have been measured in 21 controls, 33 patients with stable BEH, and 20 patients with labile BEH. Blood samples from female patients were taken between the first and sixth day after the onset of the menstrual cycle.

Mean plasma progesterone levels in the groups of patients with stable and labile BEH were significantly higher than in controls (Fig. 12).[21,27,50]

Severe sodium restriction to 10 mEq/day over four days, accelerated on the first day by furosemide causing a weight loss of more than 2 kg, with a potassium intake of 90 mEq/day resulted in a very marked increase in plasma progesterone in ten out of 12 controls studied, from a mean of 35 to that of 267 ng/100 ml for these ten subjects.[21] The same sodium restriction in a group of 15 patients with either stable or labile BEH caused a marked rise of plasma progesterone to a mean of 300 ng/100 ml in six patients, in no change in eight patients and in a major decrease in one patient. There was no apparent difference in response to sodium restriction between patients with labile or stable BEH. In these 15 patients, there was no correlation between the levels of plasma renin activity, plasma aldosterone and plasma progesterone simultaneously measured, nor was there any significant change in plasma cortisol[2 3] determined in the same plasma samples before and after four days of severe sodium restriction. Hence, changes in ACTH were apparently not responsible for the stimulation of progesterone by sodium restriction.[6,2 1]

The above results are of particular interest because many studies suggest that progesterone is involved in sodium regulation and, indirectly, in blood pressure regulation. A hypotensive effect of progesterone at high dosages in patients with BEH was first reported by Armstrong[5 1] and subsequently confirmed by our group.[3 2] In addition, progesterone was shown to possess a natriuretic effect by competitive inhibition of aldosterone at the distal tubular level,[5 2 -5 4] and the administration of high doses of progesterone stimulated aldosterone production.[5 5 -5 7] The hypothesis that placental progesterone protects the pregnant woman against the effects of high aldosterone was strongly supported by the findings of Ehrlich[5 8] that inhibition of aldosterone by a heparinoid in three pregnant women caused an exaggerated natriuresis and sodium depletion.

We must be cautious, however, in interpreting a possible interaction of a relatively small increase in plasma progesterone, as found in patients with BEH, with aldosterone activity. Several normal subjects who were maintained for up to seven days on a sodium-restricted diet, but without acceleration of sodium depletion, did not change their plasma progesterone,[2 1] while it is well known that aldosterone is strongly stimulated under similar conditions. This suggests that the stimulation of aldosterone and progesterone is mediated by different mechanisms during sodium depletion. The lack of correlation between plasma aldosterone and progesterone determined concomitantly in 65 of the above patients with BEH also speaks against the presence of such an interaction of those plasma concentrations. Lack of correlation between changes in plasma aldosterone and progesterone during the ovulatory as well as the anovulatory menstrual cycle suggests that concentrations of progesterone attained during the luteal phase, which are of the same order of magnitude as in BEH, do not affect the aldosterone and have no effect on the excretion of sodium.[2,1 4]

Low urinary pregnanediol reported[59] in patients with BEH suggests that the higher plasma progesterone could be related to lower MCR of this hormone by a mechanism similar to that for aldosterone,[12] rather than to a higher production rate.

Studies on ACTH-Dependent Mineralocorticoids

Patients with BEH and low plasma renin activity were reported by Luetscher et al[60] to have serum sodium concentrations generally higher than those with higher or normal renin activity and to have serum potassium concentrations frequently at the lower limits of normal. Other investigators found higher exchangeable sodium[61] and higher extracellular fluid volumes[62] in such patients than in normal subjects.

These findings, suggesting that hypertension in patients with low plasma renin activity was frequently associated with increased mineralocorticoid activity, stimulated our study of the metabolism of all the main mineralocorticoids in patients with different forms of BEH.[6,23,63] In untreated patients with BEH, the following were concomitantly measured: plasma aldosterone concentration and 18-OH DOC, DOC and corticosterone secretion rates, and plasma DOC concentrations. The mean DOC and corticosterone secretion rates were about the same in normal subjects (175 ± 15 SE μg/24 h and 2778 ± 232 μg/24 h ± SE), BEH patients with normal PRA (184 ± 33 and 2221 ± 254) and low-renin BEH patients (174 ± 40 and 2789 ± 364).[6,63]

However, there was a significant (p < 0.01) difference between the 18-OH DOC secretion rate in controls and patients with labile BEH (Fig. 13).

There was no correlation between the secretion rate of DOC, corticosterone and 18-OH DOC in normal-renin BEH and controls. In contrast, DOC secretion rate and 18-OH DOC secretion rate were positively correlated in patients with low-renin BEH.[63] In addition, the correlations between DOC secretion rate and corticosterone secretion rate and between corticosterone secretion rate and 18-OH DOC secretion rate were significant (p < 0.01) in patients with low PRA.

Recumbent (0800h) plasma DOC concentration was measured in control subjects and patients with normal-renin and low-renin BEH (Table 1). In patients with consistently low

TABLE 1. Plasma DOC Concentrations

	Control Subjects	I BEH Normal PRA	II BEH Low PRA	p I vs II
AGE (mean ± SE) (yr)	32.0 ± 2.0	34.2 ± 2.0	48.7 ± 1.4	< 0.001
Serum K (mEq/l)	4.5 ± 1.0	4.39 ± 0.09	3.95 ± 0.01	< 0.01
DOC (ng/100 ml)	6.8 ± 0.8	6.49 ± 0.79	9.88 ± 1.2	< 0.05

PRA, DOC levels were high. Simultaneously measured plasma aldosterone levels in patients with normal and low PRA were often in the upper limit of the normal range; they were inversely related to plasma DOC concentrations ($p < 0.05$) in the low-renin group only. Plasma concentration of aldosterone was also more significantly increased in patients with low-renin PRA ($p < 0.001$) than in patients with normal PRA ($p < 0.01$) as compared to control subjects (Fig. 2). The mean MCR of DOC, measured by continuous infusion, did not differ from that in control subjects and patients with normal PRA, which indicates that the elevated plasma DOC was not due to a decrease in the MCR. This observation is in agreement with a

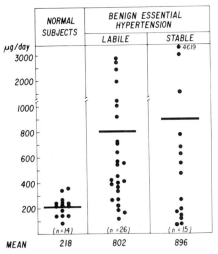

Fig. 13. 18-OH DOC secretion rate (μg/24 h) in controls and BEH patients with labile or stable BEH.

positive correlation between DOC secretion rate and 18-OH DOC secretion rate in the same patients.

Plasma DOC may thus be found in small excess in BEH and may possibly account for the low PRA among patients without elevated plasma aldosterone.

Favorable blood pressure response to spironolactones and/or dexamethasone in low-renin BEH with excessive 18-OH DOC secretion rate further points to the possibility that an enhanced mineralocorticoid activity is involved in the pathogenesis of high blood pressure. The secretion patterns of steroids in this group of patients could partially be explained by an incomplete 17α-hydroxylase deficiency.[6] An extreme example of such a disorder resembling Biglieri's syndrome[34] was studied recently[61] and the results for the purpose of illustrating the mechanism are summarized in Table 2. Plasma cortisol determinations which show a tendency to lower values in normal-renin BEH and significantly lower values in low-renin BEH (Fig. 14) are compatible with this hypothesis.

To test this hypothesis further, we again used a dynamic approach in studying the response of low-renin BEH patients to ACTH. Plasma levels of six steroids were determined simultaneously during and after an eight-hour infusion of 25 I.U. of ACTH in five control subjects and five patients (Fig. 15). The response in plasma progesterone was the same in controls and patients. Plasma DOC showed a higher basal value in some patients and an insignificant tendency to increased response to ACTH. The responses of corticosterone and 17α-hydroxyprogesterone in patients were significantly lower after four and eight hours of infusion. There were suggestions of a more pronounced response in Reichstein's compound S, an 11-deoxy-steroid, and a slightly decreased response in cortisol.

The 18-OH DOC secretion rate, already high in low-renin BEH, responded to the same infusion of ACTH normally, which resulted for some patients in very high values.[14] Dexamethasone administration decreased the 18-OH DOC secretion rate in all patients studied.[14]

The positive correlations between the corticosterone, DOC and 18-OH DOC secretion rates and the plasma DOC concentration, suggest an enhanced mineralocorticoid activity in low-renin BEH. The 18-OH DOC secretion rates were increased

TABLE 2. ♀: Age 28, 17α-Hydroxylation Deficiency
(Normal Values in Parenthesis)

Plasma Ster. (µg/100 ml)	Before Dex.	After Dex.
Compound F	0.41 (15 ± 2)	0
Compound B	10.4 (0.27 ± 0.07)	7.2
Progesterone	1.3 (0.035 ± 0.014)	0.14
Estradiol	0 (2-7)	
Testosterone	14 (275-1100)	
Secretion Rate (µg/d)		
DOC	21,600 (174 ± 14)	
Compound B	34,700 (2770 ± 232)	
18-OH DOC	8,460 (209 ± 18)	1,420
Urinary (µg/d)		
DHEA-g	<2 (270 ± 200)	
DHEA-s	<2 (3320 ± 2000)	
Etiocholanolone-g	<2 ⎱ (1650 ± 980)	
Etiocholanolone-s	<2 ⎰	
P.R.A. (ng/ml/h)	0.39 (5.26 ± 1.04)	
Plasma K (mEq/l)	3	4.9
Art. B.P. (mm Hg)	150/100	115/85
Weight (Kg)	72	69

17α-hydroxylase deficiency with hypertension and hypokalemia mimicking, prepubertal testicular feminization. Plasma progesterone and B were increased 30-fold. SR of DOC, 18-OH DOC and B were increased 100, 40 and 10-fold, respectively. Aldosterone was low. Undetectable amounts (excretion) of dehydroepiandrosterone (DHEA) glucuronide and sulfate and their urine metabolites are compatible with a marked 17α-hydroxylation deficiency. Patients with BEH show a very marked decrease in the excretion of the sulfates of the above steroids[2]; however, the values remain always measurable. The excretion of DHEA-glucuronide is unchanged in BEH. On dexamethasone 0.5 mg b.i.d. blood pressure, progesterone, B and aldosterone decreased; hyperkalemia and orthostatic hypotension requiring supplemental mineralocorticoids developed. It is suggested that a complete 17α-hydroxylase deficiency in this genetic male produced a prepubertal female phenotype due to failure of androgen synthesis. Hypertension and hypokalemia resulted from DOC, 18-OH DOC and B hypersecretion.

in low-renin BEH more consistently (in 56% of patients) than DOC secretion rates, which remain within the upper limit of the normal range. Low-renin BEH seems to be a special form of hypertension with a shift from predominantly angiotensin-dependent aldosterone toward predominantly ACTH-dependent mineralocorticoids. Under certain conditions even aldosterone can become predominantly ACTH-dependent. Our most recent observations indicate that basal plasma aldosterone concentra-

PLASMA CORTISOL CONCENTRATIONS

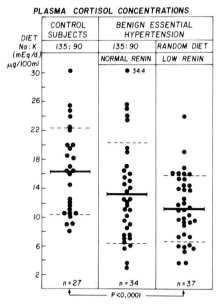

Fig. 14. Plasma cortisol concentrations were 13.1μg/100 ml ± 7.1 SD in 27 patients with BEH and normal plasma renin activity and 11.3μg/100 ml ± 4.5 SD in 37 patients with low plasma renin activity (p < 0.001) versus 16.3μg/100 ml ± 6 SD in 27 control subjects.

tions are in most cases at the upper end of the normal range and also respond excessively to ACTH.[14] A concomitant decrease in TLPF binding indicated that the increase in plasma aldosterone in response to ACTH occurred mainly in the unbound fraction while the MCR of aldosterone increased.

Conclusion

A mineralocorticoid excess leading to sodium retention and the hypertensive process, by affecting body electrolyte and fluid homeostasis and regulation of blood pressure, may be due to a combined effect of several of the above-studied steroids. Their excess results from a delicate interplay between the secretion rate and MCR. A lower MCR, probably selective for some mineralocorticoids and especially aldosterone, may be an important mechanism leading to an excess of circulating mineralocorticoids in BEH by causing delayed decreases in their plasma levels in response to sodium loading. This does not

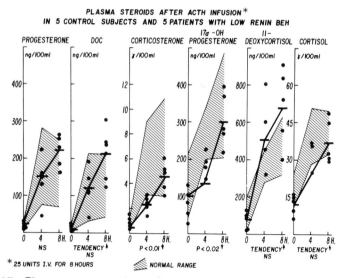

Fig. 15. Plasma concentration of progesterone, deoxycorticosterone, corticosterone, 17α-hydroxyprogesterone, 11-deoxycortisol and cortisol before and after four and eight hours of ACTH infusion (25 IU), respectively, in patients with low-renin BEH as compared to a response in control subjects (shaded area).

exclude the excessive secretion of other as yet unidentified mineralocorticoids in low-renin BEH.

A great potential interest of 18-OH DOC and other ACTH-dependent mineralocorticoids comes from the fact that those hormones are stimulated by mechanisms involving stress. At the same time, because their release is independent of the renin-angiotensin system, their secretion is not suppressible by increased dietary sodium. A possible partial deficiency of 17α-hydroxylase could be another mechanism operative in some patients with BEH.

Transient small increments in plasma concentrations of aldosterone in patients with BEH may be important, since it has been shown that a very small excess of nonsuppressible aldosterone can be a cause of curable hypertension in primary aldosteronism. In addition, the significantly increased binding of aldosterone to TLPF may be affecting the tissue activity of aldosterone in all forms of BEH under study.

The above data suggest that further studies correlating all the relevant mineralocorticoids, especially under dynamic conditions of ACTH stimulation or dexamethasone suppression (and for aldosterone the manipulation of water and electrolytes) may lead to better understanding of subtle changes in the disturbed mineralocorticoid metabolism in BEH.

Acknowledgments

The authors wish to acknowledge the active collaboration of the following research fellows during the course of these investigations: Drs. F. H. Messerli, M. Honda, S. Kubo, G. Tolis, K. Seth, J. Grose, M. Lebel and F. Ledoux.

The excellent technical assistance of Miss P. Robinson, Mrs. D. Charbonneau, Mrs. M. Monette and Mrs. F. Grégoire, as well as the skillful secretarial help of Mrs. D. L. Abastado are gratefully acknowledged.

References

1. Grollman, A., Harrison, T. R., Mason, M. F. et al: Sodium restriction in the diet for hypertension. *JAMA*, 129:533, 1945.
2. Nowaczynski, W., Kuchel, O., Lebel, M. et al: Les minéralocorticoides et l'hypertension essentielle. *Un. Méd. Canada*, 102:846, 1973.
3. Meneely, G. R.: Salt. *Amer. J. Med.*, 16:1, 1954.
4. Conn, J. W.: An overall view of primary aldosteronism. In Onesti, G., Kim, K. E. and Moyer, J. H. (eds.): *Hypertension: Mechanisms and Management*. New York:Grune & Stratton, 1973, p. 471.
5. Laragh, J. H., Ulick, S., Januszewicz, V. et al: Aldosterone secretion in primary and malignant hypertension. *J. Clin. Invest.*, 39:1091, 1960.
6. Nowaczynski, W., Kuchel, O. and Genest, J.: Aldosterone, deoxycorticosterone and corticosterone metabolism in benign essential hypertension. In Genest, J. and Koiw, E. (eds.): *Hypertension '72*. Berlin, Heidelberg, New York:Springer-Verlag, 1972, p. 244.
7. Collins, R. D., Weinberger, M. H., Dowdy, A. J. et al: Abnormally sustained aldosterone secretion during salt loading in patients with various forms of benign hypertension; relation to plasma renin activity. *J. Clin. Invest.*, 49:1415, 1970.
8. Luetscher, J. A., Camargo, C. A., Cheville, R. A. et al: Conjugation and excretion of aldosterone; testing of models with an analog computer. In Pincus, G., Nakao, T. and Tait, J. F. (eds.): *Steroid Dynamics*, Proceedings of the Symposium on the Dynamics of Steroid Hormones, Tokyo, May 1965. New York and London:Academic Press, 1966, p. 341.
9. Balikian, H. M., Brodie, A. H., Dale, S. L. et al: Effect of posture on the metabolic clearance rate, plasma concentration and blood production rate of aldosterone in man. *J. Clin. Endocr.*, 28:1630, 1968.

10. Nowaczynski, W., Sasaki, C. and Genest, J.: Radioimmunoassay for aldosterone and normal values under various physiological conditions. *J. Ster. Biochem.*, 5:123, 1974.

11. Nowaczynski, W., Kuchel, O. and Grose, J. et al: Aldosterone (A) metabolism in benign essential hypertension (BEH). Fourth Intern. Congress of Endocrinology, Washington, D. C., 18-24 June 1972. In *Excerpta Med. Intern. Congr. Ser.*, No. 256, Abstract #273.

12. Nowaczynski, W., Kuchel, O., Genest, J. et al: Further studies on aldosterone metabolism in benign essential hypertension. Submitted for publication to *J. Clin. Invest.*

13. Baulieu, E. E. and Robel, P. (eds.): *Part II, Aldosterone, A Symposium.* Oxford:Blackwell, 1964.

14. Nowaczynski, W., Kuchel, O., Genest, J. et al: Further evidence of an altered aldosterone metabolism in benign essential hypertension. Sixth meeting of the Intern. Study Group for Steroid Hormones, Rome, Italy, December 6-8, 1973. *Research on Steroids*, Vol. VI, 1974.

15. Shane, S. R., Melby, J. C. and Jones, J. E.: Prolonged upright posture and rhythms of aldosterone and electrolyte excretion. *Proc. 53rd Meeting, Endocrine Society*, San Francisco, 1971, p. A-111.

16. Gray, M. J., Strausfeld, K. S., Watanabe, M. et al: Aldosterone secretory rates in the normal menstrual cycle. *J. Clin. Endocr.*, 28:1269, 1968.

17. Katz, F. H. and Romfh, P.: Plasma aldosterone and renin activity during the menstrual cycle. *J. Clin. Endocr.*, 34:819, 1972.

18. Nowaczynski, W., Silah, J. and Genest, J.: Procedure for determination of aldosterone in human peripheral plasma by double-isotope derivative assay, and its application for measurement of secretory rate and urinary excretion. *Canad. J. Biochem.*, 45:1919, 1967.

19. Nowaczynski, W., Kuchel, O. and Genest, J.: A decreased metabolic clearance rate of aldosterone in benign essential hypertension. *J. Clin. Invest.*, 50:2184, 1971.

20. Grose, J. H., Nowaczynski, W., Kuchel, O. et al: Isolation of aldosterone urinary metabolites, glucuronides and sulfate. *J. Ster. Biochem.*, 4:551, 1973.

21. Sasaki, C., Nowaczynski, W., Kuchel, O. et al: Plasma progesterone in normal subjects and patients with benign essential hypertension on normal, low and high sodium intake. *J. Clin. Endocr.*, 34:650, 1972.

22. Mancheno-Rico, E., Kuchel, O., Nowaczynski, W. et al: A dissociated effect of amino-glutethimide on the mineralocorticoid secretion in man. *Metabolism*, 22:123, 1973.

23. Nowaczynski, W., Kuchel, O., Genest, J. et al: 18-hydroxydeoxy-corticosterone secretion rates in normotensive and essential hypertensive subjects. Presented in discussion to the paper of J. C. Melby. Laurentian Hormone Conference, 1971. (Aug. 29 to Sept. 3rd, Mont Tremblant, Quebec). *Recent Progr. Hormone Res.*, 28:343, 1972.

24. Seth, K., Nowaczynski, W., Kuchel, O. et al: Determination of the secretion rate of 18-hydroxy-11-deoxycorticosterone by a double-isotope derivative assay and studies on metabolism of 18-hydroxy-deoxycorticosterone in man. Submitted for publication to *J. Clin. Endocr.*

25. Seth, K., Nowaczynski, W., Kuchel, O. et al: Procedure for simultaneous determination of secretion rates of deoxycorticosterone and corticosterone by double-isotope derivative assay. *Canad. J. Biochem.*, 50:136, 1972.

26. Boucher, R., Veyrat, R. and DeChamplain, J. et al: New procedures for measurement of human plasma angiotensin and renin activity levels. *Canad. Med. Ass. J.*, 90:194, 1964.

27. Genest, J., Nowaczynski, W., Kuchel, O. et al: New evidences of disturbances of mineralocorticoid activity in benign, uncomplicated essential hypertension. *Trans. Amer. Clin. Climat. Ass.*, 83:134, 1971.

28. Genest, J., Nowaczynski, W. and Kuchel, O.: Mineralocorticoid metabolism in benign essential hypertension. Presented at the Sixth Meeting of the Intern. Study Group for Steroid Hormones, Rome, Italy, December 6-8, 1973. *Research on Steroids*, Vol. VI, 1974.

29. Genest, J., Boucher, R., Nowaczynski, W. et al: Studies on the relationship of aldosterone and angiotensin to human hypertensive diseases. Intern. Symposium on Aldosterone, ed. Baulieu, E. E. and Robel, P. Prague 1964, p. 393. Oxford:Blackwell, 1964.

30. Genest, J., Lemieux, G., Davignon, A. et al: Human arterial hypertension: A state of mild chronic hyperaldosteronism? *Science*, 123:503, 1956.

31. Genest, J., Nowaczynski, W., Koiw, E. et al: Participation of the adrenal glands and the kidneys in human arterial hypertension. Institution Paper, Proc. IVth World Congress of Cardiology. Tome IV-A, p. 22, Mexico:Impresor Calve, S.A., 1962.

32. Genest, J., Nowaczynski, W., Koiw, E. et al: Adrenocortical function in essential hypertension. Essential hypertension. An Intern. Symposium, ed. Bock, K. D. and Cottier, P. T., p. 126, Berlin-Gottingen-Heidelberg:Springer, 1960.

33. Nowaczynski, W., Koiw, E. and Genest, J.: Chemical method for the determination of urinary aldosterone. *Canad. J. Biochem. Physiol.*, 35:425, 1957.

34. Biglieri, E. G., Slaton, P. E., Schambelan, M. et al: Hypermineralocorticoidism. *Amer. J. Med.*, 45:170, 1968.

35. Kaplan, N. M.: Hypokalemia in the hypertensive patient. *Ann. Intern. Med.*, 66:1079, 1967.

36. Katsushima, T.: Aldosterone. *Nippon Rinsho*, 27:394, 1969.

37. Laragh, J. H., Cannon, P. J. and Ames, R. P.: Aldosterone secretion and various forms of hypertensive vascular disease. *Ann. Intern. Med.*, 59:117, 1963.

38. Laragh, J., Ulick, S., Januszewicz, V. et al: Electrolyte metabolism and aldosterone secretion in benign and malignant hypertension. *Ann. Intern. Med.*, 53:259, 1960.

39. Nowaczynski, W., Kuchel, O. and Genest, J.: A decreased MCR of aldosterone, a possible mechanism of development of hyperaldosteronism in benign uncomplicated essential hypertension. *Circulation*, 42 (suppl. 3):88, 1970.

40. Nowaczynski, W., Kuchel, O., Genest, J. et al: Dynamic aldosterone and 18-hydroxydeoxycorticosterone studies in labile and stable benign essential hypertension. In Proceedings (Symposium on Steroids

and Hypertension) of the Fourth Intern. Congress on Hormonal Steroids, Mexico, September 2-7, 1974. *J. Steroid Biochem.* 6:1975.

41. Wilkins, R. W., Culbertson, J. W. and Rymut, A. A.: The hepatic blood flow in resting hypertensive patients before and after splanchnicectomy. *J. Clin. Invest.*, 31:529, 1952.

42. Wollheim, E.: Hämodynamik und Organdurchblütung beim Hochdruck. Symposium on high blood pressure research in Feiburg i Br. The 18-19 of July 1964. In Heilmeyer, L. and Holtmeir, H. J.: *Hochdruck Forschung.* Stuttgart:Georg Thieme Verlag, 1965, p. 136.

43. Messerli, F. H., Genest, J., Nowaczynski, W. et al: Splanchnic blood flow in benign essential and renovascular hypertension. Amer. Heart Assoc. 47th Meeting, November 18-21, 1974, Dallas, Texas. (Abstract # 1122 in supplement to *Circulation,* October 1974.)

44. Cope, C. L., Harwood, M. and Pearson, J.: Aldosterone secretion in hypertensive diseases. *Brit. Med. J.,* 1:659, 1962.

45. Genest, J., Koiw, E., Nowaczynski, W. et al: Further studies on urinary aldosterone in human arterial hypertension. *Proc. Soc. Exp. Biol. Med.,* 97:676, 1958.

46. Genest, J., Koiw, E., Nowaczynski, W. et al: Study of a large steroid spectrum in normal subjects and hypertensive patients. *Acta Endocr. (Kbh),* 35:413, 1960.

47. Siegenthaler, W. E., Peterson, R. E. and Frimpter, G. W.: The renal clearance of aldosterone and its major metabolites. In Baulieu, E. E. and Robel, P. (eds.): *Aldosterone, A Symposium.* Oxford:Blackwell, 1964, p. 51.

48. Laragh, J. H.: Aldosterone in fluid and electrolyte disorders: Hyper and hypoaldosteronism. *J. Chronic Dis.,* 11:292, 1960.

49. Ross, E. J.: Aldosterone and its antagonists. *Clin. Pharmacol. Ther.,* 6:65, 1965.

50. Genest, J., Nowaczynski, W., Kuchel, O. et al: Plasma progesterone levels and 18-hydroxydeoxycorticosterone secretion rate in benign essential hypertension in humans. In Genest, J. and Koiw, E. (eds.): *Hypertension '72.* Berlin, Heidelberg, New York:Springer-Verlag, 1972, p. 293.

51. Armstrong, J. G.: Hypotensive action of progesterone in experimental and human hypertension. *Proc. Soc. Exp. Biol. Med.,* 102:452, 1959.

52. Landau, R. L., Bergenstal, D. M., Lugibihl, K. et al: The metabolic effects of progesterone in man. *J. Clin. Endocr.,* 15:1194, 1965.

53. Landau, R. L. and Lugibihl, K.: Inhibition of the sodium-retaining influence of aldosterone by progesterone. *J. Clin. Endocr.,* 18:1237, 1958.

54. Sharp, G. W. G. and Leaf, A.: Mechanism of action of aldosterone. *Physiol. Rev.,* 46:593, 1966.

55. Laidlaw, J. C., Ruse, J. L. and Gornall, A. G.: The influence of estrogen and progesterone on aldosterone excretion. *J. Clin. Endocr.,* 22:161, 1962.

56. Layne, D. S., Meyer, C. J., Vaishwanar, P. S. et al: The secretion and metabolism of cortisol and aldosterone in normal and in steroid

treated women. *J. Clin. Endocr.*, 22:107, 1962.
57. Watanabe, M., Meeker, C. I., Gray, M. J. et al: Aldosterone secretion rates in abnormal pregnancy. *J. Clin. Endocr.*, 25:1665, 1965.
58. Ehrlich. E. N.: Hepatinoid-induced inhibition of aldosterone secretion in pregnant women. *Amer. J. Obstet. Gynec.*, 109:963, 1971.
59. Vermeulen, A. and Van Der Straeten, M.: Adrenal cortical function in benign essential hypertension. *J. Clin. Endocr.*, 23:574, 1963.
60. Luetscher, J. A., Weinberger, M. H., Dowdy, A. J. et al: Effects of sodium loading, sodium depletion and posture on plasma aldosterone concentration and renin activity in hypertensive patients. *J. Clin. Endocr.*, 29:1310, 1969.
61. Woods, J. W., Liddle, G. W., Stant, E. G., Jr. et al: Effect of an adrenal inhibitor in hypertensive patients with suppressed renin. *Arch. Intern. Med.*, 123:366, 1969.
62. Jose, A., Crout, J. R. and Kaplan, N. M.: Suppressed plasma renin activity in essential hypertension. Roles of plasma volume, blood pressure, and sympathetic nervous system. *Ann. Intern. Med.*, 72:9, 1970.
63. Messerli, F. H., Kuchel, O., Nowaczynski, W. et al: Mineralocorticoid secretion in low renin benign essential hypertension. Endocrine Society, 56th Meeting, June 12-14, 1974, Atlanta, Georgia, Abstract # 16.
64. D'Amour, P., Kuchel, O., McGarry, E. E. et al: 17-hydroxylase deficiency with hypertension and hypokalemia mimicking prepubertal testicular feminization. Fourth Intern. Congress of Endocrinology, Washington, 18-24 June 1972. In *Excerpta Med. Intern. Congr. Ser.*, No. 256, Abstract # 280.

Discussion

Dr. Langford: Is the aldosterone-binding globulin-like protein inducible, either by aldosterone or by things like estrogen or cortisol, that induce other binding proteins? In general, is the progesterone secretion correlated with your aldosterone secretion? Is it affected by non-ACTH factors that affect aldosterone secretion, ie, does either sodium loading or sodium deficiency affect your progesterone secretion rate or levels?

Dr. Nowaczynski: As far as the progesterone is concerned, sodium restriction increases the plasma concentration of progesterone in normal subjects. However, the response in patients with essential hypertension was mixed. About one half responded as normal subjects and one half did not respond. Sodium restriction or loading, however, did not affect the aldosterone protein binding. Baseline plasma progesterone levels are increased in many patients with essential hypertension.

I don't think that I can answer the question as to whether the aldosterone-binding globulin-like protein is really inducible but the binding is increased in the luteal phase of the menstrual cycle, during pregnancy and in essential hypertension. As far as antihypertensive drugs are concerned, our labile hypertensives were all untreated patients, and it was in them that we had the most marked modification in this protein binding and in all of the other parameters we studied, so we can at least assume that the antihypertensive drugs were not inducing any increase in the aldosterone binding. The only steroid that we tried directly was dexamethasone which increased the aldosterone binding four- to fivefold, with a simultaneous drop in the aldosterone, plasma concentration and which occurred only in the free fraction. This means that after dexamethasone, the circulating aldosterone is mostly bound to this globulin with almost no free aldosterone. ACTH did the contrary; it decreased the binding and increased the plasma concentration of aldosterone. We have not yet tried administering progesterone or cortisol, but we are intending to do so. We did do displacement experiments in vitro with progesterone, deoxycorticosterone, 18-hydroxydeoxy-corticosterone, aldosterone and cortisol, and we can displace labeled aldosterone from its binding with aldosterone only, but we cannot displace it with other steroids or perhaps only to a very minute extent. For instance, estrogens or dehydro-epiandosterone will not displace it at all. This, in a way, indicates that it may be a specific binding. We did not do these experiments in vivo yet.

Dr. Kirkendall, Moderator: Dr. Nowaczynski, would you go over how you think the majority of patients with low renin hypertension get their hypertension? What is your hypothesis, based upon this evidence you have now?

Dr. Nowaczynski: I think that from our evidence we can probably assume that some of these patients must have a certain degree of 17α-hydroxylation deficiency, similar to that found in one patient who had a very marked decrease in 17α-hydroxylase, and in those patients we find most of the time low or low normal aldosterone values. But, as far as the majority of low renin patients is concerned, we seem to have more circulating aldosterone and more 18-hydroxydeoxycorticosterone which would indicate that there is an excess of mineralocorticoid activity coming probably from aldosterone, from 18-hydroxy-deoxycorticosterone, as well as from deoxycorticosterone and corticosterone. All three or four of these steroids seem to be slightly increased, and maybe a combination of them is enough to induce greater sodium retention.

Dr. Kirkendall: Dr. Nowaczynski, have you found many patients with rather marked degrees of 17α-hydroxylase deficiency?

Dr. Nowaczynski: This one patient that I have shown has a very marked reduction in 17α-hydroxylase. The 18-hydroxy-deoxycorticosterone is ACTH-dependent and it was very high in this patient. Many patients with low renin activity also have quite high secretory rates of 18-hydroxydeoxycorticosterone.

Dr. Kirkendall: As high as he had?

Dr. Nowaczynski: Almost. We had two or three patients who had 4 or 5 mg/day which is not far from the value of close to 8 mg/day in this patient.

Dr. Williams, Massachusetts: Do you have any feeling whether in the normal renin group, total mineralocorticoid activity was excessive or normal? Second, Dr. Tait and his group, with Brian Little, about seven or eight years ago, looked at binding of aldosterone. If I remember correctly, they found that normal plasma would bind about 50% but that, in pregnancy, something was induced, presumably by hormones that come with pregnancy, so that there was an increase in aldosterone binding. Do you have any thoughts about whether the material you are measuring is related to theirs and whether it is increased in pregnancy?

Dr. Nowaczynski: First, transient excessive plasma aldos-terone levels induced by ACTH, stress, circadian rhythm or any other stimulation seem to be present in all patients with essential hypertension because of delays in elimination of circulating aldosterone due to modifications in its metabolism, especially the clearance rate which seems to be closely related to changes in plasma protein binding. Second, the binding that we have studied is increased in the first, second, and third trimester of pregnancy, and the total aldosterone concentration is increased. Both the concentration of aldosterone bound and the total aldosterone decrease immediately postpartum. I think that probably this must be the same protein or proteins as described by Tait et al. As far as the amount bound is concerned, it was found before that about 40% was bound in normal subjects, and this was the sum of the albumin and the globulin bound fractions. We are finding that about 20% would be bound to albumin and about 15% would be bound probably to globulin-like plasma fraction in normal subjects.

Hypermineralocorticoid Hypertension

Gaddo Onesti, M.D. and Michael Fernandes, M.D.

It is now well accepted that overproduction of different mineralocorticoids by the adrenal gland may result in sustained hypertension in man.[1,2] It is also recognized that the administration of mineralocorticoids produces sustained hypertension in the experimental animal.[3] Clinical examples of hypertension caused by overproduction of mineralocorticoid hormones include primary aldosteronism (Conn's syndrome), 17-alpha-hydroxylase deficiency (Biglieri's syndrome), virilizing adrenal hyperplasia, Cushing's disease (or syndrome), non-adrenal ACTH-producing tumors and adrenocortical carcinomas (Table 1). In addition, Melby and co-workers have described excessive production of 18-hydroxy-11-deoxycorticosterone in hypertensive patients with hypertension of unknown etiology and low plasma renin.[4] Furthermore, Rapp and co-workers have reported increased production of the same hormone in genetic hypertensive rats.[5] Thus, 18-hydroxy-11-deoxycorticosterone hypertension may now represent an additional form of mineralocorticoid hypertension.

In 1940, Grollman, Harrison and Williams successfully produced hypertension in the rat by administering sterols.[6] In 1943, Selye, Hall and Rowley introduced the experimental model of deoxycorticosterone and salt hypertension.[7] Progressive elevation of blood pressure following the administration of deoxycorticosterone and salt is facilitated by previous unilateral nephrectomy.[3] Although aldosterone is the most potent mineralocorticoid, early attempts to produce experimental

---

Gaddo Onesti, M.D. *and* Michael Fernandes, M.D., *Division of Nephrology and Hypertension, Hahnemann Medical College and Hospital, Philadelphia, Pa.*

TABLE 1. Hypertension Caused by Overproduction
of Mineralocorticoid Hormones[2]

A) Primary aldosteronism (Conn's syndrome)
B) 17-alpha-hydroxylase deficiency (Biglieri's syndrome)
C) Hypertensive form of virilizing adrenal hyperplasia
   (11β-hydroxylase deficiency)
D) Cushing's disease (or syndrome)
E) Non-adrenal ACTH-producing tumors
F) Adrenocortical carcinoma
G) Iatrogenic: anovulatory pills, licorice, glucocorticoids and
   excess salt intake

---

hypertension with aldosterone administration failed.[8-10] In 1965, Hall and Hall demonstrated that d-aldosterone acetate, 0.25 mg/day, caused rapid and severe hypertensive vascular disease in the rat.[11] This was subsequently confirmed by Fregly and co-workers.[12]

Clinical observations and experimental studies have established the cause-effect relationship between mineralocorticoid excess and blood pressure elevation. However, a precise explanation of the mechanisms involved is still lacking.

Mechanisms of Experimental Mineralocorticoid Hypertension

Since the administration of sodium chloride together with the mineralocorticoid is a sine qua non for the production of hypertension, it was logical to assign to sodium chloride a major pathophysiologic role. Therefore, it has been postulated that the retention of sodium chloride and water, induced by the mineralocorticoid, resulted in swelling of the arteriolar wall, elevating resistance to flow and blood pressure.[13] Alternatively, the electrolyte composition of the arteriolar wall (increased sodium chloride content) may result in increased sensitivity of the vascular smooth muscle to neurogenic stimuli.[14] This would also lead to an increase in peripheral resistance and blood pressure. Indeed, the tail arteries in rats treated with DOCA and salt exhibit an increased responsiveness to norepinephrine.[15] In 1973, Dustin, Harris and Rand demonstrated a positive correlation between total exchangeable sodium and blood pressure in rats treated with salt and DOCA.[16] In the same study the cardiac and vascular responses to sympathetic stimulation were positively correlated with exchangeable sodium. These findings suggested that sodium retention may increase sympathetic activity.

Indeed, de Champlain and co-workers performed systematic studies of the functions of sympathetic nerve endings in regard to uptake, storage, turnover, subcellular distribution and metabolism of norepinephrine in DOCA and salt hypertensive rats.[17] The final analysis showed an increased turnover of norepinephrine in the sympathetic peripheral fibers.[18] This increase in norepinephrine turnover may play an important role in the pathophysiology of DOCA and salt hypertension, since the increase in turnover precedes the development of hypertension.[19] The sodium ion appears to be essential for this activation of norepinephrine turnover.[19,20] After two weeks of treatment with salt and DOCA, the change to a sodium-free diet for two weeks reduced the blood pressure and restored norepinephrine metabolism to normal.[19,20] Furthermore, the changes of adrenergic function induced by DOCA and salt were the opposite of those observed during periods of sodium depletion.[19,20]

Whether DOCA and salt affect the binding or the transport of norepinephrine locally at the site of the adrenergic nerve ending, or whether they influence the adrenergic activity through a direct or indirect action on the central nervous system remains to be established. According to Nakamura, Gerold and Thoenen, DOCA and salt hypertension is associated with decreased norepinephrine turnover in the brain stem of the rat.[21] Indeed, Haeusler, Finch and Thoenen have shown that the development of DOCA and salt hypertension could be prevented by destruction of central adrenergic neurons by intraventricular administration of 6-hydroxydopamine.[22] These findings support the contention that the onset of DOCA and salt hypertension is mediated by the central adrenergic neurons.

To test the hypothesis of a peripheral adrenergic dysfunction in DOCA and salt hypertension, rats whose peripheral adrenergic fibers were destroyed were studied by de Champlain[23] and by Clarke and co-workers.[24] In rats with degeneration of adrenergic nerve fibers by 6-hydroxydopamine, de Champlain reported a progressive increase in blood pressure during DOCA and salt administration. However, the blood pressure remained significantly lower than the normally innervated controls and failed to reach true hypertensive levels. In the study of Clark and co-workers, similar destruction of adrenergic nerve terminals failed to alter the onset, course and severity of DOCA and salt hypertension. The reasons for these discrepancies between the two studies are not explained at the present time.

In contrast with the theory that describes a predominant participation of the adrenergic nervous system, a theory of autoregulation explains DOCA and salt hypertension on the basis of an initial hypervolemia. DOCA and salt administration would result in an increased blood volume and a consequent increase in cardiac output. With an increase in cardiac output, the peripheral tissues would be perfused at a rate above their metabolic needs. This phenomenon causes a peripheral myogenic arteriolar constriction which would result in an increased peripheral vascular resistance and sustained blood pressure elevation.[25,26] This interpretation excludes the participation of the adrenergic nervous system and the possible direct vascular effect of the sodium ion.

The Renin-Angiotensin System in Mineralocorticoid Hypertension

Although it has been reported that the blood of animals with DOCA and salt hypertension has increased pressor activity,[27,28] it has been considered unlikely that this pressor activity is carried by the renin-angiotensin system. Administration of salt and sodium-retaining hormones is known to result in renin suppression. Gross demonstrated that deoxycorticosterone and 1% saline resulted in a significant decrease in renin content in the rat kidney[29]; similar effects were described with the administration of aldosterone.[29] It should also be noted that the administration of salt is necessary for the suppression of renin in these experimental preparations.[7] Certainly, a decrease in plasma renin activity is a well-recognized phenomenon in primary aldosteronism.[30] Precise evaluation of the components of the renin-angiotensin system in the experimental animal and man reveals that mineralocorticoids (and glucocorticoids) may exert a significant effect on renin substrate. ACTH and cortisone have been found to increase renin substrate in the rat[31] and in the dog.[32] Carretero and Gross also reported an increase in renin substrate in the experimental animal treated with mineralocorticoids.[33] This is in agreement with the elevation of substrate found in patients with primary aldosteronism.[34-36] From the pathophysiologic standpoint it is highly unlikely that the renin-angiotensin system plays any role in primary aldosteronism in man. In contrast, patients with Cushing's syndrome exhibit an elevated plasma renin activity. This is due to an increase in both renin and renin substrate.[35] At this time, despite the commonly accepted concept that renin is suppressed by mineralocorticoid excess and sodium chloride, precise studies of the components of the renin-angiotensin system (renin, renin substrate, angiotensin I, converting enzyme and angiotensin II) in experimental and clinical hypermineralocorticoid hypertension are not yet available.

Body Fluids and Systemic Hemodynamic Alterations in Human Mineralocorticoid Hypertension

Patients with primary aldosteronism have demonstrated a significant increase in extracellular water and total exchangeable sodium, while intracellular potassium is markedly decreased.[37]

The systemic hemodynamic characteristics of the hypertension of primary aldosteronism have been recently delineated by Tarazi and co-workers.[38] As compared with patients with essential hypertension, matched for age and blood pressure levels, the patients with primary aldosteronism exhibited a higher cardiac index, heart rate and left ventricular mean ejection rate. In addition, cardiac index showed a direct relationship with blood volume and an inverse relationship with diastolic blood pressure. The latter correlation stresses the predominant importance of the peripheral resistance in the maintenance of the hypertension of primary aldosteronism.[38] This hemodynamic pattern is similar to that described in renovascular hypertension[39] and end-stage renal disease.[40] These hemodynamic characteristics again emphasize the importance of the total peripheral resistance in hypertensive states associated with an increase in cardiac output.

Distler and co-workers also described the hemodynamic pattern of primary aldosteronism and showed that administration of spironolactone lowered blood pressure by decreasing cardiac output, heart rate and blood volume. At the same time, however, total peripheral resistance was also decreased.[41]

According to the work of Tarazi and co-workers, in primary aldosteronism as well as in essential hypertension, plasma volume correlated inversely with peripheral vascular resistance. However, the regression was shifted to the right in primary aldosteronism.[38] Thus, for any level of resistance, plasma volume was higher in primary aldosteronism than in essential hypertension. This is compatible with the prevailing opinion of an overexpansion of the extracellular fluid compartment (and blood volume) in primary aldosteronism. However, it should be noted that the plasma volume of primary aldosteronism, although higher than in essential hypertension, is not different from that of normal subjects.[38]

With normal intravascular volume, the high cardiac output of primary aldosteronism results from either a direct increase in myocardial stimulation[42,43] or a central redistribution of blood volume (an increase in cardiopulmonary blood volume). In primary aldosteronism, the cardiac output correlates inversely with diastolic blood pressure. This implies that peripheral vascular resistance is the primary factor sustaining blood pressure. The factors responsible for the increase of both cardiac output and peripheral resistance remain unknown. We may speculate that the "peripheral factor" responsible for the central redistribution of blood volume may also be responsible for the increase in total peripheral resistance and blood pressure.

Conclusion

Mineralocorticoid excess in man and the administration of mineralocorticoids to the experimental animal result in sustained hypertension. Despite numerous clinical observations and laboratory studies, the precise mechanism of this hypertension remains uncertain. The extensive studies of de Champlain[23] have strongly suggested the participation of the adrenergic nervous system in DOCA-salt hypertension in the rat, the experimental counterpart of human mineralocorticoid hypertension. Verification of this mechanism, however, awaits final confirmation. Although the traditional concept accepts a suppression of renin, a precise study of the various components of the renin-angiotensin system has not been accomplished. Although studies have suggested an overexpansion of the body fluids in primary aldosteronism, hemodynamic assessments have demonstrated a concomitant increase in cardiac output and total peripheral resistance in this hypertension. The simultaneous elevation of cardiac output and peripheral resistance in this situation requires further investigation. The various pathophysiologic mechanisms are not mutually exclusive. In fact, it is now well established that different pathophysiologic factors may come into play at different phases of the same hypertensive process.

Acknowledgment

The authors acknowledge the invaluable assistance of Franny Dienes in the preparation of this manuscript.

References

1. Conn, J. W.: Primary aldosteronism. *J. Lab. Clin. Med.*, 45:661-664, 1955.
2. Genest, J., Kuchel, O. and Nowaczynski, W.: Classification of hypermineralocorticoid hypertension. In Onesti, G., Kim, K. E. and Moyer, J. H. (eds.): *Hypertension: Mechanisms and Management.* New York: Grune and Stratton, 1973, p. 463
3. Hall, C. E. and Hall, O.: Sensitization to hypertensive action of desoxycorticosterone by unilateral nephrectomy: Relationship to dosage and to interval between surgery and hormone administration. *Endocrinology*, 63:329, 1958.
4. Melby, J. C., Dale, S. L., Grekin, R. J. et al: 18-hydroxy-11 deoxycorticosterone (18-OH-DOC) secretion in experimental and human hypertension. In Onesti, G., Kim, K. E. and Moyer, J. H. (eds.): *Hypertension: Mechanisms and Management.* New York: Grune and Stratton, 1973, p. 523.
5. Rapp, J. P. and Dahl, L. K.: Inheritance of 18-hydroxycorticosterone formation in genetic hypertension in rats. In Onesti, G., Kim, K. E. and Moyer, J. H. (eds.):*Hypertension: Mechanisms and Management.* New York:Grune and Stratton, 1973, p. 513.
6. Grollman, A., Harrison, T. R. and Williams, J. R.: Effects of various sterol derivatives on blood pressure in the rat. *J. Pharmacol. Exp. Ther.*, 69:149, 1940.
7. Selye, H., Hall, C. E. and Rowley, E. M.: Malignant hypertension produced by treatment with desoxycorticosterone acetate and sodium chloride. *Canad. Med. Ass. J.*, 49:88, 1943.

8. Gaunt, R. Ulsamer, G. F. and Chart, J. J.: Aldosterone and hypertension. *Arch. Int. Pharmacodyn. Ther.*, 110:114, 1958.
9. Fregly, M. J. and Arean, V. M.: Comparison of the effects of aldosterone and desoxysterone acetate on blood pressure of rats. *Acta Physiol. Pharmacol. Neerl.*, 8:162, 1959.
10. Gross, F., Loustalot, P. and Meier, R.: Vergleichende Untersuchungen uber die hypertensive wirkung von aldosteron und desoxycorticosteron. *Experientia*, 11:67, 1955.
11. Hall, C. E. and Hall, O.: Hypertension and hypersalimentation. I. Aldosterone hypertension. *Lab. Invest.*, 14:285, 1965.
12. Fregly, M., Kim, K. J. and Hood, C. I.: Development of hypertension in rats treated with aldosterone acetate. *Toxic. Appl. Pharmacol.*, 15:229, 1969.
13. Folkow, B., Grimby, G. and Thulesius, O.: Adaptive structural changes of the vascular walls in hypertension and their relation to the control of peripheral resistance. *Acta Physiol. Scand.*, 44:255, 1958.
14. Hinke, J. A. M.: In vitro demonstration of vascular hyper-responsiveness in experimental hypertension. *Circ. Res.*, 18:359, 1965.
15. Beilin, L. J., Wade, D. N., Honour, A. J. et al: Vascular hyperreactivity with sodium loading and with desoxycorticosterone-induced hypertension in the rat. *Clin. Sci.*, 39:793, 1970.
16. Dustin, G. J., Harris, G. S. and Rand, M. J.: A specific increase in cardiovascular reactivity related to sodium retention in DOCA-salt treated rats. *Clin. Sci. Molec. Med.*, 45:571, 1973.
17. de Champlain, J., Krakoff, L. R. and Axelrod, J.: The metabolism of norepinephrine in experimental hypertension in rats. *Circ. Res.*, 20:136, 1967.
18. Krakoff, L. R., de Champlain, J. and Axelrod, J.: Abnormal storage of norepinephrine in experimental hypertension in the rat. *Circ. Res.*, 21:583, 1967.
19. de Champlain, J., Krakoff, L. R. and Axelrod, J.: Relationship between sodium intake and norepinephrine storage during the development of experimental hypertension. *Circ. Res.*, 24:1, 1969.
20. de Champlain, J., Krakoff, L. R. and Axelrod, J.: Interrelationship of sodium hypertension and norepinephrine storage in the rat. *Circ. Res.*, 24:1, 1969.
21. Nakamura, K., Gerold, M. and Thoenen, H.: Experimental hypertension of the rat: Reciprocal changes of norepinephrine turnover in heart and brain-stem. *Naunyn Schmiedebergs Arch. Pharmakol.*, 268:125, 1971.
22. Haeusler, G., Finch, L. and Thoenen, H.: Central adrenergic neurons and the initiation and development of experimental hypertension. *Experientia*, 28:1200, 1972.
23. de Champlain, J.: The influence of sodium on the sympathetic system in relation to experimental hypertension. In Onesti, G., Kim, K. E. and Moyer, J. H. (eds.): *Hypertension: Mechanisms and Management.* New York: Grune and Stratton, 1973, p. 147.
24. Clarke, D. E., Smookler, H. H. and Barry, H.: Sympathetic nerve

function and DOCA-NaCl induced hypertension. *Life Sci.*, 9:1097, 1970.
25. Ledingham, J. M. and Pelling, D.: Cardiac output and peripheral resistance in experimental renal hypertension in rats. *Circ. Res.*, 2l(suppl. 2):187, 1967.
26. Guyton, A. C., Coleman, T. G. and Granger, H. J.: Circulation: Overall regulation. *Ann. Rev. Physiol.*, 34:13, 1972.
27. Dahl, L. K., Knudsen, R. D. and Iwai, J.: Humoral transmission of hypertension, evidence from parabiosis. *Circ. Res.* 24(suppl. 1):21, 1969.
28. de Champlain, J., Krakoff, L. R. and Axelrod, J.: A reduction in the accumulation of H3 norepinephrine in experimental hypertension. *Life Sci.*, 5:2283, 1966.
29. Gross, F.: Adrenocortical function and renal pressor mechanisms in experimental hypertension. In Bock, K. D. and Cottier, P. T. (eds.): *Essential Hypertension, an International Symposium.* Berlin: Springer-Verlag, 1960, p. 92.
30. Conn, J. W.: An overall view of primary aldosteronism. In Onesti, G., Kim, K. E. and Moyer, J. H. (eds.): *Hypertension: Mechanisms and Management.* New York: Grune and Stratton, 1973, p. 471.
31. Hasegawa, H., Nasjletti, A., Rice, K. et al: Role of pituitary and adrenals in the regulation of plasma angiotensinogen. *Amer. J. Physiol.*, 225:1, 1973.
32. Haynes, F. W., Forsham, P. H. and Hume, D.: Effects of ACTH, cortisone, desoxycortisone and epinephrine on plasma hypertensinogen and renin concentration of dogs. *Amer. J. Physiol.*, 172:265, 1953.
33. Carretero, O. and Gross, F.: Renin substrate in plasma under various experimental conditions in the rat. *Amer. J. Physiol.*, 213:695, 1967.
34. Rosset, E., Scherrer, J. R. and Veyrat, R.: Increased plasma renin substrate concentrations in human malignant hypertension. *Clin. Sci. Molec. Med.*, 45:219s, 1973.
35. Krakoff, C. R.: Measurement of plasma renin substrate by radio-immunoassay of angiotensin I concentration in syndromes associated with steroid excess. *J. Clin. Endocr. Metab.*, 37:110, 1973.
36. Krakoff, C. R. and Mendlowitz, M.: Plasma renin activity and plasma renin substrate in hypertension associated with steroid excess. *Clin. Sci. Molec. Med.*, 45:295x, 1973.
37. Novak, L. P., Strong, C. G. and Hunt, J. C.: Body composition in primary and secondary hypertension. In Genest, J. and Koiw, E. (eds.): *Hypertension 72.* Berlin: Springer-Verlag, 1972, p. 444.
38. Tarazi, R. C., Ibrahim, M. M., Bravo, E. L. et al: Hemodynamic characteristics of primary aldosteronism. *New Eng. J. Med.*, 289:1330, 1973.
39. Tarazi, R. C., Frohlich, E. D. and Dustan, H. P.: Contribution of cardiac output to renovascular hypertension in man: Relation to surgical treatment. *Amer. J. Cardiol.*, 31:600, 1973.
40. Kim, K. E., Onesti, G., Schwartz, A. B. et al: Hemodynamics of

hypertension in chronic end-stage renal disease. *Circulation*, 46:456, 1972.

41. Distler, A., Just, H. J. and Philipp, T.: Untersuchungen zur pathogenese des hochdrucks bei primaren aldosteronismus. *Deutsch. Med. Wschr.*, 98:100, 1973.

42. Ballard, K., Lefer, A. and Sayers, G.: The effect of aldosterone and of plasma extracts on a rat heart-lung preparation. *Amer. J. Physiol.* 199:221, 1960.

43. Tanz, R. D.: Studies of the inotropic action of aldosterone on isolated cardiac tissue preparations: Including the effects of ph, ovabain and S C-8109. *J. Pharmacol. Exp. Ther.*, 135:71, 1962.

Relationship of Multiple Variables to Blood Pressure — Findings From Four Chicago Epidemiologic Studies

Jeremiah Stamler, M.D., David M. Berkson, M.D.,
Alan Dyer, Ph.D., Mark H. Lepper, M.D.,
Howard A. Lindberg, M.D., Oglesby Paul, M.D.,
Harlley McKean, M.D., Peter Rhomberg, M.D.,
James A. Schoenberger, M.D., Richard B. Shekelle, Ph.D.
and Rose Stamler, M.A.

It has been repeatedly asserted that essential hypertension is a disease of multifactorial etiology. However, few attempts have been made simultaneously to evaluate the relationship of multiple factors of possible pathogenic significance to blood pressure. This report — based on cross-sectional and prospective epidemiologic studies in Chicago — presents data on several variables concurrently considered in relation to blood pressure. The approach is that used in the investigation of risk factors for coronary heart disease, the problem that has preoccupied cardiovascular epidemiology for over two decades. In this instance, however, instead of blood pressure serving as an independent variable, it is the dependent variable, ie, the end point. The aim is to elucidate factors that may be playing a role — even if low order — in the pathogenesis of essential hypertension.

Four methods of multivariate analysis have been used: multiple cross-classification, partial correlation, multiple logistic

Jeremiah Stamler, M.D., David M. Berkson, M.D., Alan Dyer, Ph.D., Mark H. Lepper, M.D., Howard A. Lindberg, M.D., Oglesby Paul, M.D., Harlley McKean, M.D., Peter Rhomberg, M.D., James A. Schoenberger, M.D., Richard B. Shekelle, Ph.D. and Rose Stamler, M.A., *Department of Community Health and Preventive Medicine and the Department of Medicine, Northwestern University Medical School; Division of Adult Health and Aging, Chicago Board of Health; Chicago Heart Association; the Department of Preventive Medicine, Rush-Presbyterian St. Luke's Medical Center.*

and multiple linear regression. The populations under study
have been the following:

1.   13,469 men and women, white and black, age 30-64,
     participating in a Chicago Health Department multi-
     phasic screening project based from 1965 through 1971
     in two Chicago Housing Authority public housing
     projects for low income persons;

2.   21,024 men and women, white and black, age 25-64,
     participating in the Chicago Heart Association Detection
     Project in Industry from the fall of 1967 through the
     spring of 1972;

3.   1,730 middle-aged white men employed by the Western
     Electric Company in Chicago — participants in the
     long-term prospective epidemiologic study of this labor
     force;

4.   787 middle-aged men, over 90% of whom were white,
     employed by the Peoples Gas Light and Coke Company
     in Chicago — participants in the long-term prospective
     epidemiologic study of this labor force.

Detailed descriptions of these studies, their populations and
methods, have been reported elsewhere.[1-12]

TABLE 1.
**Partial Correlation Coefficients between Blood Pressure and
Other Variables, by Age-Sex-Race
Chicago Board of Health Community Surveys, 1965-71**

	White Male Age 30-44 N=803		White Male Age 45-64 N=1,151		White Female Age 30-44 N=2,367		White Female Age 45-64 N=3,114	
	SBP	DBP	SBP	DBP	SBP	DBP	SBP	DBP
Age	.009	.082*	.193***	-.051	.117***	.138***	.244***	.042*
Heart Rate	.273***	.236***	.208***	.194***	.170***	.144***	.151***	.164*
Serum Cholesterol	.046	.092**	.017	.049	.026	.042*	.029	.031
1-Hour Plasma Glucose	.157***	.090*	.211***	.135***	.145***	.115***	.159***	.067*
Relative Weight	.272***	.304***	.219***	.243***	.318***	.359***	.266***	.298*
Hematocrit	.056	.069	.052	.112***	.016	.060**	.048**	.087*

	Black Male Age 30-44 N=630		Black Male Age 45-64 N=686		Black Female Age 30-44 N=2,515		Black Female Age 45-64 N=2,203	
	SBP	DBP	SBP	DBP	SBP	DBP	SBP	DBP
e	.108**	.082*	.145***	.029	.159***	.127***	.157***	.018
art Rate	.180***	.167***	.137***	.195***	.114***	.099***	.107***	.112***
rum lesterol	.053	.052	-.027	.001	.010	.042*	.006	.014
our Plasma cose	-.016	.019	.094*	.026	.127***	.089***	.144***	.075***
ative ght	.269***	.291***	.224***	.218***	.309***	.300***	.237***	.258***
atocrit	-.001	.007	-.049	.030	.016	.056**	.029	.066**

* $p \leq$ .05

** $p \leq$ .01

*** $p \leq$ .001

SBP is systolic blood pressure.

DBP is diastolic blood pressure.

For each partial correlation coefficient calculated, the other five variables were held constant.

Results

Chicago Health Department Community Surveys

The relationship of six variables to blood pressure was evaluated in this study: relative weight (ratio of observed weight to desirable weight for height and sex, based on actuarial tables),[13,14]* resting heart rate, plasma glucose one hour after 100 gm oral load, serum cholesterol, hematocrit and age.[1]

Partial correlation analyses. With calculation of partial correlation coefficients, ie, r's between blood pressure and each of the six independent variables adjusted for the other five, r's for blood pressure and relative weight were in the range 0.2-0.4 with p values $\leq$ .001 (Table 1). The partial r's also were highly significant for heart rate and blood pressure (range 0.1-0.3, $p \leq$ .001). For all sex-race groups except black males, partial r's were highly significant statistically for plasma glucose and blood

---

*Similar results were obtained when body mass index[15] was used rather than relative weight; only data on relative weight are presented here.

TABLE 2.
Multiple Cross-Classification Analysis of Relationship Between Four Variables and Elevated Blood Pressure by Age, Sex and Race
Chicago Board of Health Community Surveys, 1965-71

803 White Men Age 30-44 / 2,367 White Women Age 30-44

No. of Variables High	No. of Persons	DBP >95 No.	Rate/ 1,000	SBP >160 No.	Rate/ 1,000	No. of Persons	DBP >95 No.	Rate/ 1,000	SBP >160 No.	Rate/ 1,00
None	437	0	0*	2	5	1,157	4	3	4	
One Only	244	5	20	7	28	891	13	14	10	1.
Two Only	94	5	48	3	30	271	10	37	10	3.
Three or Four	28	3	65	3	101	48	3	34	3	3.
Two, Three or Four	122	8	57	6	46	319	13	39	13	3.
All	803	13	16	15	19	2,367	30	12	27	1.
Ratio: 3 or 4/None			— Δ		20.2			11.3		11.
Ratio: 2, 3 or 4/None			— Δ		9.2			13.0		12.

1,151 White Men Age 45-64 / 3,114 White Women Age 45-64

No. of Variables High	No. of Persons	DBP >95 No.	Rate/ 1,000	SBP >160 No.	Rate/ 1,000	No. of Persons	DBP >95 No.	Rate/ 1,000	SBP >160 No.	Rate/ 1,00
None	439	13	31	19	41	917	15	17	38	4
One Only	416	20	51	36	84	1,292	46	36	94	7
Two Only	224	18	82	30	129	668	38	57	75	10
Three or Four	72	12	156	16	190	237	31	143	50	21
Two, Three or Four	296	30	103	46	149	905	69	77	125	12
All	1,151	63	57	101	83	3,114	130	42	257	7
Ratio: 3 or 4/None			5.0		4.6			8.4		4.
Ratio: 2, 3 or 4/None			3.3		3.6			4.5		2.

630 Black Men Age 30-44 / 2,515 Black Women Age 30-44

No. of Variables High	No. of Persons	DBP >95 No.	Rate/ 1,000	SBP >160 No.	Rate/ 1,000	No. of Persons	DBP >95 No.	Rate/ 1,000	SBP >160 No.	Rate/ 1,00
None	321	10	28	8	24	943	26	28	16	1
One Only	202	8	41	7	35	1,045	54	51	36	3
Two Only	92	12	129	7	67	446	51	106	43	8
Three or Four	15	3	260	5	228	81	9	108	13	13
Two, Three or Four	107	15	142	12	94	527	60	107	56	9
All	630	33	51	27	40	2,515	140	54	110	4
Ratio: 3 or 4/None			9.3		9.5			3.9		7.
Ratio: 2, 3 or 4/None			5.1		3.9			3.8		5.

686 Black Men Age 45-64

None	245	20	83	21	89
One Only	266	30	111	34	130
Two Only	117	21	188	22	184
Three or Four	58	13	227	17	295
Two, Three or Four	175	34	197	39	220
All	686	84	122	94	139
Ratio: $\frac{3\ or\ 4}{None}$			2.7		3.3
Ratio: $\frac{2,\ 3\ or\ 4}{None}$			2.4		2.5

2,203 Black Women Age 45-64

None	496	36	73	35	80
One Only	924	93	101	98	110
Two Only	581	98	167	113	191
Three or Four	202	33	168	50	237
Two, Three or Four	783	131	168	163	205
All	2,203	260	118	296	137
Ratio: $\frac{3\ or\ 4}{None}$			2.3		3.0
Ratio: $\frac{2,\ 3\ or\ 4}{None}$			2.3		2.6

ΔDenominator O: ratio could not be calculated.
Cut points for variables: heart rate ⩾80 beats/min.; serum cholesterol ⩾250 mg./dl.; 1-hour plasma glucose ⩾205 mg/dl.; relative weight ⩾1.25.
*Age adjusted by 5-year age groups to the U.S. population of the same sex-race, 1960 Census data.

pressure (most p values ⩽ .001). For both hematocrit and serum cholesterol, the majority of their partial r's with blood pressure were small and statistically insignificant. Finally, 12 of the 16 partial r's for age and blood pressure — in the range 0.1-0.2 — were statistically significant, even though the analyses were for age groups of limited span (30-44 and 45-64).

Multiple cross-classification analyses. The findings of the multiple cross-classification analyses are presented in Table 2. Four independent variables were evaluated, with dichotomization — relative weight (⩾ 1.25), heart rate (⩾ 80 beats/min), one-hour plasma glucose (⩾ 205 mg/dl) and serum cholesterol (⩾ 250 mg/dl). The data are presented for four strata: none of the four variables high, any one only high, any two only high, any three or all four high; also, for the stratum, any two, three or all four high. Since mean ages tended to be higher for these latter strata for several of the overall age-sex-race groups, age-adjusted values were computed for the proportion of each stratum with elevated blood pressure (based on two cut points, diastolic pressure ⩾ 95 mm Hg and systolic pressure ⩾ 160 mm Hg). Adjustment was by five-year age groups to the U. S. population of the same sex-race, 1960 census data. Adjusted and unadjusted values for the proportions with elevated blood pressure were not sizably different.

For all age-sex-race groups, rates for elevated blood pressure were low for the stratum with none of the four variables high; in stepwise fashion, rates were progressively higher for the strata with any one only, any two only, any three or all four variables high (Table 2). This gradation was greater for the younger than the older groups, greater for whites than blacks. Thus for systolic blood pressure $\geq$ 160 mm Hg, the ratio of rates,

$$\frac{\text{persons with any three or all four variables high}}{\text{persons with none of four variables high}}$$

ranged for persons age 30-44 from 7.8 for black women to 20.2 for white men; for persons age 45-64, this ratio ranged from 3.0 for black women to 4.8 for white women.

Only a small minority of persons in any age-sex-race group — 2.0%-3.5% for the age group 30-44, 6.3%-9.2% for the age group 45-64 — had any three or all four of these variables high. A much higher percentage — 13.5%-21.0% for the age group 30-44 and 25.5%-35.5% for the age group 45-64 — had any two, three or all four variables high. Therefore, the ratio of rates,

$$\frac{\text{persons with any two, three or all four variables high}}{\text{persons with none of four variables high}}$$

was also calculated. Again for systolic blood pressure $\geq$ 160 mm Hg, this ratio ranged for persons age 30-44 from 3.9 for black men to 12.7 for white women; for persons age 45-64, from 2.5 for black men to 3.6 for white men.

Overall, for persons of both sexes and races age 30-44, 1,075 of 6,315 had any two, three or all four variables high, ie, 17.0%. Among these 17.0% were 48.6% (87 of 179) of the cases of elevated blood pressure (SBP $\geq$ 160 mm Hg). In contrast, only 30 of 179 cases, ie, only 16.8%, were present among the 2,858 persons — 45.3% of the population age 30-44 — with none of these four factors high. Therefore, this multivariable cross-classification analysis involving dichotomization of four variables — clearly a simple and crude method — was highly effective in demonstrating an association between the presence of combinations of two or more of these four factors high and elevation of blood pressure, especially in the younger age group.

Multiple logistic regression analyses. Both types of multiple regression analyses, linear and logistic, overcome the shortcoming of cross-classification analysis, ie, only limited use of the independent variables based on dichotomization. The coefficients for the multiple logistic analysis and the approxi-

TABLE 3.
Relationship Between Multiple Variables and Elevated Blood Pressure by Age-Sex-Race Coefficients for the Multiple Logistic Regression Equation and Their Statistical Significance Chicago Board of Health Community Surveys, 1965-71

803 White Males Age 30-44

Criterion for Elevated Blood Pressure	Elevated Blood Pressure No.	Rate/ 1,000	Coefficients for Multiple Logistic Regression Equation						
			Constant	Age	Heart Rate	Serum Cholesterol	1-Hour Plasma Glucose	Relative Weight	Hemato-crit
DBP >95	13	16	-22.9521	.0436	.0446	.0128	.0240***	.0236	.0826
SBP >160	15	19	-25.1627	-.0064	.0631**	-.0038	.0070	.0519**	.2121*

1,151 White Males Age 45-64

DBP >95	63	55	-11.6408	-.0533*	.0297**	.0025	.0086***	.0378***	.0565
SBP >160	101	88	-15.2385	.0854***	.0348***	-.0006	.0102***	.0207**	.0270

2,367 White Females Age 30-44

DBP >95	30	13	-21.6637	.0440	.0398**	.0058	.0110**	.0548***	.0705
SBP >160	27	11	-20.3851	.0772	.0703***	.0123*	.0122**	.0364***	-.0338

3,114 White Females Age 45-64

DBP >95	130	42	-13.7331	-.0117	.0363***	.0014	.0054***	.0336***	.0717*
SBP >160	257	83	-13.2042	.0820***	.0284***	-.0002	.0078***	.0197***	.0118

603 Black Males Age 30-44

DBP >95	33	52	-13.9547	.0339	.0398**	.0090	-.0024	.0360**	.0211
SBP >160	27	43	-12.4714	.0542	.0366*	.0103*	.0021	.0382**	-.0542

686 Black Males Age 45-64

DBP >95	84	122	- 7.2838	-.0050	.0289***	-.0040	.0009	.0220**	.0325
SBP >160	94	137	- 6.3520	.0431*	.0167*	-.0017	.0028	.0243***	-.0449

2,515 Black Females Age 30-44

DBP >95	140	56	-10.1441	.0432*	.0087	.0025	.0062***	.0231***	.0204
SBP >160	110	44	-14.7790	.0873***	.0301***	.0013	.0095***	.0211***	.0434

2,203 Black Females Age 45-64

DBP >95	260	118	- 7.5783	-.0056	.0137**	-.0008	.0015	.0249***	.0391
SBP >160	296	134	- 9.0735	.0468***	.0199***	.0016	.0047***	.0170***	-.0008

For the usual Student's t distribution:
*p≤.05; **p≤.01; ***p≤.001

mations of their statistical significance are presented for the eight age-sex-race groups in Table 3. In accordance with the findings of the partial correlation analysis, for 15 of the 16 analyses the coefficients for relative weight had t values indicating statistical significance. This was also the case for heart rate in 14 of the 16 analyses. Furthermore, it was the case for plasma glucose for seven of the eight analyses for whites, but only for three of the eight for blacks, with none of the analyses yielding coefficients with t values indicative of statistical significance for black men. In most instances, coefficients for serum cholesterol and hematocrit had t values not indicative of statistical significance. Coefficients for age had t values that were indicative of statistical significance for about half the analyses.

Data are presented in Table 4 on the ordering of whites into deciles of expected prevalence of elevated blood pressure (diastolic pressure $\geqslant$ 95 mm Hg) based on the coefficients for the six independent variables derived with the multiple logistic regression equation. See reference 1 for similar data for blacks. Sizably higher prevalence rates overall for elevated blood pressure were recorded for blacks compared to whites. This is, of course, in keeping with general U. S. experience.[4,10]

For all eight age-sex-race groups, ordering into deciles of expected prevalence of elevated blood pressure produced progressively greater rates of observed prevalence, with good correspondence between expected and observed rates (Table 4). For the age group 30-44, for whites, 38.5% (men) and 53.3% (women) of persons with observed elevated blood pressure were classified in the highest decile of expected prevalence, and 66.7% (women) and 69.2% (men) were concentrated in the highest quintile (20%) of expected prevalence (Table 4). Corresponding data for blacks were 27.3% and 27.9%, and 47.1% and 48.5%, respectively. Similar but less marked concentration of observed cases of elevated blood pressure in the highest decile and quintile was recorded for the age group 45-64.

For four of the eight analyses, chiefly for the younger age group, no cases were observed in the lowest decile of expected prevalence of elevated blood pressure. Therefore, the ratio of observed rates for the highest compared to the lowest decile could not be calculated in these four instances. For the other

Observed and Expected Prevalence of Elevated Blood Pressure (DBP ≥ 95 mm Hg), Deciles of Expected Prevalence from the 6-Variable Multiple Logistic Regression Analysis, Whites by Age and Sex, Chicago Board of Health Community Surveys, 1965-71

Decile of Expected Prevalence	803 White Men Age 30-44 Expected No.	Rate/ 1,000	Observed No.	Rate/ 1,000	1,151 White Men Age 45-64 Expected No.	Rate/ 1,000	Observed No.	Rate/ 1,000	2,367 White Women Age 30-44 Expected No.	Rate/ 1,000	Observed No.	Rate/ 1,000	3,114 White Women Age 45-64 Expected No.	Rate/ 1,000	Observed No.	Rate/ 1,000
1	0.0	0	0	0	0.8	7	0	0	0.1	1	0	0	2.1	7	3	10
2	0.1	1	0	0	1.4	12	3	26	0.2	1	1	4	3.3	11	6	19
3	0.1	1	0	0	1.9	17	0	0	0.4	2	1	4	4.4	14	3	10
4	0.1	2	1	12	2.6	22	5	43	0.5	2	0	0	5.6	18	5	16
5	0.2	3	0	0	3.3	29	7	61	0.7	3	1	4	7.1	23	8	26
6	0.3	4	1	12	4.2	36	3	26	1.0	4	1	4	9.0	29	9	29
7	0.4	5	0	0	5.4	47	4	35	1.5	6	2	8	11.7	38	11	35
8	0.7	9	2	25	7.4	64	9	78	2.5	11	4	17	15.8	51	14	45
9	1.7	22	4	50	11.1	96	12	104	4.9	21	4	17	23.2	74	25	80
10	13.6	164	5	60	26.7	230	20	172	26.0	107	16	66	52.7	167	46	146
All	17.2	21.4	13	16.2	64.8	56.3	63	54.7	37.8	16.0	30	12.7	134.9	43.3	130	41.7
Ratio: 10/1	△	—	△	—	33.4	—	△	—	260.0	—	△	—	25.1	—	15.3	—
Ratio: 9+10/1+2	153.0	—	△	—	17.2	—	10.7	—	103.0	—	20.0	—	14.1	—	7.9	—
% of All Persons with Elevated BP in 10	79.1		38.5		41.2		31.7		68.8		53.3		39.1		35.4	
% of All Persons with Elevated BP in 9+10	89.0		69.2		58.3		50.8		81.7		66.7		56.3		54.6	

△Denominator 0; ratio cannot be calculated.

four where this calculation was possible, the ratio ranged from a high of 15.3 for white women 45-64 to a low of 4.2 for black women 45-64.

Similarly, for one of the eight analyses, no cases were observed in the lowest quintile (deciles 1 and 2) of expected prevalence of elevated blood pressure, hence the ratio of observed rates for the highest compared to the lowest quintile could be calculated in seven instances. This ratio ranged from a high of 20.0 for white women age 30-44 to a low of 3.6 for black women age 45-64.

Clearly, the multiple logistic regression model is highly effective in classifying persons in regard to expectation of elevated blood pressure, based on the six variables considered.

Multiple linear regression analyses. Unlike the multiple cross-classification and multiple logistic regression analyses, it is possible with the multiple linear regression analysis to treat the dependent variable, blood pressure, as a continuous variable. The coefficients for the multiple linear regression equation for each of the eight age-sex-race groups, with diastolic and systolic pressure, respectively, as the dependent variable, are presented in Table 5, along with information on tests for statistical significance of these coefficients. Data are also given on the multiple correlation coefficient (R), on R^2 and on the F test for statistical significance of the overall multiple linear regression analysis.

The coefficients for relative weight and heart rate were all significant statistically, with $p \leqslant .001$ (Table 5). Coefficients for one-hour plasma glucose were statistically significant in 13 of the 16 analyses. Coefficients for serum cholesterol and hematocrit were statistically significant in only a minority of the analyses, 3 of 16 and 6 of 16, respectively. Coefficients for age were statistically significant in 12 of 16 analyses, with $p \leqslant .001$ in 8 of these 16.

The values for R^2 ranged from .097 to .211 for diastolic pressure; .117 to .215 for systolic pressure, ie, the six independent variables "explained" up to 21.5% of the inter-individual variation in blood pressure. R^2 values were higher for younger than older age groups for diastolic, but not for systolic pressure. R^2 values were higher for whites than for blacks. No consistent sex difference in R^2 values was noted.

Relationship between Multiple Variables and Blood Pressure, by Age-Sex-Race
Coefficients for the Multiple Linear Regression Equation, Their Statistical Significance, Values for the Multiple R and R^2, Chicago Board of Health Community Surveys, 1965-71

Age-Sex-Race Group	No. of Persons	Constant	Age	Heart Rate	Serum Cholesterol	1-Hour Plasma Glucose	Relative Weight	Hematocrit	Multiple R	R^2	F for Multiple Regression
Diastolic Blood Pressure											
White Men 30-44	803	20.471***	.1539*	.1781***	.0196**	.0139*	.1844***	.1913	.456	.208	34.91***
White Men 45-64	1,151	31.822***	-.0799	.1512***	.0113	.0201***	.1577***	.3293***	.397	.158	35.74***
White Women 30-44	2,367	24.488***	.2636***	.0960***	.0096*	.0190***	.1728***	.1548**	.459	.211	105.12***
White Women 45-64	3,114	30.218***	.0695*	.1364***	.0065	.0104***	.1571***	.2600***	.393	.154	94.31***
Black Men 30-44	630	35.103***	.1933*	.1265***	.0138	.0035	.1974***	.0226	.377	.142	17.16***
Black Men 45-64	686	43.116***	.0614	.1738***	.0001	.0048	.1566***	.0998	.312	.097	12.22***
Black Women 30-44	2,515	29.402***	.3096***	.0825***	.0111*	.0186***	.1601***	.1588**	.399	.159	78.98***
Black Women 45-64	2,203	41.023***	.0373	.0962***	.0035	.0132***	.1603***	.2265**	.315	.099	40.18***
Systolic Blood Pressure											
White Men 30-44	803	54.460***	.0245	.3052***	.0144	.0360***	.2389***	.2286	.453	.205	34.28***
White Men 45-64	1,151	24.862*	.5710***	.3011***	.0071	.0587***	.2609***	.2798	.442	.196	46.40***
White Women 30-44	2,367	56.872***	.3287***	.1683***	.0090	.0358***	.2240***	.0603	.436	.190	92.10***
White Women 45-64	3,114	16.466**	.7936***	.2394***	.0116	.0478***	.2659***	.2732**	.464	.215	141.71***
Black Men 30-44	630	66.155***	.3675**	.1956***	.0200	-.0043	.2601***	-.0034	.361	.131	15.60***
Black Men 45-64	686	73.545***	.5241***	.2018***	-.0131	.0290*	.2695***	-.2795	.342	.117	15.02***
Black Women 30-44	2,515	50.582***	.5979***	.1456***	.0041	.0410***	.2527***	.0678	.430	.185	95.02***
Black Women 45-64	2,203	42.175***	.6129***	.1693***	.0027	.0476***	.2716***	.1816	.363	.132	55.45***

Levels of Significance (F test)

* $p \leq .05$
** $p \leq .01$
*** $p \leq .001$

Chicago Heart Association Detection Project in Industry

The relationship of seven variables to blood pressure was evaluated in this study: relative weight, resting heart rate, plasma glucose one-hour after a 50 gm oral load, serum cholesterol and uric acid, cigarette smoking and age.[5]

Partial correlation analyses. With calculation of partial correlation coefficients, ie, r's between blood pressure and each of the seven independent variables adjusted for the other six, r's for blood pressure and relative weight were generally in the range 0.2 to 0.3, with most p values ⩽ .001 or ⩽ .01 (Table 6). Most of the partial r's also were highly significant for heart rate and blood pressure (range 0.1 to 0.3, p values generally ⩽ .001). Most partial r's were significant statistically for plasma glucose and blood pressure. This was also true for partial r's for serum uric acid and blood pressure. For serum cholesterol, the majority of its partial r's with blood pressure were not statistically significant. In ten of the 16 analyses, partial r's for age and blood pressure — in the range 0.1 to 0.2 — were statistically significant, even though the analyses were for age-specific groups (25-44 and 45-64). In most of the analyses, the partial r's for cigarette smoking and blood pressure were not statistically significant; the single exception was for white women age 45-64, for whom a significant negative association was recorded.

In general, these findings were similar to those of the preceding study for the common variables (relative weight, heart rate, one-hour plasma glucose, serum cholesterol, age) and their correlations with blood pressure in the major age-sex-race groups.[1]

Multiple cross-classification analyses. The findings of the multiple cross-classification analyses are presented in Table 7. Five independent variables were evaluated, with dichotomization — relative weight (⩾ 1.25), heart rate (⩾ 80 beats/min), one-hour plasma glucose (⩾ 205 mg/dl), serum uric acid (⩾ 7.0 mg/dl) and serum cholesterol (⩾ 250 mg/dl). The data are presented for four strata: none of the four variables high; any one only high; any two only high; any three, four or all five high. Since mean ages tended to be higher for these latter strata for several of the overall age-sex-race groups, age-adjusted values were computed for the proportion of each stratum with elevated blood pressure (based on two cut points, diastolic

TABLE 6.
Partial Correlation Coefficients
by Age, Sex and Race
Chicago Heart Association Detection Project in Industry, 1967-72

Variable	White Men Age 25-44 N=6,504		White Men Age 45-64 N=4,503		White Women Age 25-44 N=3,358		White Women Age 45-64 N=4,582	
	SBP	DBP	SBP	DBP	SBP	DBP	SBP	DBP
e	-.0111	.1254***	.2055***	.0623***	.1271***	.1612***	.2052***	.0636***
rt Rate	.2658***	.1540***	.2543***	.1963***	.2951***	.2345***	.2651***	.1932***
rum lesterol	.0518***	.0647***	.0367*	.0607***	.0110	.0409*	.0268	.0483**
our sma cose	.0807***	.0869***	.1479***	.1134***	.0928***	.0680***	.1203***	.1162***
ative ght	.2517***	.2240***	.2104***	.2384***	.2572***	.2044***	.2111***	.1886***
c Acid	.0532***	.0997***	.0451**	.0635***	.0443*	.0807***	.0465**	.0538***
arettes Day	.0115	-.0113	.0108	-.0165	-.0010	-.0298	-.0496***	-.0506***

ariable	Black Men Age 25-44 N=634		Black Men Age 45-64 N=280		Black Women Age 25-44 N=977		Black Women Age 45-64 N=186	
	SBP	DBP	SBP	DBP	SBP	DBP	SBP	DBP
	.0080	.0942*	.1002	-.0023	.1868***	.2275***	.0354	.0037
t Rate	.2481***	.1523***	.1042	.0944	.1655***	.1184***	.2380**	.2391**
n esterol	.0825*	.0551	-.0324	-.0068	.0035	.0341	-.0358	-.0218
ar ua se	.1434***	.1297**	.1312*	.1928**	.0953**	.0660*	.0578	.0325
ive t	.3076***	.2265***	.1498*	.1616**	.2219***	.1606***	.1983**	.2525***
Acid	.1025*	.1033**	.1913**	.1444*	.0488	.0974**	.2535***	.2233**
ettes ay	.0292	.0008	.0304	.0344	.0193	.0051	-.0741	.0347

* p ≤ .05
** p ≤ .01
*** p ≤ .001

For each partial correlation coefficient calculated, the other six variables were held constant.

pressure $\geq$ 95 mm Hg and systolic pressure $\geq$ 160 mm Hg). Adjustment was by five-year age groups to the U. S. population of the same sex-race, 1960 census data. Adjusted and un-adjusted values for the proportions with elevated blood pressure were not sizably different.

For all age-sex-race groups, particularly age 25-44, rates for elevated blood pressure were low for the stratum with none of the five variables high; in stepwise fashion, rates tended to be progressively higher for the strata with any one only, any two only, any three or more variables high. This differential was recorded consistently for the four groups of whites (Table 7), less so for blacks, possibly because of the much smaller numbers. It was consistently greater for younger than for older persons; it tended to be greater for whites than blacks. Thus, for systolic blood pressure $\geq$ 160 mm Hg, the ratio of rates,

$$\frac{\text{persons with any three or more variables high}}{\text{persons with none of five variables high}}$$

ranged for persons age 25-44 from 4.7 for black women to 45.0 for white women; for persons age 45-64, this ratio ranged from 2.6 for black men to 4.0 for white women.

Overall, for persons of both sexes and races age 25-44, 704 of 11,473 had any three or more variables high, ie, 6.1%. Among these 6.1% were 21.0% (182 of 866) of the cases of elevated blood pressure (SBP $\geq$ 160 mm Hg). In contrast, only 89 of 866 cases, ie, only 10.3%, were present among the 3,893 persons — 33.9% of the population age 25-44 — with none of these five factors high. Therefore, this multivariate cross-classification analysis involving dichotomization of five vari-ables, a simple and crude method, was again highly effective in demonstrating an association between presence of combinations of three or more of these five factors high and elevation of blood pressure, especially in the younger age group.

Multiple logistic analyses. The regression coefficients for the multiple logistic analyses and the approximations of their statistical significance are presented for the eight age-sex-race groups in Table 8. In accordance with the findings of the simple and partial correlation analysis, for 15 of the 16 analyses the coefficients for relative weight had t values indicating statistical significance. This was also the case for heart rate in 13 of the 16

TABLE 7.
Multiple Cross-Classification Analysis of Relationship Between Five Variables and Elevated Blood Pressure by Age, Sex and Race
Chicago Heart Association Detection Project in Industry, 1967-72

No. of Variables High	No. of Persons	DBP >95 No.	Rate/ 1,000	SBP >160 No.	Rate/ 1,000	No. of Persons	DBP >95 No.	Rate/ 1,000	SBP >160 No.	Rate/ 1,000
		6,504 White Men Age 25-44					3,358 White Women Age 25-44			
None	2,086	62	34*	69	37	1,253	16	14	7	6
One Only	2,394	147	65	196	81	1,542	58	38	54	35
Two Only	1,447	196	136	209	144	510	44	84	45	84
Three, Four or Five	577	150	250	147	248	53	15	266	14	270
All	6,504	555	90	621	97	3,358	133	40	120	35
Ratio: $\frac{3, 4 \text{ or } 5}{None}$			7.4		6.7			19.0		45.0
		4,503 White Men Age 45-64					4,582 White Women Age 45-64			
None	1,069	97	93	119	118	1,252	62	49	99	85
One Only	1,601	262	168	330	216	1,870	177	99	289	163
Two Only	1,196	274	229	344	292	1,054	150	140	256	244
Three, Four or Five	637	215	341	272	441	402	87	218	139	340
All	4,503	848	191	1,065	244	4,582	476	107	783	179
Ratio: $\frac{3, 4 \text{ or } 5}{None}$			3.7		3.7			4.4		4.0
		634 Black Men Age 25-44					977 Black Women Age 25-44			
None	211	8	28	5	18	343	11	49	8	39
One Only	256	40	160	33	131	454	32	86	17	48
Two Only	115	23	192	31	261	158	20	131	10	63
Three, Four or Five	52	14	257	17	340	22	2	91$^\Delta$	4	182$^\Delta$
All	634	85	140	86	140	977	65	82	39	51
Ratio: $\frac{3, 4 \text{ or } 5}{None}$			9.2		18.9			1.9		4.7
		280 Black Men Age 45-64					186 Black Women Age 45-64			
None	78	15	217	13	185	34	2	59$^\Delta$	4	118$^\Delta$
One Only	90	24	272	25	281	75	11	179	15	221
Two Only	64	28	430	24	376	61	20	313	22	347
Three, Four or Five	48	25	524	23	483	16	7	438$^\Delta$	7	438$^\Delta$
All	280	92	336	85	309	186	40	217	48	259
Ratio: $\frac{3, 4 \text{ or } 5}{None}$			2.4		2.6			7.4		3.7

$^\Delta$Not age-adjusted. N too small.
Cut points for high: - heart rate >80 beats/min.   - serum uric acid >7.0 mg./dl.
                     - serum cholesterol >250 mg./dl. - relative weight >1.25
                     - 1-hour plasma glucose >205 mg./dl.
*Age-adjusted by 5-year age groups to the U.S. population of the same age-sex-race, 1960.

TABLE 8.
Relationship Between Multiple Variables and Elevated Blood Pressure by Age-Sex-Race Coefficients for the Multiple Logistic Regression Equation and Their Statistical Significance Chicago Heart Association Detection Project in Industry, 1967-72

Criterion for Elevated Blood Pressure	Elevated Blood Pressure No.	Rate/1,000	Coefficients for Multiple Logistic Regression Equation							
			Constant	Age	Heart Rate	Serum Cholesterol	1-Hour Plasma Glucose	Relative Weight	Serum Uric Acid	Cigarettes Per Day
DBP≥ 95	555	85	-14.6776	.0488***	.0335***	.0052***	.0063***	.0356***	.0257***	-.0007
SBP≥160	621	95	-13.4769	.0083	.0554***	.0023	.0049***	.0370***	.0128***	.0040
4,503 White Men Age 45-64										
DBP≥ 95	848	188	-10.3565	.0172*	.0325***	.0028**	.0054***	.0289***	.0061*	-.0022
SBP≥160	1,065	237	-13.5616	.0780***	.0472***	.0016	.0062***	.0231***	.0053	-.0004
3,358 White Women Age 25-44										
DBP≥ 95	133	40	-16.9012	-.0405**	.0533***	.0068*	.0070**	.0325***	.0364***	-.0065
SBP≥160	120	36	-18.2391	.0470**	.0635***	.0005	.0104***	.0428***	.0275***	-.0051
4,582 White Women Age 45-64										
DBP≥ 95	476	104	-10.1758	.0192	.0376***	.0012	.0050***	.0206***	.0109**	-.0143△△
SBP≥160	783	171	-13.5489	.0804***	.0521***	.0008	.0045***	.0192***	.0070	-.0030
634 Black Men Age 25-44										
DBP≥ 95	85	134	-10.4498	.0285	.0231*	-.0008	.0092*	.0345***	.0089	.0050
SBP≥160	86	136	-13.6966	-.0089	.0568***	.0033	.0062	.0372***	.0269	.0017
280 Black Men Age 45-64										
DBP≥ 95	92	329	- 7.7725	.0303	.0175	.0015	.0066**	.0169*	.0101	.0081
SBP≥160	85	304	- 6.1497	.0281	.0152	-.0034	.0081**	.0065	.0199*	.0115
977 Black Women Age 25-44										
DBP≥ 95	65	67	-13.9111	.1359***	.0361**	-.0020	.0072*	.0173*	.0253	-.0118
SBP≥160	39	40	-16.3008	.1438***	.0249	.0047	.0145**	.0198*	.0192	-.0050
186 Black Women Age 45-64										
DBP≥ 95	40	215	- 8.4893	-.0416	.0395*	.0038	.0054	.0175*	.0474**	.0060
SBP≥160	43	258	- 6.2368	-.0427	.0441**	-.0010	.0031	.0133*	.0275	.0052

...the usual Student's t distribution: *p≤.05; **p≤.01; ***p≤.001

TABLE 9.
Observed and Expected Prevalence of Elevated Blood Pressure (DBP ≥ 95 mm Hg), Deciles of Expected Prevalence from the 7-Variable Multiple Logistic Regression Analysis, Whites by Age and Sex, Chicago Heart Association Detection Project in Industry, 1967-72

Decile of Expected Prevalence	6,504 White Men Age 25-44				4,503 White Men Age 45-64				3,358 White Women Age 25-44				4,582 White Women Age 45-64			
	Expected		Observed		Expected		Observed		Expected		Observed		Expected		Observed	
	No.	Rate/1,000	No.	Rate/1,000	No.	Rate/1,000	No.	Rate/1,000	No.	Rate/1,000	No.	Rate/1,000	No.	Rate/1,000	No.	Rate/1,000
1	6.8	10	8	12	24.8	55	31	69	1.0	3	1	3	12.8	28	13	28
2	12.2	19	13	20	37.3	83	45	100	1.9	6	1	3	19.1	42	20	44
3	17.2	26	23	35	46.5	103	37	82	2.8	8	3	9	23.8	52	23	50
4	22.8	35	27	42	56.1	125	63	140	3.8	11	2	6	28.3	62	37	81
5	30.0	46	33	51	65.9	146	70	156	5.0	15	5	15	33.5	73	43	94
6	38.9	60	37	57	77.3	172	84	187	6.8	20	14	42	39.8	87	31	68
7	51.2	79	57	88	89.8	200	80	178	9.4	28	17	51	47.7	104	45	98
8	68.9	106	66	102	106.6	237	112	249	13.6	41	16	48	58.9	129	64	140
9	100.9	155	92	142	132.3	294	130	289	22.8	68	24	72	77.7	170	73	159
10	213.8	327	199	304	208.2	460	196	433	78.5	229	50	146	138.4	301	127	276
All	562.7	87	555	85	844.8	188	848	188	145.6	43	133	40	479.7	105	476	104
Ratio: 10/1	31.4		24.9		8.4		6.3		78.5		50.0		10.8		9.8	
Ratio: 9+10/1+2	16.6		13.9		5.5		4.3		34.9		37.0		6.8		6.1	
% of All Persons with Elevated DBP in 10	38.0%		35.9%		24.6%		23.1%		53.9%		37.6%		28.9%		26.7%	
% of All Persons with Elevated DBP in 9+10	55.9%		52.4%		40.3%		38.4%		69.6%		55.6%		45.0%		42.0%	

analyses. It was the case for plasma glucose for all eight analyses for whites and for five of the eight for blacks, with neither of the analyses yielding coefficients with t values indicative of statistical significance for the small group of 186 black women age 45-64. In seven of eight analyses for whites, the coefficients for serum uric acid were statistically significant, but this was the case for only three of eight analyses for blacks. For serum cholesterol, t values of the coefficients were indicative of statistical significance in three of eight instances for whites, but in none of eight for blacks. Coefficients for age had t values that were indicative of statistical significance in six of eight analyses for whites, two of eight for blacks. None of the 16 analyses indicated a significant positive relationship between cigarette smoking and elevated blood pressure; in one instance, a significant negative association was obtained for white women age 45-64.

Data are presented in Table 9 on the ordering of whites into deciles of expected prevalence of elevated blood pressure (diastolic pressure $\geqslant$ 95 mm Hg) based on the coefficients for the seven independent variables derived with the multiple logistic regression equation. Similar data for blacks are available in reference 5. Again, sizably higher prevalence rates overall for elevated blood pressure were recorded for blacks compared to whites. This is in keeping with the findings of the preceding study and with general U. S. experience.[1,4,10]

For all eight age-sex-race groups, ordering into deciles of expected prevalence of elevated blood pressure produced progressively greater rates of observed prevalence, with good correspondence between expected and observed rates (Table 9). For the age group 25-44, for whites, 35.9% (men) and 37.6% (women) of persons with observed elevated blood pressure were classified in the highest decile of expected prevalence, and 52.4% and 55.6% were concentrated in the highest quintile (20%) of expected prevalence. Corresponding data for blacks were 27.1% and 32.3%, and 44.7% and 55.4%, respectively. Similar but less marked concentration of observed cases of elevated blood pressure in the highest decile and quintile was recorded for the age group 45-64.

For whites age 25-44, the ratio of observed rates for the highest compared to the lowest decile ranged from 24.9 to 50.0 (Table 9); for blacks, for the one of two instances where the

Coefficients for the Multiple Linear Regression Equation, Their Statistical Significance, Values for the Multiple R and R^2 ... by Age-Sex-Race
Chicago Heart Association Detection Project in Industry, 1967-72

Age-Sex Race Group	No. of Persons	Constant	Age	Heart Rate	Serum Cholesterol	1-Hour Plasma Glucose	Relative Weight	Serum Uric Acid	Cigarettes per Day	Multiple R	R^2	F for Multiple Regression
Diastolic Blood Pressure												
White Men 25-44	6,504	30.841***	.2304***	.1326***	.0189***	.0243***	.1510***	.8749***	-.0083	.408	.166	185.00***
White Men 45-64	4,503	28.671***	.1316***	.1976***	.0191***	.0259***	.1786***	.5833***	-.0135	.382	.146	109.81***
White Women 25-44	3,358	28.605***	.2666***	.2043***	.0121*	.0194***	.1085***	.7973***	-.0250	.410	.168	96.75***
White Women 45-64	4,582	35.497***	.1393***	.1875***	.0135***	.0289***	.1084***	.5534***	-.0570ΔΔΔ	.354	.125	93.68***
Black Men 25-44	634	29.135***	.1971*	.1553***	.0176	.0475***	.1602***	.9979**	.0009	.407	.166	17.75***
Black Men 45-64	280	46.943***	-.0062	.1159	-.0025	.0513***	.1345**	1.5427*	.0469	.385	.148	6.77***
Black Women 25-44	977	33.454***	.4610***	.1141***	.0107	.0195*	.0832***	1.0729**	.0066	.389	.151	24.63***
Black Women 45-64	186	22.812	.0115	.3324***	-.0079	.0090	.1720***	2.8018**	.0596	.442	.196	6.19***
Systolic Blood Pressure												
White Men 25-44	6,504	67.371***	-.0295	.3416***	.0220***	.0329***	.2489***	.6772***	.0123	.423	.179	202.43***
White Men 45-64	4,503	22.959***	.7324***	.4292***	.0190*	.0561***	.2591***	.6845**	.0146	.437	.191	151.87***
White Women 25-44	3,358	57.259***	.2886***	.3611***	.0045	.0365***	.1908***	.6025**	-.0011	.451	.203	121.88***
White Women 45-64	4,582	25.707***	.7680***	.4387***	.0126	.0502***	.2042***	.8002**	-.0935ΔΔΔ	.445	.198	161.20***
Black Men 25-44	634	45.429***	.0238	.3683***	.0377*	.0751***	.3180***	1.4129*	-.0470	.487	.237	27.84***
Black Men 45-64	280	55.944**	.4483	.2146	-.0202	.0580*	.2085*	3.4547***	.0695	.388	.151	6.90***
Black Women 25-44	977	64.948***	.5176***	.2215***	.0015	.0389**	.1606***	.7390	.0344	.403	.162	26.78***
Black Women 45-64	186	36.574	.1868	.5609***	-.0221	.0271	.2261**	5.4344***	-.2161	.443	.196	6.19***

Levels of significance (F test) * $p \leq .05$; ** $p \leq .01$; *** $p \leq .001$
ΔΔΔnegative correlation, $p \leq .001$

rate was not zero for the lowest decile, the ratio was 23.0. This ratio was also sizable, although smaller, for the age group 45-64.

Similarly, the ratio of observed rates for the highest compared to the lowest quintile for whites age 25-44 ranged from 13.9 to 37.0 (Table 9); for blacks, from 5.4 to 36.0. Again, this ratio was sizable, but smaller, for the age group 45-64.

Clearly, the multiple logistic regression model in this case, as in the preceding study,[1] proved to be highly effective in classifying persons in regard to expectation of elevated blood pressure, based on the several variables considered.

Multiple linear regression analyses. The coefficients for the multiple linear regression equation for each of the eight age-sex-groups, with diastolic and systolic pressure, respectively, as the dependent variable, are presented in Table 10, along with information on tests for statistical significance of these coefficients. Data are also given on the multiple correlation coefficient (R), on R^2 and on the F test for statistical significance of the overall multiple linear regression analysis.

The coefficients for relative weight were all significant statistically, with $p \leqslant .001$ in 14 of 16 analyses; those for heart rate were also significant, with $p \leqslant .001$ in all analyses except the two for black men age 45-64 (Table 10). Coefficients for one-hour plasma glucose were statistically significant in 14 of the 16 analyses, with $p \leqslant .001$ in 11 instances; findings were similar for serum uric acid. Coefficients for serum cholesterol were statistically significant in seven of the 16 analyses, with $p \leqslant .001$ in four of them. No statistically significant coefficients for cigarette smoking were recorded in 14 of the 16 analyses; again, the exceptions were the significant negative coefficients for white women age 45-64. Coefficients for age were statistically significant in ten of 16 analyses, with $p \leqslant .001$ in nine of these ten.

R^2 ranged in the 16 analyses from a low of .125 to a high of .237. Values for R^2 tended to be slightly higher for systolic than for diastolic pressure. They tended to be higher for younger than older age groups for diastolic, but not for systolic pressure. No consistent sex or race differences in R^2 were noted.

TABLE 11.
Relationship of Sex and Race to Systolic and Diastolic Blood Pressure, with Other Variables Simultaneously Considered, Multiple Linear Regression Analysis, Coefficients and Their Statistical Significance Chicago Health Department Community Survey (1965-71) and Chicago Heart Association Detection Project in Industry (1967-72)

Variable	Chicago Health Department Community Surveys				Chicago Heart Association Detection Project in Industry			
	6,375 Persons Age 30-44		7,154 Persons Age 45-64		11,743 Persons Age 25-44		9,551 Persons Age 45-64	
	Systolic Blood Pressure	Diastolic Blood Pressure	Systolic Blood Pressure	Diastolic Blood Pressure	Systolic Blood Pressure	Diastolic Blood Pressure	Systolic Blood Pressure	Diastolic Blood Pressure
Relative Weight	.246***	.171***	.268***	.158***	.221***	.126***	.226***	.136***
Heart Rate	.176***	.102***	.220***	.130***	.337***	.154***	.429***	.192***
Plasma Glucose	.033***	.016***	.048***	.012***	.035***	.002***	.053***	.028***
Serum Cholesterol	.009	.012***	.007	.006*	.016***	.002***	.014**	.016***
Serum Uric Acid	___	___	___	___	.780***	.914***	.909***	.657***
Hematocrit	.076	.152***	.192**	.244***	___	___	___	___
Cigarettes/Day	___	___	___	___	.001	- .001	- .021	- .026**
Age	.400***	.261***	.682***	.033	.122***	.256***	.732***	.125***
Sex	- 6.020***	- 1.706***	- 1.556**	- .705*	- 8.045***	- 2.954***	- 3.674***	- 3.346***
Race	4.893***	4.301***	5.353***	4.774***	1.698***	2.644***	4.320***	4.426***
Constant	57.060	26.006	29.700	33.624	66.324	31.771	27.557	34.748
Multiple R	.476	.477	.427	.414	.493	.443	.451	.409
R²	.226	.227	.182	.171	.243	.196	.203	.167

*p ≤ .05 **p ≤ .01 ***p ≤ .001

*Chicago Health Department Community Surveys
and Chicago Heart Association Detection Project in
Industry: Do the Several Variables "Explain" the
Race Difference in Prevalence of Hypertension?*

In both the foregoing studies, higher prevalence rates of
high blood pressure were consistently recorded for blacks than
whites, in keeping with usual American experience. Additional
multivariate statistical analyses were done to evaluate whether
the several variables considered — relative weight, heart rate,
post-load plasma glucose, serum cholesterol and uric acid,
hematocrit, cigarette smoking — account for the racial difference. For this purpose, the sex-race groups were combined for
the two age strata (< 45 and 45-64), and a code 0 was assigned
to whites, code 1 to blacks; a code 0 to men, code 1 to women.

Results with the multiple linear regression analyses are
presented in Table 11; similar results were obtained with the
multiple logistic analyses. (This table, combining sex-race
groups, serves to present a useful summary of the findings of
the preceding tables on the six-factor and seven-factor analyses,
respectively.) In both types of analyses (logistic and linear) for
both age groups of both studies, race was highly significantly
related to blood pressure independent of the several other
variables, ie, these variables did not "explain" the higher
prevalence of hypertension in blacks compared to whites. The
factors responsible for the race differential remain concealed in
the approximately 80% of the variability in blood pressure left
"unexplained" by the several variables evaluated here.

*Peoples Gas Co. and Western Electric Co. Studies:
Baseline (Prevalence) Findings*

Data on the several variables under study in this report,
including post-load plasma glucose, were initially collected in
1961 in the Western Electric Co. study and in 1965 in the
Peoples Gas Co. study, ie, some years after these long-term
prospective studies of middle-aged employed men in Chicago
were initiated in 1958.[6-12] Of the original cohorts (2,021 and
1,465 men, respectively, age 40-55 and 40-59, respectively, in
1958), complete data on the several variables under study were
available for 1,730 (85.6%) and 787 (53.7%), respectively. The
difference in percent available reflects the greater interlude

TABLE 12.
Simple and Partial Correlation Coefficients
Cross-Sectional (Baseline) Analyses
Chicago Peoples Gas Co. and Western Electric Co. Studies

Variable	787 Men -- Peoples Gas Co. Study				1,730 Men -- Western Electric Co. Study			
	Simple r		Partial r		Simple r		Partial r	
	Systolic Blood Pressure	Diastolic Blood Pressure	Systolic Blood Pressure	Diastolic Blood Pressure	Systolic Blood Pressure	Diastolic Blood Pressure	Systolic Blood Pressure	Diastolic Blood Pressure
Age	.126***	-.033	.120***	-.054	.141***	.041	.140***	.029
Relative Weight	.221***	.315***	.165***	.245***	.214***	.267***	.209***	.260***
Heart Rate	.195***	.183***	.135***	.152***	.247***	.241***	.233***	.236***
Plasma Glucose	.256***	.211***	.182***	.137***	.159***	.121***	.118***	.076**
Serum Cholesterol	.076*	.131***	.033	.090**	.100***	.109***	.055*	.066**
Serum Uric Acid	.198***	.224***	.133***	.134***				
Cigarettes/Day	.022	-.053	.044	-.038	.023	-.029	.037	-.027

Baseline data: Peoples Gas Co. Study -- 1965; Western Electric Co. Study -- 1961.

Post-load plasma glucose: Peoples Gas Co. Study -- 1-hour post-50 gm. oral load.
                                   Western Electric Co. Study -- 2-hour post-100 gm. oral load.

r -- Systolic Blood Pressure-Diastolic Blood Pressure: Peoples Gas Co. Study -- .745***
                                                     Western Electric Co. Study -- .777***

* $p \leq .05$
** $p \leq .01$
*** $p \leq .001$

(1958 to 1965) for the Peoples Gas Co. than for the Western Electric Co. cohort (1958 to 1961). For the purposes of these analyses on these two cohorts of 1,730 and 787 men, respectively, the examination data of 1961 (Western Electric Co. study) and 1965 (Peoples Gas Co. study), respectively, were defined as the baseline data. In the former study, the post-load plasma glucose was two hours after a 100 gm oral load; in the latter study, one hour after a 50 gm oral load.

Correlation analyses. The findings from the simple and partial correlation analyses of the baseline (ie, the cross-sectional or prevalence) data are presented in Table 12. In both studies, the partial r's for blood pressure (both systolic and diastolic) and relative weight, heart rate and post-load plasma glucose — while of low order — were all highly significant statistically (most p values $\leq$ .001). The partial r's for blood pressure and serum uric acid (.133 and .134 — data available from the Peoples Gas Co. study only) were similarly significant. The partial r's for blood pressure and serum cholesterol were smaller (all $<$ .10), with p values indicating significance at $\leq$ .05 in three of the four analyses.

Multiple logistic analyses. The coefficients from the multiple logistic analyses and the approximations of their statistical significance are presented in Table 13. Four blood pressure cut points were used as dependent variables — systolic pressure $\geq$ 140 and $\geq$ 160 mm Hg, diastolic pressure $\geq$ 90 and $\geq$ 95 mm Hg. For seven of the eight analyses, the coefficients for relative weight, heart rate and plasma glucose were significant statistically. This was the case only exceptionally for serum cholesterol and uric acid. None of the coefficients for cigarette smoking were statistically significant. The coefficients for age were statistically significant in five of the eight analyses, including all four with systolic pressure as the dependent variable.

Data are given in Table 14 on the ordering of men into deciles of expected prevalence of elevated blood pressure (systolic $\geq$ 140, diastolic $\geq$ 90), based on the coefficients for the several independent variables derived with the multiple logistic regression model. For both cohorts, ordering into deciles of expected prevalence of elevated blood pressure produced progressively greater rates of observed prevalence,

TABLE 13.
Relationship Between Multiple Variables and Blood Pressure — Multiple Logistic Analyses Cross-Sectional (Baseline) Findings — Coefficients and Their Statistical Significance Peoples Gas Co. and Western Electric Co. Studies

Variable	Coefficients -- 787 Men, Peoples Gas Co. Study Cutpoints for Elevated Baseline Blood Pressure				Coefficients -- 1,730 Men, Western Electric Co. Study Cutpoints for Elevated Baseline Blood Pressure			
	SBP $\geq$140	SBP $\geq$160	DBP $\geq$90	DBP $\geq$95	SBP $\geq$140	SBP $\geq$160	DBP $\geq$90	DBP $\geq$95
Age	.054***	.066**	.008	-.030	.057***	.064***	.029*	.009
Relative Weight	.019***	.008	.030***	.034***	.028***	.024***	.037***	.033***
Heart Rate	.020**	.019	.034***	.036**	.041***	.061***	.045***	.058***
Plasma Glucose	.007***	.006*	.002	.007*	.005***	.009***	.003*	.005**
Serum Cholesterol	.004	-.001	.004	.003	.003*	.000	.003*	.001
Serum Uric Acid	.008	.016	.019*	.011	—	—	—	—
Cigarettes/Day	.008	.007	.004	.008	.005	.010	-.003	.001
Constant	-10.016	-10.018	-10.615	-10.505	-11.137	-14.068	-10.874	-11.266

*p < .05
**p < .01
***p < .001

TABLE 14.

Relationship Between Multiple Variables and Blood Pressure — Multiple Logistic Analyses
Cross-Sectional (Baseline) Analyses — Deciles of Expected and Observed Prevalence of Elevated Blood Pressure
Chicago Peoples Gas Co. and Western Electric Co. Studies

Decile of Expected Prevalence of Elevated Blood Pressure	787 Men -- Peoples Gas Company Study SBP ≥140 Expected No.	Expected Rate/1,000	Observed No.	Observed Rate/1,000	DBP >90 Expected No.	Expected Rate/1,000	Observed No.	Observed Rate/1,000	1,730 Men -- Western Electric Company Study SBP ≥140 Expected No.	Expected Rate/1,000	Observed No.	Observed Rate/1,000	DBP ≥90 Expected No.	Expected Rate/1,000	Observed No.	Observed Rate/1,000
1	10.1	129	6	77	3.9	50	3	38	24.5	142	22	127	21.3	123	21	121
2	14.6	187	17	218	6.0	77	8	103	34.8	201	31	179	30.6	177	21	121
3	17.9	229	17	218	7.4	95	7	90	41.7	241	40	231	37.7	218	47	272
4	20.4	262	17	218	9.2	118	12	154	47.8	276	49	283	43.7	252	43	249
5	22.8	292	35	449	10.9	140	12	154	54.4	314	57	329	50.6	293	62	358
6	25.7	329	20	256	12.7	163	14	179	61.6	356	68	393	57.9	335	59	341
7	28.7	368	31	397	15.1	193	16	205	68.6	397	69	399	65.5	379	69	399
8	32.4	415	31	397	17.7	227	14	179	77.2	446	77	445	74.7	432	68	393
9	37.5	481	39	500	22.1	283	21	269	90.4	523	97	561	88.3	510	81	468
10	53.7	631	52	612	37.8	445	36	424	115.4	667	110	636	115.2	666	118	682
All	263.7	335	265	337	142.8	181	143	182	616.4	356	620	358	585.6	338	589	340
Ratio: 10/1	5.3		8.7		9.7		12.0		4.7		5.0		5.4		5.6	
Ratio: 9+10/1+2	3.7		4.0		6.1		5.2		3.5		3.9		3.9		4.7	
% of All With Elevated BP in 10	20.4		19.5		26.5		25.2		18.7		17.7		19.7		20.0	
% of All With Elevated BP in	?.6		34.1		41.9		39.9		33.4		33.4		34.8		33.8	

with generally good correspondence between expected and observed rates. The ratio of observed rates for the highest compared to the lowest decile of expected prevalence ranged from 5.0 to 12.0; for the highest compared to the lowest quintile, from 3.9 to 5.2. From 17.7% to 25.2% of all men with elevated blood pressure were in the highest decile of expected prevalence; from 33.4 to 39.9 in the highest quintile.

Multiple linear regression analyses. The coefficients from the multiple linear regression analyses and their statistical significance are presented in Table 15. The coefficients for relative weight, heart rate, plasma glucose and uric acid were all highly significant statistically (most p values $\leqslant$ .001). In three of four analyses, p values for the serum cholesterol coefficients were $\leqslant$ .05. None of the coefficients for cigarette smoking were statistically significant. The coefficients for age were significant in the systolic, but not the diastolic, pressure analyses. R^2 ranged from .140 to .174, ie, up to 17.4% of the interindividual variability in blood pressure was "explained" by these variables.

In summary, these cross-sectional findings in the Peoples Gas Co. and Western Electric Co. studies — highly consistent between these two studies — were also very consistent with the data from the Chicago Health Department and Chicago Heart Association surveys. In the four studies (all of them involving middle-aged white men), the multivariate analyses demonstrated with a high degree of reproducibility that relative weight, heart rate and post-load plasma glucose were significantly related to blood pressure. This was also true for serum uric acid in the two studies with data on this variable. It was inconsistently true for serum cholesterol; ie, in the multivariate analyses for middle-aged white males from some of the studies, serum cholesterol was significantly related to blood pressure, in others it was not. Consistently, cigarette smoking was not related to blood pressure in the three studies with data on this variable. Age was related much more consistently to systolic than diastolic blood pressure in these four studies of middle-aged white males.

Peoples Gas Co. and Western Electric Co. Studies:
Follow-up (Incidence) Findings

All the foregoing analyses were of the cross-sectional type. The question remains whether the specified variables relate to the *future* development of elevated blood pressure, ie, do they

TABLE 15.
Relationship Between Multiple Variables and Blood Pressure — Multiple Linear Regression Analyses
Coefficients and Their Statistical Significance — Cross-Sectional (Baseline) Findings
Peoples Gas Co. and Western Electric Co. Studies

Variable	787 Men -- Peoples Gas Co. Study		1,730 Men -- Western Electric Co. Study	
	Systolic BP	Diastolic BP	Systolic BP	Diastolic BP
Age	.418***	-.103	.579***	.068
Relative Weight	.185***	.154***	.267***	.193***
Heart Rate	.211***	.130***	.442***	.258***
Plasma Glucose	.071***	.029***	.054***	.020**
Serum Cholesterol	.014	.022*	.022*	.015**
Serum Uric Acid	.192***	.106***	_____	_____
Cigarettes/Day	.065	-.031	.056	-.023
Constant	46.060	41.693	28.269	33.763
Multiple R	.388	.418	.376	.375
R^2	.151	.174	.141	.140
F for Multiple Regression	19.7***	23.5***	47.3***	46.9***

*$p \leq .05$

**$p \leq .01$

***$p \leq .001$

truly function as prospective risk factors? More specifically, since a body of evidence exists indicating that level of blood pressure at a given point in time is a predictor of blood pressure slope,[6,16-18] the question is whether such variables as relative weight, heart rate, post-load plasma glucose and uric acid are risk factors for elevated blood pressure *over and above baseline blood pressure level.* Longitudinal data available from the Peoples Gas Co. and Western Electric Co. studies permitted an exploration of this problem. The data that follow are the initial findings.

From the Western Electric study, prospective data were available for the years 1961-1965 on 1,571 of the 1,730 men (90.8%); from the Peoples Gas Co. study, on 561 of 787

TABLE 16.
Simple and Partial Correlation Coefficients
Prospective Analyses, Cohorts with Complete Baseline and Follow-up Data
Chicago Peoples Gas Co. and Western Electric Co. Studies

Baseline Variable	561 Men -- Peoples Gas Co. Study				1,571 Men -- Western Electric Co. Study			
	Simple r		Partial r		Simple r		Partial r	
	Follow-Up SBP	Follow-Up DBP	Follow-Up SBP	Follow-Up DBP	Follow-Up SBP	Follow-Up DBP	Follow-Up SBP	Follow-Up DBP
Age	.102**	-.008	.078*	.031	.162***	.046*	.119***	.038
Systolic Blood Pressure	.652***	.537***	.626***	—	.668***	.527***	.631***	—
Diastolic Blood Pressure	.508***	.551***	—	.505***	.550***	.561***	—	.518***
Relative Weight	.127***	.201***	.001	.066	.174***	.212***	.056*	.083***
Heart Rate	.120**	.136***	.004	.045	.166***	.156***	.027	.042*
Plasma Glucose	.171***	.108**	.053	-.013	.130***	.053*	.038	-.023
Serum Cholesterol	.063	.058	.042	.007	.068**	.092***	.003	.030
Serum Uric Acid	.118**	.165***	-.039	.036	—	—	—	—
Cigarettes/Day	.029	.028	.025	.083*	.054*	-.011	.066**	.001

simple r, SBP-DBP, baseline: Peoples Gas Co. Study -- .766
                            Western Electric Co. Study -- .773

simple r, SBP-DBP, follow-up: Peoples Gas Co. Study -- .742
                             Western Electric Co. Study -- .757

*p < .05
**p < .01
***p < .001

(71.3%), for the period 1965-1970. Over the four to five year period, systolic pressure increased about 7 mm and diastolic pressure about 3 mm for both cohorts.

Correlation analyses. In accord with findings from other studies in the United States and Great Britain,[16-18] both the simple and partial correlation analyses showed a high correlation for both cohorts between baseline and follow-up blood pressures (partial r's in the range .505 to .631)(Table 16). Partial r's for each of the other baseline variables and follow-up blood pressures were of low order (with control for every other baseline variable, including baseline blood pressure). For the 1,571 men of the Western Electric Co. cohort, the partial r's for relative weight and follow-up blood pressure (both systolic and diastolic), for heart rate and follow-up diastolic pressure, for cigarette smoking and follow-up systolic pressure, and for age and follow-up systolic pressure were statistically significant. For the smaller cohort of 571 men in the Peoples Gas Co. study, the only significant partial r's (in addition to baseline and follow-up pressures) were between cigarettes and follow-up diastolic pressure and between age and follow-up systolic pressure.

Since these two cohorts encompassed both men with normal and elevated blood pressure at baseline, they could not appropriately be used for prospective analyses (cross-classification or multiple logistic) of *incidence* of elevated blood pressure (see below). However, it was appropriate to do multiple linear regression analyses, with actual level of follow-up blood pressure as the dependent variable (Table 17). Coefficients for baseline pressure regressed against follow-up pressures were found to be highly significant statistically in these multiple linear regression analyses (p values consistently $\leqslant$ .001). Of the additional baseline variables, coefficients for relative weight were still statistically significant for the Western Electric Co. cohort, as well as the coefficient for cigarettes in relation to follow-up systolic pressure and for age in relation to follow-up systolic pressure. R^2 values ranged from .313 to .323 for follow-up diastolic pressure as the dependent variable and from .432 to .458 for follow-up systolic pressure as the dependent variable, ie, it was possible to "explain" as much as 45.8% of the interindividual variability in follow-up blood pressure with the specified baseline variables, principally baseline blood pressure.

TABLE 17.
Relationship Between Multiple Variables and Blood Pressure —
Multiple Linear Regression Analyses
Coefficients and Their Statistical Significance —
Prospective Analyses, Cohorts with Complete Baseline and Follow-Up Data
Chicago Peoples Gas Co. and Western Electric Co. Studies

Baseline Variable	561 Men -- Peoples Gas Co. Study		1,571 Men -- Western Electric Co. Study	
	Follow-Up Systolic BP	Follow-Up Diastolic BP	Follow-Up Systolic BP	Follow-Up Diastolic BP
Age	.265	.067	.419***	.084
Relative Weight	.001	.039	.058*	.055***
Heart Rate	.006	.036	.042	.043
Plasma Glucose	.017	-.003	.015	-.006
Serum Cholesterol	.015	.002	.001	.006
Serum Uric Acid	-.047	.028	————	————
Cigarettes/Day	.031	.066	.083**	.001
Systolic BP	.657***	————	.694***	————
Diastolic BP	————	.558***	————	.556***
Constant	33.009	24.567	13.989	25.185
Multiple R	.658	.559	.676	.568
R^2	.432	.313	.458	.323
F for Multiple Regression	52.5 ***	31.4 ***	188.3 ***	106.4 ***

To assess relationship of these variables to risk of developing
elevated blood pressure, cohorts normotensive at baseline
(defined as systolic pressure less than 135 and diastolic less than
85 mm Hg) were identified. These numbered 733 men from the
Western Electric Co. study (42.4% of the baseline cohort of
1,730 men) and 327 men from the Peoples Gas Co. study
(41.6% of the baseline cohort of 787 men). Again, the
dependent variables were systolic and diastolic pressure after
four to five years of follow-up. At follow-up, systolic pressures
were on the average about 9-10 mm Hg higher than at baseline
(from 119 and 120 to 129); diastolic pressures, 4-5 mm Hg
higher (from 74 and 76 to 78 and 81).

Correlation analyses. Partial correlation coefficients between baseline and follow-up pressures — in the range .206-.383
— were highly significant statistically for both studies

(p ⩽ .001) (Table 18). In three of the four analyses, the partial r's for relative weight and blood pressure — in the range .062-.126 — were statistically significant (p ⩽ .05). Partial r's for heart rate and blood pressure of .078 were statistically significant for the Western Electric Co. cohort (p ⩽ .01). One partial r of .106 for systolic pressure and plasma glucose in the Peoples Gas Co. study was statistically significant (p ⩽ .05). One of the two available partial r's for uric acid and blood pressure — .107 — was significant (p ⩽ .05). Three of the four partial r's for cigarette smoking and blood pressure — in the range .070-.115 — were significant (p ⩽ .05). None of the four low order partial r's for serum cholesterol and blood pressure were significant. The two partial r's for age and systolic pressure were significant.

Multiple logistic analyses. Coefficients for both baseline systolic and diastolic pressure had p values indicating statistical significance for all eight analyses, ie, for all four cut points for follow-up blood pressure as the dependent variable for both studies (Table 19). The only other coefficients with p values indicating statistical significance were two for relative weight, one for plasma glucose and three for age.

The coefficients from the multiple logistic regression analyses were applied to each man to compute his expected risk of developing elevated blood pressure, and the men were then ordered into deciles of expected risk. Data are presented for two of the four cut points for elevated blood pressure, one systolic (⩾ 140 mm Hg) and one diastolic (⩾ 90 mm Hg) (Table 20). For all four analyses, there was good correspondence between expected and observed incidence rates of elevated blood pressure. The ratio of the observed incidence rate for the highest compared to the lowest decile of expected incidence ranged from 5.4 to 12.5 for the three of the four analyses for which this statistic could be calculated; for the highest compared to the lowest quintile, from 3.4 to 25.0. From 14.8% to 30.5% of men with elevated blood pressure were in the highest decile of expected incidence; from 29.7% to 50.0% in the highest quintile.

Multiple linear regression analyses. In the multiple linear regression analyses, as in the multiple logistic, the coefficients for baseline blood pressures as independent variables — re-

TABLE 18.
Simple and Partial Correlation Coefficients, Prospective Analyses
Cohorts with Baseline Systolic Pressure < 135, Diastolic Blood Pressure < 85 mm Hg
Chicago Peoples Gas Co. and Western Electric Co. Studies

Baseline Variable	327 Men -- Peoples Gas Co. Study				733 Men -- Western Electric Co. Study			
	Simple r		Partial r		Simple r		Partial r	
	Follow-Up		Follow-Up		Follow-Up		Follow-Up	
	SBP	DBP	SBP	DBP	SBP	DBP	SBP	DBP
Age	.095*	.010	.100*	.028	.121***	-.016	.120***	-.011
Systolic Blood Pressure	.416***	.340***	.383***		.337***	.190***	.323***	
Diastolic Blood Pressure	.259***	.289***		.227***	.219***	.224***		.206***
Relative Weight	.128**	.219***	.024	.126*	.087**	.104**	.062*	.082*
Heart Rate	.132**	.115*	.043	.057	.115***	.101**	.087**	.087**
Plasma Glucose	.180***	.131**	.106*	.050	.054	-.013	.032	-.041
Serum Cholesterol	.034	.035	.031	.014	.024	.061*	-.027	.038
Serum Uric Acid	.083	.151**	.035	.107*				
Cigarettes/Day	.051	.027	.095*	.115*	.044	.010	.070*	.012

Baseline Systolic Blood Pressure and Diastolic Blood Pressure: Peoples Gas Co.: .574; Western Electric Co.: .542

Follow-up Systolic Blood Pressure and Diastolic Blood Pressure: Peoples Gas Co.: .710; Western Electric Co.: .660.

*p < .05
**p < .01
***p < .001

TABLE 19.
Relationship Between Multiple Variables and Elevated Blood Pressure — Multiple Logistic Analyses
Prospective Findings, Cohorts with Baseline Systolic Pressure < 135 and Diastolic Blood Pressures < 85 mm Hg
Coefficients and Their Statistical Significance
Chicago Peoples Gas Co. and Western Electric Co. Studies

Baseline Variable	Coefficients -- 327 Men, Peoples Gas Co. Study				Coefficients -- 733 Men, Western Electric Co. Study			
	Cutpoints for Elevated Follow-up Blood Pressure				Cutpoints for Elevated Follow-up Blood Pressure			
	SBP ≥140	SBP ≥160	DBP ≥90	DBP ≥95	SBP ≥140	SBP ≥160	DBP ≥90	DBP ≥95
Age	.069*	.113	.019	.076	.047*	.097*	.030	-.006
Systolic Blood Pressure	.118***	.102**	.128***	.165***	.067***	.079***	.059***	.066*
Diastolic Blood Pressure	____	____	.022*	.006	____	____	.014*	.012
Relative Weight	.006	-.012	.002	-.031	.012	-.002	.011	.012
Heart Rate	.008	.019	.003	.009	.015	-.002	-.002	.008
Plasma Glucose	.002	.030***	.004	-.010	-.003	.006	.001	-.004
Serum Cholesterol	.003	-.004	.009	.009	-.001	-.003		-.005
Serum Uric Acid	-.004	.017	.024	.011	____	____	____	____
Cigarettes/Day	.023	.024			.005	.013	.007	.002
Constant	-21.710	-27.219	-17.537	-18.111	-13.499	-17.449	-9.626	-7.941

*p ≤ .05
**p ≤ .01
***p ≤ .001

Prospective Findings, Cohorts with Systolic BP < 135 and Diastolic BP < 85 mm Hg
Deciles of Expected Incidence of Elevated Blood Pressure
Chicago Peoples Gas Co. and Western Electric Co. Studies

Decile of Expected Incidence of Elevated Blood Pressure	327 Men -- Peoples Gas Co. Study								733 Men -- Western Electric Co. Study							
	Follow-up SBP ≥140				Follow-up DBP ≥90				Follow-up SBP ≥140				Follow-up DBP ≥90			
	Expected		Observed		Expected		Observed		Expected		Observed		Expected		Observed	
	No.	Rate/1,000	No.	Rate/1,000	No.	Rate/1,000	No.	Rate/1,000	No.	Rate/1,000	No.	Rate/1,000	No.	Rate/1,000	No.	Rate/1,000
1	1.1	34	2	63	.7	21	0	0	6.3	87	4	55	8.9	120	5	68
2	2.3	72	1	31	1.3	41	1	31	9.2	125	7	96	11.6	158	11	151
3	3.6	112	2	63	1.9	59	2	63	11.6	159	11	151	13.6	186	18	247
4	4.8	151	4	125	2.6	82	1	31	13.9	190	17	233	15.6	214	18	247
5	5.8	183	7	219	3.2	99	2	63	16.2	222	16	219	17.1	234	19	260
6	7.5	233	5	156	4.1	127	7	219	19.1	262	29	397	18.7	256	14	190
7	9.1	283	11	344	5.1	161	7	219	22.0	302	21	288	20.6	283	21	288
8	11.1	346	11	344	6.6	207	5	156	25.5	349	17	233	22.2	304	22	301
9	14.2	445	14	438	8.6	270	10	313	29.3	401	30	411	24.2	331	27	370
10	23.1	593	25	641	15.8	406	15	385	36.4	479	37	487	29.8	392	27	355
All	82.6	253	82	251	49.9	153	50	153	189.5	259	189	258	182.1	248	182	248
Ratio: 10/1	21.0		12.5		22.6		Δ		5.8		9.3		3.3		5.4	
Ratio: 9+10/1+2	11.0		13.0		12.2		25.0		4.2		6.1		2.6		3.4	
% of All with Elevated BP in 10	28.0		30.5		31.7		30.0		19.2		19.5		16.4		14.8	
% of All with Elevated BP in 9+10	45.2		47.6		48.9		50.0		34.7		35.4		29.7		29.7	

ΔDenominator zero. Ratio cannot be computed.

gressed against follow-up blood pressures as dependent variables — were all highly significant statistically for both studies (.507 and .676 for systolic, .325 and .336 for diastolic, all p values ≤ .001) (Table 21). Coefficients for relative weight with diastolic pressure as the dependent variable were statistically significant for both studies (p≤ .05). Coefficients for heart rate were statistically significant for the Western Electric Co., but not the Peoples Gas Co. cohort (p≤ .05). Two of the four coefficients for cigarettes were statistically significant (p≤ .05). The coefficient for age for follow-up systolic pressure as the dependent variable was significant for the Western Electric Co. cohort (p≤ .001).

TABLE 21.
Relationship Between Multiple Variables and Blood Pressure —
Multiple Linear Regression Analyses Coefficients and Their Statistical
Significance,Prospective Analyses — Cohorts with Baseline Systolic
Blood Pressure < 135, Diastolic Blood Pressure < 85 mm Hg
Chicago Peoples Gas Co. and Western Electric Co. Studies

Baseline Variables	327 Men -- Peoples Gas Co. Study		733 Men -- Western Electric Co. Stu	
	Follow-up Systolic BP	Follow-up Diastolic BP	Follow-up Systolic BP	Follow-up Diastolic BP
Age	.308	.056	.370[***]	-.022
Relative Weight	.020	.070[*]	.063	.053[*]
Heart Rate	.051	.044	.133[*]	.089[*]
Plasma Glucose	.032	.010	.012	-.011
Serum Cholesterol	.010	.003	-.008	.007
Serum Uric Acid	.041	.082	____	____
Cigarettes/Day	.112	.087[*]	.083[*]	.009
Systolic Blood Pressure	.676[***]	____	.507[***]	____
Diastolic Blood Pressure	____	.336[***]	____	.325[***]
Constant	14.727	30.754	33.102	44.331
Multiple R	.453	.360	.375	.257
R^2	.205	.130	.141	.066
F for Multiple Regression	10.2[***]	5.9[***]	17.0[***]	7.3[***]

R^2 varied from .066 to .205, ie, up to 20.5% of the interindividual variability in follow-up blood pressures was "explained" by the several baseline variables entered into the analyses (Table 21). R^2 values were higher for follow-up systolic than for follow-up diastolic pressure as the dependent variable.

Discussion

The findings presented here from four cross-sectional studies in Chicago are highly consistent. With use of three multivariate statistical procedures (partial correlation, multiple logistic regression and multiple linear regression), three variables — relative weight, resting heart rate, and plasma glucose one hour after an oral load — were repeatedly found to be independently related to both diastolic and systolic blood pressure and to elevated pressure, with p values generally of $\leq .01$ or $\leq .001$. This was also true for serum uric acid in the two studies in which this measurement was made.

The fifth variable considered, serum cholesterol, was significantly related to blood pressure in some but not all of the multivariate analyses. The significant relationships were found for the most part for white males, both under age 45, and 45 and older, but with greater consistency in the former.

No positive association emerged in any of the analyses between cigarette smoking and blood pressure, or elevated blood pressure.

The seventh variable, age, was significantly related to blood pressure (particularly systolic pressure) independent of the other six variables in a majority of the analyses, more consistently for the younger than for the older age groups. Thus, even within the relatively narrow 15- to 20-year bands used in these analyses, there apparently was an independent contribution of age to blood pressure, not accounted for by the low order significant associations between age and such variables as relative weight and plasma glucose.

With both the techniques of multiple cross-classification and multiple logistic, simultaneously using the several independent variables, it was repeatedly possible to concentrate a high proportion of all cases of elevated blood pressure in a small substratum of each age-sex-race group, more so for the younger than the older ones. For example, when the coefficients from the multiple logistic regression analyses for the Chicago Heart Association study were used to estimate expectation of elevated blood pressure for individuals in the eight age-sex-race groups, and persons were then ordered into quintiles of *expected* prevalence of high blood pressure (eg, diastolic pressure ≥ 95 mm Hg), for persons age 25-44 from 45% to 56% of *observed* cases of elevated blood pressure were in the highest quintile (20%) of expected prevalence. The observed prevalence of elevated blood pressure was many times greater for the highest quintile of expected prevalence than for the lowest. A similar but less effective concentration of cases of elevated blood pressure was obtained with the multiple cross-classification method, eg, by dichotomizing five of the independent variables and identifying the substratum with any three, four or all five high.

These extensive data demonstrate that in cross-sectional analyses multiple biologic variables are independently related to blood pressure and elevated blood pressure.

Availability of four- to five-year prospective data from the Chicago Peoples Gas Co. and Western Electric Co. studies permitted exploration of the further questions: Are these variables also *prospectively* related to susceptibility to elevated blood pressure? In particular for persons originally normotensive, are such variables as relative weight, heart rate, post-load plasma glucose, uric acid, serum cholesterol, cigarette smoking independent risk factors for subsequent development of elevated blood pressure, independent of baseline level of blood pressure (within the generally accepted range of normal, since this variable itself is apparently highly related to risk of elevated pressure)?

First, initial analyses bearing upon these questions consistently showed that level of baseline pressure within the normal range is highly related to level of blood pressure four to five years later and is the most significant known factor indicating risk of subsequent development of elevated blood pressure. These findings confirm other reports to this effect.[16-18] In addition, they indicate that at least two of the other variables, relative weight and heart rate, and possibly post-load plasma glucose and serum uric acid, may be risk factors for elevated blood pressure independent of baseline blood pressure level. Furthermore, although none of the four cross-sectional studies yielded evidence of a positive relationship between cigarette smoking and blood pressure, the prospective data from both the Peoples Gas Co. and Western Electric Co. studies suggest that cigarette smoking may be a risk factor longitudinally for elevated blood pressure.*

In these prospective analyses, using the several variables (including baseline blood pressure), it was possible to identify in the upper quintile (20%) of expected incidence as many as 50% of the originally normotensive men who actually developed elevated blood pressure over the four- to five-year follow-up period. Incidence of observed elevated blood pressure ranged from as high as 349 per 1,000 in five years for the highest quintile of expected incidence to as low as 16 per 1,000 in five years for the lowest quintile of expected incidence, a more than 20-fold difference.

To place these positive findings in balanced perspective, it is at the same time appropriate to note that in the prospective analyses, much of the ability to identify the risk of subsequently developing elevated blood pressure lies in the level of the original (baseline) pressure; the other variables enhance this ability only modestly. Moreover, in both the cross-sectional and prospective analyses, the variables under investigation "explain" no more than 20% or 25% of the interindividual variability in blood pressure. The major portion of this variability remains unexplained as part of the continuing riddle of the pathogenesis of essential hypertension. Nor is there any real understanding of the mechanisms whereby such variables as relative weight, heart rate, plasma glucose, uric acid, serum cholesterol and cigarette smoking relate to blood pressure. The importance of these continuing uncertainties is well illustrated by the data presented in Table 11, forcefully indicating that the seven variables considered here do not account for the major black-white difference in prevalence of hypertension.

Despite these major remaining issues and, therefore, the limitations of the findings reported here, they may have practical implications, particularly in the crucial area of approaches to the primary prevention of high blood pressure. With a set of data simple to collect en masse among young people — eg, blood pressure, weight and heart rate (plus family

*A detailed review of other work along these lines is presented in references 1 and 5.

history) — it becomes possible even without collection of blood to identify hypertension-prone persons as early as the teens and twenties. In addition to long-term surveillance, safe nutritional-hygienic measures can then be instituted (even though their efficacy remains to be confirmed) — eg, correction or avoidance of obesity, moderation in salt usage, rhythmic exercise to achieve and maintain optimal cardiopulmonary fitness with its concomitant bradycardia and avoidance of cigarettes. While no evidence as yet permits a statement that such measures will be effective, findings do indeed suggest the *possibility* of primary prevention of at least a proportion of the millions of cases making up the present-day mass epidemic of hypertensive disease. Certainly, controlled prospective studies, ie, field trials to assess this matter are urgently needed. And — in view of the safety of the nutritional-hygienic measures — there appear to be good reasons for physicians to apply these approaches in practice for their hypertension-prone families. Prevention is often possible long before etiology and pathogenesis have been clarified. So it may well be with hypertension!

Summary

1. Cross-sectional (prevalence) analyses of the relationship of multiple variables to blood pressure were done using data from four Chicago epidemiologic surveys: Chicago Board of Health Community Surveys involving 13,469 men and women, white and black, age 30-64; the Chicago Heart Association Detection Project in Industry, encompassing 21,024 men and women, white and black, age 25-64; 1,730 middle-aged white men of the Western Electric Co. study; 787 middle-aged men (over 90% of whom were white) of the Peoples Gas Co. study.

2. Four multivariate statistical methods — partial correlation, multiple cross-classification, multiple logistic regression and multiple linear regression — were used to evaluate the relationship between the several variables and blood pressure. The analyses were carried out separately for specific age-sex-race groups. The variables included relative weight, resting heart rate, plasma glucose after oral glucose load, serum uric acid and cholesterol, current cigarette smoking habit, hematocrit and age.

3. In all four populations, the first three of these variables — relative weight, heart rate, and plasma post-load glucose — were independently related to blood pressure with a high degree of consistency, with p values for statistical significance ≤ .01 or ≤ .001 in the great majority of analyses.

4. Serum uric acid — a variable evaluated in two of the four populations — was also independently related to blood pressure in a great majority of the analyses, with p values of ≤ .01 or ≤ .001.

5. The findings with respect to the relationship of serum cholesterol to blood pressure were generally negative, except for white males; for this one sex-race group, a high proportion of the multivariate analyses indicated a statistically significant relationship.

6. No positive relationship was found between cigarette smoking and blood pressure in the three of the four populations with data on this variable.

7. In the one study yielding data on hematocrit (the Chicago Board of Health Community Surveys), this variable was independently related to diastolic — but not to systolic — pressure for four age groups of men.

8. Although the analyses were age-specific for all four populations, encompassing an age band of either 15 or 20 years, age was often significantly related to blood pressure, especially to systolic blood pressure, independent of the several other variables studied.

9. In all four studies, when the multivariate logistic regression model and its coefficients, computed from the experience of an entire age-sex-race group, were used to calculate an expectation of elevated blood pressure for each person, and then persons were ordered from low to high in expectation, a high proportion of all persons with recorded elevations of blood pressure were in the highest decile and quintile of expected prevalence. The observed prevalence of elevated blood pressure was consistently several times as high for the highest decile or quintile of expected prevalence as for the lowest. A similar but less effective concentration of cases of elevated blood pressure was obtained with the multiple cross-classification method, by dichotomizing four or five of the independent variables and identifying the substratum with multiple variables high.

10. Findings of the multiple linear regression analyses indicated that about 20% to 25% of the interindividual variability in blood pressure at these survey examinations was "explained" by the several variables considered.

11. Prospective data involving four to five years of follow-up were available for two of the populations, ie, the middle-aged males of the Peoples Gas Co. and Western Electric Co. studies. The aforementioned multivariate statistical methods were used to evaluate relationships between several baseline variables and blood pressure at the four- to five-year re-examinations (ie, follow-up blood pressure). Baseline (initial examination) blood pressures were included as dependent variables in these analyses.

12. Among the baseline dependent variables, blood pressure was found to be the measurement most powerfully related prospectively to follow-up blood pressure and risk of developing elevated blood pressure in four to five years for men originally normotensive.

13. With baseline blood pressure so related in a highly significant way to follow-up blood pressure, results from some of the multivariate analyses indicated that relative weight, heart rate, post-load plasma glucose, serum uric acid, serum cholesterol and cigarette smoking may make an additional low-order independent contribution to follow-up blood pressure and risk of elevated blood pressure.

14. With use of these several variables in these multivariate analyses, it was possible to identify strata of these populations (eg, highest quintile of expected risk of elevated blood pressure) with very high incidence rates of elevated blood pressure over four to five years, contrasting markedly with men in the lowest quintile of expected risk, with low rates of observed incidence.

15. The possibility exists that these findings may be applied in an effort to accomplish the primary prevention of hypertension. Thus, the risk factors for elevated blood pressure may be useful for the early identification of hypertension-prone persons, eg, in young adulthood. Use can be made of safe nutritional-hygienic methods for control of these risk factors for possible prophylactic purposes.

Acknowledgments

The work of the Chicago Health Department Community Surveys was successfully pursued thanks to the cooperation and support of Eric Oldberg, M.D., President, Chicago Board of Health, and Chairman, Board of Directors, Chicago Health Research Foundation. It is also a pleasure to pay tribute to the entire staff of the Heart Disease Control Program, Division of Adult Health and Aging, Chicago Health Department, and of the Chicago Health Research Foundation, aiding in this research, especially Howard Adler, Ph.D., Willie Reedus, R.N., and Raymond Restivo; also Juanita Chestang, Jean Civinelli, Roberta Crawford, Nancy Dalton, Sammie Ellis, Gail Pacelli, Edna Pardo, Frances Petersen, Peggy Powell, R. Raphaelson, Margie Shores, Eve Smolin and Ika Tomaschewsky. It is also a pleasure to express appreciation to the Chicago Housing Authority for its cooperation in this effort.

The work of the Chicago Heart Association Detection Project in Industry was accomplished thanks to the invaluable cooperation of almost 100 Chicago companies and organizations, their officers, staffs and employees whose volunteer efforts made this project possible. Acknowledgment is also gratefully extended to all those in the Chicago Heart Association — staff and volunteers — serving the Project: Louis DeBoer, Executive Director (retired) and Kay Westfall, Program Director; the Chicago Heart Association Detection Project in Industry Staff: Susan Shekelle, Coordinator; Pamela Bessmond, Thelma Black, Clarice Blanton, Joan Carothers, Arlene Dungca, Mary Ann Foelker, Susan Forkos, Carol Fulgenzi, Harold Gram, Jean Graver, Inger Hansen, Cherry Latimer, Karen Strentz, R.N., and Suzann Ward, R.N.; also, the volunteer members of the Heart Disease Detection Committee of the Chicago Heart Association and its Subcommittees: Howard Adler, Ph.D., Rene Arcilla, M.D., Robert Arzoecher, Ph.D., Richard A. Carleton, M.D., Angelo Cottini, Edwin Duffin, Ph.D., Morton B. Epstein, Ph.D., Robert E. Fitzgerald, M.D., Philip Freedman, M.D., Burton J. Grossman, M.D., Robert R. J. Hilker, M.D., Robert S. Kassriel, M.D., Clinton L. Lindo, M.D., Gerald Masek, Ph.D.,

Richard McNamara, Robert A. Miller, M.D., Robert Mosley, Jr., M.D., Milton H. Paul, M.D., Wallace Salzman, M.D., Robert Sessions, Howard H. Sky-Peck, Ph.D., Donald Singer, M.D., Lachichida Sinha, M.D., Grace Smedstead, Ralph Springer, J. Martin Stoker, M.D., Carl Vogel, Ira T. Whipple, M.S., and Quentin D. Young, M.D.

It is also a pleasure to express appreciation to the Officers and executive leaderships of both the Peoples Gas Company and the Western Electric Company in Chicago; their continuous cooperation and support over the years since the late 1950s made these two studies possible. Thanks are also due to the research staff of the Peoples Gas Company Study, Elizabeth Stevens, R.N., research assistant, Wanda Drake and Celene Epstein; also to Patricia Collette, M.A.; and to the staff of the Company Medical Department, Patricia Benson, R.N., Carl Checchia, M.D., Luis Evangelista, M.D., John Finch, M.D., Mary Ann Guzik, R.N., Gerald Holtz, M.D., Ruth Jaffke, Aaron Kerlow, M.D., Robert Matthews, M.D., Hermine Mizelle, R.N., H. Bates Noble, M.D., Harry Petrakos, M.D., Henry Ruder, M.D., Grace Smith, Elsie Traina, R.N., and David Trish.

The following physicians were active in the Western Electric Company Study and their invaluable assistance is gratefully acknowledged: Maurice Albala, Harry Bliss, Herschel Browns, Marvin Colbert, Henry De Young, Peter Economou, Sanford Franzblau, Robert Felix, John Graettinger, Buford Hall, Wallace Kirkland, Joseph Muenster, Hyman Mackler, Adrian Ostfeld, Robert Parsons, Charles Perlia, Norman Roberg, Marvin Rosenberg, George Saxton, Armin Schick, John Sharp, Jay Silverman, Donald Torun and Walter Wood.

The biochemical analyses for the Chicago Health Department, Chicago Heart Association and Peoples Gas Company studies were done in the research laboratories of the Chicago Board of Health and Chicago Health Research Foundation, under the direction of Morton B. Epstein, Ph.D., and Howard Adler, Ph.D.; we are also pleased to acknowledge the fine contribution of the two chief technicians, Dana King and Ika Tomaschewsky.

It is also a pleasure to express appreciation to the computer programming staff of the Department of Community Health and Preventive Medicine, Northwestern University Medical School — Dan Garside, Tom Tokich and Julia Wannamaker — who generated the data from all four studies.

These research endeavors were supported by the American Heart Association, Chicago Heart Association, Illinois Heart Association and the National Heart and Lung Institute of the U. S. Public Health Service. The Western Electric Company Study was also aided by grants from the Otho S. Sprague Foundation, the Research and Education Committee of the Presbyterian-St. Luke's Hospital and The Illinois Foundation. The Chicago Heart Association Detection Project in Industry was principally supported by the Illinois Regional Medical Program. The investigators are also pleased to acknowledge the support of many private donors.

References

1. Stamler, J., Stamler, R., Rhomberg, P. et al: Multivariate analysis of the relationship of six variables to blood pressure: Findings from Chicago Community Surveys, 1965-71. *J Chronic Dis.* (In press.)
2. Stamler, J., Schoenberger, J. A., Lindberg, H. A. et al: Detection of susceptibility to coronary disease. *Bull. N. Y. Acad. Med.*, 45:1306, 1969.
3. Schoenberger, J. A., Stamler, J., Shekelle, R. B. et al: Current status of hypertension control in an industrial population. *JAMA*, 222:559, 1972.
4. Stamler, J., Schoenberger, J. A., Shekelle, R. B. et al: Hypertension: The Problem and the Challenge. *The Hypertension Handbook*, West Point, Pa.:Merck, Sharp and Dohme, 1974, p. 3.
5. Stamler, J., Rhomberg, P., Schoenberger, J. A. et al: Multivariate analysis of the relationship of seven variables to blood pressure: Findings of the Chicago Heart Association Detection Project in Industry, 1967-72. *J. Chronic Dis.* (In press.)
6. Stamler, J.: On the natural history of hypertension and hypertensive disease. In Cort, J.H., Fencl, V., Hejl, Z. et al (eds.): *The Pathogenesis of Essential Hypertension.* Proceedings of the Prague Symposium. Prague:State Medical Publishing House, 1960, p. 67.
7. Stamler, J.: On the epidemiology of hypertensive disease. In Cort, J.H., Fencl, V., Hejl, Z. et al (eds.): *The Pathogenesis of Essential Hypertension.* Proceedings of the Prague Symposium. Prague:State Medical Publishing House, 1960, p. 107.
8. Stamler, J., Berkson, D. M., Lindberg, H. A. et al: Relationship of weight to hypercholesterolemia, hypertension and electrocardiographic abnormalities in middle-aged Chicagoans. *Memorias Del IV Congreso Mundial de Cardiologia*, IV-A:474, 1963.
9. Stamler, J., Berkson, D. M., Lindberg, H. A. et al: Socioeconomic factors in the epidemiology of hypertensive disease. In Stamler, J., Stamler, R. and Pullman, T.N. (eds.): *The Epidemiology of Hypertension.* New York, N. Y.:Grune and Stratton, 1967, p. 289.
10. Stamler, J.: *Lectures on Preventive Cardiology.* New York, N. Y.: Grune and Stratton, 1967.

11. Stamler, J., Berkson, D. M. and Lindberg, H. A.: Risk factors: Their role in the etiology and pathogenesis of the atherosclerotic diseases. In Wissler, R.W. and Geer, J.C. (eds.): *The Pathogenesis of Atherosclerosis.* Baltimore, Md.:Williams and Wilkins, 1972, p. 41.
12. Paul, O., Lepper, M. H., Phelan, W. H. et al: A longitudinal study of coronary heart disease. *Circulation,* 28:20, 1963.
13. *Build and Blood Pressure Study, 1959,* Vol. I. Chicago, Ill.:Society of Actuaries, 1959.
14. New Weight Standards for Men and Women. *Statist. Bull. Metrop. Life Insur. Co.,* 40, 1, Nov.-Dec. 1959.
15. Keys, A., Fidanza, F., Karvonen, M. J. et al: Indices of relative weight and obesity. *J. Chronic Dis.,* 25:329, 1972.
16. Harlan, W. R., Osborne, R. K. and Graybiel, A.: A longitudinal study of blood pressure. *Circulation,* 26:530, 1962.
17. Miall, W. E. and Lovell, H. G.: Relation between change of blood pressure and age. *Brit. Med. J.,* 2:660, 1967.
18. Paffenbarger, R. S. Jr., Thorne, M. C. and Wing, A. L.: Chronic disease in former college students. VIII. Characteristics in youth predisposing to hypertension in later years. *Amer. J. Epidem.,* 88:25, 1968.

Discussion

Dr. Langford: Dr. Stamler is a great scientist and he is also a bit of a lay preacher! Dr. Stamler, I wish to rise in objection to the pathogenetic implications of the last few minutes of your presentation, because it might appear that the elevated glucose and the elevated uric acid have some pathogenetic blood pressure-raising effect, but the alternate possibility that these are markers for something else seems to me at least equally tenable right at this moment.

Dr. Stamler: Dr. Langford, that is absolutely correct. I go to my friends in metabolism and I say to them, "Why is it that there are these correlations among such variables as plasma glucose (a carbohydrate metabolic marker), serum uric acid (a protein metabolic marker), serum triglycerides (a fat metabolic marker)?" And the best people to whom I ask this question are not able to give me much of an explanation, beyond cautioning that maybe alcohol has something to do with it! Our cross-sectional data indicate that these variables are related to blood pressure independent of relative weight. That "something else" may be related metabolically to all of this is certainly possible. But it is also possible that preventing and correcting obesity, controlling rapid heart rate by moderate frequent rhythmic exercise, stopping cigarettes — all safe nutritional-hygienic measures — may achieve primary prevention of hypertension in identifiable hypertension-prone young people. All these possibilities need to be researched; they are all testable hypotheses.

Dr. Hoobler, Michigan: Dr. Stamler, I want to address myself to your slide which referred to the diastolic blood pressure as a predictor of future hypertension. What puzzles me, when you do these studies, is: Why don't you look at the increment in blood pressure over a time period and relate that to the initial blood pressure? I think it would be much better to look for an incremental rise, because it is probably just as important whether the blood pressure goes from 80 to 86, or from 88 to 94.

Dr. Stamler: If I understand what I have heard from our colleagues in the 1,000 Aviators Study, even within a narrow range of blood pressure recorded at age 20 or so (when these men were inducted into the Air Force as healthy and normotensive), a few millimeters difference in this baseline pressure predicts the *slope* of blood pressure rise over subsequent decades, ie, the degree (amount) of the increment. Miall's data and ours indicate a similar phenomenon. The baseline level predicts the extent of the rise. One could make the dependent variable either the prospective blood pressure (eg, diastolic five years post baseline) or the increment; I doubt the result would be different. We'll take a look at it that other way.

Dr. Kass: I am a little perturbed because some of the carefully developed epidemiologic data of other studies have not received enough attention with respect to this question. These studies show quite clearly that the greatest single determinant of later rise in blood pressure was the blood pressure level at the first measurement. So, I don't think it is as critical as we once thought to study increment; it is necessary only to determine the resting blood pressure, in relation to the ranking order in the peer group. In Framingham, Massachusetts, this rise of blood pressure with time wasn't observed. What they did observe was that each individual tended to remain in his or her own quintile during many years of observation, more or less saying the same thing, although why the rise didn't occur I am not sure (perhaps the methodology was enough different in the two studies). Along those same lines, we have a few other predictors, which we should be discussing, and I should like to hazard the possibility that one of the reasons the multiple R values aren't higher is that we are not looking at the best predictors, and this is a function of future research. Finally, if we built up a multiple regression in which we use blood pressure plus weight plus a dietary factor do we not, in fact, absorb all of the glucose and uric acid data?

Dr. Stamler: I think that that question can be answered only rhetorically at this point. It is a valid question. We should reiterate that our main purpose here was to see if any of these factors added anything to prediction over and above blood pressure at baseline. The answer is that they add something, very little quantitatively, but something intriguing in terms of possible preventive approaches. One of our problems is that within our populations — eg, the Peoples Gas Co. and Western Electric Co. men, for whom diet data are available — differences between individuals in diet variables are small, difficult to measure and of questionable reproducibility and validity; the intra-individual variability is as great as the interindividual variability. When that is the case — as Keys, Fidanza and their colleagues have pointed out — great difficulties exist in relating nutritional variables to an end point, eg, blood pressure, for purposes of interindividual comparison within a population. And on a variable like salt intake, we have almost no data. We need work on methodology for that variable. Incidentally, family history needs to be "plugged in" to these multivariate analyses.

Dr. Miller, Maryland: I have two very simple questions. First, how did you handle the problem of dropouts in your prospective study, using your logistic-type functions and (2) I am sure that many people here don't quite understand what we mean when we say "logistic function." Second, approximately what proportion of the hypertensive problem can be accounted for by the constellation of precursors that you spoke about?

Dr. Stamler: As to people available at baseline in the prospective studies but not available four and five years later for a follow-up blood pressure (our end point of concern), we just left them out of the analysis, of necessity. The only people on whom blood pressure can be measured are those around at the time of follow-up exam. The main reasons for such loss to follow-up were death and retirement.

As to the multiple logistic analysis, I refer you to the *Journal of Chronic Disease* (20:511-524, 1967) by Truitt,

Cornfield and Kannel. It is essentially a method in which the dependent variable is a zero-one variable, not a continuous one, eg, risk of becoming hypertensive (vs. remaining normotensive), risk of dying (vs. remaining alive), risk of having a coronary (vs. not having one). In our analyses, the dependent variable was risk of being hypertensive (in the cross-sectional analyses), of becoming hypertensive (in the prospective analyses). Based on the experience of the entire population, coefficients are computed for each of the several variables, for the multiple logistic equation. There are at least two methods of generating the coefficients: (1) a discriminant function method, originally described by Truitt, Cornfield and Kannel and (2) an iterative method. They are both good. The iterative method is probably better because it has fewer assumptions. The only problem connected with it is that it costs ten times as much as the discriminant function method on the computer. Therefore, in these studies we used the less expensive method although it is sometimes fraught with problems. Once the coefficients that best fit that whole experience have been generated, those coefficients and the values for each person are used in the multiple logistic equation to calculate his probability of having elevated blood pressure. People are then ordered from low to high based on these estimated probabilities, and this array is divided in deciles or quintiles. Comparisons are then made of how close the actual observed rates of elevated blood pressure correspond to the estimated — eg, in the lowest quintile of expectation, do you have the lowest rate of observed prevalence (or incidence)?

Dr. Dollery: Dr. Stamler, I would like to focus on what you were saying about heart rate. In the last two sessions, we have been discussing essentially etiological factors and we have given a lot of attention to salt, renin, weight, and so forth. One area which we have not discussed as adequately as we might have is the area of adrenergic activity and the sympathetic nervous system. There seems to be a lot of evidence that this is involved in essential hypertension, namely, the evidence of heart rate, the fact that the plasma volume tends to be down a little, that the hematocrit tends to be up a little, and the work showing that apparently plasma noradrenalin is correlated with blood pressure positively. It does seem to me that we must not forget the role of the central nervous system and, particularly, the adrenergic circuits in the control of blood pressure. For my money, it is at least as likely that the problem of essential hypertension's origin lies there as it does in any of the other things that we have discussed.

Dr. Stamler: I agree. I think all of you know that we have repeatedly said, in discussing the black-white difference in hypertension prevalence, that there are three reasonable hypotheses: (1) it is population genetics — this I frankly doubt; (2) it has something to do with nutrition; and (3) it has something to do with the central nervous system, and specifically the higher nervous activity — the significance of being a black person in a society of segregation and discrimination. Those are not mutually exclusive hypotheses. Dr. Peiss pointed out here at the First Symposium ten years ago that heart rate is a reflector, if you will, of the level of central nervous system arousal. This certainly is in line with what you are saying. I still regard as highly viable the hypothesis that the higher nervous system activity has something to do with the fundamental problem. On the other hand, the heart rate phenomenon may be a response, effect not cause. That is one of the big reasons why we are so interested in the prospective data. One can also speculate that heart rate relates somehow to body fluid volumes, if not plasma volume, then maybe to total extracellular fluid or total body water, the old idea that hypertension is a state of occult edema. I think that we have an important phenomenon that needs to be pursued actively, but I frankly have no definitive explanation for it and I can only speculate.

Dr. Labarthe, Minnesota: A footnote to the question about heart rate can be added, based upon another component of the Chicago Gas Company experience, which has been under study quite recently. The problem was to assess intra-individual variation in blood pressure over a series of approximately five years of periodic examinations. When relative weight, cigarette smoking, cholesterol and heart rate were considered in relation to various measures of intra-individual blood pressure variation, heart rate was the one which very strongly associated with one of these, ie, the slope of the systolic reading over that five-year period.

IV
Pediatric Aspects

Familial Aggregation of Blood Pressure and Urinary Kallikrein in Early Childhood

Edward H. Kass, M.D., Ph.D., Stephen H. Zinner, M.D.,
Harry S. Margolius, M.D., Ph.D., Yhu-Hsiung Lee, M.D.,
Bernard Rosner, Ph.D. and Allan Donner, Ph.D.

It is commonplace to stress that we know little about the etiology of hypertension and, therefore, are uncertain of when the disorder begins, what its natural history is and how best to prevent or treat it. It is reasonable to assume that with better information concerning etiology, we will have improved prospects for prevention and will also have improved the likelihood of developing drugs which, by being more narrowly directed toward specific etiologic features of the disorder, may give greater therapeutic benefit with less toxicity. One is mindful that it is not necessary to understand the etiology of a disease in order to control it, but it does help.

In exploring the problem of etiology of hypertension, we have made two basic assumptions. The first, which we all implicitly recognize, is that blood pressure changes that we are studying are merely manifestations of an underlying metabolic disorder, whatever etiologic factors are responsible for those metabolic changes. Therefore, it would be wise to look for these changes before we recognize elevated blood pressure. The

Edward H. Kass, M.D., Ph.D., *William Ellery Channing Professor of Medicine and Director, Channing Laboratory, Harvard Medical School and Departments of Medicine and Medical Microbiology, Boston City Hospital, Mass.;* Stephen H. Zinner, M.D., *Department of Medicine, Roger Williams General Hospital and Division of Biological and Medical Sciences, Brown University, Providence, R.I.;* Harry S. Margolius, M.D., Ph.D., *Departments of Pharmacology and Medicine, Medical University of South Carolina, Charleston;* Yhu-Hsiung Lee, M.D., Bernard Rosner, Ph.D. and Allan Donner, Ph.D., *Channing Laboratory, Harvard Medical School.*

second assumption, flowing from the first, is that if the factors leading to elevated blood pressure precede the actual blood pressure changes, then searching for etiology in those with established hypertension may be frustrating, simply because of the possibility that the search may be occurring too late in the natural history of the disease. If, for example, events marking the onset of hypertension can be identified in early childhood, then looking for etiologic factors only in the middle-aged adult may not be as rewarding as would be hoped.

It seemed appropriate in our search for etiologic factors to look for the earliest evidence of elevation of blood pressure and then, if possible, for still earlier evidence of metabolic findings that could be associated with elevated blood pressure. First, then, how early in life can the characteristics of hypertensive individuals be identified with confidence? Two epidemiologic findings were employed. Both are important recent contributions to the epidemiology of hypertension, and both of them are discussed elsewhere in this symposium.

The first finding is the well-known familial aggregation of blood pressure, whereby age- and sex-corrected blood pressures of adult first order relatives can be shown to aggregate at all levels of blood pressure, with a regression coefficient of 0.2-0.3.[1] The second epidemiologic observation that seems relevant is the tracking phenomenon in which, in adult populations, those who have entered long-term longitudinal studies of blood pressure have tended to retain their blood pressure rank relative to other adults studied. Those whose pressures were high at the beginning of a 10- or 15-year study, whether clinically in the so-called abnormal or in the so-called normal range, tended to remain high throughout the period of observation, and such persons experienced excess morbidity and mortality from cardiovascular illness.[2,3]

These two facts have not received the recognition they merit in the world of practical affairs, although they have been recognized by insurance companies. Many companies now rate at excess risk young people, even at blood pressures of 130/85, if they are young enough, because this level of blood pressure for age is associated with excess risk.[4]

Our interest in the problem was aroused as we were examining blood pressure data in relation to the problem of bacteriuria, which at that time was being studied in collaboration with Miall and Stuart in the populations in Jamaica and Wales.[5] If hypertension was a disease of the middle or later years, as was conventionally taught, then the familial aggregation of blood pressure in older individuals should be quite different from that in younger adults, after suitable age correction. However, when this was tested, it became apparent that the familial aggregation effect was not sensitive to age in adults. This could best be interpreted by assuming that younger people whose blood pressures had not yet passed the arbitrary levels of 140-150/90-100 mm Hg nevertheless were ranked so that those with high blood pressures for their age were particularly likely (within the constraints of the regression coefficient of 0.2-0.3) to have older relatives who were frankly hypertensive. Thus, the familial aggregation of blood pressure in first order relatives could be used as a marker, and these data indicated that the familial aggregation effect was already well established by age 16, which was the youngest age group in studies of Miall et al.[6]

At this time, we were preparing to carry out a ten-year follow-up of those women who had initially been studied for the effect of bacteriuria on pregnancy and Dr. Zinner undertook this study. The population for follow-up consisted of consecutive women who had originally been studied during pregnancy, some with bacteriuria and some as controls without bacteriuria. These mothers and their children, aged 2-14, were studied for familial aggregation of blood pressure.

Taking blood pressures of members of a family, and particularly of small children, seemed to pose problems. There was fear that observer bias might arise since the observer would know the familial relationship. Therefore, a blood pressure recording device was developed[7] in collaboration with Professor Erik Mollo-Christensen of the Massachusetts Institute of Technology and modified by Dr. Roger Mark. This device contains an ordinary mercury manometer in which electrodes are embedded at 5 mm intervals. Alternate intervals are wired to set off a 5 kilohertz signal, which allows easy marking. All of the sounds arising from the antecubital fossa are picked up in a microphone, and these are either stored on a tape for later playback through a standard electrocardiograph or played out

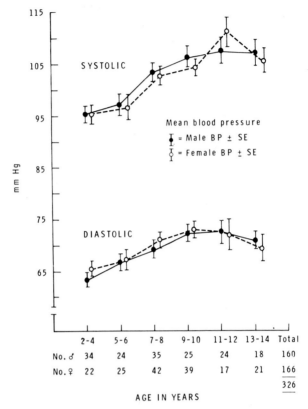

Fig. 1. Blood pressure of children aged 2-14. (From Zinner et al.[8])

directly through a recorder built into the apparatus. Standard cuff sizes, following the recommendations of the American Heart Association, are used in relation to arm girth. With this device, objective blood pressure recordings are obtained and can be tested for variance within and between observers. It is usually quite easy to detect systolic sounds, muffling, or total disappearance of the Korotkoff sounds. Paired blinded readings show that inter- and intraobserver errors are under 2 mm for systolic and diastolic readings of the tapes.[7]

The second concern was that blood pressures would be difficult to measure in small children who would not be cooperative. This fear proved to be unwarranted. All blood pressures were taken in the home, beginning with the mother and working down to the youngest child. The young usually

TABLE 1. Familial Aggregation of Blood Pressures in Children
in Successive Surveys

Survey	Age	Blood Pressure (SDU*)	Degrees of Freedom	F Ratio	Regression Coefficient Sib-Sib §
1968	2-14	Systolic			
		Among families	175	3.08†	0.336
		Within families	531		
		Diastolic (K4)			
		Among families	175	2.68†	0.319
		Within families	530		
1972-3	6-18	Systolic			
		Among families	162	1.971‡	
		Within families	446		
		Diastolic (K4)			
		Among families	162	2.019‡	
		Within families	445		

*SDU (Standard Deviation Unit) = [X-X']/SD in which X represents blood pressure of child, X' means blood pressure of his/her age and sex group and SD the standard deviation of blood pressure of that group.
†$P < 0.01$.
‡$P < 0.001$.
§For comparison, the regression coefficients observed by Miall and Oldham[6] were 0.303 for systolic and 0.252 for diastolic pressures of adult siblings.

waited rather impatiently for their turn, and there were no difficulties.

The blood pressure data obtained were smooth, and the variances were small. These data were clumped in two-year age intervals because at that time, the numbers were rather small (Fig. 1). More data have now been obtained and can be stratified by single years, with the same intrafamilial aggregation effects. In order to standardize for age, the Z score or standard deviation unit (SDU) was used.[8] Deviations from normal distribution are negligible in children of this age group. In the Z score, the mean blood pressure of the relevant age and sex groups is subtracted from the blood pressure of the propositus and the difference divided by the standard deviation for the group. A positive score indicates a pressure higher than the mean, a negative score a pressure lower than the mean for the age and sex group involved, and the degree of deviation is a function of the standard deviation.

It was found that intrafamilial aggregation of blood pressure for siblings aged 2-14 was significantly greater than random expectation and that the sib-sib and mother-sib relations were in the order of magnitude previously observed by Miall and Oldham for adults (Table 1).

The initial data were insufficient to permit study of aggregation for each year of age separately, but house-to-house studies in East Boston have since demonstrated that by age 2 there is significant familial aggregation. Sib-sib regression coefficients for 2-year-olds, against their older siblings, are of the same order of magnitude as those for older children and, in turn, of the same order of magnitude as those seen for adults. Studies now in progress in newborn infants are not yet complete but so far show only weak aggregation effects between mother and infant. Therefore, an answer should soon be forthcoming at what age in early life the familial aggregation of blood pressure becomes established.

Other noteworthy features of this first study were that there were no differences in blood pressure between white and black children, and that mean family blood pressure scores reflected the altered distribution from the expected that would come from the familial aggregation effect seen in individuals. The excess in familial mean blood pressures above two standard deviations is quite in agreement with expectation based on adult blood pressure measurements.[8]

The next step was to reexamine these same children four years later to determine if the familial aggregation effect was still detectable and to determine the stability of blood pressure rank in these children (Table 1). When the follow-up blood pressure measurements were plotted against the initial readings for systolic and diastolic pressures, there was a significant correlation between the initial and follow-up pressures, indicating a substantial degree of stability of blood pressure in these children (Fig. 2). Thus, the ranking or tracking effect within families is significantly stable. Once again, in the follow-up, black and white children had similar blood pressures, and of course, the familial aggregation of blood pressures continued to be significantly manifest.

It now seemed appropriate to seek some evidence of biochemical change comparable to the changes found in adult hypertensives. This is not easy to do at epidemiological levels.

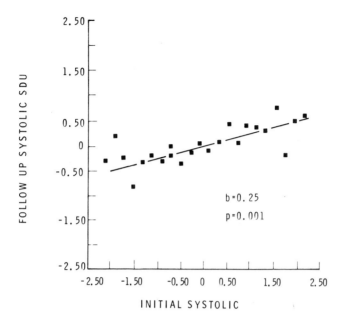

Fig. 2. Stability of blood pressure in children in two measurements in the home, made four years apart. Initial cohort aged 2-14 and blood pressures given as Z scores or standard deviation units (see text). (From Zinner et al. *Amer. J. Epidemiol.* [In press.])

We chose urinary kallikrein as the parameter that might lend itself best to this, since it could be performed on a casual urine specimen and, therefore, was more acceptable to the general population for initial epidemiological purposes than were studies that required 24-hour urine collections or withdrawal of blood and the like. Margolius, Geller and their colleagues had demonstrated that in adults with fixed hypertension, urinary kallikrein levels were significantly lower than in normotensive individuals and those with primary aldosteronism.[9] It appeared that kallikrein, an enzyme of renal origin which liberates a potent vasodilator from an alpha-globulin substrate, might possibly counterbalance pressor effects and seemed to be under mineralocorticoid control, so it probably belongs in the cycle of mechanisms that relate to the control of blood pressure. Casual urine specimens in large populations have not been studied extensively for kallikrein. All of the previous work had been performed under rigorous metabolic conditions.

TABLE 2. Variables Affecting Urinary Kallikrein Concentration in 601 Children by Single Regression Analysis

	Regression Coefficient	Std. Error	P
Urinary potassium concentration	+ 0.736	0.064	< .001
Urinary creatinine concentration	+ 0.657	0.061	< .001
Mother's kallikrein concentration	+ 0.335	0.038	< .001
Race	+ 0.720	0.073	< .001
Sex (Male < Female)	- 0.161	0.077	< .05
Time of Day (AM)	+ 0.221	0.084	< .01
Season (Summer)	- 0.208	0.078	< .01
Mother's blood pressure (K4)*	- 0.180	0.037	< .001
Child's blood pressure (K4)*	- 0.093	0.039	< .02

*In Standard Deviation Units.
(From Zinner, et al, submitted for publication.)

Urine specimens were collected in the children who were studied in the follow-up examination. Several findings of note have now emerged despite the early stage in the development of these data. First, the concentration of kallikrein in the urine was familially aggregated significantly and in the same order of magnitude as familial aggregation of blood pressure.[10] Second, kallikrein was found to be strongly related to the potassium concentration of the urine, and the effect of potassium was stronger than the effect of sodium, which was rather a surprise. Third, black children had significantly lower kallikrein levels than did white children, despite the similarities of their blood pressures. The race effect persisted at all levels of electrolyte concentration. Fourth, there was a significant effect of body weight.

The single correlations for the factors that have shown to be significant are listed in Table 2. Many of the findings are to be expected. However, the variables dealing with time of day and season were a surprise. In further analysis, children with the highest 10% and those with the lowest 10% of kallikrein concentrations had correspondingly significant inverse blood pressure relations, so that those with the 10% highest kallikreins had significantly lower blood pressures than those with the 10% lowest kallikreins.[10] When multiple regression was applied to these data, the significant factors, in order of importance, were

TABLE 3. Multiple Regression Analyses of Variables
Affecting Urinary Kallikrein Concentration*

Variable	Contribution to R^2
Urinary potassium concentration*	0.181
Urinary creatinine concentration*	0.102
Race	0.086
Weight	0.024
Season	0.016
Sex	0.009
Time of day	0.006
Urinary sodium	0.004
Multiple correlation (R^2) =	0.428

*As logarithm.
(From Zinner, et al, submitted for publication.)

urinary potassium, urinary creatinine, race, weight, season, sex, time of day and urinary sodium. These gave a multiple correlation (R^2) of 0.428, so that almost half of the variance was accounted for by this small group of metabolic parameters (Table 3). The confounding effects that were uncovered clearly require a great deal of further study. The curious effect of season and time of day needs standardization, and only further work will supply us with the kind of baseline information that we need. How much standardization of electrolyte effect is needed and how much can be accomplished at epidemiologic levels remain to be determined.

What does all this suggest? First, it seems likely that urinary kallikrein is only one of several biochemical markers of hypertension in the adult that are destined to be found also in unusual concentration in the child, in relation to blood pressure. Therefore, a systematic search is needed and should help us to determine which metabolic changes precede and which follow changes in blood pressure. It has been suggested here that the kallikrein effect precedes the divergence of blood pressure between black and white children. In Boston, as elsewhere, adult blacks, in careful household surveys, tend to have higher blood pressures than adult whites. Whether the difference in kallikrein concentration in children indicates a precursor metabolic change or suggests that in the growing generation of young blacks the black-white differences can no longer be detected remains to be seen. However, the latter hypothesis would leave unexplained the differences in kallikrein concentration that have been observed.

The data seem to provide a way in which the earliest metabolic events associated with changes in blood pressure can be detected and to offer an approach to the perplexing genetic-environmental problem. None of us is likely to doubt that given environmental events that may affect blood pressure are particularly likely to do so in certain individuals and that the particular susceptibility of certain individuals will probably best be explained on some type of genetic background. On the other hand, the effective isolation of significant environmental factors that may be necessary, if not sufficient, to account for increases in blood pressure would be an obvious target for preventive and therapeutic action.

It appears then that familial aggregation of blood pressure occurs in early childhood and that certain metabolic events that are characteristic of the adult hypertensive are also discernible in early childhood. Until a direct relation between adult hypertension and these facts, by longitudinal study, is clearly established, these data are presented only as a basis for a theoretical structure. But should the hypothesis become validated, a number of hypotheses that are currently in use start to become less attractive. Tensional changes associated with adult occupation or adult migration, dietary and other conditions imposed or studied during adulthood, and related ideas would need to be modified to encompass effects occurring during the earliest stages of life. Furthermore, the earlier in life a disease state begins, the more likely it becomes that etiological factors relevant to the disease are limited in number. A reasonable alternative to the multifactorial approach is the possibility that we may find a single or few necessary if not sufficient factors that lead to the elevation of blood pressure in later life. The prospects for understanding the problem of hypertension become considerably brighter with the possibility that it can be identified as a disorder that begins in the earliest stages of life.*

---

*Several contributions to the present symposium have added significantly to the present hypothesis concerning the origin of hypertension. The contributions presented by Holland, Biron and Beaglehole have demonstrated familial aggregation in school-age children from London,

References

1. Pickering, G.: *High Blood Pressure*. London:Churchill, 1968.
2. Miall, W. E.: Follow-up study of arterial pressure in the population of a Welsh mining valley. *Brit. Med. J.*, 2:1204, 1959.
3. Kannel, W. B., Dawber, T. R., Kagan, A. et al: Factors of risk in the development of coronary heart disease — six year follow-up experience: The Framingham Study. *Ann. Intern. Med.*, 55:33, 1961.
4. *The Underwriting Significance of Hypertension for the Life Insurance Industry*. Publication V.(NIH) 74-426, Department of Health, Education and Welfare, U. S. Public Health Service, Bethesda, Md., 1974.
5. Kass, E. H., Miall, W. E. and Stuart, K. L.: Relationship of bacteriuria to hypertension: An epidemiological study. *J. Clin. Invest.*, 40:1053, 1961.
6. Miall, W. E. and Oldham, P. D.: The hereditary factors in arterial blood pressure. *Brit. Med. J.*, 1:75, 1963.
7. Kass, E. H. and Zinner, S. H.: How early can the tendency toward hypertension be detected? In *Preventive Approaches to Chronic Disease*. Milbank Mem. Fund Quarterly, Vol. 47, No. 3, July 1969.
8. Zinner, S. H., Levy, P. S. and Kass, E. H.: Familial aggregation of blood pressure in childhood. *New Eng. J. Med.*, 284:401, 1971.
9. Margolius, H. S., Geller, R. and Pisano, J. J.: Altered urinary kallikrein excretion in human hypertension. *Lancet*, 2:1063, 1971.
10. Zinner, S. H., Margolius, H. S., Rosner, B. et al: Familial aggregation of urinary kallikrein in childhood. To be published.

Discussion

Dr. Langford: What is the correlation between the sodium concentrations of your sib pairs?

Dr. Kass: It hasn't been studied in quite that way. It has only been part of the regression. In the multiregression matrix, it is down near the bottom of the list at 0.008.

Montreal and the Polynesian islands. These would seem to leave no doubt of familial aggregation in childhood. Biron's study indicates that the familial aggregation effect is limited to natural siblings and is absent or small in adopted members of a family. However, there is some increasing aggregation effect with time, and the relation of aggregation to the age at which adoption occurred is still under investigation by the Montreal group. The presentation by Blumenthal indicated that sib-sib aggregation in a cohort of black families was absent in the newborn infant and was detectable by the first month of life. The Boston group indicated that newborn infants in their study had only a weak correlation of blood pressure to maternal blood pressure. It thus appears that the familial aggregation effect may be measurable during the first month or months of life, and it remains to be seen whether this is true in different population groups and in relation to metabolic changes of the type herein discussed.

Dr. Langford: I wanted you to comment upon the possibility that your kallikrein correlations were not at all primary movers but purely matters of the correlates of their food habits, their sodium and their potassium, that, indeed, maybe your kallikrein was an indicator of sodium excretion.

From some of our pairs, in our 18-year-old cases, sodium excretion correlation was 0.427, salt taste threshold 0.445, and systolic pressure 0.373. You know, kallikrein is affected by sodium load as well as potassium load. I would like you to argue your way out of the box in which I am trying to put you, Dr. Kass.

Dr. Kass: I don't believe that it needs much argument at this point because the data aren't complete, Dr. Langford. I think what one would have to say is that the effect of urinary potassium on kallikrein was contrary to expectations. Beyond that, we will just have to wait for the rest of the data to develop. What has come out quite clearly is that potassium is a much stronger regulator of kallikrein than is sodium. Sodium, in fact, has moved down nearer the bottom of the list, and we will just have to wait and see what that means.

Dr. Zweifler, Michigan: Since, in general, the blood pressure in adult blacks is higher than it is in adult whites, I am surprised that the children don't show any blood pressure difference, if there is a familial aggregation of blood pressure.

Dr. Kass: You see, that is exactly the point! Let me enlarge on that. What we are suggesting as an hypothesis is that there will be a time in the natural history of hypertension, when the blood pressure effect will not have shown up, although the metabolic changes will already have appeared. Many studies of children don't show a black-white difference, but then, as you get into the adolescent period, just as Dr. Langford showed, the divergence begins to show up. Yes, the metabolic change is already there is what we would like to believe.

Dr. Tobian: We have been discussing this subject in the last two days of this symposium. By the time that Dr. Langford is studying his adolescents, which are about 18 years old, a black-white difference is clearly present. By the time you are studying them, which is 2, 3, 4, 5 years old, they are not different. But you actually have studied all of the ages in between 2 and 18, so could you tell us when the difference really manifests itself?

Dr. Kass: From our data, we can't say. All we can say is that, by age 14, a difference is not apparent. But I think that Dr. Langford has studied this much more carefully than we have and I think he should have some data on this point.

Dr. Langford: I just want to suggest that under the socioeconomic conditions that you are studying, the black-white difference might not emerge.

Dr. Kass: It doesn't look that way, because in the adults it is clearly there, in our same community.

Dr. Williams, Massachusetts: I think that Dr. Langford's question is an important one, in view of the balance studies that Dr. Margolius as well as our own group have completed. The question is what does change the level of urinary kallikrein. There is significant correlation, as you probably know, between urinary sodium and kallikrein excretion when you change dietary intake on a metabolic unit. The higher the level of dietary sodium intake, the lower the level of urinary kallikrein. The reverse would be the case if you restrict sodium. When we looked at our data in relationship to potassium intake, there really was not the same sort of correlation. While potassium would change kallikrein excretion, dietary sodium seemed to have a much more profound effect. Therefore, I wouldn't dismiss the possibility that maybe the changes you observed in kallikrein, even though you couldn't show it in your own data, may be related to the dietary intake of sodium in the two groups of patients.

Dr. Kass: Before I comment, I know that Dr. Zinner has some important data relative to your observations, Dr. Williams, and after Dr. Zinner makes his remarks, perhaps then I could comment.

Dr. Zinner, Rhode Island: Actually, the correlations that are presented in these data that Dr. Kass showed are perfectly consistent with those animal experimental data, as well as the clinical patient material that Dr. Margolius has reported in *Circulation Research*, namely, that as Dr. Williams has mentioned, a low sodium intake over a period of days results in a gradual but definite rise in urinary kallikrein excretion and this response is blunted but nevertheless present in patients with hypertension. On the other hand, and in our multiple regressions that Dr. Kass presented, there was an inverse relationship of urinary sodium and kallikrein concentration. In addition, Dr.

Margolius has some unpublished animal experiments in which he has infused potassium salts into dogs and measured urinary kallikrein. There was a prompt and very rapid rise in urinary kallikrein excretion. So, all of these data aren't inconsistent with the findings in the experimental animal and in patients studied in the metabolic unit. In addition, there may be diurnal variations as hinted at in the data presented, consistent with some role of sodium-retaining steroids and possibly relating to urinary kallikrein. It is also possible that a role for urinary kallikrein might be found relative to the control of blood pressure.

Dr. Kass: I don't believe that there is a conflict. What we are seeing here is one of the many examples of how epidemiologic research and clinical investigative data have to be put together. One can focus on sodium and make it the key, but this doesn't seem to be the way that Mother Nature is operating.

Dr. Simpson, New Zealand: I noticed that the excretion of kallikrein was closely related to excretion of creatinine. Does this not suggest that perhaps the amount of fluid lost by the child is affecting the urinary kallikrein concentration? And could there not be familial variations in actual fluid intake?

Dr. Kass: Yes, it is entirely possible. Until one can do 24-hour studies, it will be very difficult to answer this question. Such studies are now being planned.

Dr. Miller, Maryland: I am not quite sure that we all understand what we are talking about when we say kallikrein in the urine. Is there a natural process by which it gets there? If not, what stimulates kallikrein release and what do you think forces it to go into urine?

Dr. Kass: The kallikrein workers should answer this. Let me merely give you my view. Dr. Geller is here and he can give you an authoritative correction. The enzyme is of renal origin. It has been correlated inversely with blood pressure levels, much as many of the other things we have talked about: the renin-angiotension system, the aldosterone system. It is simply one more of the many biochemical markers that we link to the hypertension problem. It happens not to have been a very fashionable one, so it is perhaps a little less familiar. But fashions change and it will become familiar over the next year or two. Then, everybody will know all about it. Its variation with blood pressure seems to be so striking that we can't really afford to leave it out.

Dr. Geller, Maryland: The enzyme is probably of kidney origin. Studies trying to correlate or identify or characterize urinary kallikrein with kidney kallikrein suggest that they are one and the same. There is an enzyme in plasma, plasma kallikrein, which has characteristics which are completely unlike those of the urinary enzyme. The enzyme in urine is "active," in that the enzyme when injected into plasma or acting upon a plasma substrate will generate a kinin. The enzyme in plasma does not exist in an active form and has to be activated through some other mechanism, whether it be plasmin or complement or Hagemann factor or contact with glass. It is an enzyme which is in urine, but why it is there, I do not think anyone can answer. It would be interesting to speculate that the apparent deficiency of urinary kallikrein in patients with essential hypertension could lend some credence to a theory that hypertension is a function of the deficiency of the vaso-depressor system. Recently, with the studies on prostaglandins, there is more evidence that hypertension has to be looked at from a "deficiency of the vasodepressor" mechanism, in addition to the preponderance of data studied on the vaso-constrictor side.

Dr. Cassel: As usual, I have much admiration for your findings. I must disagree with your interpretations.

Dr. Kass: That is in the best of academic traditions.

Dr. Cassel: We have been discussing for the last few minutes whether kallikrein as an enzyme is a particular substance influencing blood pressure status or whether kallikrein is but a proxy indicator of changes in potassium and sodium and things of that nature. I don't believe that that question will be answered by looking at the relationships of potassium or sodium to kallikrein, but it may be answered by looking at the relationship of kallikrein to substantive blood pressure levels.

Dr. Kass: In adults under careful metabolic study, this question has been answered. This is what led to the use of it in children. When adults with sustained hypertension were com-pared to normotensives in a total metabolic study, the kallikrein excretion was greatly depressed in the hypertensives. Here, there was no question of variation due to other factors.

Dr. Cassel: Were there variations in potassium levels?

Dr. Kass: No. I think that this should be made perfectly clear. The only problem involved is the variation in the epidemiologic study in childhood.

Dr. Cassel: Don't you agree that it would be better if it had been done in a prospective fashion, so we know which came first, the kallikrein or the change in blood pressure? Now, assuming that you would find in these studies that kallikrein levels at one point in time are clues to the blood pressure levels in a second point in time, that does not necessarily mean that you have discovered a new etiologic model. I think that your mention of the tuberculosis model is inappropriate in this regard. I think it is more likely that if the secretion of kallikrein is related in any way to blood pressure, it probably advances the susceptibility of that individual with the low kallikrein levels to the effects of a variety of environmental stimuli. There may be a very modest relationship between kallikrein levels and blood pressure at this age. You are not necessarily finding an etiologic specific agent but merely a tracer.

Dr. Kass: In my presentation, I evidently confused the issues, but I didn't mean to do this. I was in no way trying to imply that I thought that kallikrein was the etiologic factor. There is no reason at all to think so now, nor was I trying to imply that whatever factor or factors we discovered necessarily operated exclusively from the kallikrein system. That seems right now a completely premature speculation. On the other hand, in discussing etiology, I was hoping to imply that we might in fact, using kallikrein or other biochemical markers, find the earliest times when these move toward what we consider abnormal ranges and then try to track back. This might in turn allow us to uncover some etiologic factors which may have been disregarded in the past.

Factors Influencing Blood Pressure in Children

W. W. Holland, M.D. and S. A. A. Beresford, M.A.

Many studies in adults have demonstrated the importance of social and environmental factors in influencing levels of blood pressure. Miall et al[1] have drawn attention to the effects of genetic and environmental factors on levels of blood pressure in adults in the United Kingdom. Zinner et al,[2] in a selected population of children in Boston, showed the importance of familial aggregation on levels of blood pressure in children aged 2 to 14 years.

Recent suggestions that levels of blood pressure in children influence the level of blood pressure attained as adults led us to consider further the investigation of blood pressure among children. The present study was designed to determine the variation in levels of blood pressure in a group of children and to see whether we could explain the variation in levels by environmental, social and genetic factors.

A suitable population of children was available. We had undertaken a prospective investigation of a group of families in which a child had been born between July 1, 1963 and June 30, 1965. The families at that time lived in six of the electoral wards of Harrow, a northwest suburb of London. The area chosen covered a considerable range of social and environmental conditions. We had obtained reasonably complete information on family size and social conditions in this group and had

These studies have been supported in part by a grant from the Department of Health and Social Security.

W. W. Holland, M.D., B.Sc., F.R.C.P., F.F.C.M., *Professor*, and S. A. A. Beresford, M.A., M.Sc., *Lecturer, Department of Community Medicine, St. Thomas's Hospital and Medical School, London, England.*

maintained contact with over 90% of the original group up to 1970.

A random sample of 568 families was taken from this list. This sample was stratified by size of family and social class so that there would be sufficient numbers in each category for comparisons to be made on the effect of these two factors. As described in an earlier paper,[3] home visits were made during 1970 and 1971 and blood pressure measurements were obtained for each family member. Readings were taken twice, using the left arm of the subject while seated. In order to eliminate as much observer bias as possible, a Wright modification of the Garrow random zero sphygmomanometer was used.[4] To overcome the problem of the effect of arm size on the recording of blood pressure in children, we had previously investigated the influence of different cuff sizes on blood pressure readings in the same child.[5] We postulated that this effect might be due to the dissipation of the excess pressure produced by the smaller cuff into the surrounding flesh. In this present study, we adopted the suggestion of Long and colleagues, and we used the largest cuff that would comfortably encircle the arm. In practice, this depended upon the length of the arm from the acromion process to the olecranon. The blood pressure reading obtained was then adjusted for cuff size assuming that a large cuff (size 5) has no bias and that overestimation due to a smaller cuff is the same whatever the age, weight or blood pressure of the child.

Of the 568 families in the sample, 38 had moved from the area before we could visit them and 29 refused to take part. The remaining 501 families were visited by a field worker who obtained blood pressure measurements for each family member living at home. Some mothers and some fathers had either left the home or died. There were also ten index children from whom blood pressure readings were not obtainable. This left 491 of the index children with completed forms. The number of families for whom blood pressure information was available for mother, father and index child was 455 or 91% of the families visited.

Table 1 gives the mean systolic blood pressure of the index child after adjustment for cuff size. It shows that between the ages of 5 and 8, the mean levels of blood pressure were between 88 and 93 mm Hg. Figure 1 illustrates the range of systolic blood pressure of the index child and siblings included in our

TABLE 1. Mean Systolic Blood Pressure (mm Hg) of Index Child,
Adjusted for Cuff Size

| | Age (Years) | | | | |
	5	6	7	8	Overall
Male	88.0	88.5	88.7	93.3	88.8
Female	89.8	89.5	90.2	91.9	90.0
Numbers in each age group	77	214	160	40	491*

*There were ten index children for whom one or other blood pressure reading
was not obtained.

study. The distribution of blood pressure of the index children
is shown in Figure 2. The distribution of mean systolic pressure
was slightly skewed to the right and the best normal distribution which fitted the data had a mean of 89 mm Hg. We also
fitted two normal distributions to the data (Fig. 3); their
combined distribution was a significantly better fit than the
single normal distribution. However, when differences in blood
pressure due to age, height and weight were removed, the single
normal distribution fitted as well as the two normal distributions. Transforming the data by a logarithmic transformation
and then fitting a normal distribution gave no better fit.

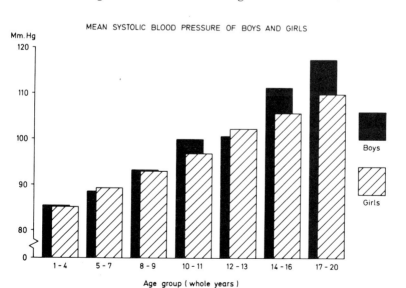

Figure 1.

MEAN SYSTOLIC BLOOD PRESSURE OF INDEX CHILDREN, ADJUSTED FOR CUFF SIZE

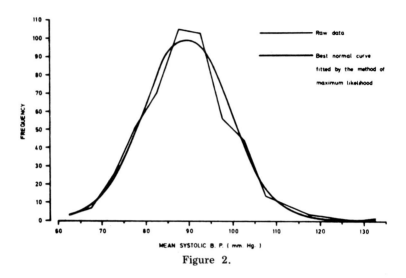

Figure 2.

MEAN SYSTOLIC BLOOD PRESSURE OF INDEX CHILDREN, ADJUSTED FOR CUFF SIZE

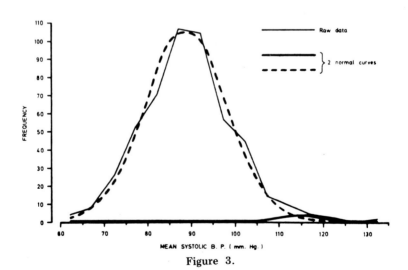

Figure 3.

Using multiple regression and covariance analyses, we attempted to see what factors influenced the differences between children. Although there were slight differences in blood pressure between the boys and girls, these were not statistically significant. Analyzing the effects of height, weight and age, we found that only weight had an effect on levels of blood pressure independent of the effect of height and age. When the effects of parents' systolic levels of blood pressure were considered in the regression equation, the independent effect of weight remained very highly significant. We thus found that the major determinants of levels of blood pressure in index children were their weight and the level of blood pressure of the mother and father. We also examined the influence of other environmental factors such as social class. We found that social class differences did influence levels of blood pressure in the children. In general, levels of blood pressure were higher in lower class than in the upper class groups. However, these differences could be explained by the variations of blood pressure in the parents. If adjustment was made for level of blood pressure of parents on the blood pressure of children, no significant difference between social class groups was found. We were also unable to find any effect of area of residence, family size, race or season of the year. We considered the importance of the influence of a one parent family on the blood pressure of the child by looking at variations in blood pressure in children with only a father or with only a mother. However, the numbers were too small to show any difference, and the variations were not remarkable.

Variations in levels of blood pressure are obviously also seen in parents. We found that the major factors that influenced the level in parents of the index child were their weight and their age.

The fact that the interviewing was done by three different field workers had some effect. Children interviewed by field worker 3 were a little older, taller and heavier on average than those interviewed by field worker 1. Thus, comparisons of the results obtained by the three field workers are not simply a test of observer variation. In fact, the results of the three differed significantly even after adjustment for age, height and weight (for the index children only). No simple explanation could be found for this, but the differences were adjusted for in other analyses. Figure 4 attempts to demonstrate the differences that can be accounted for by a variety of factors in levels of systolic blood pressure in the mothers, fathers and index children.

Finally, one of the factors influencing levels of blood pressure in the child was pulse rate, perhaps because of excitement or previous activity. We thus found four factors associated with level of blood pressure in the index child: weight, social class, pulse rate and the level of blood pressure in the parents. We were unable to find any independent effects due to age, sex, height, area of residence, race, family size, skinfold thickness, season, past history of kidney disease, one or two parent family or birth order.

In an attempt to determine the importance of familial factors in the inheritance and levels of blood pressure, we examined the influence of blood pressure of the siblings. These, of course, are the least homogeneous group and hence the most difficult to analyze. Their ages range from a few months to 30 years. About half of the very young could not be measured because they were too upset. About a fifth of the older siblings were no longer living with the family.

The factors associated with the levels of blood pressure of the siblings were, again, pulse rate, weight and height. Classically, studies of the inheritance of blood pressure have not made any adjustment for environmental factors in calculating the coefficient of resemblance between relatives (Table 2). This approach assumes there is no interaction between genetic and environmental factors, but the recognition that blood pressure increases with age in a way which differs between men and women has led Pickering[6] and Miall[7] to use age-sex adjusted scores. Acheson and Fowler[8] question the suitability of such scores for genetic comparisons, observing that they do not correct the skewness of the distribution of blood pressure. Ignoring the effect of environmental factors temporarily, we first examined the correlations between actual level of systolic blood pressure of members of a family. The mother-daughter and father-son correlations are higher than those reported by the Tecumseh study[9] but the mother-son, father-daughter correlations are comparable. Each coefficient is highly significant. If there were no random environmental influence, no contribution from a shared environment and the mode of

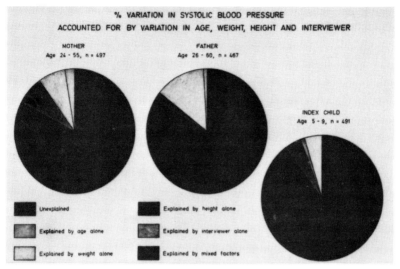

% VARIATION IN SYSTOLIC BLOOD PRESSURE
ACCOUNTED FOR BY VARIATION IN AGE, WEIGHT, HEIGHT AND INTERVIEWER

MOTHER
Age 24 - 55, n = 497

FATHER
Age 26 - 60, n = 467

INDEX CHILD
Age 5 - 9, n = 491

Unexplained

Explained by age alone

Explained by weight alone

Explained by height alone

Explained by interviewer alone

Explained by mixed factors

Figure 4.

inheritance was ~~simple~~ *additive*, ie, no dominance, with either a single gene or many genes acting independently, the expected correlation between first degree relatives would be 0.5. The number of siblings of an index child varied between 0 and 8. In order to give each family an equal chance of contributing to the sib-sib comparison, only one sibling's blood pressure was compared with that of the index child. For convenience, this was chosen to be the oldest sibling. Again, each correlation coefficient is significantly greater than zero, but less than the so-called

TABLE 2. Correlations of Systolic Blood Pressures (mm Hg)
(Adjusting for Cuff Size Only)

Parent-Offspring		*Mother*	*Father*	
Index Child	Girl	.19	.17	Expected value = 0.5
	Boy	.16	.29	
Sibling-Sibling		*Oldest Sib*		
		Girl	*Boy*	
Index child	Girl	.28	.29	Expected value = 0.5
	Boy	.32	.27	

expected value. The correlations are larger than the interclass correlation coefficient in the Tecumseh study of 0.17.

Another way of circumventing the differing numbers of children in families is to compare those families with the same number of children. Table 3 shows the results of such comparisons using age-sex adjusted scores. Correlation coefficients were similar to those obtained by using the actual blood pressures. The majority of coefficients were significantly different from zero, but also significantly less than the expected value. Correlation between the father's score and that of the child in a one child family was consistent with the expected value. If the environment shared by the members of a family has an effect on blood pressure, the correlation between their pressures will be greater than that due to genetic resemblance alone. These environmental factors are likely to operate through the home environment of the relatives and also between spouses who have been married for an appreciable time. Assuming random mating, the genetic resemblance between spouses is zero, and any correlation between their blood pressures must be due to shared environment. Indeed, one may use this correlation as an estimate of the effect of shared environment on the blood pressures of other family members. Since the correlation between the blood pressure scores of parents is 0.05, which is not significantly different from zero, it may be deduced that the contribution of shared environment to the coefficients of resemblance between parents and children is negligible.

To summarize therefore, these studies clearly demonstrate that weight, pulse rate and level of blood pressure of parents influence the blood pressure level of children. It would also appear from these studies that the effect of environmental and

TABLE 3. Correlations Using Age-Sex Adjusted Scores
Mean Score of Children

| | Number of Children in Family | | | | |
	One	Two	Three	Four	Five
Mother	-.16	.17	.17	.41	-.03
Expected value	.50	.58	.61	.63	.65
Father	.35	.12	.30	.24	.40
Mid-parent	.07	.22	.31	.46	.27
Expected value	.71	.82	.87	.89	.91

social factors on level of blood pressures of a relatively homogeneous group of families living in one part of northwest London is relatively small, compared with the effects of genetic factors and weight. The effect of genetic factors and weight on the determination of blood pressure is not large, but it is highly significant. It would thus appear that we can at least identify (at a relatively early age) a group of individuals who perhaps ought to remain under greater surveillance than other members of the population. In preventive medicine, particularly in relation to blood pressure, individuals must be identified *before* they develop lesions. In view of the increasing frequency of measurement of levels of blood pressure in adults, it would appear logical that where we know that parents have raised levels of blood pressure, their children should be included in any system of surveillance that is initiated. It is this group of children who should be warned not to become overweight. Thus, weight and level of blood pressure in parents are important in determining the levels of blood pressure of the next generation.

References

1. Miall, W. E., Bell, R. A. and Lovell, H. G.: *Brit. J. Prev. Soc. Med.*, 22:73, 1968.
2. Zinner, S. H., Levy, P. S. and Kass, E. H.: *New Eng. J. Med.* 284:401, 1971.
3. Beresford, S. A. A. and Holland, W. W.: *Proc. Roy. Soc. Med.*, 66 (10):1009, 1973.
4. Wright, B. M. and Dore, C. F.: *Lancet*, 1:337, 1970.
5. Long, M., Dunlop, J. R. and Holland, W. W.: *Arch. Dis. Child.*, 46:636, 1971.
6. Hamilton, M., Pickering, G. W., Roberts, J. A. F. et al: *Clin. Sci.*, 13:273, 1954.
7. Miall, W. E., Heneage, P., Khosla, T. et al *Clin. Sci.*, 33:271, 1967.
8. Acheson, R. M. and Fowler, G. B.: *J. Chronic. Dis.*, 20:731, 1967.
9. Johnson, B. C., Epstein, F. H. and Kjelsberg, M O.: *J. Chronic. Dis.*, 18:147, 1965.

Discussion

Dr. Hoobler, Michigan: Dr. Holland's last suggestion prompts me to bring up a piece of work that Dr. Richard Remington and I did some years ago, which may be of some interest to those of you who may be trying to identify early hypertension.* Our plan was to measure the blood pressure and the variability of blood pressure of the teenage offspring of parents attending the hypertension clinic and matching it with 50 teenagers from the local school system whose parents' blood pressure was considered to be normal. There was no difference in the variability of the blood pressure between the offspring of one hypertensive and the offspring of no hypertensive parentage. However, there was about a 2 mm difference in the systolic blood pressure which turned out to be significant, of course being higher for the offspring of the marriages containing one hypertensive individual. The diastolic blood pressure was not different. The pulse rate, oddly enough, was slower in the offspring. The main gist of this discussion is that in 50 individuals, you can only get a 2 mm systolic difference. We are certainly not going to pick up that difference in the clinic. We are going to have to use a marker such as kallikrein or something else. We will not get it by picking up the blood pressure of a child being a little higher than the average.

Dr. Borhani: I have two questions. One, I seem to misunderstand or, at least, miss what you say in terms of the effect of shared environment. Is it negligible between the entire membership of the family or just the parents to children? Second, have you been looking into the husband and wife correlation?

Dr. Holland: Yes, I am sorry, I did say that to look at the effect of the shared environment, we looked at the correlation between the mother and the father. We did not find any significant correlation. We have looked at this also in relationship to duration of marriage, in view of some of the comments that various people have made earlier, and we cannot find any difference between those who have been married for a short time and those married for a long time.

Dr. Langford: I am theoretically surprised about the failure to find any spouse aggregation of blood pressure. Maybe Cupid is blind, but his arrows probably have a fairly short range. As

---

*Remington, R., Lambarth, B., Moser, M. et al: Circulatory reactions of normotensive and hypertensive subjects and of the children of normal and hypertensive parents. *American Heart J.*, 59:58, 1960.

long as there is a social class gradient of blood pressure, and I shall bet that there is, is it just too weak of an effect to see? Is that the explanation for it?

Dr. Holland: I cannot explain it. We can't find an effect of social class on blood pressure, independent of weight in the adult. There is, of course, an effect of weight on marriage patterns in that fat women tend to marry fat men. We have corrected for that. (If you take that out of the equation, we are unable to find anything.) The correlation coefficients are of the order of 0.02.

Dr. Winkelstein: I think that the most interesting observation in the Buffalo Spouse Aggregation Study was that in the limited number of families who had children over the age of 15, parent-child aggregation was limited to those families where spouse aggregation occurred. The data which you have just reported, to my knowledge, are the first data set since we reported this phenomenon about six or seven years ago, which would allow one to test that hypothesis, but it will require a different form of analysis in which the families are classified according to the degree of aggregation between parents. It is interesting to note that in the Buffalo Spouse Aggregation Study, when we used the scoring technique which you use, we, too, found no aggregation between spouses. Although I am not a statistician, I would wonder whether it might not be conceivable, when one looks at the families and classifies them according to the degree of similarity between parents, that you may find the same pattern. At any rate, as far as I know, this is the first set of data which could really be used to test exhaustively the hypothesis of familial aggregation due to environmental factors.

Dr. Holland: Dr. Sackett who is in our department may be able to convince Miss Beresford, who is the statistician who has done all of this work, to change her ways!

Dr. Sackett: I think that the failure to show spouse aggregation is quite consistent with spouse concordance for blood pressure, because the nature of your sampling, as you pointed out, was such that these were all families which had a new birth a relatively short time earlier. Therefore, the likelihood of having individuals married for a sufficient period of time that the concordant spouse pairs would be uncovered due to dissolution of discordant spouse pairs is small. This is what we would expect in the face of assortative marriage.

Dr. Holland: I am not absolutely certain of that because there were 87 of these families who had children aged 15 years and over, and there were only 414 families who had no child over age 15 years. I am afraid that we did not have any families with lengthy marriages. So, I am not sure that your explanation is correct, but I cannot answer it from the analysis that we have done.

Longitudinal Studies of Blood Pressure in Offspring of Hypertensive Mothers

Barbara E. Klein, M.D., Charles H. Hennekens, M.D.,
Mary Jane Jesse, M.D., Janet E. Gourley, B.S.N.
and Sidney Blumenthal, M.D.

Significant gaps exist in our understanding of the natural history of essential hypertension, particularly its early stages. It is a rare diagnosis in the pediatric age group. Most children diagnosed by present standards as having hypertension have identifiable causes of their elevated pressures.

Frequent reports of the existence of familial aggregation of essential hypertension have appeared in the literature and the possible role of inheritance of this disease has been emphasized.[1-3] Familial resemblance of arterial pressure among first degree relatives not only at hypertensive but at all levels of pressure was reported by Miall and his colleagues[4] and by Johnson, Epstein and their colleagues.[5] Although most of their observations were made upon an adult population, they did include some data from children. Zinner, Levy and Kass[6] extended these observations to a childhood population ranging in age from 2 to 14 years, with a mean of 8.3 years.

An understanding of the determinants of blood pressure at all levels and the quantitative or qualitative differences in those

Supported by U. S. Public Health Service Research Grant (HL 14141) from the National Heart and Lung Institute.

Barbara E. Klein, M.D. and Charles H. Hennekens, M.D., *Department of Epidemiology and Public Health;* Mary Jane Jesse, M.D., *Professor of Pediatric Cardiology,* Janet E. Gourley, B.S.N. and Sidney Blumenthal, M.D., *Professor of Pediatric Cardiology, University of Miami School of Medicine, Fla.*

determinants across the range of blood pressure levels is a necessary first step in studies of the natural history of hypertension. Studies of the arterial pressure of infants, children and their parents which are longitudinal rather than cross-sectional in nature would shed light on these blood pressure determinants.

Those levels must be described prior to any attempt to consider those factors associated with arterial pressure levels and their variability in infants and children. This is now under investigation in a longitudinal study at the Specialized Center of Research program at the University of Miami.

A number of questions have been posed, including:

1. Is sibling aggregation demonstrable in families with children under 2 years of age?

2. If the answers is yes, is it present when the sibling group includes a newborn?

3. Is family aggregation demonstrable in young families — that is, when young parents are included with their young children?

4. If family aggregation exists, does it persist over time?

5. Does the individual child remain at or near the same arterial pressure level for his age and sex over time?

6. Are arterial pressure levels of a newborn or the tendency toward familial aggregation different if the mother is chronically hypertensive, pre-eclamptic or normotensive?

The purpose of this preliminary report is to describe the methodology utilized in one ongoing study and to present data concerning aggregation of blood pressure in sibships younger than those previously reported.

Methods of Procedure

Population Studied

Patients were recruited from the Jackson Memorial Hospital's Obstetrics Clinic. Pregnant women who were married, living with the father of the expected child and willing to participate were enrolled in the study. Blood pressure measurements were obtained on the siblings and father of the expected newborn during the third trimester of the pregnancy.

Methods of Blood Pressure Determination

From age 2 through adulthood, blood pressures were measured using a mercury manometer. Cuff size for all individuals, regardless of age, was at least one half of the length of the upper arm. With the arm supported comfortably at heart level, the cuff was applied firmly to the upper arm, approximately 1 inch above the antecubital space. Korotkoff sounds I, IV and V were recorded.

Blood pressures of children under the age of 2 were measured with the Arteriosonde 1010, utilizing the Doppler technique. The infant was positioned on its back with the right arm extended. Gelisonde, a coupling medium which aids in sound transmission, was applied to the transducer. The cuff was placed firmly around the upper arm above the antecubital space. Korotkoff sounds I, IV and V were recorded.

Methods of Data Analyses

Mean values of two blood pressure readings per subject recorded at five-minute intervals were used in the analyses. Blood pressure values were expressed in standard deviation units to adjust for age and sex. SDU equals the subject's pressure reading minus the mean for his age and sex group divided by the standard deviation of blood pressures in that group. Age groups were stratified by two- and three-year intervals. Statistical procedures included analysis of variance and single regression analysis. The regression coefficient was calculated by the random selection of one child in each family as a propositus and performance of the regression analysis of the siblings' scores on that of the propositus.

Results

Blood pressures were obtained on 157 of 159 siblings. Figure 1 shows mean blood pressures by sex within age groups for these 157 children age 1-14 years. Systolic pressures for males ranged from a mean of 101.0 mm Hg in the 1 to 3 year age group to 102.0 in the 12 to 14-year-olds. For females, the range was from 102.5 mm Hg in the 1 to 3-year-olds to 104.2 in

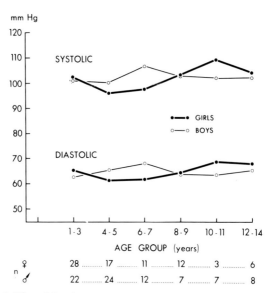

Fig. 1. Mean blood pressures of 157 progeny by age and sex.

TABLE 1. Aggregation of Blood Pressure for All Sibships

	Degrees of Freedom	Mean Square	F	p
Systolic				
Among	43	1.278		
			1.88	< .025
Within	79	.681		
Diastolic				
Among	43	1.179		
			1.56	< .05
Within	79	.755		

TABLE 2. Aggregation of Blood Pressure for Black Sibships

	Families	Siblings	F	p
	32	94		
Systolic			2.24	< .005
Diastolic			1.96	< .02

TABLE 3. Correlation Coefficients
of Blood Pressures for Black Sibships

	r	p
Systolic	.28	< .02
Diastolic	.26	< .03

the 12 to 14-year-olds. Diastolic pressures ranged from 62.9 to 65.4 in males; the range in females was from 65.5 to 67.8.

An analysis of variance was done on 124 children from 44 families containing at least two siblings. Of these 44 families, 32 were black. Table 1 shows a significant aggregation for systolic ($p < .025$) and diastolic ($p < .05$) pressures. The mean age for these children was 6.2 years.

Because of the small number of white families, the analysis of variance was repeated for 94 children from 32 black families. As shown in Table 2, this analysis showed aggregation of blood pressure which was more significant than noted previously, at the level of $p < .005$ for systolic pressure and $p < .02$ for diastolic pressure.

The correlation coefficients among these 32 black sibling groups were .28 for systolic pressure ($p < .02$) and .26 for diastolic pressure ($p < .03$) (Table 3).

Discussion

Longitudinal data are being obtained from newborn infants, their siblings and their parents which will allow comparisons of levels of their arterial pressure over time as well as determination as to whether those arterial pressure levels are a function of the levels of their parents. This study demonstrates blood pressure aggregation within sibships in a younger group of children than has been previously reported. The regression coefficients between the blood pressures of a randomly selected child and his siblings were statistically significant and consistent in magnitude with the results of other studies in older sibships.

The evidence that sibling aggregation of blood pressure is demonstrable in early childhood does not shed light on the relative causal roles of heredity and environment. Determination of the youngest age at which aggregation occurs should be of value. Aggregation present in the newborn would suggest either genetic or intrauterine influences. Such data would supplement studies of twins or of adopted children compared with other members of their households.

The aggregation of arterial pressure within sibling groups of children at all levels of arterial pressure has important connotations if supported by additional data such as aggregation in families and its persistence at the same level over time. Miall[4] has reported that those adults with the highest initial pressures experience the greatest rises in pressure over the years. The possibility that this applies to children as well requires documentation. Data are not yet available concerning the influence if any of the mother's pressure on the level of the newborn or whether there is a greater correlation in those sibling groups with the highest levels of pressure.

Longitudinal studies of parents and their progeny, including the pregnant mother and her newborn child, will aid in elucidating the relative roles of heredity and environment in blood pressure control and provide practical assistance to the clinician responsible for the care of children.

Conclusion

The protocol of a longitudinal study of arterial pressure in the offspring of hypertensive, pre-eclamptic and normotensive mothers is described and sibling aggregation of arterial pressure at a younger age than has been previously reported is documented.

The significance of this study is discussed relative to the potential elucidation of environment and heredity as controlling factors in all levels of blood pressure in children and their possible practical clinical implications.

References

1. Ayman, D.: Heredity in arteriolar (essential) hypertension: A clinical study of the blood pressure of 1,524 members of 277 families. *Arch. Intern. Med.*, 53:792, 1934.
2. Hamilton, M., Pickering, G. W., Roberts, J. A. F. et al: The aetiology of essential hypertension. IV. The role of inheritance. *Clin Sci.*, 13:273, 1954.
3. Chazan, J. A. and Winkelstein, W., Jr.: Household aggregation of hypertension: Report of preliminary study. *J. Chronic Dis.*, 17:9, 1964.

4. Miall, W. E. and Oldham, P. D.: The hereditary factor in arterial blood pressure. *Brit. Med. J.*, 1:75, 1963.
5. Johnson, B. C., Epstein, F. H. and Kjelsberg, M. O.: Distributions and familial studies of blood pressure and serum cholesterol levels in a total community — Tecumseh, Michigan. *J. Chronic Dis.*, 18:147, 1965.
6. Zinner, S. H., Levy, P. S. and Kass, E. H.: Familial aggregation of blood pressure in childhold. *New Eng. J. Med.*, 284:402, 1971.

Discussion

Dr. Schoenberger: Wouldn't it have been more consistent to compare blood pressures in the older sibs, using the Arteriosonde than with the two different methods that you used?

Dr. Blumenthal: This came up for a good deal of discussion and perhaps you are correct. However, using the mercury manometer in the older children is more comparable to the method utilized in daily practice. In addition, we are in the process of comparing the Arteriosonde and the mercury manometer. There is ample evidence in the literature that if one compares direct arterial pressures with the Arteriosonde to the mercury manometer, that these are compatible. We are now in the process of comparing not the direct intra-arterial pressure, but Arteriosonde and the mercury manometer.

Dr. Zinner, Rhode Island: You may not have had time to analyze these data, but was there any consistent difference in blood pressure, either raw or in age-adjusted score, in black versus white children?

Dr. Blumenthal: Charles, can you answer that?

Dr. Hennekens, Florida: We were reluctant to include the analyses on the very small number of families (12) who were white. However, we did do analyses of variance which showed no significant aggregation for systolic or diastolic pressure in the small group of white families. Both the product moment and intraclass correlation coefficients showed essentially no association between sibling groups.

Dr. Feinleib: Could you tell us what the correlation was between the infant's blood pressure at one day, and his blood pressure at one month, and also with blood pressure at one year?

Dr. Hennekens: The data that we have available are on correlations between newborn and one-month-old pressures on these same infants, and the correlation coefficients were of the order of magnitude of 0.49 for systolic and 0.38 for diastolic pressures.

Dr. Kass, Moderator: Could I just add one bit of data before calling Dr. Blackburn? Dr. Lee has been doing the same type of thing and we hope soon to send the manuscript to Dr. Blumenthal and his associates for examination. But also it looks as though, with the Arteriosonde, one gets quite coherent data. The mother-child correlation on the second or third day of life looks to be significant in the diastolic, although not in the systolic blood pressures. This has not yet been analyzed for all of the confounding variables, so I hope that you will look upon this as preliminary data. But it looks as though something has happened between mother and child that is not yet reflected in sib-sib. We are not yet certain that this mother-child effect is the same one that is seen later in life.

Dr. Blumenthal: I would just like to make a comment about the diastolic pressure. We are insecure about the diastolic pressure using the Arteriosonde. The comments I made had to do with systolic pressure. We have noted marked variability in the newborn period in diastolic pressures which may be biological, but it also may be instrumental.

Dr. Blackburn, Minnesota: I think we are pushing you too far, Dr. Blumenthal, on data and conclusions about these 44 families, but it is so very interesting. Do you know whether the children at one month were weaned or suckled?

Dr. Blumenthal: I think they were weaned.

Dr. Hennekens: Yes, all on formulas.

Dr. Kass: Again, just a small piece of information. It appears that breast vs. formula feeding wasn't a significant variable in Dr. Lee's study.

Dr. Miller, Maryland: Your conclusion was that you didn't find any aggregation in sibs?

Dr. Blumenthal: With the newborns.

Dr. Miller: Did you really have a chance to, with that small number of families?

Dr. Hennekens: We examined the power of our F test for a family size of three siblings and found a sample of between 30 and 50 families to be associated with a beta error of between 0.1 and 0.2.

Dr. Lovell: These data are concentrated very much on the newborn. Have you any information on the effect of the birth of a child on the siblings with whose pressures you are making comparisons?

Dr. Blumenthal: Do you mean the nature of the delivery? No, we have no information on that. I should say that to the best of our knowledge, these were healthy newborns. Whether they had some underlying other condition we cannot tell. Does that answer your question?

Dr. Lovell: That answers part of it. The main point of my question was: Does the arrival of a new infant in the family influence the blood pressure of the siblings?

Dr. Blumenthal: I do not know. It is a superb point. All we can say is that the other sibs, as well as the other members of the family, are being followed longitudinally. We do have measurements on those sibs before that baby was born, but not before the mother was pregnant. Maybe that pregnancy makes a difference.

Familial Aggregation of Blood Pressure in Adopted and Natural Children

Pierre Biron, M.D., Jean-Guy Mongeau, M.D.
and Denise Bertrand, M.Sc.

Introduction

In February 1971, Zinner et al[1] reported the existence of the phenomenon of familial aggregation of blood pressure among 721 children from 190 natural families. The children's ages ranged from 2 to 14 years. Maternal-child correlation coefficients were respectively 0.16 for systolic and 0.17 for diastolic pressures; sib-sib correlation coefficients were 0.34 and 0.32, respectively. Within-families variance of children's blood pressure was significantly lower than between-families variance (F=3.08 and 2.68, respectively). The distribution of mean family childhood pressures was flatter (platykurtic) than the Gaussian distribution.

Since no attempt had been made to determine the relative contribution of home environment or genetic factors underlying this phenomenon, in 1972 we undertook a comparable cross-sectional survey of 274 families with adopted children.

What follows is a preliminary report of our findings.

Supported by the Quebec Heart Foundation, and by the Kidney Foundation of Canada (73-74).

Pierre Biron, M.D., M.Sc., *Associate Professor of Pharmacology; Clinical Pharmacologist, Hypertension Clinic, Hôpital du Sacré-Coeur;* Jean-Guy Mongeau, M.D., F.R.C.P., *Associate Clinical Professor in Pediatrics; Chief, Nephrology Service and Hypertension Clinic, Hôpital Sainte-Justine, and* Denise Bertrand, M.Sc., *Research Associate, Biomedical Engineering Program, Ecole Polytechnique and Faculté de Médecine, Montreal, Canada.*

Methodology

Between 1972 and 1974 home visits were made to 274 families having at least one adopted child in the Montreal area. The population studied was composed of 129 natural children (65 boys, 64 girls), 379 adopted children (197 boys, 182 girls) and 538 parents (264 fathers, 274 mothers). Among adopted children, 297 (78%) may be considered as early adopted (ie, prior to their first anniversary) and 82 may be considered as late adopted. The homes were visited only once by an experienced nurse, on a weekday evening, at least one hour after supper, a few days after prearranging the visit by telephone. Permission to be visited had previously been sought through the *Société d'Adoption et de Protection de l'Enfance de Montréal.* The adoptive parents were of French-Canadian descent; the real parents of the adopted children, unknown to us, were of the same ethnic background. Two fathers receiving drug therapy for hypertension and eight who were absent from home were eliminated from the survey. Families with children under 1 year old were not surveyed, nor were those with children adopted for a period of less than one year.

Blood pressure was taken with a standard mercury sphygmomanometer fitted with a constant deflation valve. Cuffs of appropriate widths were used in children. The first and fourth Korotkoff sounds were used. During each visit, the members of the family were usually asked to sit around a table while the nurse noted the age, sex and status (adopted or natural) of each child and then proceeded to measure height and weight. The blood pressure was taken in the sitting position, in the following order: parents first (fathers first on even days, mothers first on odd days), then the children; the children were measured in a sequence counterbalanced with respect to status and randomized for individuals within a status. Then blood pressure was taken a second time, using the same sequence. The two readings were averaged to yield a single value for the systolic and a single value for the diastolic.

The blood pressure of each individual was transformed into an age and sex adjusted score expressed in standard deviation units (SDU). An SDU score is the reading of an individual, in millimeters of mercury, minus the mean pressure for his age and sex group, over the standard deviation for that group. An average parental score was obtained by averaging the father's and the mother's score for each family. In the ten families without father's readings, the mother's score was used as the average parental score. In children, 3-year age groups were formed; the group 4-6 years includes children aged from 4 years to 6 years and 11 months, etc. Ten-year age groups were used for the parents. A preliminary grouping of children according to status revealed no significant differences between mean blood pressures of the two statuses within the same age and sex group; the data from children of both statuses were therefore pooled within each of these age and sex groups.

We used statistical analyses similar to those used by the Kass group so that our results would be comparable; additional alternatives are presently being considered. To estimate parent-child aggregation, the correlation coefficient r of Pearson was computed, using the blood pressure score of each natural child against the average score of his natural parents, and the score of each adopted child against the average score of his adopted parents. This method has the advantage of using the information from every child, but introduces a slight bias because parents with more than one natural or more than one adopted child are represented more than once. In this paper, the coefficient of determination (r^2) multiplied by 100 was used to describe the percentage of association between children's blood pressure scores and those of their parents. Statistical tests, of course, were carried out on the square root r.

Two methods were used to estimate child-child aggregation. First, a variance analysis was carried out to determine if the variations of the mean family childhood scores were significantly greater than the variations of the within-families individual childhood scores. A one-way analysis of variance on the childhood scores was carried out on the data from 89 families with two or more adopted children, another one on the data from 39 families with two or more natural children. Another method was applied to the same families; a propositus was randomly selected among the natural children, and his score was compared with the score of the other natural child (if there were only two natural children) or with the average score of the other natural children (if there were more than two natural children in the family). A comparison of the same type was made between adopted children, and the correlation coefficient r of Pearson was used.

Results

Population Description

Figure 1 shows sample sizes after grouping children according to status, age and sex. There were no adopted children over 15, whereas 31 natural ones were 16 or over. The modal class was 7-9 years for natural children and 1-3 years for adopted children. Thus, the natural children had been exposed to their

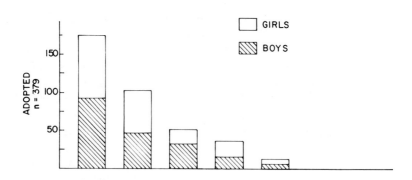

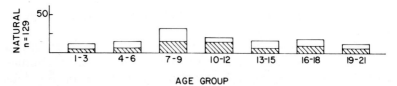

Fig. 1. Frequency distribution of adopted and natural children by age and sex groups. By virtue of their higher average age, the natural children had been exposed to their familial environment for a longer period than the adopted children. The majority (78%) of the adopted children had been adopted before their first birthday. There were 278 (73.3%) adopted children aged 6 years or under against 101 (26.7%) over that age. In contrast, there were 25 natural children (19.4%) 6 years old or under as against 104 (80.6%) over that age.

home environment for a longer period than the early adopted children (78%) and even more than the late adopted ones. The mean blood pressures of each age and sex group of natural siblings were not significantly different from those of adopted children, a finding in line with the identity of ethnic background and living area (Montreal).

Parent-Child Resemblance

The overall resemblance between parents and children is shown in Figure 2 and detailed in Table 1. Despite the larger sample size, no significant correlation was found to exist (at the 5% level) between adoptive parents and adopted children. We

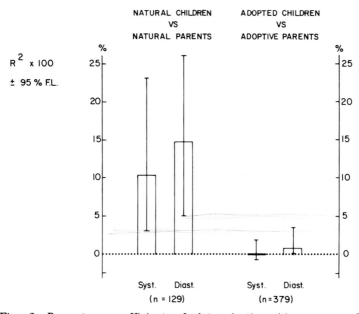

Fig. 2. Percentage coefficient of determination (the square of the coefficient of correlation of Pearson, multiplied by 100) between the systolic and diastolic pressure scores of each natural child and the average score of his two natural parents, and between the blood pressure scores of each adopted child and the average of his two adoptive parents. The correlation for adopted children is nonsignificant; the 95% fiducial limits include zero. Although the fiducial limits of the correlation for natural children are relatively wider, due to a smaller sample size, the correlation is very highly significant ($p < 0.001$). The scores consisted of standard deviation units, adjusted for age and sex.

TABLE 1.

Status	Natural	Adopted
Sample size	129	379
Degrees of freedom	127	377
Systolic pressure		
Correlation coefficient r	0.3370	0.0332
Upper 95% fiducial limit	0.4815	0.1322
Lower 95% fiducial limit	0.1693	-0.0678
t value of r	4.0338	0.6442
Significance of r	$p < 0.001$	N.S.
Regression equation	$Y = -0.0808 + 0.2455X$	$Y = -0.0519 + 0.0237X$
Significance of b	$p < 0.001$	N.S.
Diastolic pressure		
Correlation coefficient	0.3816	0.0897
Upper 95% F.L.	0.5205	0.1887
Lower 95% F.L.	0.2241	-0.0110
t value of r	4.6530	1.7495
Significance of r	$p < 0.001$	N.S.
Regression equation	$Y = -0.0448 + 0.3013X$	$Y = -0.0692 + 0.0660X$
Significance of b	$p < 0.001$	N.S.

Correlation and regression coefficients of blood pressure scores of children versus the average parental scores:

Y = children score   X = parental score

have not made a statistical comparison between the r for natural and the r for adopted children because the population of adopted children had been exposed to their home for a shorter period of time on the average. The diastolic pressure shows more resemblance between parent and child than the systolic in both status groups.

Child-Child Aggregation

Table 2 shows that the between-families variation of childhood pressure scores is significant at the 5% level for children of both statuses. However, the level of significance of the difference is much higher for natural children.

The correlation between randomly selected natural propositi and the other siblings in families with more than one natural child was as follows: for systolic pressure, r=0.20 ($r^2 \times 100 = 4\%$) and for diastolic pressure, r=0.30 ($r^2 \times 100 = 9\%$). The same correlations among adopted children

TABLE 2.

Children	B.P.	S.V.	D.F.	S.S.	M.S.	F	P
Natural	Systolic	Between families	38	59.20	1.56	2.96	< 0.001
		Within families	54	28.41	0.53		
	Diastolic	Between families	38	62.72	1.65	3.08	< 0.001
		Within families	54	28.89	0.53		
Adopted	Systolic	Between families	88	96.01	1.09	1.59	≃0.010
		Within families	115	78.74	0.68		
	Diastolic	Between families	88	91.30	1.04	1.52	≃0.025
		Within families	115	78.60	0.68		

Analysis of variance of childhood blood pressure scores, showing that the coefficient of Fisher is twice as great for natural children as for adopted ones, and that the p value is at least 10 and 25 times greater, respectively, for systolic and diastolic. SDU score = $(x_i - \bar{x})/s$ where x_i = blood pressure in mm Hg. of an individual; $\bar{x}$ = mean blood pressure of age and sex group; s = standard deviation of age and sex group.

were much lower: for systolic pressure, $r=0.08$ ($r^2 \times 100 = 0.64\%$) and for diastolic pressure, $r=0.12$ ($r^2 \times 100 = 1.44\%$).

Both of these analyses were carried out on a limited number of families: 39 with two or more natural children and 89 with two or more adopted children.

Discussion

Our data for natural children are grossly similar to those of Kass' group.

The phenomenon of parent-child correlation does not seem to be significant in adopted children, since the r coefficient was not significant between 379 adopted children and their adoptive parents. However, a larger sample may eventually reveal some small but significant difference.

The phenomenon of child-child resemblance among the adopted is not entirely absent, but is much smaller than among the natural ones. By variance analysis, the Fisher coefficient is twice as small and the p values 10-25 times smaller in adopted children. By correlation analysis, the percentage coefficients of determination are six times smaller in adopted children. It is probable that this small degree of child-child resemblance is proportional to the length of the adoption period, a factor that has not been controlled in the present preliminary study.

A valid comparison of r values between natural and adopted groups could be made if we had a sufficient sample size in each age group for each status and if the late adopted were excluded. A total of nearly 1,000 families may have to be surveyed to achieve this end. Results from 398 families (256 natural and 553 adopted children) are presently being analyzed; preliminary analyses confirm the trends of the present report.

We conclude that the familial aggregation of blood pressure, whether between parent and child, or between children, is almost entirely the result of heredity.

Three other characteristics considered to be related to the risk of developing obstructive coronary disease have been measured: body weight, height, and weight/height ratio. These three characteristics also seem to show very little familial aggregation in adopted children.

Acknowledgments

We are thankful to Dr. Edward H. Kass for encouraging us to undertake this study; to Dr. Fernand Roberge, Dr. Jean-Claude Panisset and Miss Juliette Ducros for their help in the computerization of the data; to the *Société d'Adoption et de Protection de l'Enfance de Montréal*, especially to Dr. Gaétan Nolin, Dr. Bernard Méthot, Miss Claire Rochon and Mr. René Erhardt; to Mrs. Suzanne Couet-Hudon, Miss Lise Audet, Mrs. Lucette Dallaire and Mrs. Diane Lapierre for carrying out the home visits; to Mr. Jean-Marc Picard for statistical advice; to Miss Ninon Dagenais for secretarial assistance and to all the adoptive parents who cooperated in our study.

References

1. Zinner, S. H., Levy, P. S. and Kass, E. H.: Familial aggregation of blood pressure in childhood. *New Eng. J. Med.*, 284:401-404, 1971.

Discussion

Dr. Cassel: This was a most refreshing presentation, Dr. Biron. May I ask what seems to be the obvious question: Why could you not compare these natural and adopted children at specific ages?

Dr. Biron: It is really a question of numbers. I didn't have enough children in each age group. If I separate them into three-year age groups, the comparisons would have a too high risk of Type II (beta) error.

Dr. Cassel: And it was not even possible to take, for example, the adopted children for 1, 2 and 3 years and compare them with the natural children for 1, 2 and 3 years of age?

Dr. Biron: I did a lot of comparisons. However, since my individual sample sizes are still small, I just don't dare to present them to you. When there is no difference in a sample, that does not mean that there isn't one in the population.

Dr. Kass, Moderator: As I recall, Dr. Biron, you were looking also at length of time a child lived in the family as one of the variables. Do you have any information here?

Dr. Biron: In some additional statistical analyses, I have removed the late adopted and when I do that I realize that there is a small influence of length of adoption. There is a very small although not significant positive correlation if I take the age group of, say, 12 to 15, among the adopted.

Dr. Kass: So there does appear to be some influence that comes on with time, which is fascinating, of course.

Hypoth₀ - no dif 3 co adopted & nal. childer.
he rejects this because he finds sig dif

Blood Pressure Studies in Polynesian Children

R. Beaglehole, M.D., Clare E. Salmond, M.Sc.
and I. A. M. Prior, M.D.

In this paper results are presented from studies of two groups of Polynesian children: Tokelau Islanders and New Zealand Maoris.

The three atolls which comprise the Tokelau Islands lie 480 km north of Samoa. The Tokelauan society is composed of a number of interlocking social groups which form a structurally complex but egalitarian society. Although the rate of social change toward "modernization" is increasing, life in the islands in 1971 still very largely followed the traditional pattern.[1] The way of life and the environment are in marked contrast to that which characterizes New Zealand and other Western countries.

The Maoris have been resident in New Zealand for ten centuries. Although there have been many changes in their society, especially the recent urbanization, some of the fundamentals of their original culture remain. The mean blood pressure levels of the Maoris are similar to those of the Caucasian majority.[2]

Two sets of results are discussed. The major section deals with a family study of blood pressure in Tokelauan children. It is preceded by an examination of the differences in the blood pressure levels by place of residence of Polynesian children in an attempt to establish whether the levels in these children exhibit similar patterns to those in the adult population. The blood

R. Beaglehole, M.D., Clare E. Salmond, M.Sc. *and* I. A. M. Prior, M.D.,
Epidemiology Unit, Wellington Hospital, Wellington, New Zealand.

pressure levels of Tokelau Island adults living in their home islands are substantially lower than those of New Zealand Maoris and show only a small increase with age.[3] The reasons for these differences in adults have not yet been elucidated, although it is possible that differences in body mass, salt intake and social environment may be involved.

The relevant evidence concerning male children is shown in Figure 1 in which mean systolic blood pressures for Tokelauan children aged 5-6 and 14-15 years are contrasted with Maori

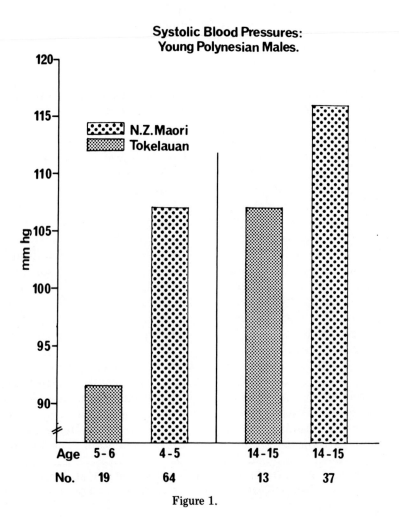

Figure 1.

children aged 4-5 and 14-15 years. All blood pressure readings were taken by members of the same Unit. In both young children and teenagers, the mean systolic pressures are significantly higher in the Maoris than in the Tokelauans. The Quetelet Index is the best index of body mass in both groups of children and its role in these blood pressure differences was examined. For the young children, the pressure differences cannot be attributed to the known differences in body mass because in neither group is there a correlation between body mass and blood pressure. In the teenagers, however, after controlling for the Quetelet Index by analysis of covariance, no significant differences remain between the Tokelauans and the Maoris.

A different pattern emerges in the females (Fig. 2). Young Tokelauan girls again have significantly lower systolic pressure than the Maoris, and this cannot be attributed to the known differences in body mass. In the teenagers, however, there are no significant differences in pressure between the Tokelauans and the Maoris.

Thus, we have evidence which suggests that the known differences in blood pressure of Polynesian adults according to place of residence are also apparent in children. Although we cannot explain the differences in pressure in young children, those that exist in teenage males can be explained by differences in body mass.

The family study of blood pressure in Tokelau Islanders utilizes data from the Tokelau Island Migrant Study.[3] The first stage of the family study, the results of which are presented here, involves an analysis of data collected on children and their parents living on their home islands. The second stage will be a replication of these analyses using data collected on children and their parents from the same islands but resident in New Zealand.

The Tokelau population was examined in the islands in March and April 1971. It consisted of all children aged 5-15 years and their parents. Five hundred and two (97%) of the 518 children on the census list had recorded systolic and fourth phase diastolic blood pressures. The children were linked through their parents into 210 different sibling groups. (Seven children were not allocated a sibship number because of lack of information about their parents.) It is worth noting that unlike

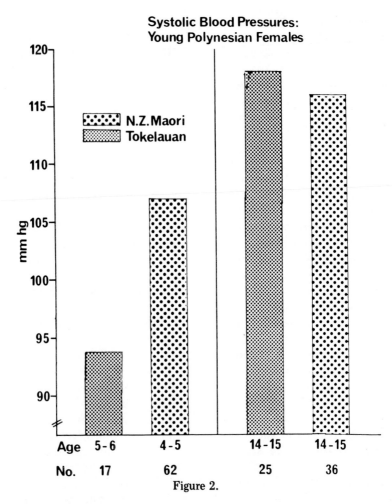

Figure 2.

other Polynesian societies, "siblings" are children who live in the same household and with their natural parents; very few children are adopted either formally or informally in the Tokelau Islands.[4]

The data collected on the children included height, weight and one casual blood pressure which was estimated after about five minutes rest using a random zero sphygmomanometer. All blood pressures were estimated by one observer without knowledge of the family relationships. Two different cuff sizes were available and the one that most comfortably encircled the child's arm was used. No adjustment was made for cuff size.

The adults underwent a more extensive examination which included two blood pressure estimations with the same type of sphygmomanometer. The average of these two estimates is used in our analyses.

The mean systolic and diastolic blood pressures for the total group of Tokelau children are shown in Figure 3. Both systolic and diastolic pressures increase with age in both sexes and are higher in girls than in boys. Since the Quetelet Index (Fig. 4) increases with age in both sexes and after the age of 10 is higher in girls than in boys, its influence on blood pressure was examined. The partial correlation of systolic blood pressure with Quetelet Index controlling for age was first examined in each yearly age group. All but one of the significant positive associations were in the 9-14 year-old children and these groups were pooled for the subsequent analyses. In this latter age group, there is a significant positive correlation between systolic blood pressure and Quetelet Index of 0.27 (n = 145) in boys and

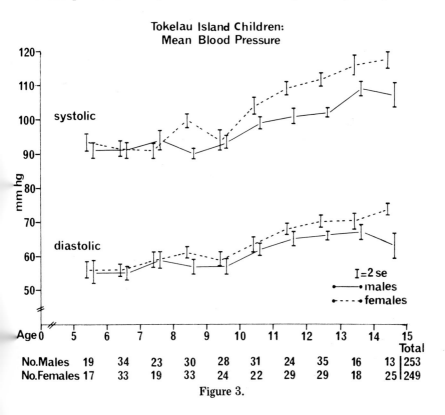

Figure 3.

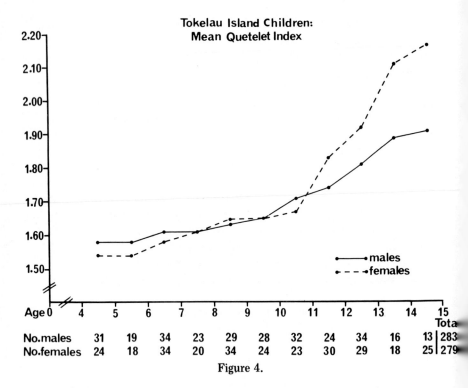

Figure 4.

0.19 (n = 147) in girls. In the younger groups, there is no significant correlation and in neither sex is there a significant relation between diastolic pressure and Quetelet Index.

The increase of systolic pressure with age is significant at the 1% level in both sexes in children aged 9-14 years and cannot be explained by the increase in Quetelet Index with age. The sex difference in systolic pressure is also significant in those aged 9-14 years and cannot be explained by the known sex differences in the Quetelet Index.

The sibship similarity of blood pressure z scores adjusted for year of age and sex was examined by analysis of variance between and within sibships in the 133 sibships with between two and seven siblings. The results show that for both systolic and diastolic pressure, the variance within sibships is significantly less at the 1% level than that between sibships in the age group studied. There is a sibship similarity of blood pressure in these children.

The influence of family size (number of siblings) on this familial similarity of blood pressure was assessed by estimating the variances within sibships for each sibship size. The similarity of these estimates of variance supports the conclusion that the sibship similarity of blood pressure is independent of family size.

To investigate the influence of blood pressure level on sibship similarity of pressure, one index child from each of the 133 sibships was chosen at random, and the regression of the remaining siblings' systolic blood pressure z score on the index child's z score was calculated. The regression line (Fig. 5) has a slope of 0.141 with standard error 0.057, and the correlation coefficient is 0.141 (p = 0.017). The linear component of

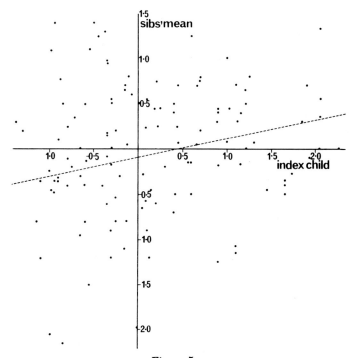

Regression of Siblings' systolic blood pressure score on Index child's score.

Figure 5.

regression is significant, and no evidence for a nonlinear component was found. We thus conclude that the same relationship between the index children's score and the mean score of the remaining siblings holds at all levels of the index children's scores.

To examine the influence of parental variables on a child's blood pressure, one index child was chosen at random from each of the 210 original sibships. Complete parental data were available for 136, or 78%, of the index children with living parents. No significant differences in the age distribution, systolic blood pressure z scores or in Quetelet Index were found between those index children with and those without complete parental data. Controlling for mother's age and the Quetelet Index of both child and mother, there is a significant correlation between child's systolic z score and mother's systolic pressure only in boys aged 5-8 years ($r = 0.33$, $p = 0.03$, $n = 46$).

Overall, the best predictor of a child's systolic blood pressure in the stepwise regressions is the child's age. To control for the effect of a child's age, systolic blood pressure z scores adjusted for year of age and sex are used in the analyses which relate parental variables to a child's blood pressure.

For boys 5-8 and girls 9-14, and for the pooled age and sex groups, the mother's systolic blood pressure is the best predictor of a child's systolic z score (for the pooled groups the significant multiple R^2 is 0.034). In fact, no other variable, either child or parental, significantly improves the prediction obtained by the mother's systolic pressure.

Controlling a child's blood pressure for age, sex and body mass, the predictive power of the mother's systolic pressure remains significant in boys 5-8 years and girls 9-14. For the pooled age and sex groups, however, we cannot predict a child's z score by knowledge of the mother's systolic pressure any better than by chance.

Finally, the correlation between the systolic pressure of mothers and fathers was examined; 152 pairs of parents were available for this analysis. Controlling for both the age and Quetelet Index of the spouses, no significant association between their pressures was found.

Discussion

The pattern of blood pressure in Polynesian children from two points of view was examined. First, the mean blood pressure levels in young children and in teenagers living in two contrasting environments were presented. There is no obvious explanation for the significant differences in the blood pressures of the young children. In teenagers, however, the differences that exist can be explained in terms of the known differences in body mass.

The second section described a family study of blood pressure in Tokelau Island children living on their home islands. A sibship similarity of blood pressure, which held at all levels of pressure and was unrelated to family size, was demonstrated. The best and only predictor of a child's systolic pressure z score was the mother's systolic pressure, although it explained only a small proportion of the total variation in the child's pressure.

The level of pressure in the Tokelauan children, although lower than in the New Zealand Maori, is higher than that reported for children of similar ages by Zinner et al[5] and Beresford and Holland.[6] This difference between the general level of pressure in Tokelauan children and these other populations is a reflection of technical differences in the estimation of blood pressures between the child studies. The Tokelau/Maori comparisons are of more value in that the blood pressure estimates were made by members of the same Unit with appropriate care. In both sets of teenagers, but not in the younger children, blood pressure is significantly correlated with body mass. The fact that differences in body mass explain the differences in pressure in teenage males highlights an area in which intervention, even at this young age, may prove useful. The lack of relationship between blood pressure and body mass in young children may relate to the lack of correction of blood pressure for cuff size.

The family study of blood pressure in Tokelauan children produced no new results. The confirmation of the work of others is not without interest, especially since the genetic make-up and physical environment of the Tokelauans are in marked contrast to those of the American children on whom similar studies have been conducted.

The sibship similarity results are exactly as found by Zinner et al[5] and indicate that in the Tokelauan society, a familial tendency to elevated blood pressure is established relatively early in life. The fact that the relationship between siblings holds at all levels of pressure suggests that in this population (as in others), arterial pressure is determined by graded polygenic inheritance. The similarity of these results to those of Zinner et al suggests that genetic factors may be responsible for the family aggregation of blood pressures. That the similarity present among siblings was not present between spouses also suggests that genetic, rather than environmental, factors may be responsible for the sibship similarity.

The differences between our results and those of Beresford and Holland[6] in the relationship between parental variables and child's pressure are difficult to interpret but may relate to our smaller sample. The only parental variable we found to be related to a child's systolic pressure z score was the mother's pressure. In contrast, the English study found that the father's pressure and parental weight were also significant.

Two groups of Tokelau children have now been examined in two different environments — their home islands and New Zealand — and it is possible that by holding the force of heredity constant, these studies will further elucidate the relative importance of genes and environment on the familial similarity of blood pressure.

Acknowledgments

The authors wish to acknowledge the support and guidance received from the Tokelau Island Project Committee of the South Pacific Research Committee of the Medical Research Council of New Zealand, the Medical Research Council of New Zealand, the Cardiovascular Disease Unit of the World Health Organization, the Wellington Hospital Board, the Department of Health and the Tokelau communities in New Zealand and in the Islands.

Support from Merck Sharp & Dohme (N.Z.) enabled Robert Beaglehole to attend the Symposium and this is gratefully acknowledged.

References

1. Hooper, A. and Huntsman, J.: A demographic history of the Tokelau Islands. *J. Polynesian Soc.*, 82:366, 1974.
2. Prior, I. A. M.: Cardiovascular epidemiology in Polynesians in the Pacific. *Singapore Med. J.*, 3:223, 1973.
3. Prior, I. A. M., Stanhope, J. M., Evans, J. G. et al: The Tokelau Island Migrant Study. *Int. J. Epidem.*, 3:225, 1974.
4. Hooper, A.: Personal communication, 1974.
5. Zinner, S. H., Levy, P. S. and Kass, E. H.: Family aggregation of blood pressure in childhood. *New Eng. J. Med.*, 284:401, 1971.
6. Beresford, A. A. and Holland, W. W.: Levels of blood pressure in children: A family study. *Proc. Roy. Soc. Med.*, 66:1009, 1973.

Discussion

Dr. Lovell: If I have followed the proceedings rightly, I think that Dr. Holland provided us with evidence that the children's pressures were related to those of both parents. Dr. Beaglehole, you have provided us with evidence that there is a relationship only with the mother. Can you make any suggestion as to the reason for the difference? Specifically, is there a promiscuity problem in the Polynesian Islands?

Dr. Beaglehole: I really have no explanation for the difference. Our study population was smaller. This may be one factor involved. Regarding the promiscuity problem, illegitimate births are known to occur and we know of them. They were excluded from the sibship studies. There were half a dozen, possibly. There were only one or two children on whom we did not have any information at all about their parents and, of necessity, they were also excluded. The children lived with their first degree relatives and with their natural parents.

Dr. Holland: This is a very interesting study that you have done. However, one major difference between our study and yours is that you have used the Quetelet Index. Is there any reason why you haven't looked at height and weight separately, rather than the Quetelet Index? One of the problems is that the Index may be appropriate in children aged 5 and 6, but not at 14 and 15 years of age. I think that there are different relationships at different ages. Certainly, we have found that in Kent school children.

Dr. Beaglehole: We did in fact look at weight separately initially and then, to remove the effect of height, we used the Quetelet Index. We found that the Quetelet Index was the best index of body mass in that it was least correlated with height at all age groups.

Dr. Kass, Moderator: Just to clarify the point: Was there a relationship between blood pressure and weight in the younger children?

Dr. Beaglehole: No, there wasn't.

Dr. Neutra, Massachusetts: For the record, please repeat your observation about the differences between the average levels of blood pressure of the Polynesian children and adults versus the ones in Dr. Holland's study. Also, what was the score between sibs and the index children which results from the scattergram that you showed? It seems it would be very small, smaller than the levels that have been reported from American and European families.

Dr. Beaglehole: To answer the first question, the blood pressure levels in the Polynesian Islanders in adults are lower than that reported for New Zealand or American adults. Yet, I have figures that show that the blood pressure levels of children tend to be higher in our children than in the studies conducted by Kass and Holland. I am sure this latter discrepancy is due to technical differences.

Dr. Neutra: What is the order of difference?

Dr. Beaglehole: About 10 mm higher on average, although we used a random zero sphygmomanometer and we had two cuff sizes. We didn't adjust for cuff size, as Dr. Holland did. We certainly didn't use the same device as Dr. Kass. The similarity between siblings is lower than that reported in other studies.

Dr. Neutra: What was the value?

Dr. Beaglehole: The correlation coefficient is 0.14.

Dr. Cassel: Would you agree, would the people here at this symposium today agree, with the premise that because there is a similarity in sib-sib relationship or parent-child relationship found in many different ethnic groups across the world, with different levels of blood pressure, and with different personal-social relationships and with different environmental circumstances, this would clearly suggest that, insofar as those similarities are due to genetic similarities, the distribution of genes responsible for those factors is the same in different ethnic groups? Therefore, we cannot explain the differences in blood pressure levels between different ethnic groups on the basis of different genetic predispositions. This is not to say that genetic factors are not important in blood pressure, but they do not explain the differences in ethnic groups.

Dr. Kass: I certainly would subscribe to that view. Dr. Holland and Dr. Sackett also agree. Dr. Beaglehole, also. It must be wrong, because we are all agreed.

V
Therapeutic and Preventive Trials

Medical Research Council Trial Material

Colin T. Dollery, M.B.

The two Veterans Administration cooperative trials in the treatment of hypertension[1,2] were a landmark in the understanding of the efficacy of antihypertensive therapy, but inevitably they left a number of important questions unanswered. Among the most important are the efficacy of treatment in very mild hypertension in women and in the elderly. To try to answer the first of these questions, and in part the second, the Medical Research Council in Britain convened a Committee under the chairmanship of Professor W. S. Peart to investigate the desirability and practicality of a trial of treatment in mild hypertension. The Committee reported that a trial was both desirable and practical, and a pilot phase was begun, coordinated by Dr. W. E. Miall at the Epidemiology and Medical Care Unit, Northwick Park Hospital. The pilot trial has been in progress for a year, but it is much too early to draw any conclusions from it, apart from some tentative ones concerning the efficacy of the antihypertensive regimes which are being used. However, some of the major decisions made in designing the trial are of general importance and deserve discussion.

Hospital or Community Based?

I had thought that the trial might be based upon hospital hypertension clinics, for reasons of simplicity and economy. Large numbers of individuals discovered to have mild asymptomatic hypertension at preemployment or insurance examinations are referred to hospital hypertension clinics for investigation and advice about treatment. They would have formed a convenient and motivated study group. Further

Colin T. Dollery, M.B., *Professor of Clinical Pharmacology, Royal Postgraduate Medical School, Hammersmith Hospital, London, England.*

consideration showed that to operate from hospital hypertension clinics was probably impractical and almost certainly undesirable. The impracticality became obvious when calculations showed that the number of patients to be admitted to the trial would probably be between 10,000 and 20,000. The number of individuals presenting themselves at particular clinics within the required pressure range was not more than one or two a week. Even with a very large number of cooperating clinics, it would have been impractical to obtain the numbers within any reasonable span of time. Patients who attend a specialist hospital clinic are unlikely to be fully representative of those with that disease entity in the community at large. They are more likely to have complications which have caused them to seek medical advice. This is one of the main problems in interpreting the Veterans Administration data because many of the patients had cardiac, cerebral or renal complications of hypertension when they were entered into the trial. A public health policy for the control of hypertension in the community should be based on a representative sample of hypertensive patients drawn from that community. The decision was taken to recruit patients by screening in general practice, in industrial clinics and through organizations screening whole communities. The number of individuals recruited from each source by August 1974 is shown in Table 1.

Criteria for Admission to the Trial

Ethical considerations dictated that the trial could not include patients with pressure levels at which benefits of treatment had been demonstrated beyond reasonable doubt. In the Veterans Administration study, significant benefits of treatment were demonstrated for individuals with diastolic

TABLE 1. Recruitment of Patients up to August 1974

Source	Men	Number Women	Total
General practices	146	242	388
Industrial clinics	50	21	71
Screening organizations	79	59	138
Totals	275	322	597

pressures in the range 105 mm Hg and higher, but there was not a significant difference between the treated and control groups in the range 90-104 mm Hg. It must also be remembered that the pretreatment pressure levels quoted in the Veterans Administration trial are the average of the last two readings after a period of six to eight weeks on placebo. To compare these readings with the first casual diastolic blood pressure reading, it is probably necessary to add 10-12 mm Hg.

The patients were selected on the basis of two screening examinations. At the first screen if the mean of duplicate readings equals or exceeds 200 systolic or 90 diastolic, the patient is recalled one week later but otherwise is dismissed. At the second screen, if the mean of four readings (two of the first visit and two of the second) is less than 200 systolic and 90 diastolic, the patient is reassured and dismissed. If the mean equals or exceeds 200 systolic or 110 diastolic, the patient is not entered in the trial but referred for treatment. If the mean of the four readings equals or exceeds 90 diastolic but does not exceed 109, provided that the systolic does not exceed 200, the patient is recalled for an entry examination by a physician. The patient must remain within the entry criteria of blood pressure at this examination, and there are a number of excluding criteria such as evidence of accelerated hypertension, psychiatric illness, contraindications to the drugs used in therapy, or unwillingness of the general practitioner to sanction entry to the trial.

Choice of Therapeutic Regimes

There are many different types of antihypertensive drug, each with distinct advantages and disadvantages. The major requirements for a drug to be used in mass treatment in the community are ease of use, proven efficacy, low toxicity and, if possible, low cost. As the trial was planned to last five to ten years, this ruled out any very recently introduced agent whose long-term toxicity was still to be established.

These considerations suggested that thiazide diuretics should form the basis of the therapeutic regime. Thiazides have a flat dose-response relationship, a predominantly nonpostural effect and cause few symptoms. Their efficacy is limited. The majority of patients reported in the literature show a fall in mean blood pressure of about 12 mm Hg.[3] Several untoward effects of thiazides are known, including hypokalemia, hyperglycemia, hyperuricemia and calcium retention, but none has so far proved to be of major concern in the treatment of hypertension. The MRC Committee decided to adopt bendrofluazide in a dose of 10 mg daily as the basis of one of its drug regimes as this thiazide diuretic is the cheapest available in the United Kingdom. If blood pressure control is inadequate on bendrofluazide alone, methyldopa can be added.

The next question was whether there should be one drug regime or two. Several arguments were advanced against a total commitment to thiazides: (a) Existing studies on the drug treatment of hypertension suggest a favorable effect in preventing cerebral hemorrhage and cerebral infarction, heart and renal failure, but show little or no effect upon the incidence of myocardial infarction. It was just possible that this lack of effect on myocardial infarction could be a consequence of the therapeutic regime used, almost all of which contained thiazides. (b) The University Group Diabetic Program in the United States suggested that tolbutamide, another sulfonamide, might increase the incidence of myocardial infarction.[4] (c) The tendency of the thiazides to elevate plasma renin and the suggestion that renin itself might damage blood vessels.[5]

None of these arguments, by itself, was substantial but collectively they were sufficient to convince the Committee to recommend a second main drug regime that would not include a thiazide. It was decided to use propranolol in a dosage of up to 240 mg daily, there being some evidence that this was roughly equipotent with the thiazides.[6] Propranolol also has a low incidence of side effects and a nonpostural effect upon blood pressure. Guanethidine was chosen as the drug that could be added to this regime if propranolol alone was inadequate.

Control of Blood Pressure

Early results show that the two regimes are of roughly equivalent efficacy in the control of blood pressure. Side effects of treatment have been few and, for the most part, trivial. The main problem has been that the separation of blood pressure in the treated and control groups has not been as large as was hoped. In the treated group the average diastolic pressure at 12 weeks was approximately 13 mm Hg lower than the entry level of pressure; the comparable difference for systolic pressure was approximately 24 mm Hg. However, the placebo group showed a fall in pressure from the entry level which was a little over half as great as this. Thus, the difference in systolic pressure between treated and control groups was approximately 10.5 mm Hg and the diastolic 5.5 mm Hg at 3 months and had changed very little in the smaller number of patients followed for 12 months.

Dropouts

At 12 months 17.9% of the patients in the treated group had been withdrawn from randomized treatment and 7.5% of the controls. These figures are disturbingly high, but the corresponding percentage of patients withdrawn from the trial is only 5.9% in the treated group and 4.4% in the control group at 12 months. The main reason for withdrawal from randomized treatment is drug side effects and the patients are then switched to the other regime. Patients in the control group are withdrawn from randomized treatment with placebo if their diastolic pressure exceeds 115 mm Hg.

Trial Size

The numbers required to be admitted to the trial have been calculated by Dr. Miall and Professor Cochrane. They considered casual diastolic IV pressures and took as end points cerebrovascular and myocardial infarction morbidity and mortality, and hypertensive, heart and renal disease mortality. Assuming that the age and sex distribution in the main trial will be similar to that in the pilot phase and using South Wales data on morbidity and mortality, and taking into account the separation of blood pressures achieved in the pilot trial, they calculated that 19,200 individuals would have to be admitted to the trial to give a 95% chance of detecting a difference significant at the 1% level using a two-tailed test.

Cost

It is not easy to make a reliable estimate of the total cost of the trial. Some costs are met out of existing budgets for the

Epidemiology and Medical Care Unit and elsewhere, but estimates have to be made of the annual costs to be met from research funds for a trial of 20,000 patients lasting five years. The figure is £360,000 per annum (U. S. $864,000 per annum).

This is between 1% and 2% of the annual budget of the Medical Research Council of the United Kingdom. The MRC has so far authorized only the pilot phase of the trial which is likely to include up to 2,000 patients.

The cost of the trial can be compared with the cost of the treatment or the saving in not treating if the results were negative. The annual cost of the drug regime for each patient at current prices quoted in the Monthly Index of Medical Specialties would be £4.15 for bendrofluazide 10 mg daily and £27.08 for propranolol 240 mg daily. If the results of screening the British adult population in the age range of 35 to 64 years were similar to that obtained in the screening to date, approximately 1 million people would fulfill the criteria. The annual cost of treating them would thus be approximately £4 million with bendrofluazide and £27 million with propranolol. Although the costs of the trial are high, the cost of drifting into a form of treatment whose efficacy is unproved is clearly much higher.

Discussion

The trial design has proved satisfactory and the two drug regimes have similar effects upon the blood pressure. It is to be hoped that no serious toxic effect of either drug will be disclosed during the trial, such as the problems that have arisen recently with reserpine and practolol.[7]

The trial is large, complex and costly, but the question asked is one of substantial importance to the public health. The cost is small compared with that likely to be incurred if the decision were taken to treat this group of patients without further evidence.

The main concern lies in the small separation of blood pressure between the placebo and treated groups. In the course of time the two groups should separate further as the placebo group resumes an upward trend of blood pressure, but there is no more than a hint of this in the small number of patients who have been followed for 12 months. One possibility would be to combine the two drug regimes as there is evidence that propranolol and benzothiadiazine diuretics have an additive effect upon blood pressure.[8] However, this would negate the aim of studying the effects of the individual drugs as well as the effect of blood pressure reduction, and no final decision has been made.

Acknowledgments

The Medical Research Council Trial of Treatment in Mild Hypertension is a multicentered cooperative venture managed by a Committee involving the work of a great many people. This paper is a report by one Committee member concerning the progress of the trial to date. I am grateful to the Chairman, Professor Peart, and the coordinator, Dr. Miall, for permission to refer to some of the preliminary results.

References

1. Veterans Administration Cooperative Study: *JAMA*, 202:1028, 1969.
2. Veterans Administration Cooperative Study: *JAMA*, 213:1143, 1970.
3. Cranston, W. I., Juel-Jensen, B. E., Semmence, A. M. et al: *Lancet*, 2:966, 1963.
4. Prout, T. E., Knatterud, G. L., Meinert, C. L. et al for the University Group Diabetic Program: *Diabetes*, 21:1035, 1972.
5. Brunner, H. R., Laragh, J. H., Baer, L. et al: *New Eng. J. Med.*, 286:441, 1972.
6. Paterson, J. W. and Dollery, C. T.: *Lancet*, 2:1148, 1966.
7. Boston Collaborative Drug Surveillance Program: *Lancet*, 2:669, 1974.
8. Richardson, D. W., Freund, J., Gear, A. S. et al: *Circulation*, 37:534, 1968.

Bibliography

Gavras, H., Brown, J. J., Lever, A. F. et al: *Lancet*, 2:19, 1971.

Discussion

Dr. Shaper: I noticed that the estimates for the number of events to be expected are based on the data from South Wales which is a very soft water area. As there are tremendous regional variations in the United Kingdom, with approximately a 40% difference in mortality, between the very hard and the very soft areas, has this been taken into account?

Dr. Dollery: No, it hasn't.

Dr. Freis, Moderator: It is very striking, Dr. Dollery, that the pressures fell so much in the control group. The placebo effect was truly remarkable and quite the opposite of what we had. I wonder whether the difference was due to the fact that we had a prerandomization trial period of two to four months, in which the patients were on known placebos and their pressures at entry, then, were the averages of the last two readings during that placebo control period.

Dr. Dollery: I think that is the main reason for the difference. We have discussed whether we should not have a three month period on placebo and admit only those who still fulfill the criteria at the end of that time. From the point of view of producing an end point to the trial, that probably would be desirable and the decision has not finally been taken about it. There are, however, some objections. I believe that in your own trial, you did during that period also tests for compliance and discarded about one half of the individuals for failing to comply.

Dr. Freis: Yes, that is right.

Dr. Dollery: In our trial, we are concerned that the results should be applicable to the community at large and, therefore, wouldn't wish to discard people simply for that reason. Second, we also wanted to do a study which at least in some way resembled the way people might be handled in the community at large. It isn't usual practice to have a placebo period of this duration.

Dr. Meneely, Louisiana: Am I correct that you excluded individuals with a potassium level below 3.4?

Dr. Dollery: Yes, at entry, that is one of the exclusion criteria. Not many people have been dropped for that reason.

Dr. Meneely: What explanation do you offer for the early fall in the placebo group?

Dr. Dollery: I don't offer an explanation of it. It certainly was unexpected to me in its magnitude and over the period for which it has been sustained. I think that anybody who looks at antihypertensive medications is aware of placebo effects of the order of 5 mm Hg in mean pressure. These are somewhat larger than that and are surprisingly well sustained.

Dr. Freis: I think that it is the difference between casual and "basal" blood pressure. As your patients come back, they get more acclimated to the physicians. This is the reason why phenobarbital was considered to be a successful antihypertensive agent for 20 or 30 years.

Dr. Dollery: Our readings, of course, are based on the mean of six readings at three interviews, so this isn't just purely the difference between an initial casual reading and a subsequent casual reading. I remember reading a paper by Dr. Geoffrey Rose in the *Lancet* some years ago, reporting a study in which pressures were taken at three successive interviews. There was a big drop between first and second and some drop between second and third, but not a very big drop thereafter.

Dr. Kass: I should like to reinforce this general discussion by recalling what we all know but which I think sometimes gets overlooked. We don't have any information to indicate what the risks are in those people who enter a trial with a high pressure and then because of the so-called placebo effect have their pressures fall. The only information we have is that the first blood pressure is still a very powerful indicator of morbidity and mortality. I think that the implication that these people whose pressures have fallen during a series of successive visits are in fact spared an excess morbidity and mortality has nothing to support it.

Dr. Freis: I would like to challenge that. I may be wrong, but it seems to me that when you take a group of people in whom you have measured the blood pressures at one time, that you have a heterogeneous mix; and in the heterogeneous mix, you have a high risk group who have persistent elevation of blood pressure and a much lower risk group who have labile hypertension. When you look at the average result out of that heterogeneous mix, you find that the risk is high, but still there may be subgroups mixed in whose risk is very low. There have been a few studies done on labile hypertension. Storm-Mathisson has done a ten-year follow-up of labile versus nonlabile hypertensive patients. He finds about an eight times difference in morbidity and mortality between those who remain hypertensive after being hospitalized, as opposed to those who become normotensive after being hospitalized over a ten-year period of follow-up. So that it may be that lability is a very important indicator of risk.

Dr. Kass: Let me clarify what I think are two different streams to this conversation. I don't think that anyone would

seriously question that those with fixed elevated blood pressures have a greater risk than those whose blood pressures are
more labile. The fact that those who have higher pressures in
the hospital had greater risks later has been reaffirmed doesn't
alter anyone's basic thought about the process. The query is
whether those who were labile hypertensives had a greater risk
than those who never had an elevated pressure. That is what
hasn't been answered. I am merely suggesting that, given what
we know about long-term follow-up studies, there is reason to
suppose that those whose pressures are sometimes elevated in
these measurements in fact have a somewhat greater risk,
although surely not as great as you point out, as those with a
fixed pressure.

Dr. Dollery: We don't know the answer to that.

Dr. Freis: We don't know the answer, I would agree. But we
shouldn't assume an answer.

Dr. Kass: We shouldn't assume it, in either direction.

Dr. Freis: In either direction.

Dr. Shansky, Illinois: I am wondering, especially with
reference to your worries about the thiazides inducing an
increase in the renin, what sort of laboratory work-up was done
on these patients and did it indeed include a renin sampling?

Dr. Dollery: No, not in the main trial. Within the trial, there
are various subsidiary studies and Dr. Lever's laboratory in
Glasgow is going to measure renin in a sample of these patients,
just as my laboratory in London is going to measure the plasma
concentrations of the drugs used in a sample of the patients. It
would increase the cost and complexity considerably to have
done this in everyone.

Dr. Lawton, Iowa: Dr. Dollery, I would like to ask you
about the magnitude of change in blood pressure from visit to
visit and mention an experience that we have had this summer
in conjunction with our mild hypertension study. We screened
10,000 patients in eastern Iowa, of whom approximately 1,000
have met the criteria of mild hypertension (diastolic 90-104 mm
Hg). From a community "prescreen" to the first clinic visit, we
have found two thirds have dropped below a diastolic pressure
of 90 mm Hg. Then, from the first clinic visit to the second
visit, only 20% of the subjects had diastolic pressures below 90
mm Hg. We were surprised by the magnitude of two thirds of
mild hypertensives having normal pressure on a repeat check. I

wonder if we should really have been so surprised.

Dr. Dollery: I am interested to hear about that study. The proportion of patients who are fulfilling our entry criteria in relation to the numbers screened is between 5% and 10% in the different centers, but it is averaging nearer 5% overall.

Dr. Lovell: Dr. Dollery, is there any possibility that your control group might be getting some treatment or approach to treatment by their physicians that distinguishes them from the patients in the treatment group, for example, different advice about weight, about dietary factors, and so on?

Dr. Dollery: I don't think so. The patients are being seen by the same individuals. Their blood pressures are being taken by specially trained nurses. We will keep a check on various aspects of these individuals to see if there are changes in things like body weight with time, which would indicate that there is some other independent variable.

Dr. Stamler: I wanted to make a comment about lability and to pick up the remarks that were made earlier. First, we do know some of the answers. If we take pressures over a few years' time, and take a mean, the mean is quite predictive. The first blood pressure is highly correlated with subsequent individual pressures (r = about 0.6) and with the mean. As Dr. Labarthe has shown in working with the data from our study of the Chicago Peoples Gas Co. labor force, the intra-individual standard deviation, which reflects lability around that mean, is totally nonpredictive. In using the term lability, two things are being confused: a tendency with successive blood pressure measurements over short periods of time for the pressure to go down (an adaptation or acclimatization phenomenon, if you will) and the degree of long-term fluctuation around a mean. I think that we should be careful not to speak about the degree of fluctuation around a mean as having any predictive power at all.

Dr. Freis: Dr. Stamler, you mean "predictive of risk"?

Dr. Stamler: Yes, that is right.

Dr. Dollery: I think that the word lability is not an entirely appropriate one to describe what we are observing.

Trials of Therapy for Mild Hypertension in the United Kingdom

W. W. Holland, M.D. and M. W. Adler, M.B.

A number of randomized controlled trials have demonstrated some reduction in morbidity and mortality from stroke, renal and cardiac failure as a result of hypotensive treatment. However, most of these trials have limitations and their results must be interpreted with caution. The real problem has been the selection of individuals for inclusion. First, the studies have tended to use individuals with some existing abnormality; second, the subjects have been selected from patients already attending hospital clinics who continued to be treated from a hospital base.

In this paper we will describe two trials (one hospital, one community-based) of symptomless individuals with raised blood pressure undertaken by our department. They illustrate some of these problems as well as other difficulties we encountered.

Hospital-based Trial

The first study[1] was designed to test the hypothesis that effective lowering and maintenance of diastolic pressures from levels between 100 and 120 mm Hg to levels below 100 mm Hg reduces morbidity and mortality from cardiovascular disease. We also studied the incidence of side effects from drugs used in treatment and observed the willingness of all the patients to

These studies have been supported in part by a grant from the Department of Health and Social Security.

W. W. Holland, M.D., B.Sc., F.R.C.P., F.F.C.M., *Professor, and* M. W. Adler, M.B., M.R.C.P., *Lecturer, Department of Community Medicine, St. Thomas's Hospital and Medical School, London, England.*

continue taking drugs for any length of time. Most were free of symptoms attributable to raised blood pressure.

The study took place in Cardiff and in London. In Cardiff it was carried out by the Medical Research Council Epidemiological Research Unit and Department of Medicine, United Cardiff Hospitals; in London by the Departments of Medicine and Clinical Epidemiology and Social Medicine, St. Thomas's Hospital. Patients were drawn from two sources: surveys of random samples of the general population and hospital patients. The study was carried out in both centers from July 1967 to December 1970 and was continued for a further year at St. Thomas's Hospital. The criteria for selection were that patients should be men and women between 45 and 69 years with two casual sitting diastolic blood pressures between 100 and 120 mm Hg on two occasions separated by an interval of at least two weeks. Blood pressure throughout the trial was recorded by the Wright modification of the Garrow random zero sphygmomanometer. The patients selected had to be willing to join the trial and to attend a clinic regularly. Certain exclusion criteria were also laid down.

The patients were allocated at random to either a control or treatment group. The control group received calcium lactate. Those in the treatment group were given any one of three regimens. The aim of treatment was to reduce the diastolic blood pressure below 100 mm Hg as far as was consistent with the patient's comfort. Progression from one regimen to the next depended upon the blood pressure response and incidence of side effects. Reasons for withdrawal from the trial were death, persistent poor cooperation or attendance for either social or medical reasons, and, in the control group, a rise of diastolic pressure above 130 mm Hg on one occasion or other clear indications for antihypotensive treatment. The physicians knew which treatment the patient was being given, but the random zero sphygmomanometer eliminated bias in measurement.

One hundred and sixteen patients were admitted to the trial. Figure 1 shows the changes in levels of blood pressure throughout the course of the trial. The mean levels of blood pressure in the treated group fell in the first six months, and this fall was maintained. The control levels remained around the mean on entry for 18 months. By this time six of the nine

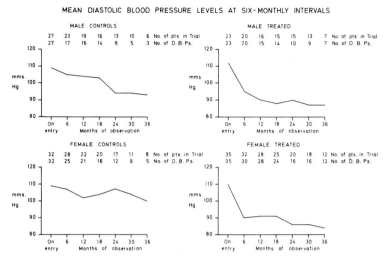

Figure 1.

controls whose diastolic pressures rose above 130 mm Hg had
been withdrawn from the trial, and comparison of mean levels
of blood pressure in the two groups was no longer possible.

Table 1 shows the treatment given. The treatment group
consisted of 58 patients; 31 were treated with bendrofluazide
with potassium, 4 with alpha-methyldopa alone, 12 with
alpha-methyldopa and bendrofluazide and 11 with debrisoquine
with bendrofluazide. No patient had to be withdrawn from the
trial as a result of drug side effects, but two refused to continue
drug taking and there was one report of possible postural

TABLE 1. Type of Treatment Given

Drugs Used	Males	Females	Total
Bendrofluazide	13	18	31
Bendrofluazide and Methyldopa	5	7	12
Bendrofluazide and Debrisoquine	2	9	11
Methyldopa	3	1	4
Total	23	35	58

Figure 1 is reproduced with permission from the *British Medical
Journal* (3:434-436, 1973).

TABLE 2. Medical Indications for Leaving Trial

Group	Indication	No. of Patients	Total
Controls:			
Men	Diastolic blood pressure rose above 130 mm Hg	5	
	Died – cause unknown	2	8
	Myocardial infarct and pulmonary embolus	1	
Women	Diastolic blood pressure rose above 130 mm Hg	4	
	Died infarct of cardiac septum	1	6
	Developed cardiac failure	1	
Treated:			
Men	Admitted to geriatric hospital – senility	1	1
Women	Died of fractured skull	1	2
	Myocardial infarct	1	

TABLE 3. Mean Diastolic Pressures During Trial
Figures in Parentheses Are Numbers in Each Group

Group	On Entry	Remained in Trial	Left for Medical Reasons	Left for Management Reasons	Left Area
Controls:					
Men	109 (27)	103 (13)	124 (8)	96 (5)	96 (1)
Women	109 (31)	105 (20)	129 (6)	96 (4)	90 (1)
Total	109 (58)	104 (33)	126 (14)	96 (9)	93 (2)
Treated:					
Men	112 (23)	91 (15)	100 (1)	99 (6)	103 (1)
Women	110 (35)	89 (29)	99 (2)	84 (4)	-
Total	110 (58)	90 (44)	100 (3)	92 (10)	103 (1)

Tables 2 and 3 are reproduced with permission from the *British Medical Journal* (3:434-436, 1973).

hypotension. Seventeen patients were withdrawn from the trial for medical reasons, 14 in the control and 3 in the treated group (Table 2). Nine of the controls left because the diastolic pressures rose above 130 mm Hg, two died, two developed a myocardial infarct and one cardiac failure. In comparison, in the treated group, one patient died, one was admitted to a geriatric hospital and one developed a myocardial infarct. The mean diastolic pressures of all patients entering, remaining and withdrawing from the trial for either medical or management reasons are shown in Table 3. The 19 who left for nonmedical reasons either defaulted or were uncooperative; of these, ten left the trial within a year of entry.

The trial does not provide any clear answer as to the results of treatment of raised blood pressure. This is due to four factors, namely, the small number of patients included at the outset, the deterrent effect of investigations, the loss of patients from the control group and, last, the fact that supervision was provided from within the hospital.

The problem of the small numbers was partly related to the fact that the patients were virtually all free of any symptoms and were therefore very unwilling to take part in any long-term treatment program. Several patients found intravenous pyelography unpleasant and their subsequent management on admission to the trial was difficult. It would seem from the results of our investigations that such tests are neither necessary nor justified as a routine in symptom-free patients and should be carried out only when indicated. These findings reinforce those of Gifford[2] who reported that 4.5% of nearly 5,000 patients with raised blood pressure seen at the Cleveland Clinic had evidence of renal vascular disease, but only 0.13% were treated surgically.

Most of the patients in the trial were controlled by use of bendrofluazide alone. However, the main difficulty in interpreting the results lies in the disappearance of increasing numbers of patients from the control group due to diastolic pressures rising above 130 mm Hg. However comparable the two groups may have been at the outset, within 18 months this comparability had disappeared. On the present evidence, it is clear that the main function of treatment is to prevent the rise of blood pressure. It cannot be concluded that treatment effectively reduces the risks of death or morbid events due to cardiovascular disease.

This trial also brought the realization that it was impossible to obtain sufficient numbers of individuals for inclusion in a randomized controlled trial to be undertaken in the hospital atmosphere of either St. Thomas's or the Cardiff Royal Infirmary. Furthermore, the number of individuals to be recruited from epidemiological random sample surveys or from invitations to outpatients attending hospital for other reasons was insufficient to conduct the sort of trial necessary to establish whether the reduction of blood pressure reduces morbidity or mortality.

Community-based Trial

It. was for these reasons that we decided to try to devise a different form of management for symptomless individuals with moderately raised blood pressure. Within the context of medical practice in the United Kingdom, it seems obvious from our experience that we are unlikely to be able to answer the question by using specialized hospital clinics. In the United Kingdom, every individual is registered with a general practitioner to whom he can turn when he has any medical problems. The general practitioner normally refers to hospital only about 2% of all patients seen.[3] We felt that it was important to carry out a study within general practice for two closely related reasons. First, all past studies have been hospital based and thus unable to give answers relevant to the "unselected hypertensive" at large in the community. Second, the general practitioner is most likely to identify the symptomless patient and maintain contact once treatment has been instituted in the normal medical care situation.

The original intention was to use a number of different general practices. However, it was extremely difficult to obtain full general practitioner cooperation, since we were unable to answer the very pertinent question of how much work would be involved and how much it would cost. The only practice willing to perform the study without this information was our own teaching practice at St. Thomas's. We were aware that this practice was by no means typical of others without teaching

TABLE 4. Randomized Controlled Trial of Treatment
of Moderate Hypertension

Objectives:
1. To measure the effect of antihypertensive treatment on subsequent
   mortality and morbidity of subjects with moderate hypertension.
2. To measure:
   a. The number of subjects with hypertension previously unknown to
      the practice.
   b. The number of subjects with hypertension who are receiving
      treatment.
3. To see whether subjects with moderate hypertension are willing to start
   and continue therapy over a number of years within the context of
   general practice.
4. To assess the feasibility of screening and treatment for hypertension
   from general practice.
5. To measure the cost of screening for moderate hypertension in general
   practice and entering suitable patients into the treatment trial.

and research responsibilities. Therefore, in June of this year we
succeeded in persuading another practice in southern England
to take part.

It should be emphasized that our major purpose was to
conduct a pilot investigation to determine the feasibility of
undertaking a randomized controlled trial of treatment of
moderately raised blood pressure within the context of general
practice. The study examines various aspects of hypertension
apart from those directly related to the question of whether
treatment reduces mortality and morbidity (Table 4). Thus, we
will be interested in measuring the number of hypertensive
subjects previously unknown to the practice *and* the number of
patients who are receiving treatment for their disease. Of equal
importance to showing a reduction in sickness and death will be
the question of whether symptomless patients are prepared to
maintain treatment for five years. It is quite obvious that to
show the former without the latter, even if this is possible, will
mean that more effort must be concentrated on making this
prophylactic treatment acceptable. Finally, we hope to get
some idea of the cost of screening for moderate hypertension in
general practice. Our present protocol differs from that of the
study which is being carried out by Miall and his group of the
Medical Research Council Epidemiology and Medical Care Unit

at Northwick Park. Our trial does not attempt to assess the value of treatment by drug a, b or c on the level of blood pressure, but it is concerned with comparing management of blood pressure by whatever means necessary to lower it.

The scheme of the study is shown in Figure 2. We used the age/sex register as our sampling frame. This has created problems which will be discussed later. The register identified 1,612 men between 35 and 64 years who were invited to attend screening clinics. Blood pressure was taken using a Wright modification Garrow random zero sphygmomanometer. On the first visit, blood pressure was taken twice on the same arm after the patient had been sitting for at least five minutes. All those with a mean of two diastolic pressures (Diastolic V) of 90 mm Hg or above were asked to return for a second measurement at a later date. Patients with blood pressures below this level were not considered for entry into the trial.

The second set of measurements on those with levels of 90 mm Hg and above was performed after an interval of at least one week and not more than one month. If the mean of the

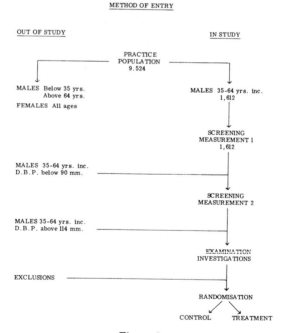

METHOD OF ENTRY

Figure 2.

four diastolic pressures — that is, the combination of the first and second visits — was 90-114 mm Hg, the patients were considered suitable for entry into the trial. Those with levels above 114 mm Hg were excluded.

Patients with the required levels then were given a full physical examination. We also obtained baseline information about symptoms and smoking history, performed electrocardiograms and took blood for urea and electrolytes, cholesterol, serum creatinine and uric acid measurements.

The study began in June 1972. If a patient failed to attend after the initial letter of invitation, a second one was sent. If there was no response, the individual was designated a nonrespondent. As mentioned earlier, we used the practice's age/sex register as our sampling frame. Table 5 illustrates some of the problems this created. The original number of men aged 35-64 years was supposedly 1,612. Twenty of these were incorrectly registered in that they appeared twice or were, in fact, women; a further 129 were no longer on the list when the study started. The list was, in fact, 9% inflated, which is a little below average for England and Wales. During the course of the 18-month screening, 153 more patients were removed from the list. This meant that the actual number of patients left for possible screening was 1,310. We have now identified 1,008 men, giving us a response rate of 77%. We are at present making personal visits to all the nonrespondents.

We would now like to discuss some of our findings on the patients seen so far. Even though we have identified 1,008 men,

TABLE 5.

Original age/sex register	1,612
Incorrectly registered	20
Off the list at start of the study	129
Off the list during the screening	153
Data collected	1,008
Unaccounted for	25
Nonresponders	277
Original age/sex register inflated by (149/1612)	9.2%
Response rate (1008/1310)	76.9%

TABLE 6. Proportion of Patients With Different
Levels of Diastolic Blood Pressure
(Men Aged 35-64 Years)

Level DBP	Patients	
	Number	Percentage
89 mm Hg or below	680	73.0
90-114 mm Hg	229	24.5
115 mm Hg or above	23	2.5
Total	932	100.0

76 of these were excluded without measurements since they were bedridden or chronically ill. Thus to date we have measured the blood pressure twice on at least one occasion on 932 patients. The results take the mean of the two readings and Table 6 shows how the measurements fall into three categories: 89 mm Hg or below; 90-114 inclusive; and 115 and above. Seventy-three percent of the patients had diastolic pressures below 90 mm Hg and 24.5% between 90 and 114 mm Hg. One hundred and two patients, or 10% of the base population screened, were eventually entered into the trial. Patients were stratified by age and randomly allocated to either treatment or control groups.

The control group receive a placebo tagged with Riboflavine which is given as a fixed dose. The design is single blind so that the patients are unaware that the tablets are inactive. The treatment group is started on a diuretic also tagged with Riboflavine. The aim of treatment is to reduce and maintain diastolic blood pressure below 90 mm Hg. If the diuretic fails to achieve this degree of control, we add a hypotensive agent. In addition to checking for urine fluorescence we make pill counts, since we feel that it is important to acquire some idea of patients' cooperation in a treatment trial of this nature. As mentioned previously, to show a reduction in mortality and morbidity by treatment leaves unanswered the problem of whether those offered treatment can tolerate the long-term commitment, both in terms of remembering to take the tablets and of tolerating side effects should they arise.

Of the patients so far randomized to the treatment group, 85% are controlled on Navidrex K once or twice a day. Looking at those patients who have been in the treatment or control group for at least six months — namely, 37 in the former and 39 in the latter — the fall of mean diastolic pressure in the controls was from 99.2 mm Hg to 96 mm Hg and in the treatment group from 99.8 mm Hg to 90.1 mm Hg. The aim of treatment is to reduce diastolic blood pressure to below 90 mm Hg. It is clear that we have not been totally successful in this and will have to increase treatment slightly more rapidly or develop a more rigid regimen of stepwise care.

This trial then has highlighted a number of problems. The first of these has been the response rate and the number of individuals to be included in the study. We used the age/sex register which is supposed to identify all individuals on the practice list. Our experience has shown that this is overly optimistic. This may imply that we shall require using more practices than we thought necessary in designing the proper study. One of the other problems has been that fewer patients were admitted to the trial by the criteria used than would normally be expected from epidemiological evidence of blood pressure distribution. Presumably, this is because we only admitted individuals who had appropriate levels of blood pressure on four occasions, and because the general practitioners excluded more patients on medical grounds than we had expected. The practitioners had some anxiety about lowering blood pressure too rapidly even when moderate and were also uneasy about lowering it much below 90 mm Hg. It is obvious that in such a trial using the average general practitioners, more supervision and exhortation will be required to achieve satisfactory levels of maintenance of blood pressure for those on treatment.

In the future design of a trial of treatment of moderately raised blood pressure in general practice in the United Kingdom, therefore, three main points must be considered carefully. These may be summarized as follows:

1. Size of group to be studied.

2. Training and cooperation of general practitioners. Many general practitioners are unwilling to undertake the rigors of a properly controlled trial and the sort of treatment that is necessary.

3. Measurement of adherence to the medication. We do not yet know whether patients are willing to continue to take drugs

for the period required in such long-term therapy. Certainly our experience in general practice is more encouraging than our experience in hospitals. Of those entered into the community-based trial, more than 75% are still present after 18 months.

It is likely that we shall have to educate general practitioners far more extensively about the problems of such trials and the difficulties of treatment before we can undertake the sort of trial required to answer the question in the United Kingdom. An alternative, of course, would be to pay the general practitioners for doing such an investigation, but this raises complex ethical issues.

This paper has attempted to highlight some of the problems facing workers undertaking research in the field of hypertension and its treatment. It is clear from our own experience that to attempt to solve the problems of performing studies using hospital populations by moving out into the community is only partially successful and that it creates new dilemmas that must be faced and coped with.

References

1. Departments of Medicine and Clinical Epidemiology and Social Medicine, St. Thomas's Hospital Medical School, London, and Department of Medicine, United Cardiff Hospitals, and the Medical Research Council Epidemiological Research Unit, Cardiff: Control of moderately raised blood pressure. Report of a co-operative randomised controlled trial. *Brit. Med. J.*, 3:434-436, 1973.
2. Gifford, R. W.: Milbank Memorial Fund Quarterly XLVII, 170, 1969.
3. Morrell, D. C., Gage, H. G. and Robinson, N. A.: *J. Roy. Coll. Gen. Pract.*, 21:77, 1971.

Discussion

Dr. Borhani: Do I understand you correctly that the general practitioners, once they screened and identified hypertensives, treated these patients themselves without any intervention on your part, in terms of either education or direction?

Dr. Holland: The results that I have given you are from one group practice of four doctors who met with us for about 15 months, in 1966-1967, to decide on the criteria for treatment and the treatment to be given once an individual has been detected as having an abnormality. This included hypertension. We did not control whether they gave the appropriate treatment. We are now going through their records to find out what drugs, if any, they had used. In our other studies we have not seen any major side effects.

Dr. Winkelstein: While you have said that there were no side effects, could there be side effects that we are not accustomed to seeking out? Are you making any effort to ascertain the reasons for a discontinuation?

Dr. Holland: We certainly looked at this in detail in the hospital-based study with a questionnaire. We were unable to detect many more in the treatment group than in the control group. Maybe there were. But the people who dropped out from the trial were the controls.

Dr. Hoobler, Michigan: Yes, I think that there is a side effect that we don't know enough about. In our personal experience in Ann Arbor there is impotency. When you really look into it you find that a substantial number of people on thiazides are affected. I would like to ask those of you who presented papers how often you really did search for this tactfully, of course, and tried to find out whether this might provide a relationship to noncompliance.

Dr. Holland: We did ask and we found one case — but he was in the control group!

Dr. Dollery: I just wanted to comment on the question of drug side effects. There are few data from the M.R.C. trials, but for some time Christopher Bulpitt of our group has been using symptom questionnaires in hypertensive patients on long-term treatment. Essentially, what Bulpitt found in this study was a high complaint rate for many of the apparently drug-related side effects even among those who were apparently healthy and not on drugs.

Dr. Holland: However, I think there is a difference if the majority of patients are only on diuretics.

Dr. Smith: A further comment on the side effect issue. It is very clear that one not only has to ask the question as to how patients feel in general in order to get at side effects, but also to query on a number of specific items repeatedly, beginning with *prior* to the onset of treatment. In the Public Health Service trial, in which all subjects in the treatment group have been on thiazides, this procedure for assessing side effects has been followed and incidence of male lack or loss of potency has been identical in the control and treated group.

The Veterans Administration Cooperative Study

Edward D. Freis, M.D.

The goal of the Veterans Study was to determine whether reduction of blood pressure with antihypertensive agents would protect against the major complications of essential hypertension. The study was begun in 1963 and comprised 523 male veteran patients in 16 Veterans Administration Hospitals whose prerandomization blood pressures, as measured in the outpatient clinics, averaged between 90 and 129 mm Hg.

Characteristics of Patients and Plan of Trial

Since the patients presented at the hospital with some sort of complaint, they exhibited a higher prevalence of cardiovascular abnormalities than would be the case if case finding had been carried out by screening asymptomatic individuals in the community. Thus, 58% had some cardiovascular abnormality detectable either by history, physical examination or laboratory studies. Approximately 25% had cardiomegaly by x-ray and 16% had left ventricular hypertrophy by electrocardiogram; 7% had a history of myocardial infarction, 8% of prior congestive heart failure and 5% had a prior cerebral thrombosis.[1] Patients with a history of malignant hypertension, cerebral or subarachnoid hemorrhage or azotemia were excluded.

The median age was 49.2 years for the control group and 48.1 years for the treated series. Fourteen percent of patients were below 40 years of age and 21% were age 60 or older. The average known duration of hypertension was five years, but the actual duration of hypertension probably was considerably longer than this.

Edward D. Freis, M.D., *Senior Medical Investigator, Veterans Administration and Chairman of the Veterans Administration Cooperative Study on Antihypertensive Agents, Washington, D. C.*

Before entering the study, all patients were admitted to the hospital for work-up and for measurement of basal blood pressure which was taken three times daily. Those whose diastolic blood pressures averaged below 90 mm Hg from the fourth through the sixth hospital day were rejected, thereby excluding patients with labile hypertension.

Because of the factors indicated above, the patients in the Veterans Administration trial were at considerably higher risk than the average patient with essential hypertension. Target organ damage was detectable in nearly 60% of the group, the hypertension was of long duration and the blood pressure remained elevated during hospitalization.

A further selection of patients was carried out with respect to compliance. Prior to randomization the patients entered a prerandomization trial period in which they were given known placebos containing riboflavin. Pill counts were done and urinary fluorescence produced by riboflavin was tested under ultraviolet light. Only those patients whose fluorescence was positive and whose pill counts were within the acceptable range for two successive clinic visits were admitted to the trial. It should be emphasized that the question being asked in the trial was whether antihypertensive agents protect against major complications. To answer this question it was essential that all patients on active drugs take their medications. Quantitatively different results probably would have been obtained in an unselected population where some patients would be compliant and others would not.

The patients were randomly assigned, double-blind, to either a combination of active drugs or to placebos. The active combination of drugs consisted of hydrochlorothiazide 50 mg twice daily plus 0.1 mg reserpine twice daily plus 25 or 50 mg hydralazine three times daily. Provision was made for reducing drugs or dosage in the event of hypotensive symptoms.

Results in Patients With Initial Diastolic
Levels of 115-129 mm Hg

The results are best reported in two subsets. The first comprises 143 patients with initial diastolic blood pressures between 115 and 129 mm Hg and the second, 380 patients with diastolic levels between 90 and 114 mm Hg. The trial was terminated in the more severe group after an average post-randomization follow-up of only 15.7 months in the placebo treated patients and 20.7 months for the active drug group.[2] The briefer period of follow-up of patients in the placebo group was caused by the high incidence of severe complications necessitating their early removal from the trial.

Whereas during the postrandomization period there was no significant change in blood pressure in the placebo group, there was a marked reduction in the active drug group. For example, at eight months following randomization, the diastolic among the actively treated patients averaged 29 mm Hg below the prerandomization level as compared to no essential change in the placebo group.

As indicated in Table 1, of the 70 patients randomized on placebos, 27 developed major complications. By contrast, only

TABLE 1. Morbid Events by Diagnosis
(115-129 mm Hg)

| Diagnosis | Control Group | | Treated Group |
	Total	Terminating	Total
Accelerated hypertension	7	7	0
Strokes	4	2	1
Congestive heart failure	4	2	0
Renal damage	3	3	0
Myocardial infarction	3	1	0
High diastolic pressure	3	3	0
Aortic rupture	3	3	0
Total	27	21	1

one cardiovascular complication occurred among the 73 patients treated with active drugs. One other actively treated patient had to be removed from the study because of a depression presumably related to reserpine and hyperglycemia secondary to the thiazide diuretic. The morbid events occurring in the control group were predominantly those associated with severe hypertension. The most frequent complication was "accelerated hypertension" with the appearance of hemorrhages, exudates or papilledema in the optic fundi, dissecting aneurysm in two of the four fatal cases and congestive heart failure. Stroke or early renal failure occurred in a few patients.[2] Atherosclerotic complications were uncommon.

Results in Patients With Initial Diastolic
Levels of 90-114 mm Hg

Mortality and Morbidity

The remaining 380 patients whose clinic diastolic blood pressures averaged between 90-114 mm Hg prior to randomization were followed for an average period of 3.3 years, the longest period of follow-up being 5.5 years.[3] As in the more severe patients, blood pressure was significantly reduced in the treatment group and was unaffected in the placebo treated patients. Nineteen of the patients in the control group died of cardiovascular complications as compared to eight in the treated group. Of the deaths in the control group, seven were due to stroke as compared to one in the actively treated patients. Myocardial infarction and sudden death combined represented the most frequent cause of death occurring in 11 of the control patients and 6 of the actively treated group (Table 2).

The incidence of all cardiovascular complications, nonfatal as well as fatal, is best presented by the life-table method of analysis (Fig. 1). By this method, the cumulative incidence rate at five years for the control group rises to 55%, whereas for the treated group the incidence is only 18%, an approximate 3:1 difference in favor of treatment. The significance of the difference yielded a t-value of 5.0 which is highly significant. In addition to the patients who developed cardiovascular complications there were 20 patients who were removed from the trial because their blood pressures rose to 125 mm Hg or higher and remained elevated for three weekly clinic visits. All 20 were in

TABLE 2. Causes of Death in Patients with Initial
Diastolic Blood Pressures of 90-114 mm Hg

Cause	Placebo Group	Treated Group
Hemorrhagic stroke	4	0
Thrombotic stroke	3	1
Sudden death	8	4
Myocardial infarction	3	2
Dissecting aneurysm	1	0
Atherosclerotic aneurysm	0	1
Total cardiovascular deaths	19	8

ALL MORBID EVENTS

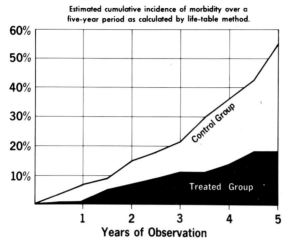

Fig. 1. Cumulative percentage incidence of morbidity over a five-year period as estimated by the life-table method of analysis in the control group as compared to the actively treated group of patients with prerandomization diastolic blood pressures averaging between 90 and 114 mm Hg.

the control group. If they had been retained in the trial, the incidence of morbid events in the control group probably would have been higher than that actually observed.

Diagnostic Categories

When the events were classified into diagnostic categories, it was evident that all of the various cardiovascular complications associated with hypertension appeared to be prevented or at least reduced by treatment except those complications associated with coronary artery disease. The incidence of myocardial infarction was essentially the same in the two groups as was the occurrence of heart blocks and atrial fibrillation. On the other hand, stroke was only one fourth as common in the treated patients while congestive heart failure, accelerated hypertension and renal damage were limited exclusively to the control patients. Whereas the incidence of atherosclerotic complications was low in the patients with diastolic levels of 115-129 mm Hg, such complications predominated in the patients with the lower initial diastolic pressures of 90-114 mm Hg.

Blood Pressure, Age and Race

When the group with initial diastolic blood pressures of 90-114 mm Hg were subdivided into those with levels of 90-104 and those with levels of 105-114 mm Hg, it was evident that the benefit of treatment was greatest in the latter group. Specifically, in the 105-114 subset, the incidence of morbid events was four times greater in the control group as compared to the treated patients. However, in the 90-104 subset, the incidence ratio of control to treated patients was only 1.5:1.0. The former was a significant difference whereas the latter was not. Almost all of the complications occurring in the treated patients with initial diastolic levels of 90-104 were those associated with coronary artery disease.

The incidence of complications in both the control and treated patients rose with age and was very high above age 60. However, the benefit of treatment was apparent at all ages. While there appeared to be little protection against myocardial infarction or disturbances in cardiac rhythm or conduction in the age group above 60, there was considerable difference in the incidence of stroke and a complete absence of congestive heart failure in the treated patients. Approximately 42% of the patients were black. The effectiveness of treatment was the same in the black as in the white patients.

Electrocardiogram

Electrocardiograms were taken in 280 of the 380 patients before and at yearly intervals during treatment.[4] In patients who had no signs of left ventricular hypertrophy prior to randomization, the incidence of abnormal QRS voltage, ST-segment depression or T wave flattening or inversion was only one fourth that found in the control group. Also, in patients with signs of left ventricular hypertrophy prior to randomization, the reversion to normal of QRS voltage or ST-segment depression was approximately 2.5 times greater in the treated than in the control patients. No effect of treatment was noted on the electrocardiographic manifestations of coronary artery disease such as Q and QS patterns, conduction defects or arrhythmias.

Degree of Blood Pressure Reduction

The data also were analyzed with respect to the importance of normalizing the blood pressure in preventing major complications.[5] Blood pressures recorded on the treated patients at the four month visit after randomization were used to select two subgroups. Subgroup A comprised 67 treated patients who exhibited diastolic levels of 90 or higher after four months of active treatment (partial control) while subgroup B included 62 patients with diastolic levels of 80 mm Hg or less (good control). In subgroup A, 14.9% developed morbid events during an average follow-up of 3.2 years while in subgroup B, 9.7% developed complications. The incidence of morbid events in subgroup A was significantly less than the 28.9% of patients in the untreated control group who developed major complications. These results suggest that while treatment is somewhat more effective when the blood pressure is controlled at normotensive levels, considerable therapeutic benefit still can be obtained with only partial control of the hypertension.

Discussion

The results of the Veterans Administration trial leave no doubt that antihypertensive drug treatment is effective in patients with diastolic blood pressures averaging 105 mm Hg or above. All of the patients were men and it is not certain that these results can be applied directly to women. In patients with diastolic blood pressures below 105 mm Hg, the results of the present study were equivocal in that the incidence of events was somewhat but not significantly less in the treated as compared to the control group.

The failure to find a significant difference between control and treated patients with mild hypertension was associated with the fact that the majority of their complications were related to coronary artery disease and that treatment appeared to have no effect on this condition. However, due to the long natural history of atherosclerosis and the relatively short duration of the trial it is possible that many of the patients who developed such complications already had extensive atherosclerosis of their coronary arteries prior to randomization. Therefore, they would not be expected to achieve a preventive effect from treatment. It is possible that a trial carried out in younger individuals in an earlier stage of their hypertensive disorder might yield different results.

In the patients with the highest diastolic blood pressures, the predominant complications were those specifically related to hypertension such as the accelerated phase of hypertension, congestive heart failure and renal damage. Treatment was most effective in preventing these complications. In the patients with mildest elevations of diastolic blood pressure, the predominant complications were associated with atherosclerosis for which treatment was the least effective. Hypertension aggravates and accelerates atherosclerosis. The two disorders go hand in hand. It appears likely that further advance in the prevention of complications in hypertension will depend upon the development of effective measures for reducing or arresting the rate of progression of atherosclerosis, particularly of the coronary arteries.

References

1. Veterans Administration Cooperative Study Group on Antihypertensive Agents: Effects of treatment on morbidity in hypertension. III. Influence of age, diastolic pressure, and prior cardiovascular disease; further analysis of side effects. *Circulation*, 45:991-1004, 1972.
2. —— I. Results in patients with diastolic blood pressures averaging 115 through 129 mm Hg. *JAMA*, 202:1028-1034, 1967.
3. —— II. Results in patients with diastolic blood pressure averaging 90 through 114 mm Hg. *JAMA*, 213:1143-1152, 1970.
4. Poblete, P. F., Kyle, M. C., Pipberger, H. V. et al: Effect of treatment on morbidity in hypertension. Veterans Administration Cooperative Study on Antihypertensive Agents. Effect on the electrocardiogram. *Circulation*, 48:481-490, 1973.
5. Taguchi, J. and Freis, E. D.: Partial reduction of blood pressure and prevention of complications in hypertension. *New Eng. J. Med.* (Scheduled for publication August 15th.)

Discussion

Dr. Tyroler: I wonder if you have had the opportunity to look at the control group. If I saw your data correctly, approximately one third of the untreated group also had a drop in blood pressure over time, and this speaks again to the question that you raised earlier about the heterogeneity of populations of this type which may well have subpopulations.

Did you look at the incidence of morbid events in the untreated group stratifying them in the same fashion as you did the treated group in relation to change of blood pressure?

Dr. Freis: We are in the process of actually doing that, and we are also interested in the question of possible seasonal variations in blood pressure and rhythmic variation in blood pressure over a time.

Dr. Hoobler, Michigan: You are very familiar with our particular stroke study, but perhaps some in the room are not, so I will make a few points about it. This is a cooperative study and the results were recently published in *JAMA*.* We selected people with diastolic blood pressures of between 90 and 115 who had had one stroke in the past year; half were treated and half were not treated. We had comparable changes in blood pressure to Dr. Freis' study. Treatment had little influence on the recurrence rate, which was curiously not related to the blood pressure of the group, whether the higher tertile or the lower tertile. However, in some subgroups that were subjected to high natural recurrence rates there was some but not a significant reduction in the new events. It shows that at a certain point, control of blood pressure, after vascular complications have occurred, has a diminishing effect on the occurrence of new events. I am particularly interested in the 5% individuals who had a prior stroke. Do you know how many had strokes in the follow-up period?

Dr. Freis: The secondary strokes were so few that we could not do much with them.

Dr. Marienfeld, Missouri: I wonder if we are not overlooking a basic difference in Dr. Dollery's patient population group and yours, in that you used a placebo. The expectation for successful outcome of any treatment including a placebo on the part of the general practitioner's private patient compared to the VA patient may be totally different.

Dr. Dollery: It is reassuring to hear the National Health Service referred to as private practice. The comment I wanted to make was about comparability of different studies in terms of pressure criteria. The point is a very obvious one but, nevertheless, most of us repeatedly overlook it. Dr. Freis, your

*Hypertensive — Stroke Cooperative Study Group: Effect of anti-hypertensive treatment on stroke recurrence. *JAMA*, 229:409-418, 1974.

pressure criteria were the means of the last two readings in a period of placebo therapy, whereas the MRC entry criteria, if it had been adapted in that way, would have been about 5.5 mm lower. Indeed, if one's entry criteria had been the initial reading, you would have almost doubled that difference. This does have a very major implication for public health policy and hypertension control programs. We all talk about a particular range of diastolic pressures as being the range in which a particular action should be taken to do something, or nothing, or to further follow and observe. But we don't mean the same thing.

Dr. Freis: Another point is that the patients had been in the hospital before they even entered the prerandomization outpatient trial period, and they were receiving placebos. So that they were almost like the Dollery group after they had been randomized.

Dr. Curry, District of Columbia: I am curious about the type of morbid event that occurred in the 90-104 mm Hg group. In looking at 262 black patients in the Washington, D. C. area, who had experienced myocardial infarction, Dr. S. K. Chun in our department noticed that patients with the highest blood pressures had the lowest mortality. Among that group of patients in your study, were the morbid events mostly coronary events?

Dr. Freis: Yes, they were. In the treated group they were almost exclusively events related to coronary disease. It might be atrial fibrillation or heart block or something like that, but myocardial infarction and atherosclerotic events, if you consider a thrombotic stroke an atherosclerotic event, accounted entirely for the events.

Dr. Hatano: This question is particularly directed to Dr. Dollery. Is the difference between the treated group and the placebo group only attributable to the type of drug and to no other kind of intervention such as instruction about changing life styles, etc.?

Dr. Dollery: The answer is that there is no other difference and the design of the trial is that there should be no other difference.

Dr. Simpson, New Zealand: It is obvious that in many studies there is a problem with dropouts and failure to comply. Did you ever follow up the 54% who dropped out who never started to take part in the study? The corollary of these dropout rates is that if we are going to move to treat very mild hypertension, I think we have an obligation to be very efficient in our treatment and I doubt if any of us really are very efficient in our treatment at this stage.

Dr. Freis: I do not know. We are experimenting with hypertension detection follow-up clinics in the Veterans Administration now in which patient education is a large component of the program. I do not know what is really going to work out the best. I think this is a research area all of its own.

Dr. Hatano: Coming back to the same question, the reason I raise it is that in Japanese studies they use a lot of other types of instruction to regulate life style. The evaluation of such intervention is not the purpose of the British study, but there may be an effect by a change of life style of the patient under placebo.

Dr. Holland: Obviously there will be some effect because the patients are being seen regularly by their doctors who, if they have a cough, will tell them to stop smoking and if they are overweight will tell them to reduce their weight; but the active therapy is different, and the other methods of treatment are the same for both treatment and control groups.

Intervention Trial in Mild Hypertension
U.S. Public Health Service Hospitals
Cooperative Study Group[*]

W. McFate Smith, M.D., M.P.H.,
Willard P. Johnson, M.D. and Louis Bromer

Data of the Society of Actuaries,[1] the Framingham experience[2] and the Pooling Project of the Council on Epidemiology of the American Heart Association[3] leave no doubt that excess morbidity and mortality are experienced by both sexes, at all ages, and in direct proportion to the elevation of their blood pressure above diastolic levels of 80 mm Hg.

The treatment of hypertension has been guided by the presumption that intervention which lowers pressure would prevent the cardiovascular complications. Support for this hypothesis began to accumulate over a decade ago — first, in the case of the malignant phase of hypertension and, subsequently, for severe but benign primary hypertension. The reports of Hamilton,[4] Leishman[5] and Bjork[6] are noteworthy in this regard. Whereas only Hamilton's study was prospective and included concurrent controls, all demonstrated consistently an improved prognosis when pressure was lowered.

By inference, it was logical to expect that lowering the blood pressure should also improve the prognosis for less severe

*Baltimore, Boston, New Orleans, San Francisco, Seattle, Staten Island.

W. McFate Smith, M.D., M.P.H., *Chairman, U. S. Public Health Service Cooperative Study Group; Clinical Professor of Medicine, University of California School of Medicine, San Francisco;* Willard P. Johnson, M.D., *Director, EKG Center, U. S. Public Health Service Hospital, Seattle, Wash.; and* Louis Bromer, *Biostatistician, Public Health Service, Division of Hospitals, West Hyattsville, Md.*

and mild hypertension. However, in view of the natural history of the disease, which includes a long, relatively asymptomatic, uncomplicated phase, we anticipated that it might be exceedingly difficult to demonstrate.

Nonetheless, since we shared a general reluctance to commit such individuals to a lifetime of medication, which is itself not without hazard, expense and inconvenience, the Cooperative Study Group of the Public Health Service Hospitals concluded there was need for a well-designed, long-term prospective intervention trial to evaluate the influence of blood pressure control on the complications of mild to moderate hypertension.

Planning for such a study began in 1964 with the first subjects being entered in September 1966. This turned out to be less than a year after the beginning of the Veterans Administration prospective trial[7,8] with similar objectives, which confirmed the findings of Hamilton for those with diastolic blood pressures in the 115-129 mm Hg range and subsequently extended these observations of benefit to their group of subjects in the range of 90 to 114 mm Hg.

The Public Health Service intervention trial differs in a number of significant ways from the Veterans Administration study. A baseline report describing the protocol in detail and characterizing the study population has been published,[9] and only a summary of the key features and significant differences from the Veterans Administration trial will be presented here.

Selection of Cases

The investigation was designed as a primary prevention study; that is, every reasonable effort was made to exclude individuals who had already sustained demonstrable target organ damage. Also excluded were those who had known or recognizable predisposition to degenerative vascular disease.

Subjects being screened for inclusion in the study were taught to measure their own blood pressures, with accuracy being carefully checked by physicians, nurses or trained technicians. Pressures were recorded twice daily (6-12 hours apart) in the sitting position after ten minutes of quiet rest. Such measurements were recorded for four to six weeks while the subjects were off all antihypertensive medication. Pressures recorded during the final week of this period were averaged as the qualifying control. "Clinic basal" pressure, determined at each pretreatment visit, was defined as that pressure recorded after the subject sat quietly for ten minutes.

Male and female subjects up to age 55 were qualified for admission to the study if their average diastolic blood pressure during the control period was between 90 and 114 mm Hg and their "clinic basal" diastolic pressures were 90 mm Hg or greater.

Those thus qualified were admitted to the study if not excluded for the following reasons:

1. Diabetes mellitus, renal insufficiency or hypercholesterolemia ($>$ 350 mg/dl).

2. Abnormal electrocardiogram, including single or double Master's test.

3. Radiographic cardiomegaly.

4. Grade III or IV retinopathy.

5. Clinical history or findings of (a) previous arterial thrombosis or vascular insufficiency, whether coronary, cerebral or peripheral; (b) congestive heart failure; (c) angina pectoris; (d) valvular heart disease or (e) secondary or correctable hypertension.

6. Known sensitivities to the intervention agents.

Placebo Trial Period

Qualified subjects were then started on a three-month trial period on placebo medication, during which time additional baseline blood pressures and chemistries were obtained. Subjects were excluded whose diastolic pressures fell to less than 90 mm Hg on two or more of the three clinic visits during the period.

Treatment Program

At the conclusion of the trial period, subjects were randomly assigned either active or placebo treatment, and this medication was substituted for the identical placebo of the trial period and administered in double-blind fashion. Active therapy consists of chlorothiazide 500 mg plus rauwolfia serpentina 100 mg in one tablet taken twice daily, a regimen which controls blood pressure in up to 80% of such cases.[10-12]

Follow-up Procedures

Subjects are followed at bimonthly intervals with determination of blood pressure and heart rate. A pill count is made and a side effects query carried out.

Semiannually, a limited physical examination which includes funduscopy is conducted. ECG, urinalysis and determination of serum creatinine and potassium are also carried out at that time.

Annually, in addition to the above, an exercise ECG, cardiac series, creatinine clearance, serum cholesterol, triglycerides and a two-hour post-glucose serum glucose are recorded.

Morbidity Observations

The statistical end points were defined in terms of specified cardiovascular complications classified conventionally into primary, secondary and tertiary (Table 1). They have also been categorized into those morbid events considered direct complications of the elevated blood pressure and those which are predominantly arteriosclerotic complications (Table 2). The term "treatment failure" was applied only to those individuals whose blood pressure levels rose progressively or precipitously to sustained diastolic levels of 130 mm Hg or more. Such subjects were removed from the protocol and treated expeditiously using appropriate antihypertensive drugs.

Statistical Design

The design provides for both sequential (truncated binomial boundaries) and life table analysis, the former in order to recognize the earliest possible stopping point should results favor either group. Only primary end points are being used in the sequential analysis. Subjects were randomly assigned to treatment or placebo and then matched by race and sex for two broad age groups (under 46 and 46-55). This stratified randomization was carried out within each of the six participating clinics.

Morbidity data on which to base sample size and duration of follow-up were not available in the literature, so published *survival rates* were used. These were available both for mild to

TABLE 1. Classification of End Points

Primary
    Cerebral hemorrhage or thrombosis
    Myocardial infarction
    Death
        Cardiovascular disease
        Sudden
Secondary
    Coronary insufficiency
    Cerebrovascular arterial insufficiency
    Peripheral arterial insufficiency or occlusion
    Renal insufficiency
    Encephalopathy and/or malignant hypertension
    Congestive heart failure
Tertiary
    Cardiac enlargement
    ECG abnormality
        LVH/LVI
        Positive exercise test
        Arrhythmias and conduction disturbances
Treatment failure
    Accelerated hypertension

TABLE 2. Classification of Complications

Hypertensive
    Cerebral hemorrhage
    Aortic dissection
    Renal insufficiency
    Encephalopathy or retinopathy Grade III or IV
    Malignant or accelerated hypertension
    Cardiac enlargement
    Left ventricular hypertrophy
Atherosclerotic
    Cerebral thrombosis
    Myocardial infarction
    Coronary insufficiency
        Angina pectoris
        ECG abnormality − ischemia, arrhythmias,
        and conduction disturbances
    Claudication syndromes

moderate hypertension[13-16] and for the general male population of the same age groups not dying of cardiovascular
diseases.[17] Curves fitted to the survival rates for the two groups
(Fig. 1) reveal that after ten years of follow-up, mild to
moderate hypertensive patients had a survival rate of 65%
compared to 85% for the general male population.

It was calculated that in order to demonstrate with a high
degree of confidence (α 0.05, β 0.05) that the survival rate of
treated hypertensives was comparable to that of the normotensive population, 328 subjects (164 matched pairs) would be
required in this truncated sequential design.[18] This assumes
that the magnitude of difference to be expected between the
treated and nontreated groups would be of the same order of
magnitude as illustrated in Figure 1.

Morbidity rates were expected to be somewhat higher than
fatality rates, giving rise to a projection that the desired degree
of difference would be seen earlier. Seven years was estimated,
and on the basis of anticipated dropouts over that period of
time, a final sample size of 400 to 450 subjects was considered
desirable.

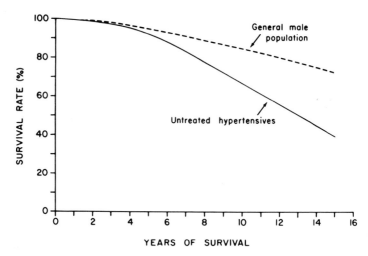

Fig. 1. Survival rates of mild to moderate hypertensive patients and general
male population of initial age 45 to 49 who did not die of cardiovascular
diseases.[13,21] This figure was previously published by the same authors[9]
and is published here by permission of the American Heart Association.

Characteristics of the Study Population

Of the 422 subjects admitted to the study, 33 were subsequently disqualified as misadmissions, leaving 389 for follow-up and analysis.[9]

The subjects averaged 44 years of age with minimal variation of the distribution by race or sex. Only 20% of the sample under study is female, which reflects a characteristic of the beneficiary population of the Public Health Service Hospitals. Non-whites constitute 23% of the group. Fifty-nine percent of the participants had received no prior therapy for hypertension, and of those who had, 90% appeared to have responded satisfactorily. Approximately one third had never smoked cigarettes, but another 25% were previous smokers, so that at the time of entry nearly one half were smokers.

The pretreatment home control blood pressure averaged 148/99 mm Hg with the highest frequency distribution of systolic pressures in the range of 140 to 149 and diastolics 90 to 95 (Table 3).

TABLE 3. Control Blood Pressure

Pressure (mm Hg)	Total No.	%	Active Treatment No.	%	Placebo Treatment No.	%
Subjects	389	100.0	193	100.0	196	100.0
Systolic						
<140	105	27.0	52	26.9	53	27.0
140-159	216	55.5	111	57.5	105	53.6
160-179	60	15.4	29	15.0	31	15.8
180-199	6	1.5	1	0.5	5	2.6
>199	2	0.5	–	–	2	1.0
Average	147.8		146.8		148.7	
S.D.	13.5		12.4		14.5	
Diastolic						
90-95	152	39.1	77	39.9	75	38.3
96-100	91	23.4	41	21.2	50	25.5
101-105	66	17.0	31	16.1	35	17.8
106-110	41	10.5	23	11.9	18	9.2
111-115	39	10.0	21	10.9	18	9.2
Average	99.3		99.5		99.1	
S.D.	6.9		7.1		6.9	

TABLE 4. Electrocardiographic Data in 389 Subjects

	No.	%
Hypervoltage (LVH)		
$S_{vl} + R_{v5}$ or $R_{v6} > 35$ mm	53	13.6
Deepest S_v + tallest $R_v > 45$ mm	43	11.1
R_{v5} or $R_{v6} > 26$ mm	23	5.9
Total by at least one	63	16.2

It is important to note that 79.5% of the participants have pretreatment diastolic blood pressures in the range of 90-105 mm Hg.

Left ventricular hypertrophy (LVH) defined as electrocardiographic hypervoltage was found in 16.2% of subjects by at least one of three separate criteria (Table 4).

Using Scheie's criteria for optic fundi grading[19] in which "hypertensive" and "sclerotic" changes are graded separately on a scale of 0 to IV, over 90% had Grade I or less "hypertensive" changes and only 8.2% had sclerotic changes greater than Grade I.

As reported earlier,[9] the average serum cholesterol level was 224 mg% with only 14% exceeding 260 mg%. The mean triglyceride level was 165 mg%, and the mean value for serum glucose two hours after a 100 gm load was 106.4 mg%. Serum uric acid averaged 6.2 mg% with 14.4% exceeding 8.0 mg%. Eight subjects had a clinical diagnosis of gout.

The distribution of all pretreatment characteristics into the active drug and placebo groups was uniform.

The Veterans Administration study was not a primary prevention trial in that subjects with known or demonstrable target organ disease or previous cardiovascular complications were not excluded.[20] For example, over 50% (Table 5) had a cardiac, CNS or renal abnormality. One in five had either a prior myocardial infarction, a stroke or previous congestive failure. Three times as many subjects (more than one in four) had Grade II hypertensive changes in the optic fundi.

These abnormalities were more frequent in the older patients. For example, 46% of those under age 50 had one or more compared to 65% of those age 50-59 and 78% of the patients above age 59 years. This is particularly notable in

TABLE 5.

	U.S. Public Health Service	Veterans Administration
Average age	44.4 years	51 years
Under age 50	80%	53%
Under age 46	49.4%	–
Over age 55	0	–
Age 60 or more	0	21.3%
Black	23.1%	41%
Male	80%	100%
Control systolic pressure	148 mm Hg	157 mm Hg
Control diastolic pressure	99 mm Hg	101 mm Hg
Duration known hypertension	–	4.5 years
Duration 5 years or more	2.8%	48%
Cardiac enlargement	0	25%
LVH	*16.2%	**16.3%
Cholesterol	224 mg/dl	247 mg/dl
Optic fundi – Grade II	8.7%	27.9%
Any cardiac, CNS or renal abnormality	0	57.6%
Myocardial infarction	0	7.1%
Congestive heart failure	0	7.6%
Cerebral thrombosis	0	5.0%

*Hypervoltage; **Hypervoltage plus ST & T abnormality.

comparisons with the Public Health Service study population which averaged six years younger and included no one over age 55. Twenty-one percent of the Veterans Administration patients were age 60 or more.

In further contrast, 16.3% of the Veterans Administration subjects had definite LVH by ECG and 25% had radiographic cardiac enlargement. In the Public Health Service trial, none had either cardiac enlargement or definite LVH by ECG. Hypervoltage without ST or T wave abnormalities was present in 16.2%.

Two points deserve emphasis: first, the VA population was at significantly greater risk of developing cardiovascular complications; second, most of the morbid events (42 of 56 in the control group) occurred in those at greatest risk as a result of preexisting target organ damage. In fact, 37.3% of control subjects with prior abnormalities sustained subsequent morbid events, while only 16.1% of those without prior abnormalities had complications during the trial. The strong association of

this greater risk with age is evident when one notes that 41 of
the 56 events in the control group occurred in subjects age 50
or older, with nearly half of all events (27) occurring in the
group over 59 years of age.

One final comparison deserves mention. As Dr. Freis has
emphasized since publishing these data in 1970,[8] most of the
events occurred in the group of subjects whose diastolic blood
pressure was in the range of 105 to 114 mm Hg. This group
constituted over 54% of the study population. This stands in
marked contrast to the PHS trial where nearly 80% of subjects'
pressures were in the 90-104 mm Hg range. Even so, both age
and the presence of cardiovascular abnormalities at entry had a
greater influence on subsequent attack rates than did entry level
of blood pressure. Indeed, it has been concluded that patients
with pretreatment diastolic blood pressures in the range of 90
to 104 mm Hg derived very little benefit from therapy unless
they had cardiovascular abnormalities at entry or were over 50
years of age, and that a longer period of observation would be
needed in order to assess the value of treatment in lower risk
subgroups.

Results

In view of the foregoing, it should come as no surprise to
anyone that after an average follow-up period of over five years,
based on the primary end points of myocardial infarction,
stroke and death, a stopping point has not been reached. On the
other hand, considerable new data on the incidence of
secondary and tertiary end points and their preventability with
antihypertensive agents are emerging. These end points are
themselves known to be associated with increased risk when
present.

Of equal importance to the question of whether to employ
drugs in the management of mild hypertension is the extensive
experience and data base being accumulated concerning the
long-term side effects and toxicity of the drugs employed.
Particularly in the lower risk subgroups, side effects and
long-term toxicity assume greater weight in the cost/benefit
equation.

The results presented here will describe the present status of
all admissions, the drug effects and side effects, the morbidity

TABLE 6. Status of Admissions – Average Follow-up – 64 Months

	Total		Treatment		Control	
	No.	%	NO.	%	NO.	%
Admissions	422	–	211	–	211	–
Misadmissions	33	–	18	–	15	–
Net admissions	389	100.0	193	100.0	196	100.0
Terminations (of coded therapy)	159	40.9	66	34.2	93	47.4
Withdrawal from study	43	11.1	19	9.9	24	12.2
Lost to follow-up	59	15.2	28	14.5	31	15.8
Alive	36	–	16	–	20	–
Status unknown	23	–	12	–	11	–
Drug intolerance	19	4.9	16	–	3	–
Morbid events	21	5.4	3	–	18	–
Deaths	(4)	–	(2)	–	(2)	–
Treatment failure	17	4.4	0	–	17	4.4
Remain on coded therapy	230	59.1	127	65.8	103	52.6
Remain under follow-up	312	80.2	155	80.3	157	80.1

experience of the control group (with some comparisons to the Veterans Administration experience) and ECG changes observed in the treatment and control groups.

Follow-up time ranges from three to eight years with a mean of 64 months. One hundred fifty-nine have been terminated from their assigned regimen (Table 6). Fifty-nine (15.2%) of these have been lost to follow-up. Drug intolerance necessitated termination in 19 cases and major morbid events in 21, four of which were deaths. At present, 80.2% remain under active follow-up and 59.1% are still on their assigned regimen.

Drug Effects

The active drug treatment group continues to show a decrease in mean serum potassium of approximately 0.5 mEq/liter compared to no change in the control group. However, overt or clinically significant hypokalemia remains to be seen. An attempt has been made to correlate hypokalemia (serum $K < 3.5$ mEq/liter) with central ECG readings of changes consistent with hypokalemia. Sixty percent of subjects with "hypokalemia" ECGs had serum potassium values in excess of 3.5 mEq/liter, and 65% of subjects with serum hypokalemia had normal ECGs. Approximately 25% of all subjects have had one or more serum potassium values below 3.5 mEq/liter.

Serum uric acid values in the treatment group have shown an average rise of approximately 1.0 mg/dl compared to no change in the control group. However, only three subjects have developed clinical gout during the study and two of these were in the control group.

The tendency reported earlier for the treatment group to have higher post 100 gm load serum glucose levels than the controls has diminished, and in the cohort followed 48 months, no difference is present.

Side Effects

Over half (55.4%) of all subjects on active therapy have reported side effects, while in the placebo group, similar effects were reported in one third. The side effects of rauwolfia, namely, nasal congestion, lethargy and drowsinesss, and alteration of sleep habits, have been most frequent, with nasal congestion being the dominant voluntary complaint. However, intolerable side effects have occurred in only 19 subjects, two of which were in the control group. In only two cases has the medication been terminated because of mental depression, although 14% have acknowledged some depressive symptoms. Such symptoms have occurred in the active treatment group twice as frequently as in the controls. Impotence has been reported in equal numbers of the active and placebo treatment groups.

Morbidity in the Control Group

Seventy-five subjects (38.3%) have sustained 103 morbid events (Table 7) for an event rate per 100 subjects of 52.6. The age and pretreatment blood pressure level of these subjects did not differ significantly from that of those without events. There was also no higher rate of events in those with diastolic blood pressures greater than 105 mm Hg compared to those below that level.

Seventy-one of the events were classified as "hypertensive," but only three of those were primary end points (cerebrovascu-

TABLE 7. Morbid Events in Control Group
USPHS Cooperative Study
64 Months Follow-up

	No.	Rate Per 100 Subjects
Total subjects	196	–
Total with events	75	38.3
Total events	103	52.6
Total hypertensive	71	36.2
CVA	3	1.5
LVH (possible)	23	11.7
LVH (definite)	13	6.6
LVI	17	8.7
Cardiomegaly	10	5.1
Retinopathy	5	2.6
Total atherosclerotic	32	16.3
Myocardial infarct	7	3.6
Sudden death	2	1.0
Other CHD	23	11.7
Treatment failures	17	8.7

lar accidents). Thirty-two were "atherosclerotic" complications, nine of which were primary end points. There were 17 treatment failures (progressive rise in blood pressure).

The highest event rate was 11.7 per 100 subjects and occurred for electrocardiographic hypervoltage (possible LVH) and for manifestations of coronary heart disease (CHD) other than myocardial infarction or sudden death.

Definite left ventricular hypertrophy (LVH) and left ventricular ischemia (LVI) were the next most frequent morbid events; when combined, they accounted for an event rate of 15.3/100 subjects.

Table 8 lists the 56 morbid events by category that occurred in the control group of the VA study II who were followed for approximately 40 months. Also shown is the incidence of comparable events in the control group of the PHS Study at 64 months observation. This comparison underscores the significant differences in risk between the subjects in the two studies and lends further pertinence to the question of whether mild uncomplicated hypertension requires drug therapy in its management.

TABLE 8. Morbid Events in Control Subjects

Observation Period	VA (II) 40 Months		USPHS 64 Months	
	No.	%	No.	%
Strokes	20	10.3	3	1.5
Coronary heart disease	13	6.7	9	4.6
Congestive heart failure	11	–	0	–
"Accelerated" hypertension or renal damage	7	–	0	–
Dissecting aneurysm	2	–	0	–
Atrial fibrillation	2	–	2	–
Conduction defect	1	–	1	–
	56	28.9	15	7.6
Treatment failure	20	10.3	17	8.6
Total subjects	194	100.0	196	100.0

Electrocardiographic Changes

ECG voltage, when examined as a single variable within our total population of hypertensives, distributes itself with respect to age in the same way as has been reported for normotensives.[21] Thus, total ECG amplitude tends to decrease with age (Fig. 2).

Since the duration of hypertension might be construed as an important determinant of the development and amount of LVH, it is interesting that the older hypertensive, who presumably has had hypertension longest, tends to have lower voltage than the younger hypertensive whose myocardium has presumably had the least exposure to elevations of pressure and pressure-work.

QRS voltage dropped in the group of patients given active drug and remained unchanged in the group given placebo (Fig. 3). This phenomenon was apparent at the first six months of follow-up and has not changed after nearly six years. It is interesting to note that placebo patients as a group have not developed higher voltage with time.

If the Sokolow voltage criteria (S_{v1} and R_{v5} or $R_{v6} > 35mm$) are used to define hypervoltage, a total of 33 have developed it since entering the study (Table 9). Twenty-three of these were on placebo and 10 were on active drugs. An additional 59 had hypervoltage at entry into the study, 25 of whom received active drugs and 34 placebo. Nearly one half of the latter

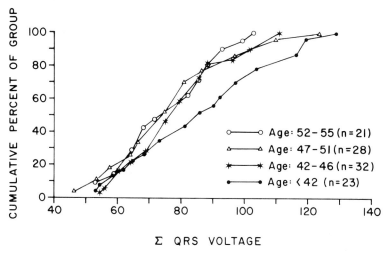

Fig. 2. Relationship of QRS voltage to age in 104 hypertensive subjects. A method has been devised for assessing QRS amplitude that minimizes the effect of body build and direction of QRS vector. QRS voltage is expressed as the sum of the R in AVL, the largest R in any of the limb leads, the deepest limb lead S wave, the S waves of precordial leads V_1 and V_2, and the R waves of V_5 and V_6. The resulting sum (Σ QRS) has the advantage of being a single value which incorporates most published criteria in common usage.

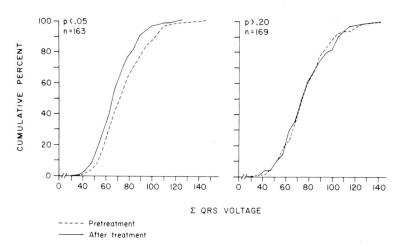

Fig. 3. QRS voltage changes in 163 drug treated subjects and 169 controls after six or more months.

TABLE 9. Left Ventricular Hypertrophy – ECG Hypervoltage

	Pretreatment						Developed During Study			
	Total	%	Treatment	%	Control	%	No.	Treatment	Control	%
Patients	59		25		34		33	10	23	
Events	19	33.1	4	16.0	15	44.1	7	1	6	26.0
Myocardial infarction	1		1		0		2	1	1	
Death	1		1		0		1	0	1	
CVA	0		0		0		0	0	0	
CHF	0		0		0		0	0	0	
Enlarged heart	3		0		3		1	0	1	
Other	14		2		12		3	0	3	

experienced subsequent morbid events, while only 16% of those on active drugs did so. Of those who developed hypervoltage, only one of the 10 on active drugs sustained an additional event, compared to six of 23 who were on placebo. This suggests that if untreated, subjects with hypervoltage are more likely to have other events, and subjects without hypervoltage are more likely to develop it. However, its presence or development has not been associated with a greater incidence of stroke, myocardial infarction, death or congestive heart failure.

Left ventricular ischemia (LVI) has developed in 40 subjects in 18 of whom it was associated with hypervoltage (Table 10). Thirty of these subjects were in the placebo group. Whether or not associated with hypervoltage, the incidence of LVI was tripled in the control group.

Twenty-eight subjects developed a positive double Master's test (DMT) after entry into the study (Table 10). Seventeen of these were on active drug; 11 on placebo. Several of the early cases developing positive DMT had resting ECGs suggestive of hypokalemia, with the abnormal DMT reverting to normal after oral potassium supplements. The protocol was therefore modified to require the retesting of all positive DMT after three weeks of oral K supplementation.

It can be seen that nearly two thirds of all subjects retested after K supplementation reverted to normal, and this was equally true for the treatment and control groups. Only five of 23 retested proved not to be reversible.

TABLE 10. Left Ventricular Ischemia – ECG

	No.	Treatment	No.	Control
Total subjects		193		196
With hypervoltage		5		13
Without hypervoltage		5		17
Total events		10		30
Abnormal Double Master's Test				
Initially positive	17	100%	11	100%
Not retested	3		2	
Retested (1 or more times)	14		9	
Reverted to normal	11	65%	7	64%
Irreversible	3		2	

Summary and Conclusions

The Public Health Service intervention trial is addressing the question of whether significant benefit derives from the drug treatment of mild, relatively early, uncomplicated hypertension. The Veterans Administration study did not directly address this question, but to the extent that the data permitted, suggested that such patients derived very little benefit from therapy. It was logically concluded that a longer period of observation would be required to assess the value of treatment.

The PHS trial is set up as a seven to ten year study with a sequential design which employs the primary end points of myocardial infarction, stroke and death in the determination of the stopping point. After 64 months of observation, the stopping point has not been reached.

The experience to date is that whereas morbid events are occurring at a significant rate, they are preponderantly of the secondary or tertiary category and would have to be considered minor in terms of clinical severity. In the control group, the most interesting observations are the rates of development of electrocardiographic LVH and LVI which had a combined rate of 27.0 per 100 subjects. These changes and coronary disease other than myocardial infarction are themselves significant elements of risk for premature death or disability from degenerative vascular disease and cannot, therefore, be dismissed lightly. It may be significant that these events occur less frequently in the treated group and that, when already present, they are associated with fewer other complications when the blood pressure is being treated. It is fortunate that although side effects are frequent, toxicity per se has been rare and intolerable side effects requiring discontinuance of drugs uncommon.

Overt or clinical hypokalemia has not occurred and acute gout has been rare despite a significant change in the serum values of these substances in the treated group.

The lowering of ECG voltage seen early in the treated group and the lack of change in either direction in the placebo group are interesting and associated with appropriate degrees of change in blood pressure. However, the possibility that it is purely a drug effect, eg, depletion of myocardial potassium, cannot be ruled out. The observation of the reversibility of abnormal double Master's ECG tests by oral potassium administration adds to the intrigue of this matter.

The PHS trial will continue for a minimum of two more years unless a statistical stopping point is reached earlier. The relative value of the drug treatment of mild, uncomplicated hypertension should be much clearer at that time.

References

1. Society of Actuaries: Build and blood pressure study. New York, Society of Actuaries, 1959.
2. Kannel, W. B., Schwartz, M. J. and McNamara, P. M.: Blood pressure and risk of coronary heart disease; Framingham Study. *Dis. Chest,* 56:43, 1969.
3. Paul, O.: Risks of mild hypertension: Ten-year report. *Brit. Heart J.,* 33(suppl):116, 1971.
4. Hamilton, M., Thompson, E. N. and Wisniewski, T. K. M.: Role of blood pressure control in preventing complications of hypertension. *Lancet,* 1:235, 1964.
5. Leishman, A. W. D.: Merits of reducing high blood pressure. *Lancet,* 1:1284, 1963.
6. Bjork, S., Sannerstedt, R., Falkheden, T. et al: Effect of active drug treatment in severe hypertensive disease. *Acta Med. Scand.,* 169:673, 1961.
7. Veterans Administration Cooperative Study Group on Anti-hypertensive Agents: Effects of treatment on morbidity in hypertension. *JAMA,* 202:1028, 1967.
8. Veterans Administration Cooperative Study Group on Anti-hyperensive Agents: II. Results in patients with diastolic blood pressure averaging 90 through 114 mm Hg. *JAMA,* 213:1143, 1970.
9. Smith, W. M., Bouchard, R. J., Bromer, L. et al: Morbidity and

mortality in mild essential hypertension. *Circ. Res.* (suppl. 2):30, 31:11-110, 1972.

10. Smith, W. M., Damato, A. N., Galluzzi, N. J. et al: Evaluation of antihypertensive therapy — cooperative clinical trial method: I. Double-blind control comparison of chlorothiazide, rauwolfia serpentina, and hydralazine. *Ann. Intern. Med.*, 61:829, 1964.

1-1. Smith, W. M., Damato, A. N., Garfield, C. F. et al: Evaluation of anti-hypertensive therapy: II. Double-blind controlled evaluation of mebutamate. *JAMA*, 193:727, 1965.

12. Smith, W. M., Bachman, B., Galante, J. G. et al: III. Double-blind control comparison of alpha methyldopa and chlorothiazide, and chlorothiazide and rauwolfia. *Ann. Intern. Med.*, 65:657, 1966.

13. Palmer, R. S., Loofbourrow, D. and Doering, C. R.: Prognosis in essential hypertension: Eight year follow-up study of 430 patients on conventional medical treatment. *New Eng. J. Med.*, 239:990, 1948.

14. Sokolow, M. and Perloff, D.: Prognosis of essential hypertension treated conservatively. *Circulation*, 23:697, 1961.

15. Simpson, F. O. and Gilchrist, A. R.: Prognosis in untreated hypertensive vascular disease. *Scot. Med. J.*, 3:1, 1958.

16. Frant, R. and Groen, J.: Prognosis of vascular hypertension. *Arch. Intern. Med.* (Chicago), 85:727, 1950.

17. National Center for Health Statistics: *Vital Statistics of the United States, 1964.* Vol. II, Mortality, part A, Washington, D. C., DHEW Public Health Service, 1966.

18. Armitage, P.: *Sequential Medical Trials.* Springfield, Ill.:Charles C Thomas, 1960.

19. Scheie, H. G.: Evaluation of ophthalmoscopic changes of hypertension and arteriolar sclerosis. *Arch. Ophth.*, 49:117, 1953.

20. Veterans Administration Cooperative Study Group: Effects of treatment on morbidity in hypertension. III. Influence of age, diastolic pressure and prior cardiovascular disease. *Circulation*, 45:991, 1972.

21. Harlan, W. R., Jr., Oberman, A., Graybiel, A. et al: Serial electrocardiograms: Their reliability and prognostic validity over a 24 year period. Bur. of Med. and Surg., MFO 22.03, Q2-5007.13, March 2, 1967.

Appendix

Participants in the PHS Cooperative Study

Protocol Committee:

W. McFate Smith, M.D., M.P.H. (Chairman); Richard J. Bouchard, M.D., Louis Bromer, B.A., Anthony N. Damato, M.D., Willard P. Johnson, M.D., Richard H. Thurm, M.D., John A. Vaillancourt, M.D., J. Richard Warbasse, M.D.

Advisory Board:

Thomas R. Dawber, M.D., Walter M. Kirkendall, M.D., John R. McDonough, M.D., H. Mitchell Perry, M.D., Warren Winkelstein, M.D.

Coordinating Center:

W. McFate Smith, M.D., M.P.H. (Director), Stanley Edlavitch, Ph.D., John A. Vaillancourt, M.D., Frances Mohr, Louise Lee.

Statistical Unit:

Louis Bromer (Director); Julie Wagner, Lyla Rosloff, Annie Brown, Steven Schwab, Dr. Jerome Cornfield (Consultant).

ECG Center:

Willard P. Johnson, M.D.

Cardiac Series Center:

S. Erik Carlsson, M.D., Professor of Radiology, University of California Medical Center.

PHS Supply Service Center:

Salvatore D. Gasdia, Officer in Charge

Principal Investigators, PHS Hospitals:

Baltimore: J. Richard Warbasse, M.D., Richard J. Bouchard, M.D.

Boston: Richard H. Thurm, M.D.

New Orleans: Christfried Urner, M.D.

San Francisco: John A. Vaillancourt, M.D., Thomas T. Yoshikawa, M.D., Charles R. McElroy, M.D.

Seattle: Willard P. Johnson, M.D., Robert Wills, M.D.

Staten Island: Anthony N. Damato, M.D.

Morbidity Referees: Nicholas J. Galluzzi, M.D., PHS Hospital, Staten Island, New York; Claude R. Garfield, M.D., PHS Hospital, Norfolk, Virginia.

Discussion

Dr. Stamler: I would like to ask a few questions about the original design and the experience. First, I do not think I heard the precise way the blood pressure at baseline was characterized. Since this has a lot to do with determining the type of population, I would like to know a little more about it. Second, what about the cigarette smoking habit? I do not think I saw that on the slides. Finally, I was puzzled by the group taken off the protocol. On one slide, a sizable percentage (49%) was no longer in the study and was lost to follow-up.

Dr. Smith: Our subjects were selected on the basis of having diastolic pressures between 90 and 114 as the average of the final two weeks of pressures measured at home during a period of four to six weeks off all antihypertensive agents. The majority, 80% or so, had never been treated, so they were virgin in that regard. They then were brought in and, if they were not excluded for other causes, were entered into a three month placebo control period. They also had a set of clinic measurements, so-called basal clinic pressures, in which they rest for 10 to 20 minutes before measurement. These determinations were made prior to the home blood pressure phase and again, while on placebo. Incidentally, about 22% fell out after having passed the original screen by having diastolic less than 90 at home. We have followed this group to see how many of them subsequently would qualify or develop the need for therapy and it has been a very insignificant, low number. So the blood pressures that were used for selection were home blood pressures. The baselines for estimating response to therapy are the clinic controls.

The answer to your second question having to do with cigarette smoking is that approximately one third had never smoked. Another 25% were previous smokers, leaving over 40% who smoked at baseline. No specific effort to obtain a reduction or cessation of smoking was made.

I believe the third question had to do with dropouts. The 40% figure you referred to is the total in whom coded therapy was discontinued and includes subjects who withdrew voluntarily (11%), those in whom intolerance to medications developed (5%) and those in whom it was terminated after a morbid event was sustained or loss of control of blood pressure supervened (10%). The number lost to regular follow-up over the five years is 59 or 15.2%, and for half of these we have current information that they are alive.

Dr. Hoobler, Michigan: When you mentioned coronary CHD in general, I assume this means the development of angina or positive Master's test as apart from ECG changes.

Dr. Smith: The "other coronary disease" was angina with or without a positive exercise test, and arrhythmias or conduction defects.

Dr. Hoobler: The second question has to do with your ECG high voltage. Did it correlate with blood pressure?

Dr. Smith: Did the 16% of subjects who entered with high voltage have higher blood pressures?

Dr. Hoobler: Right.

Dr. Smith: I have not looked at that.

Dr. Hoobler: The last question, would you make any more comments about the difference between the average clinic blood pressures on the placebo and the home blood pressures? We do not know what to do with a patient who goes home and has blood pressures below 90 but is always 95 or above in the clinic.

Dr. Smith: This experience is based on far more than this trial because we have used the home blood pressures in all of our previous drug trials as well. We have observed about an 8.0 mm Hg lower pressure taken at home when compared to the more or less casual clinic pressure. That drops off to about 5.0 mm difference when you use a placebo control.

Dr. Hoobler: Is that across the board or are there some who have the same blood pressures at home and in the clinic?

Dr. Smith: That is an average for the group. Incidentally, the pressures in our treated group dropped immediately on the fixed regimen and reached their lowest point within four months time. There has been no tendency for them to rise or fall since that time over five years of observations. The same is true for the placebo group. Their pressures, although there was again an initial small fall, have remained at that level subsequently without any tendency to rise.

Dr. Meneely: I am most interested in the potassium piece. What is the explanation why the potassium supplementation worked in the control group with regard to the reversion of the Master's test?

Dr. Smith: Our reason for giving it in the first place was that the control tracing suggested hypokalemia and we felt that as a baseline it should be corrected before an exercise test was done and interpreted. That was based on a gut feeling. We knew of no data to suggest that hypokalemia was associated with false positive exercise tests, and I do not know that any data have been generated subsequently to establish or refute that.

Hypertension in Holmes County, Mississippi

James A. Schoenberger, M.D., Marion Carter, B.A.,
Edward J. Eckenfels, B.A., Dennis Frate, M.A.,
Eddie Logan, M.A., Kenrad Nelson, M.D.,
William Peltz, B.S., Richard Roistacher, Ph.D.
and Demitri B. Shimkin, Ph.D.

Introduction

Hypertension has repeatedly been described by many observers[1] as the major public health problem of blacks, yet this widely accepted view is based on surveys of relatively small numbers of individuals. The data in this paper are derived from a large-scale assessment of the distribution of blood pressures in a poor, rural black community in Mississippi, where an opportunity existed to observe a larger number of individuals than has been studied previously. The unique circumstances of this community, organized to determine its own health needs, provided the ideal setting for these investigations. The Milton Olive III Memorial Corporation, a nonprofit organization made up of representatives of the black community, had received a grant from the National Center for Health Services Research and Development, Department of Health, Education and

Supported in part by Grant #HS00422, National Center for Health Services Research and Development, Department of Health, Education and Welfare.

James A. Schoenberger, M.D *and* Edward J. Eckenfels, B.A., *Department of Preventive Medicine, Rush-Presbyterian-St. Luke's Medical Center, Chicago, Ill.;* Eddie Logan, M.A., *Holmes County Health Research Project, Milton Olive III Memorial Corporation, Lexington, Miss.;* Kenrad Nelson, M.D., *Department of Preventive Medicine, University of Illinois Abraham Lincoln School of Medicine, Chicago;* Dennis Frate, M.A., Richard Roistacher, Ph.D., William Peltz, B.S., Demitri B. Shimkin, Ph.D. *and* Marion Carter, B.A., *Center for Advanced Computation and the Department of Anthropology, University of Illinois at Urbana.*

Welfare. This grant permitted the Corporation to undertake a biosocial assessment of its health problems, to relate these to the demographic and cultural characteristics of the community and to develop new programs for dealing with major health needs. Since 1969, assisted by consultants from a number of institutions, studies have been conducted under the control of community representatives and staffed largely by community people trained by the consultants in the skills necessary to conduct the research. This arrangement has assured nearly total community cooperation in the baseline assessments of population census and housing survey and has made feasible random sampling for specific studies. Pilot programs have received virtually complete cooperation from the residents.

In 1971 a nutritional survey[2] was conducted in a stratified random sample of 500 households. Determination of blood pressures in 692 persons aged 18-79 showed the magnitude of the prevalence of hypertension and its importance as a major health problem. Definite hypertension, defined as a blood pressure of 160 mm Hg systolic and/or 95 mm Hg diastolic, rose steadily with age from 14.3% in men aged 25-34 to 52.2% in those aged 65-74 and in women, from 20% to 50.9%, respectively. The overall prevalence was 33.3% in men and 39.8% in women in contrast to 27.6% for both sexes in the National Health Survey of 1960-1962.[3]

These preliminary findings were the impetus to initiate a demonstration project in the community control of hypertension making maximum use of the meager resources in professional personnel, a limited supply of free drugs which were available and the community workers who had been trained to carry out field surveys. In this report, the prevalence of hypertension in 4,272 black individuals will be reported and related to the demographic and biosocial characteristics of the population and other environmental factors. These data were derived from door-to-door screening of the community. The results of referral to a community health center for diagnostic evaluation and treatment have been presented elsewhere.[4]

Materials and Methods

Holmes County, located in the center of the state, is the third poorest county in Mississippi and one of the poorest in the

United States. The 1970 U. S. Census estimated the population at 15,743 blacks and 7,345 whites. There are no large cities in the County, the larger towns having between 1,000 and 1,500 blacks. It is, in a very real sense, a microcosm of the black belt of the United States. Figure 1 is a map of the area showing the major geographic divisions of the 769 square miles of the County: the Delta occupying the western third and the Hills, the eastern two thirds. The soil in the Delta is alluvial, characterized by a high organic content and a low electrolyte content. The Hills consist of two distinct soil types. One is loess, a deposited soil, which extends eight to ten miles east of the bluff separating the Hills from the Delta. Loess is the lowest of the three soils in electrolytes and organic matter. The other Hill soil, a red-yellow podzolic, characterized by a prominent

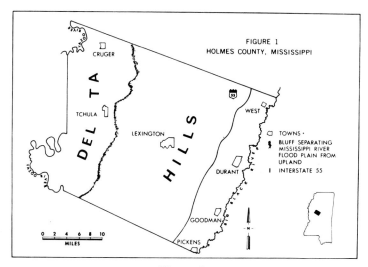

Figure 1.

TABLE 1. Soil Analyses in Holmes County, Mississippi
(Expressed as % by Weight)

	Upland (Clay)	Bluff (Loess)	Delta (Alluvial)
Fe_2O_3	4.42	4.64	6.44
MgO	.92	.88	1.37
CaO	.61	.38	.67
Na_2O	1.31	.95	.58
K_2O	1.82	1.87	1.73

subsurface layer of clay, has the highest electrolyte content. One consequence of these characteristics of the physical environment has been a higher prevalence of parasitoses and hepatitis in the Delta area, since a substantial amount of food, grown in small garden plots, is exposed to this organic milieu. An analysis of the mineral content of the three soil types is shown in Table 1. The most striking difference is the higher sodium content in the upland clay area. This finding may be reflected in the sodium content of the water supply, much of which is derived from shallow wells. Unfortunately, no comparable data on the electrolyte content of the water are currently available for the three geographic subdivisions of the County.

Holmes County is very poor; United States Census data give a 1969 mean per capita income of $632 for blacks and $2,277 for whites. The data show that over half of the black households had no one employed. Generally, in the urban areas people are older, unemployment is higher and more households are headed by a female. In the rural areas a quarter of the land is owned by black farmers, about 300 of whom are substantial and about 500 of whom are part-time farmers. In addition, almost all rural families own or rent a subsistence plot, on which much of the vegetable, poultry and pork supply of the County people depends. Our data show housing in the County to be generally poor. Window and door screening is often absent or in disrepair. Farm animals are frequently penned in close proximity to houses and wells. According to our housing survey, piped water is available to 53% of the 3,947 black homes in the County; in some black communities as many as 90% of the houses are dependent upon shallow wells. Indoor toilet facilities are found in only 44% of black households. Outdoor privies, often close to and above grade from the well, are present in over half the black households.

The population census conducted in the winter of 1969-1970 enumerated 16,591 persons in 3,741 households. The true population, corrected by standard demographic techniques, is estimated at 18,000. Of these persons, about 3,000 are in-migrants from nearby counties, while some 30,000 black Holmes Countians have migrated out, especially to Chicago, Detroit, Jackson and Los Angeles. In the cohorts aged 25-44, 80% of the men and 65% of the women have migrated. Return migration is typical for the older age groups.

The effects of migration upon hypertension prevalence are uncertain in the absence of control studies among the out-migrants. Nevertheless, it should be noted (Table 2) that relatively higher levels of hypertension are evident in Holmes County at early, pre-migration ages.

Beginning in April 1972, and for a period of 17 months until August 1973, the population was evaluated for the prevalence of hypertension by a field staff of community workers. These individuals had been trained in the techniques of measuring blood pressure using a mercury manometer and the

TABLE 2. Hypertension in Blacks in Holmes County, Mississippi Expressed as Percent Compared With Blacks in the National Health Survey, 1960-62.

MALES

Age	Borderline*	Definite**	Blacks National Health Survey**
10-17	4.9	1.5	–
18-24	13.9	6.6	1.9
25-34	17.9	34.5	12.5
35-44	25.7	32.7	26.5
45-54	18.2	43.2	30.8
55-64	21.6	50.5	44.6
65-74	23.0	57.8	66.0
75+	25.2	56.1	59.8
All 18-79	21.1	43.5	27.6

FEMALES

Age	Borderline*	Definite**	Blacks National Health Survey**
10-17	5.1	1.5	–
18-24	7.9	3.5	3.4
25-34	15.9	23.9	8.5
35-44	19.8	31.5	25.6
45-54	25.4	42.6	41.9
55-64	24.6	52.1	41.0
65-74	25.0	57.6	71.0
75+	27.2	57.0	69.4
All 18-79	21.2	39.5	27.6
Both Sexes 18-79	21.2	40.0	27.6

*Blood pressure 140-159/90-94
**Blood pressure $\geq$ 160/95
Males = 1669, 1042 aged 18-79
Females = 2566, 1776 aged 18-79

first and fifth phase Korotkoff sounds as denoting systolic and diastolic blood pressures, respectively. Training included use of a double stethoscope so that accuracy could be monitored by the instructors and use of special training film.[5] Blood pressure measurements in the sitting position were made on 4,272 individuals 5 years of age and over. Blood pressures and demographic data were obtained in the home by the community staff workers who systematically went out to houses assigned on a daily basis from work maps prepared in the population census and housing survey of all black homes in the County. About 83% of the households were contacted at least once. In only 7% of the households were field workers not permitted to measure blood pressures. Despite all of the efforts made, the population sampled by the hypertensive survey proved to be significantly different in composition by age and sex from the uncorrected results of the Health Research Project census (Table 3). A small part of this difference, notably the larger proportions of women aged 65 and over, reflects better coverage in the hypertension survey. In general, however, there is no reason to believe that the nature or magnitude of the biases thus introduced affect the hypertension prevalence data significantly.

Results

The mean blood pressures stratified by age and sex are shown in Table 4 for females and in Table 5 for males. For both sexes, there is a steady rise with age in both systolic and diastolic blood pressures. The correlation of 0.42 between systolic blood pressure and age was better, perhaps because the measurement of systolic blood pressure is more reliable. Systolic blood pressure rose an average of 0.89 mm Hg per year of age.* The correlation between diastolic blood pressure and age was 0.18. A tendency to low values, especially in the younger age groups, gave rise to a greater variance. The mean systolic blood pressure in males was 130.9 and in females, 131.2. The mean diastolic blood pressure in males was 73.3 and in females, 77.5. The difference in diastolic blood pressure was significant (F value 4.34, p value 0.05).

---

*The regression of systolic blood pressure with age was age x 0.89 + 96.73; for diastolic blood pressure the regression was age x 0.51 + 56.07.

The data are particularly noteworthy because of the large number of measurements in younger individuals aged 5-19. In this age group there are little published data and, hence, no clear definition of normal limits has been possible to date.

Hypertension in this study was defined as borderline when the systolic blood pressure values were 140-159 mm Hg and/or the diastolic values were 90-94 mm Hg. Definite hypertension was defined as greater than or equal to 160 mm Hg systolic and/or greater than or equal to 95 mm Hg diastolic. Using these criteria, the prevalence of hypertension in this population sample is shown in Table 2, stratified by age and sex, and compared with data reported for blacks in the National Health Survey of 1960-1962. A strikingly high prevalence of definite hypertension in both men and women was confirmed in this large sample. Compared to the National Health Survey data, the prevalence is noticeably higher in Holmes County throughout all age strata except those 65 and older. For the younger ages from 10-24, a surprisingly high percentage had systolic blood pressure values of 140-159 and/or diastolic values of 90-94, perhaps already indicative of definite hypertension.

The high prevalence of hypertension in the County and the wealth of demographic and biosocial data previously obtained from the population census and housing surveys encouraged the testing of a number of hypotheses regarding possible relation-

TABLE 3. Age and Sex Distribution in the Hypertension Sample Compared to the Total Census, Holmes County, Mississippi

	FEMALES				MALES			
	Hypertension Survey		Census		Hypertension Survey		Census	
Age	No.	%	No.	%	No.	%	No.	%
5-9	229	9.0	1,150	15.7	210	12.6	1,140	17.9
10-14	325	12.8	1,156	15.8	246	14.8	1,130	17.8
15-19	321	12.6	1,029	14.0	215	13.0	1,000	15.7
20-24	115	4.5	441	6.0	67	4.0	376	5.9
25-34	201	7.9	591	8.1	84	5.1	388	6.1
35-44	257	10.1	625	8.5	113	6.8	424	6.7
45-54	291	11.5	661	9.0	148	8.9	497	7.8
55-64	338	13.3	691	9.4	208	12.5	551	8.7
≥65	462	18.2	982	13.4	367	8.7	850	13.4
TOTAL	2,539	60.0% of total	7,326	53.5% of total	1,658	40.0% of total	6,356	46.5% of total

TABLE 4. Mean Blood Pressure of Black Females
Holmes County, Mississippi

Age	No.	Systolic (mm Hg)		Diastolic (mm Hg)	
		Mean	Std. Dev.	Mean	Std. Dev.
5-9	227	94.3	17.4	52.3	16.2
10-14	325	107.0	14.1	60.8	15.8
15-19	321	111.2	14.8	65.0	15.6
20-24	115	112.6	16.9	68.0	17.8
25-29	102	125.9	22.3	80.1	17.7
30-34	99	129.6	22.5	89.7	24.7
35-39	104	129.1	24.3	84.2	20.2
40-44	153	142.4	26.6	86.1	17.8
45-49	147	142.4	28.2	89.4	18.4
50-54	142	147.0	24.5	91.6	20.7
55-59	160	149.9	25.5	88.3	19.8
60-64	177	156.3	28.9	89.4	18.8
65-69	163	156.4	28.0	88.0	17.5
70-74	141	160.8	27.7	92.1	22.7
75-79	86	156.7	25.6	86.2	23.0
80-84	41	159.7	28.8	88.5	28.2
85-89	13	164.8	30.1	81.7	14.0
90-94	10	165.3	26.6	78.4	26.4
≥95	8	165.3	28.6	95.8	28.8

TABLE 5. Mean Blood Pressure of Black Males
Holmes County, Mississippi

Age	No.	Systolic (mm Hg)		Diastolic (mm Hg)	
		Mean	Std. Dev.	Mean	Std. Dev.
5-9	208	93.6	13.7	49.9	16.7
10-14	246	106.6	15.0	57.3	18.9
15-19	215	117.5	16.6	60.0	19.6
20-24	67	123.6	16.3	69.9	18.3
25-29	41	128.8	18.7	72.2	22.0
30-34	43	143.8	29.4	87.5	24.2
35-39	41	135.6	20.9	86.7	14.9
40-44	72	137.3	19.7	84.9	16.3
45-49	70	142.1	26.3	87.5	19.5
50-54	78	144.5	27.5	86.2	18.2
55-59	98	147.3	28.7	87.4	20.5
60-64	110	155.5	30.8	89.6	21.9
65-69	143	156.7	26.4	86.4	20.7
70-74	101	159.3	26.9	84.4	22.7
75-79	56	157.7	24.7	85.6	20.5
80-84	35	154.2	25.3	80.1	16.0
85-89	22	165.5	23.0	91.7	28.8
90-94	8	156.5	23.0	86.8	24.0
≥95	2	138.0	-	91.0	-

ships between environmental or social factors and hypertension. A Delta-Hill contrast was expected, given the Delta's alluvial soils, evidently more significant pathogen reservoirs (streptococcus, Ascaris, etc.), later population entry, multiple origins and greater social heterogeneity (plantations, larger black farms, urban poor) and weaker extended families. Table 6 shows that the highest diastolic blood pressures are found in the rural Delta area. These differences are highly significant.

TABLE 6. The Effect of Living in the Delta or Hill, Urban or Rural, on Mean Blood Pressure, Holmes County, Mississippi (Analysis of Covariance: Age as a Covariate)

			SYSTOLIC*	*DIASTOLIC**
Female	Hill	Urban	146.5	87.8
		Rural	141.6	84.0
	Delta	Urban	146.1	84.5
		Rural	145.0	90.0
Male	Hill	Urban	148.2	83.6
		Rural	146.3	81.7
	Delta	Urban	155.2	87.1
		Rural	143.6	89.1

*Mean blood pressures in mm Hg, age adjusted

Effect	Degrees Freedom	*Multivariate*	F RATIO *Systolic*	*Diastolic*
Urban-Rural	2	.7465	1.3227	.0015
Hill-Delta	2	11.2951**	7.6734**	21.2075**
Sex	2	4.1292*	.0567	6.6679**
Urban-Rural x Hill-Delta	2	7.6150**	2.4555	15.2102**
Urban-Rural x Sex	2	0.0035	0.0049	0.0060
Hill-Delta x Sex	2	1.9443	1.1291	1.3529
Urban-Rural x Hill-Delta x Sex	2	1.8413	3.6573*	0.7242

*P < .05
**P < .01

Their interpretation is elusive however. It will be recalled that the electrolyte content of the soil is lowest in the Delta, particularly in respect to sodium. Moreover, the physical condition of dwellings in regard to adequate screening, indoor plumbing, or the proximity of animals proved to have no effects on mean blood pressures. On the other hand, as seen in Table 7,

TABLE 7. Effect of Source of Water Supply on Mean Blood Pressure
Holmes County, Mississippi
(Analysis of Covariance: Age as a Covariate)

		SYSTOLIC*	DIASTOLIC*
Well Water	Female	140.9	86.9
	Male	146.4	86.3
Piped Water	Female	144.0	82.8
	Male	144.6	77.9

*Mean blood pressure in mm Hg, age adjusted

Effect	Degrees Freedom	Multivariate	F Ratio Systolic	Diastolic
Sex	2	4.3422*	0.3443	6.1537**
Well	2	16.3093**	0.0286	28.9886**
Sex x Well	2	2.3506	3.2948	3.1092

*P < .05
**P < .01

significantly higher diastolic blood pressures are found in those homes in which the water supply is derived from shallow wells. The F value of 29 gave this a high degree of significance ($p < .01$). No significant difference between the Hill and Delta regarding the source of the water supply could be demonstrated.

The analysis of social factors yielded important results, both negative and positive. Basic measures of relative poverty — the quality of housing, household crowding and employment vs. unemployment (Table 8) — all failed to show any association with blood pressure. The years of schooling did not show any association with the prevalence of hypertension in either sex, nor did the number of persons per household.

Three correlates with hypertension were identified. As Table 9 shows, those individuals listed as the head of a

TABLE 8. Effect of Employment on Blood Pressure in Black Adults
Age 18 and Over, Holmes County, Mississippi
(Analysis of Covariance: Age as a Covariate)

			SYSTOLIC*	DIASTOLIC*
Unemployed	Female	Hill	143.5	84.7
		Delta	144.4	87.7
	Male	Hill	145.3	87.2
		Delta	149.3	89.5
Employed	Female	Hill	140.5	85.0
		Delta	145.6	88.1
	Male	Hill	147.4	82.4
		Delta	144.3	87.9

*Mean blood pressure in mm Hg, age adjusted

Effect	Degrees of Freedom	F VALUES		
		Multivariate	Univariate	
			Systolic	Diastolic
Employment	2	0.6	1.14	0.33
Sex	2	3.73	0.007	6.66**
Employment & Sex	2	0.37	0.74	0.03
Hill-Delta	2	10.88**	7.29**	20.42**
Employment x Hill-Delta	2	0.39	0.78	0.11
Sex x Hill-Delta	2	1.95	0.15	2.77
Employment x Sex x Hill-Delta	2	0.816	1.59	0.07

*P < .05
**P < .01

household, whether male or female, had significantly higher blood pressures ($p < .01$). Place of birth was also significantly related to the prevalence of hypertension. Whereas 21% of the native-born residents of the County had definite hypertension, 29.9% of those born elsewhere in the South (almost all in nearby counties) were hypertensives. Finally, both farm and nonfarm laborers had higher blood pressures than did workers in other occupations.

TABLE 9. Effect of Status as Head of Household
and Mean Blood Pressures in Blacks
Age 18 and Over, Holmes County, Mississippi
(Analysis of Covariance: Age as a Covariate)

			SYSTOLIC*	DIASTOLIC*
Not Head	Female	Hill	140.0	83.9
		Delta	142.8	85.3
	Male	Hill	128.9	67.7
		Delta	127.9	80.3
Head	Female	Hill	149.8	87.4
		Delta	150.5	93.1
	Male	Hill	149.7	84.5
		Delta	150.3	90.3

*Mean blood pressure in mm Hg, age adjusted

Effect	Degree of Freedom	F VALUES Multivariate	Univariate Systolic	Diastolic
Hill-Delta	2	10.81**	8.52**	19.61**
Head of Household	2	5.66**	1.05	11.28**
Sex	2	3.003*	0.2	4.9**
Hill-Delta x Head of Household	2	0.31	0.13	0.27
Hill-Delta x Sex	2	2.67	0.66	2.99
Head of Household x Sex	2	2.40	0.0049	4.10**
Hill-Delta x Head of Household x Sex	2	2.45	0.003	4.37**

*p < .05
**p < .01

Discussion

The manifestation of high blood pressure is considered to be the result of environmental influences acting over time on the genetically predisposed individual.[6] The black community in Holmes County, Mississippi, provided an ideal location for studying these environmental factors because hypertension is very prevalent in this relatively homogeneous population.

The environment is marked by all-pervasive poverty and social deprivation. The population reached its peak in 1910 and has fallen progressively since. World War I and the Depression were the impetus for accelerated migration of blacks to the north. Land owned or rented by blacks has declined from two thirds of the County total in 1910 to a quarter today.[7]

Agricultural displacements due to mechanization have forced former sharecroppers and plantation hands into urban slums. Loss of income derived from farm labor has reduced an increasing number to subsistence gardening and reliance on food stamps. By 1970 only one third of the black population aged 16 and over was employed and in half the households there was no employed individual at all.[8, 9]

The extensive out-migration of young men and women has resulted in an extreme imbalance in the sex ratio in the critical ages of 20-49, with fewer than three men to four women. As a correlate, only two thirds of all black families have both husband and wife present.

Socioeconomic conditions in the County were rated by the U. S. Bureau of the Census[9] as very poor for blacks and poor for whites. Marked educational differences between the two races exist. Forty-three percent of black men and 22% of black women had fewer than five years of schooling contrasted to 9% and 4%, respectively, for whites. Full-time employment is exceptional for blacks, 78% of whom were at poverty-level incomes. Corresponding differences in housing between blacks and whites reflected the over threefold higher per capita income of whites. Death rates for blacks were 50% above those expected for whites in the southeastern states. For whites, the excess mortality was only 7%.

These stressful conditions were the setting, then, for the social background of hypertension among black people of Holmes County, Mississippi. The results of this investigation show that even under conditions of great poverty and presumed sociopsychological stress, the associations with hypertension appear to be complex. The strongest indication is that specific social roles define the subpopulations particularly at risk. Holmes County black society places critical responsibilities upon the heads of households, who are the decision-makers and managers of extended families, as well as their own immediate kin.[8] Conversely, children, the elderly and other dependents can call upon support from a network of relatives; the fosterage of children by grandparents is a common way of reducing strains in large families.

At another level, black-white relationships are the tensest. It is not surprising that laborers, who are almost all highly dependent on whites and whose status among blacks is low, should be most hypertensive.

Finally, local in-migrants have largely come to Holmes County from even more deprived areas, for example, to take advantage of Head Start. This is in accordance with migration theory on selection by "minus factors."[10]

The fact that higher mean diastolic blood pressures were found in the Delta where the soil content is lowest in sodium is discordant with the extensive evidence linking salt with hypertension.[11] It was assumed that soil sodium would be reflected in the sodium content of water derived from shallow wells and vegetables grown in gardens. Unfortunately, data on the sodium content of the food and water and electrolyte excretion studies are not available at this time. Although diastolic blood pressures were higher among those who obtained water from a well, no consistent relationship could be shown for those living in the Delta vs. the Hills in this regard.

Conclusions

Blood pressures were measured in a community-wide door-to-door screening of 4,272 black residents of Holmes County, Mississippi. Mean systolic and diastolic blood pressures rose with age, the former in a more correlated fashion. In males, age-adjusted diastolic blood pressure was significantly lower.

Hypertension was very prevalent. Definite hypertension was found in 43.5% of the males and 39.5% of the females aged 18-79; these values are 50% higher than those reported for blacks in the National Health Survey of 1960-1962.

Among the environmental factors associated with elevation of diastolic blood pressure was residence in the Delta region of the County, even though the soil in this area has the lowest sodium content. On the other hand, higher blood pressures were found in those depending upon shallow wells as a water source. Social factors associated with higher diastolic blood pressures in this poverty-stricken, socially deprived area were head of household status, work as a laborer and in-migration from elsewhere in the South. If poverty is the common factor underlying the strikingly high prevalence of hypertension, these preliminary studies should be invaluable in further investigation of the precise mechanisms by which it asserts its action.

References

1. Stamler, J.: High blood pressure in the United States — an overview of the problem and the challenge. In *Proceedings of the National Conference on High Blood Pressure Education.* National Heart and Lung Institute. U. S. Department of Health, Education and Welfare publication number (NIH) 73-486, 1973.
2. Nelson, K.: Unpublished data.
3. U. S. Department of Health, Education and Welfare: Blood pressure of adults by race and area, United States, 1960-1962, National Health Survey, National Center for Health Statistics Series II: Number 5, 1964.
4. Eckenfels, E., Schoenberger, J., Shumway, D. et al: The community control of hypertension in a poor, black rural population. Paper delivered at the Annual Meeting of the Council on Epidemiology, American Heart Association, San Diego, California, March 4-5, 1974.
5a. Wilcox, J.: Observer factors in the measurement of blood pressure. *Nursing Res.,* 10:4-17, 1961.
5b. Film M1582, Blood Pressure Reading, National Audiovisual Center, General Services Administration, Washington, D. C.
6. Pickering, G.: The inheritance of arterial pressure. In Stamler, J., Stamler, R. and Pullman, T. (eds.): *The Epidemiology of Hypertension.* New York:Grune and Stratton, 1967, p. 18.
7. Shimkin, D.: Black migration and the struggle for equity: A hundred year record. In Eaton, J. (ed.): *Migration and Social Welfare.* New York:National Association of Social Workers, Inc., 1971.
8. Shimkin, D., Louie, G. and Frate, D.: The black extended family: A basic rural institution and a mechanism of urban adaptation. Ninth International Congress of Anthropological and Ethnological Sciences, Inc., Chicago, 1973.
9. U. S. Bureau of the Census: 1970 census of population: Characteristics of the population, Mississippi. Part 26. Washington, D. C.: U. S. Government Printing Office. January, 1973.
10. Lee, E. S.: A theory of migration. *Demography,* 3:47-57, 1966.
11. Knudsen, K. D., Iwal, J. and Dahl, Z. K.: Salt, heredity and hypertension. In Onesti, G., Kim, K. E. and Moyer, J. H. (eds.): *Hypertension: Mechanisms and Management.* Twenty-sixth Hahnemann Symposium. New York:Grune and Stratton, 1973, p. 111.

Discussion

Dr. Benjamin Johnson, Illinois: I was struck by the fact that in your means by age there seemed to be no sex difference at all, which is not the usual thing in either blacks or whites. Do you have any ideas why?

Dr. Schoenberger: All we can tell you is that this is what we found. The data represent a sample of about one fourth of the black population with no bias in the way we attempted to obtain the data.

Dr. Shansky, Illinois: Do you have any data on the dietary factors involved in this population?

Dr. Schoenberger: This will be reported in another study. The nutritional study was done on a random, stratified sample of the population. It revealed some interesting data on obesity. The women on the average were extremely obese with an average weight of 165 pounds and a height of 5 feet 3 inches. The men weighed the same and were 5 feet 8 inches tall; so obesity is limited to the women. In future studies we will evaluate the nutritional status more fully, but I am not prepared to report on that at the present time.

Dr. Dollery: I can understand the way you feel about the terrible poverty of these people, but I wonder if the conclusion that you came to at the end, that the high incidence of high blood pressure is in some way related to it, is supported by your data. The data you presented in employed versus unemployed people showed no difference at all. Presumably there would be a substantial difference in per capita income in those groups.

Dr. Schoenberger: I advance only as a hypothesis that poverty may in some way be a stressful condition and that we should try to quantitate it and try to understand it better. I cannot prove it conclusively. Further studies are needed to try to break down the socioeconomic classes to see whether there is any difference in the prevalence of hypertension.

Dr. Stamler: This is one of the few studies of the black belt counties in our country. It is the only recent one I know and I want to congratulate all the people on it. We should note in regard to the question raised that there is a body of data in our country indicating that among whites the least educated and the lowest income groups in our country have more high blood pressure. Moriyama, Krueger and I summarized the data on this in our APHA monograph of a few years ago. Few of us are aware of this or think much about it. I believe that the British social class data are not very different, although I am not quite sure.

Dr. Roistacher, Illinois: I would say two things: first, systolic pressure correlates with age in Holmes County; second, diastolic pressure seems to correlate with some psychosocial stress. I think that we cannot now abandon the hypothesis that somehow psychosocial stress has to do with hypertension.

Dr. Miller, Maryland: When I was being taught preventive medicine, one of the cardinal laws was you never identify somebody in a survey and not do anything about it. You have a lot of people there that are sick. What did you do about it?

Dr. Schoenberger: At the time we were doing this survey, we had an on-going program for referral of all hypertensives into a community center and clinic where we had free drugs and were providing treatment. The problem was that the support for the program ran out. When it did, we did a follow-up and called all the hypertensives and told them that the program was terminating because of lack of funds and urged them to seek medical care through the usual sources. We were acutely aware of the moral issue here and had not started the screening program until we had the clinic fully equipped and staffed and ready to go. The problem was lack of financial support to carry on the program.

Therapeutic Trials
in Renovascular Hypertension

Norman M. Simon, M.D.

Renal arterial stenosis has been recognized as an important cause of remediable hypertension in man. Nevertheless, the proper management of patients with renovascular hypertension remains open to question. Early enthusiasm for surgery was tempered by the sobering report of Homer Smith[1] in 1956, who noted that only 26% of patients treated by nephrectomy were normotensive for as long as one year after surgery. It was in this climate that the large-scale Cooperative Study of Renovascular Hypertension[2] was organized in the United States in 1961 in an effort to study hypertensive patients carefully and to select patients with renal arterial lesions for surgical treatment.

Fifteen institutions, including Northwestern University Medical Center, participated in the Cooperative Study over the eight-year period from 1961 to 1969.

The Cooperative Study

All patients enrolled in the study were evaluated according to a standard protocol which included demographic data, historical information, findings on physical examination and the

Dr. Simon was a member of the Executive Committee of the Cooperative Study of Renovascular Hypertension. His work was supported in part by grants HE 06652 and AM-0564 from the National Institutes of Health and by the Otho S. A. Sprague Foundation. Certain studies were carried out in the Clinical Research Center at Passavant Memorial Pavilion, Northwestern University Medical School, supported by grant RR48 from the National Institutes of Health.

Norman M. Simon, M.D., F.A.C.P., *Associate Professor of Medicine, Northwestern University Medical School, Chicago, Ill.*

results of laboratory tests: urinalysis, blood chemistries, chest x-ray, electrocardiogram, rapid-sequence intravenous pyelogram, radioisotope renogram, individual kidney function tests and renal arteriography.[2]

During the course of the study, 2,442 patients were evaluated, of whom 884 had renal arterial lesions demonstrated on arteriography. No attempt was made to develop uniform criteria for selection of treatment for patients enrolled in the study. These decisions were left to the discretion of investigators at the participating centers. By and large, surgical treatment was preferred over medical therapy. Thus, 570 patients underwent vascular reconstructive surgery and/or nephrectomy. Sixty-eight of the 570 patients who underwent operative treatment were suspended from the study for various reasons. The results of surgery in the remaining 502 patients will be reviewed in this report.[3]

The primary procedure was unilateral or bilateral renal artery reconstruction in 315 patients, nephrectomy in 168, partial nephrectomy in 10 and reconstruction with contralateral nephrectomy in 9 patients. Sixty-seven patients had two operative procedures and four had three procedures. Thirty-four patients expired as a result of surgery for an operative mortality rate of 6.8%. Classification of the blood pressure response 12 months or more after surgery was made in 384 cases. Patients were classified as *cured* if the average diastolic blood pressure was 90 mm Hg or less with at least a 10 mm Hg decrease from the preoperative level. Patients were considered to be *improved* if the average diastolic blood pressure was between 90 and 110 mm Hg, but at least 15% lower than the preoperative level. *Failure* included those cases with an average diastolic blood pressure greater than 90 mm Hg and less than a 15% decrease in diastolic pressure, and all patients with a diastolic blood pressure greater than 110 mm Hg.

The results are presented in Table 1. Fifty-one percent of patients were cured of hypertension while an additional 15% improved after surgery. Patients with unilateral disease showed a significantly higher rate of cure and improvement than patients with bilateral disease. In patients with unilateral disease, those with fibromuscular lesions benefited from surgery more often than patients with atherosclerotic lesions (80% vs. 63%), and primary nephrectomy resulted in cure or improve-

TABLE 1. Cooperative Study of Renovascular Hypertension

	Cured	Improved	Cured and Improved	Failure	Operative Death
Overall results	51%	15%	66%	34%	6.8%
Atherosclerosis vs.	46	17	63	37	9.3
fibromuscular hyp.	58	13	71	29	3.4*
Unilateral vs.	55	15	70	30	5.8
bilateral disease[1]	39	17	56*	44	10.2
Unilateral athero vs.	48	15	63	37	7.3
unilateral fibro.	64	16	80**	20	3.7
Bilateral athero vs.	40	23	63	37	13.8
bilateral fibro.	38	5	43	57	2.3
Nephrectomy vs.	54	15	69	31	3.3
reconstruction[2]	46	10	56*	44	3.2

[1] Etiologies other than atherosclerosis or fibromuscular hyperplasia excluded.
[2] Treatment of atherosclerotic or fibromuscular lesions as primary procedure.
*p-value less than 0.05.
**p-value less than 0.01.

ment of hypertension more consistently than primary arterial reconstruction (69% vs. 56%). Secondary nephrectomy, undertaken in 31 patients who responded poorly to vascular surgery, was as equally effective as primary nephrectomy in alleviating hypertension.

These findings suggested that technical failure of arterial reconstruction was an important factor. Functional significance of the arteriographic lesion demonstrated by preoperative studies or by intraoperative renal arterial pressure gradients was also found to be significant. Thus, in 26 patients with unilateral disease who had technically successful surgery but who showed no evidence of functional disparity between the two kidneys, cure or improvement of hypertension after surgery occurred in only 12%.[3] When technical failures of surgery and patients who did not demonstrate any functional correlates of stenosis were excluded, vascular reconstruction was significantly more effective than nephrectomy (87% vs. 72% cured and improved), and results in patients with unilateral disease were not significantly better than in patients with bilateral lesions.

Operative mortality rates in the various groups are listed in Table 1. The death rate following surgery was significantly greater in patients with atherosclerotic disease than in those with fibromuscular lesions, 28 of the 34 deaths occurring in the former group. Renal failure, hemorrhage and myocardial infarction accounted for more than 80% of the primary causes of death. In patients with atherosclerotic lesions, coronary artery disease and impaired renal function were associated with greater surgical mortality, while surgical failure was related to hypertension of longer duration and left ventricular hypertrophy.[4] Age, severity of hypertension and history of previous cerebrovascular or peripheral vascular disease were not found to be of prognostic significance.

The mortality rates of various surgical procedures[5] are listed in Table 2. The rates after unilateral nephrectomy or simple unilateral arterial reconstruction were similar but increased sharply when unilateral reconstruction was complicated, bilateral surgery was performed, or extrarenal procedures (repair of an aortic aneurysm or aorto-iliac occlusive disease) were added. There was no correlation between mortality rate and technique of vascular reconstructive surgery.

Other Studies

Contemporaneous with the Cooperative Study, a number of other centers in the United States and Europe began to

TABLE 2. Mortality After Surgery

Procedure	No.	Deaths	Mortality Rate
Unilateral nephrectomy	240	8	3.3%
Unilateral reconstruction	250	8	3.2
Simultaneous attempted reconstruction followed by ipsilateral nephrectomy or second reconstructive procedure	25	7	28.0
Simultaneous bilateral reconstruction	35	2	5.7
Simultaneous reconstruction and contralateral nephrectomy	8	2	25.0
Simultaneous renovascular operations with extra-renal surgery	16	4	25.0
Miscellaneous	3	3	
Total	577	34	

investigate the efficacy of medical treatment of patients with renovascular hypertension and to compare the results of medical therapy with those of surgery. The results of these clinical trials[6-12] are summarized in Table 3.

Dustan and co-workers[6] at the Cleveland Clinic reported their experience with 131 patients with renal arterial disease who were followed from one to six years after the start of treatment. Ninety-nine patients were selected for surgery while 32 patients in whom "operative treatment seemed contra-indicated" were given hypotensive durgs. The latter group was older, had a longer duration of hypertension, presented symptoms of coronary or cerebral arterial disease more frequently and had greater impairment of renal function. Blood pressure responses to treatment were assessed in relation to normal

TABLE 3. Comparison of Surgical and Medical Treatment
of Renovascular Hypertension

Investigator	Period of Follow-up (Years)	Group[1]	No. of Cases	Cured & Improved	Failure	Deaths Total	Operative
Dustan (1963)	1-6	S	99	58%	20%	22%	10%
		M	32	41	28	31	
Peart (1967)	0-8	S	46	44	21	35	13
	0-6	M	42	45	36	19	
Shapiro (1969)	1-6	S	43	49	16	35	7
		M	72	variable control		40	
Bergentz (1969)	½-10	S	74	56	19	25	11
Kjellbo (1970)		M	165	46	24	30	
Owen (1973)	0-5	S	59	58	15	27	10
		M	83	35*	31	34	
Hunt (1973)	1-8	S	63	89	9	2	0
Fibromuscular		M	70	84	16	0	
Atherosclerosis		S	37	76	24	0	0
		M	44	75	18	7	
Fibromuscular	7-14	S	63	86	6	8	0
		M	70	62**	21	17	
Atherosclerosis		S	37	65	5	30	0
		M	44	20**	18	62**	

[1]S – Surgical treatment; M – Medical treatment
*p-value less than 0.05; **p-value less than 0.01

blood pressure levels adjusted for age. Surgery resulted in cure or improvement of hypertension in 58% of cases while medical therapy was effective in 41%. The operative mortality rate was 10% and the total mortality in the surgical group during the period of observation was 22%. Thirty-one percent of the poorer risk medical group died. Deaths in both groups occurred largely in patients who were treatment failures, resulting primarily from the complications of atherosclerosis. In nine of ten medical patients who recorded blood pressure readings at home, excellent control of arterial pressure was achieved with conventional hypotensive drugs.

Peart[7] reported his findings in 88 patients with renovascular hypertension who were observed for periods up to eight years. Selection of treatment was made on an individual basis. Age, severity of hypertension, number of preceding complications and predominance of atherosclerotic lesions were apparently comparable in both treatment groups. Forty-four percent of patients in the surgical group can be classified as cured (diastolic blood pressure less than 100 mm Hg) or improved (diastolic pressure less than 110) as compared to 45% of medically treated patients. One of the effects of surgery even when it failed to lower blood pressure was to make the hypertension more responsive to drug therapy. The operative mortality was 13% and total mortality in patients treated surgically 35% as compared to 19% in the medical treatment group. Athero-sclerotic events accounted for almost all of the deaths. Fatal and nonfatal vascular complications occurred in both groups without relation to the degree of control of hypertension and were more common in patients with signs of antecedent vascular disease.

Owen,[8] apparently including some of the same patients reported by Peart, presented somewhat different results in comparing medical and surgical treatment in a series of 142 patients who were followed over a five-year period. The medical treatment group was older and included patients who were considered to be unfit for surgery. Fifty-eight percent of surgically treated patients were classified as cured or improved in contrast to 35% of medically treated patients. The operative mortality rate was 10% and total mortality rate in the surgical group, 27%. Thirty-four percent of the medical group died during the observation period. The mortality rate was related to age, increasing sharply after the fourth decade. Deaths occurred even when the blood pressure was controlled at normal levels.

Shapiro and associates[9] summarized the findings obtained at the University of Pittsburgh in a series of 115 patients followed from one to six years. The surgical treatment group was significantly younger, had better renal function, showed left ventricular hypertrophy less often, but had more severe retinopathy than the medical treatment group. The renal artery lesions were predominantly atherosclerotic in etiology. Twenty-eight percent of patients were normotensive or markedly improved after surgery while an additional 21% were labeled as "slightly improved." Variable control of hypertension was achieved with hypotensive drugs. The mortality rates were comparable in the two groups, 35% in surgical patients and 40% in medically treated patients. The operative mortality was 7%. The majority of deaths resulted from vascular complications in the brain, heart and kidneys. Factors associated with a more favorable response to surgery included younger age, shorter duration of hypertension, better renal function and nephrectomy as opposed to vascular reconstruction.

Bergentz and Kjellbo and their co-workers[10,11] presented the results of surgical treatment of 74 patients and medical treatment of 165 patients with renal arterial lesions observed for periods up to ten years. Patients were selected for surgery on the basis of a variety of criteria which included age, severity and duration of hypertension, degree of control with hypotensive drugs, extent of target organ damage and other factors suggesting a favorable response to surgery. Accordingly, medically treated patients were older and showed greater target organ damage than surgically treated cases. Fifty-six percent of patients were normotensive or had greater than a 20 mm Hg decrease in diastolic blood pressure after surgery as compared to 46% with comparable responses after medical therapy. The mortality rates were 25% in the surgical group, including 11% postoperatively, and 30% in the medical group. Almost all deaths in both groups occurred in patients with atherosclerotic lesions, frequently with good control of hypertension, and resulted from atherosclerotic complications.

In contrast to the previous studies based primarily on retrospective analysis, Hunt and associates[12] at the Mayo Clinic carried on a prospective investigation of 214 patients with renal arterial hypertension who were evaluated during the interval from 1958-1965 and were followed for periods of 1 to 14 years. Patients were largely between the ages of 15 and 60 years. Those with more than one vascular complication or with significant impairment of renal function (glomerular filtration rate less than 50 ml/min) were excluded. All patients except for some in the pediatric age group or those with accelerated hypertension were assigned to medical treatment. Blood pressure control was considered satisfactory if the standing diastolic blood pressure could be maintained at levels of 100 mm Hg or less in adults and 90 mm Hg or less in children. One hundred fourteen patients were treated medically for six months or longer. One hundred patients were subjected to surgical treatment, 18 without trial of hypotensive drugs and 82 because of failure of medical therapy involving at least three antihypertensive drugs in combination. Patients in the medical treatment group had less severe hypertension but were three to five years older than those treated surgically.

Adequate numbers of patients permitted analysis of the results according to the two major etiologies of the renal arterial lesions — atherosclerosis and fibromuscular hyperplasia. Findings were presented at three different periods of observation. At the initial evaluation period one to eight years after beginning treatment, surgery and medical therapy were equally highly effective while mortality rates were extremely low. After 7 to 14 years 86% of patients with fibromuscular lesions continued to benefit from surgery while the number of patients responding to medical treatment decreased significantly to 62% and medical deaths increased correspondingly. The changes were more striking in patients with atherosclerosis. Sixty-five percent of surgical patients continued to be cured or improved as compared to only 20% of patients under medical treatment. The marked decrease in response to medical treatment was balanced by an increase in mortality to 62%, a level significantly greater than 30% in the surgical group. Cardiovascular causes accounted for the majority of deaths in all treatment categories.

Knowledge of the natural history of renal arterial disease provides important information in arriving at a decision regarding medical or surgical treatment. Stewart and co-workers[13] at the Cleveland Clinic reported their findings in 88 patients who did not undergo surgery and were followed by serial renal angiography for periods of one to eight years. Of 36 patients with atherosclerotic lesions, 36% showed signs of progressive obstruction often with secondary complications of dissection or thrombosis. It was not possible to predict by angiography which lesions would progress. Wollenweber et al[14] reported definite progression of atherosclerotic renal artery disease in approximately half of the involved arteries and the appearance of new lesions in three arteries in 30 patients, selected for repeat angiography because of an increase in blood pressure, reduction in renal size or function or development of aorto-iliac disease.

Harrison and McCormack,[15] representing investigators at the Mayo Clinic and Cleveland Clinic, summarized evidence that fibromuscular hyperplasia was not a uniform entity and could be divided into subtypes based on distinctive pathologic and angiographic characteristics. Utilizing the combined pathologic-angiographic classification in the study of 62 patients with fibromuscular hyperplasia, Stewart[13] noted that medial fibroplasia, identified by the typical string-of-beads pattern on angiography, was the most common lesion and rarely progressed. By contrast, subadventitial fibroplasia, intimal fibroplasia and fibromuscular hyperplasia, which together accounted for only 25% of fibrous lesions, frequently showed progressive obstruction, thrombosis or dissection and might affect previously uninvolved vessels. Sheps et al[16] reported progression of stenosis in 19 of 55 patients with fibrous lesions. In addition, two patients developed atherosclerotic changes involving the renal arteries. Multifocal lesions with large beads or with large and small beads, corresponding to medial fibroplasia in Stewart's terminology, progressed infrequently.

The efficacy of hypotensive drug therapy in the management of renovascular hypertension was reevaluated recently by Chassin and Sullivan.[17] These investigators treated 24 patients who were subsequently cured or improved by surgery with conventional antihypertensive drugs. The mean diastolic blood pressure in patients with fibromuscular lesions decreased from a level of 128 to 106 mm Hg with an average of two hypotensive drugs, while three hypotensive agents (usually a diuretic, hydralazine and either methyldopa or reserpine) were required to lower the mean diastolic pressure from 127 to 107 mm Hg in patients with atherosclerotic lesions. These findings supported the earlier observations of Dustan and co-workers concerning the utility of pharmacologic treatment of renal arterial hypertension.

On the other hand, Buhler and co-workers[18] claimed that propranolol was the drug of choice in treating patients with renovascular hypertension because of its renin inhibiting property. In eight patients with unilateral renal artery disease, propranolol decreased blood pressure in proportion to the degree of suppression of plasma renin levels, having greatest effect when control renin levels were elevated. The response to propranolol correlated well with the change in blood pressure produced by surgery.

Conclusions and Comments

Based on the short-term results of surgery issuing from the Cooperative Study of Renovascular Hypertension and the longer term results comparing surgical and medical treatment at a number of centers in the United States and Europe, we may arrive at the following conclusions:

In patients followed for one year or more after surgery in the large-scale Cooperative Study, hypertension was cured or improved in about two thirds of the cases. The mortality rate of surgery was approximately 7%. In a number of smaller series, the operative mortality rate ranged from 0 to 13%.

Surgery was more effective in patients with unilateral disease, especially fibromuscular lesions, than in patients with bilateral disease. Primary nephrectomy produced a more consistent lowering of blood pressure than primary vascular reconstruction. The better results in unilateral disease and the superiority of nephrectomy could be attributed to the occurrence of technical failures after vascular reconstructive procedures.

Surgical mortality rates increased sharply when arterial reconstruction was complicated or coupled with extrarenal surgery.

Surgical deaths occurred more often in patients with atheromatous lesions. Coronary artery disease and impaired renal function were associated with significantly increased operative mortality. In the presence of either of these conditions, the mortality rate exceeded 20%.

In all studies comparing the long-term results of surgical and medical treatment, the two treatment groups were not comparable. Patients assigned to medical therapy were poorer risks than patients subjected to surgery. The medical patients were older, showed a longer duration of hypertension and had greater vascular damage in the target organs of brain, heart and kidney.

Surgery was significantly more effective than medical therapy in producing a sustained lowering of blood pressure in two of six therapeutic trials, those reported by Owen[8] and Hunt.[12] However, the therapeutic efficacy of surgery varied widely — from a level less than 50% to a value of 89%.

The prospective study at the Mayo Clinic[12] involved somewhat better risk patients. At the initial evaluation period one to eight years after beginning treatment, surgery was no more effective than hypotensive drug therapy. However, differences between the two treatment groups became apparent after 7 to 14 years of observation, as the number of patients whose hypertension was controlled by drug therapy sharply decreased and deaths in the medical group markedly increased. Several possible explanations of these results must be considered. First, surgery might produce a greater and more protracted hypotensive response than drug therapy. The mean blood pressure in the surgical treatment group was almost 20 mm Hg lower than that in patients treated medically. Second, the deterioration of results in the medical treatment group might reflect greater antecedent vascular disease which became manifest over the longer period of observation. Third, the findings could be attributed to an increasing failure of adherence to drug therapy as the trial progressed.

In the various trials, deaths in both surgical and medical treatment groups resulted primarily from atherosclerotic complications. Of all cardiovascular deaths, 37% occurred in patients deemed to have a good response to surgical or medical therapy. The presence of significant vascular disease before the start of treatment could account for this disturbing finding.

Atherosclerotic lesions of the renal arteries showed angiographic progression in about one third of the patients treated medically. The most common fibromuscular lesion, medial fibroplasia, rarely caused progressive obstruction. The less common lesions, involving fibroplasia of the intima or adventitia and true fibromuscular hyperplasia, frequently produced progressive stenosis, thrombosis or dissection. Careful follow-up of patients with renal arterial lesions by intravenous pyelography, renal angiography and assessment of individual kidney function is warranted in an effort to search for progression. The effects of vascular reconstructive surgery in modifying the natural history of arteriographic lesions remain to be clearly defined.

Conventional combination hypotensive drug therapy was usually effective in reducing the blood pressure in patients with renal arterial lesions. Propranolol might be of particular value in these patients because of its ability to suppress renin production.

Selection of surgical or medical treatment of renovascular hypertension involves consideration of a number of important factors (Table 4). Surgery is preferred for the young patient, the patient with hypertension of short duration or the patient with accelerated hypertension, in whom vascular disease is absent and renal function is normal. Surgery is more likely to succeed when renal arterial disease is unilateral and functionally significant. It is urgently needed when progression of an arterial lesion with loss of renal function is likely. If vascular reconstruction is feasible, surgery is indicated in an effort to conserve

TABLE 4. Important Factors in Selection of
Surgical or Medical Treatment

	Surgical	Medical
Age	Under 30 years	Over 60 years
Duration of hypertension	Less than 3 years	More than 5 years
Severity of hypertension	Accelerated	Nonaccelerated
Coronary artery, cerebrovascular, peripheral vascular disease	Absent	Present
Renal function	Normal	Impaired
Location of lesion	Unilateral	Bilateral
Type of lesion	Progressive forms of fibromuscular hyperplasia	Nonprogressive: medial fibroplasia
Reparability of lesion	Amenable to vascular reconstruction	Requires nephrectomy
Functional ischemia	Present	Absent
Response to hypotensive drugs	Poor	Satisfactory

renal function. Finally, surgery may be selected to supplant medical therapy when the response to hypotensive drugs is poor or drug toxicity is disabling.

Medical therapy is advisable for the older patient, the patient with hypertension of long duration or the patient with benign hypertension associated with significant vascular disease and impaired renal function. Drug therapy is worthy of trial when renal arterial lesions are bilateral, stable or are not amenable to vascular reconstruction. Medical treatment is clearly indicated for patients in whom the rapid sequence intravenous pyelogram, individual kidney function tests, or renal vein renin assays fail to establish the functional significance of an arteriographic lesion.

References

1. Smith, H. W.: Unilateral nephrectomy in hypertensive disease. *J. Urol.*, 76:685, 1956.
2. Maxwell, M. H., Bleifer, K. H., Franklin, S. S. et al: Demographic analysis of the study. *JAMA*, 220:1195, 1972.
3. Foster, J. H., Maxwell, M. H., Franklin, S. S. et al: Results of operative treatment of renovascular occlusive disease. *JAMA.* (In press.)
4. Simon, N. M., Franklin, S. S., Bleifer, K. H. et al: Clinical characteristics of renovascular hypertension. *JAMA*, 220:1209, 1972.
5. Franklin, S. S., Young, J. D., Jr., Maxwell, M. H. et al: Operative morbidity and mortality in renovascular disease. *JAMA.* (In press.)
6. Dustan, H. P., Page, I. H., Poutasse, E. F. et al: An evaluation of treatment of hypertension associated with occlusive renal arterial disease. *Circulation*, 27:1018, 1963.
7. Peart, W. S.: Treatment of hypertension associated with renal artery stenosis. In Engel, A. and Larsson, T. (eds.): *Stroke: Thule International Symposium.* Stockholm: Nordiska Bokhandelns Forlag, 1967.
8. Owen, K.: Results of surgical treatment in comparison with medical treatment of renovascular hypertension. *Clin. Sci. Molec. Med.*, 45:95s, 1973.
9. Shapiro, A. P., Perez-Stable, E., Scheib, E. T. et al: Renal artery stenosis and hypertension: Observations on current status of therapy from a study of 115 patients. *Amer. J. Med.*, 47:175, 1969.
10. Bergentz, S. E., Kjellbo, H., Hansson, L. O. et al: Renal artery stenosis and hypertension. I. Surgical treatment. *Scand. J. Urol. Nephrol.*, 3:229, 1969.
11. Kjellbo, H., Lund, N., Bergentz, S. E. et al: Renal artery stenosis. III. Follow-up observations in operated and non-operated patients. *Scand. J. Urol. Nephrol.*, 4:49, 1970.

12. Hunt, J. C. and Strong, C. G.: Renovascular hypertension: Mechanisms, natural history, and treatment. *Amer. J. Cardiol.*, 32:562, 1973.
13. Stewart, B. H., Dustan, H. P., Kiser, W. S. et al: Correlation of angiography and natural history in evaluation of patients with renovascular hypertension. *J. Urol.*, 104:231, 1970.
14. Wollenweber, J., Sheps, S. G. and Davis, G. D.: Clinical course of atherosclerotic renovascular disease. *Amer. J. Cardiol.*, 21:60, 1968.
15. Harrison, E. G., Jr. and McCormack, L. J.: Pathologic classification of renal arterial disease in renovascular hypertension. *Mayo Clin. Proc.*, 46:161, 1971.
16. Sheps, S. G., Kincaid, O. W. and Hunt, J. C.: Serial renal function and angiographic observations in idiopathic fibrous and fibromuscular stenosis of the renal arteries. *Amer. J. Cardiol.*, 30:55, 1972.
17. Chassin, M. R. G. and Sullivan, J. M.: Pharmacologic management of renovascular hypertension. *JAMA*, 227:421, 1974.
18. Buhler, F. R., Laragh, J. H., Vaughan, E. D., Jr. et al: Antihypertensive action of propranolol: Specific antirenin responses in high and normal renin forms of essential, renal, renovascular and malignant hypertension. *Amer. J. Cardiol.*, 32:511, 1973.

Discussion

Dr. Freis, Moderator: Dr. Simon, that was an excellent review. I wanted to ask you about your opening statement that renovascular hypertension is an important cause of remedial hypertension in man. To make such a statement, it would seem to me, you need to know what is the prevalence of this disorder in the general population, not just what is the prevalence in specialized clinics where patients are funneled in from all over the state. Have you any answer to that? What is the cure rate where patients have relief of their hypertension and do not have to go on medical therapy?

Dr. Simon: In answer to your first question, being a nephrologist primarily, Dr. Freis, of course I consider renovascular disease an important cause of hypertension. But in terms of frequency, you are quite right, we were dealing with quite a selected population, even in the Cooperative Study. Thirty-six percent of patients in the Cooperative Study had renal artery hypertension. I would agree with you that in unselected series the figure is well below 10% and probably on the order of 1% to 2%.

Dr. Freis: That is a big difference, 10% and 1%, especially when you are talking about 23 million hypertensives and I really would like to know the answer to that.

Dr. Holland: I cannot give you the answer to that question except that from two population studies, one in South Wales and one in Lambeth, there was one possible case out of 300 to 400 individuals with hypertension. As a pupil of Sir Austin Bradford Hill, I was taken aback by the use of tests of statistical significance in comparing these two groups. Were these randomized control trials? The conclusions that you draw are very important, but they may not be applicable if the two groups are not comparable.

Dr. Simon: That was the very point that I was trying to make, that none of the trials that were carried out were controlled. There was no random allocation of patients to medical or surgical treatment. Patients treated medically were by and large much poorer risks and I was only attempting to use statistics to show certain differences which might look to be significant. For example, in the Dustan series, 58% versus 41% was by no means statistically significant. In those cases where statistical significance was achieved, one could question the meaning of the results based on the very problem that you have raised.

Dr. Freis: I think you also said that there was a big difference in age between the two groups.

Dr. Simon: In most series the medically treated patients were older than the surgically treated patients.

Dr. Dollery: I would have thought the only conclusion that you can draw from the data is that no conclusion is possible about the relative merits of medical and surgical treatment. I would say, perhaps unfairly, one could summarize your final slide by saying that if a patient was young enough to withstand surgery that he should have surgery, that if he was too old and ill then medical treatment would be what you would apply. That is pretty well what has been done and any kind of comparison between groups under those circumstances is invalid.

Dr. Simon: I would wholly agree and that is the implication I would like to leave with you, that I do not think there has been one adequate therapeutic trial to answer the question whether medical or surgical therapy is appropriate.

Dr. Carolyn McCue, Virginia: Could you tell us more specifically about the distribution in age groups? You have alluded to the younger children or the older patients.

Dr. Simon: I cannot precisely answer your question but in almost all series the vast majority of patients could be considered to be in the adult age range, most being above the age of 20 and almost all being above the age of 15, with very few patients in what could be called the pediatric age.

Dr. Labarthe, Minnesota: A question of central importance is whether the evidence available so far is sufficient to warrant a trial, in view of estimates of the extent of the problem of renovascular hypertension in the population. Would Dr. Simon be in a position at this point to recommend, in fact, that a controlled trial should be done?

Dr. Simon: We are probably in the same stage that we are in in terms of bypass surgery for coronary artery disease. These studies were done earlier with the clear supposition that surgical therapy was going to be vastly superior to medical therapy. Obviously, such has not turned out to be the case. Yes, in terms of clear thinking about the problem, I would think that a careful, prospective trial of medical versus surgical therapy of renal artery hypertension is in order. I think we now understand what variables are important, which ones must be controlled. This would take a large-scale cooperative effort. Whether this is a wise allocation of limited medical resources, considering the greater importance of the patient with essential hypertension, is certainly debatable.

Dr. Haynes, Canada: I would like to hear the answer to Dr. Freis' other question, what proportion of those people who have been treated surgically for renovascular hypertension were controlled without any medication? I believe from one of your statements that there was a considerable chance of contamination and that the surgical group could have been on medical treatment as well.

Dr. Simon: I can only speak from the results in the Cooperative Study. Patients who were classified as cured of their hypertension were patients who had diastolic blood pressure levels below the 90 mm Hg and who were off all antihypertensive therapy. This figure was about 50%. However, you must realize that this is at one particular period, approximately one year or so after surgery. Whether the blood pressure will continue to remain at normal levels without the use of drugs we cannot answer at this time from the Cooperative Study. In many other studies patients were considered to be cured if their blood pressures could be maintained below 90 with mild hypotensive therapy. I would not consider that to be a cure.

Dr. Freis: In that regard I would say that I saw data from a series from France where over a five-year period there was a gradual return. At one year the results looked very good but over a five-year period there was gradual return so that at five years nearly all were hypertensive again. I am not saying that is representative, but I do not think one year is long enough for a follow-up in such a chronic disease.

Dr. Hoobler, Michigan: I was not going to say anything, but I am almost forced to by the generally negative conclusion. In the first place a 6%-8% mortality rate really involves a lot of very tough bilateral surgical cases. Most of us in practice think about unilateral renal disease with a clear-cut angiographic abnormality and a good surgical team. Using that approach in Michigan, at least, I would doubt we have had any deaths. We have not had any recrudescence of hypertension in the very simple case which particularly in younger people calls for surgery. Let us put on the record the other side, too. Many of the statistics were obtained in the early years of the study in which we were developing techniques. I think if you were to analyze the results in the last year of the study, the mortality rate would be less and the cure rate would probably be higher.

VI
Community Studies and Programs

Sequels to Screening for Hypertension

R. R. H. Lovell, M.D.

At the symposium on the Epidemiology of Hypertension,[1] held here ten years ago, much time was devoted to discussing population surveys undertaken to establish facts about blood pressure in different communities. Screening means more than fact-finding. In the context of this symposium, it describes the measurement of blood pressure (with or without other things) in a community, with the intention that people showing abnormalities have a further check-up which may result in treatment being advised.

Sequels to screening will be influenced by the primary purpose for which the screening is undertaken. In many studies, special arrangements are made for check-ups on subjects screened positive and for their subsequent management. This is so when the primary object of screening is to find patients for therapeutic trials. It is also the case when the process of regularly repeated screening is itself being evaluated as in the Permanente study.[2]

In Australia, and perhaps in other countries, if widespread community screening for hypertension were initiated as a measure of preventive medicine, reasons could be advanced for having subjects who need to be checked, and possibly treated, handled within the existing health care system. In order to judge if this method of dealing with subjects picked up by screening is to be commended, it is necessary to find out what happens when it is used.

Reports bearing on this from the United States[3-5] give the impression that the handling of notified subjects has been considered disappointing. I am going to present and discuss

R. R. H. Lovell, M.D., *Professor and Chairman, University of Melbourne Department of Medicine, The Royal Melbourne Hospital, Victoria, Australia.*

some findings that are more encouraging. The observations
arose from a screening study done with Drs. R. J. Prineas and
W. B. Stephens in a provincial city in Australia. The primary
object was to discover the prevalence of hypertension and the
extent to which it was being diagnosed and treated.

The Screening Study

The design and findings of the screening study have been
described in detail elsewhere.[6] The screening was done in
September 1971. The subjects were people aged 50-59 living in
the central part of the provincial city of Albury, New South
Wales (pop. 25,000). From a census-defined population, 1,515
were screened (an overall response of 79%). Only blood pressure
(BP), weight and height were measured. Only subjects with
diastolic blood pressure (DBP) ⩾ 110 mm Hg were notified.
These people received a single letter advising them to have a
further check-up from their local doctor, who was also notified.

The Follow-up

Follow-up so far has included searches of the local registry
of deaths and of the admission and discharge records of the two
local hospitals, and postal inquiries addressed to the 21 local
doctors, 3 and 18 months after the screening. The focal point of
the follow-up was a postal inquiry about treatment directed to
participating subjects 21 months after screening, ie, after they
had attended at a central place in Albury to have their BP
measured.

Our experience has been that a postal inquiry about
treatment for hypertension brings quite accurate replies.[6] In
this study, in a subsample of cases in which this was tested,
there was agreement between doctors and patients in 85% of
cases. The most frequent disagreement was in the 12% of cases
in which the patient denied treatment which the doctor said
was being prescribed, so that the rate of treatment reported
here may be an underestimate.

The Sequels

The sequels discovered by these inquiries are described in
detail elsewhere[7, 8] and may be summarized as follows:

At 3 months: Of 200 subjects notified with DBP ≥ 110 mm Hg, 90% had seen their doctor and treatment had been started or changed in 45% of them.

At 21 months: Information was obtained on 98% of 1,514 in the original screened sample.* There had been 17 deaths (4 in the notified group). The rate of treatment in the screened sample had risen from 12% to 21%. The rate of treatment in the notified group had risen from 27% to 50%. Two thirds of the newly treated subjects in the screened sample were not among those who had been notified as having DBP ≥ 110 mm Hg. The numbers of new strokes occurring in Albury in people aged 50-64 were 13 in 1970-1971, 12 in 1971-1972 and 4 in 1972-1973.

The outstanding sequel to the screening was the increased treatment rate in the screened sample from 12% to 21% 21 months after screening. A detailed comparison of the status of the screened sample in 1971 and 1973 is shown in Table 1. Altogether, 3% of subjects did not reply, had left the district or had died. The patients newly on treatment in 1973 were 135 subjects who had never been told they had high blood pressure in 1971 and a smaller number, 38, who had previously been told but who were not on treatment in 1971.

TABLE 1. Comparison of Status in 1971 and 1973 of Subjects
Whose Blood Pressure Was Measured in 1971

| | Status in 1971 | | | | |
| | | Previously Told BP Was High | | | |
Status in 1973	Never Told BP Was High	Not on Treatment	On Treatment	Total	Percent
No reply	1		2	3	0.2
Left district	20		6	26	1.7
Dead	12	2	3	17	1.1
Not on treatment	1,009	115	27	1,151	76.0
On treatment	135	38	144	317	21.0
Total	1,177	155	182	1,514	100.0
Percent	77.8	10.2	12.0	100.0	

*Records of one original subject were lost.

Table 1 also shows that of the 182 patients who were on treatment in 1971, 27 said they were no longer under treatment in 1973. This suggests that in Albury, as elsewhere, treatment once initiated is not always sustained.

It has already been indicated that two thirds of the subjects newly started on treatment by 1973 were not among those notified in 1971. In other words, two thirds of them in 1971 had diastolic pressures on screening of less than 110 mm Hg and so no comment was made to them or to their doctors.

Diastolic blood pressures in 1971, in relation to 1973 treatment status, are illustrated in Figure 1. It shows the distributions of the 1971 DBPs of the 1,178 subjects (1,177 with records in 1973) who in 1971 said they had never been told they had high blood pressure. The hatched columns show the DBPs of the 135 subjects newly on treatment in 1973. (Means and standard deviations: 103.8±16.3 mm Hg for 64 males and 99.1±18.4 mm Hg for 71 females.) The clear columns show the DBPs of the other 1,043 subjects in the group, 1,009 (97%) of whom were known to be alive and not on treatment in 1973 (Table 1). (Means and standard deviations: 89.8±13.6 mm Hg for 523 males and 89.0±13.0 mm Hg for 520 females.)

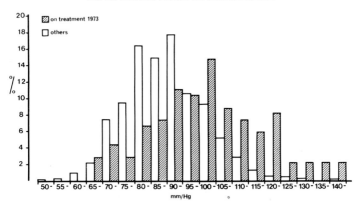

Fig. 1. Distribution of 1971 diastolic blood pressures of subjects who in 1971 had never been told they had high blood pressure. Hatched columns show distribution of pressures of 135 subjects newly on treatment in 1973. Clear columns show distribution of pressures of the 1,042 others.

Clearly, the people newly on treatment were not just a random sample of everyone screened, for their pressure distribution was significantly different from that of people who had not been started on treatment.

From these distributions, it seems highly probable that many of the subjects newly started on treatment by 1973 would have had DBPs when treatment was initiated well below the level of 110 mm Hg that we used as the cutoff point for notification. This would accord with the fact that many local doctors indicated, before they knew the results of the survey, that they would generally treat patients with DBP $\geq$ 110 mm Hg, and also with the fact that our early follow-up showed that the doctors' stated intentions were in good agreement with their actual practice.[7]

Discussion

It is evident from these findings that the frequency of treatment in the subjects screened was strikingly increased in the 21 months after screening and that this increase occurred within the ordinary local health care system. Most people in Australia can identify one general practitioner whom they regard as their personal doctor and whom they pay a fee for service. The health care system is based on voluntary insurance, the benefits from which are subsidized by government. At the time of this study, most of the Albury 50-59 year age group would have been insured and after reimbursement from their insurance fund the cost to the patient of a consultation with a general practitioner would have been about 80 cents Aust. ($1.20 US). Under the Pharmaceutical Benefits Scheme, a prescription would have cost them $1.00 Aust. ($1.50 US).

An increased rate of treatment in a community is not necessarily an indication of benefit. Some benefit may be presumed to have been conferred as a result of increasing the rate of treatment in those notified as having DBP $\geq$ 110 mm Hg from 27% to 50%. Among the 46 subjects concerned there were several who, on further checks made by their doctors, proved to have sustained very high pressures. But these 46 made up only one third of the total of those newly treated, and there is less certainty that those symptomless subjects who were started on treatment with lower pressures would have benefited — an uncertainty which is the basis of the controlled trials of treatment in mild hypertension at present being conducted. The test of benefit in a community must be reduced hypertension-associated morbidity and mortality which is not outweighed by illness or death from other causes, nor by spoiling the quality of people's lives. Our study permits no conclusion on this. As already indicated, there were fewer strokes in the 50-64 age group in Albury as a whole after the screening; this change was not paralleled in other age groups, but with the small numbers it could have happened by chance.

Whether or not the increased treatment rate following screening was a good thing, it is worth considering the factors that might have been responsible for it. They may be relevant to future planning; anyway, the etiology of a disturbance in a community following screening demands explanation.

The possibility was considered that the increase might simply have reflected a change in the country as a whole. A nationwide increase of this order would have been reflected in a sharp increase in the number of prescriptions written for hypotensive drugs under the Pharmaceutical Benefits Scheme. The numbers have been increasing over many years, but figures supplied by the Commonwealth Department of Health show that the increase between 1971 and 1972 and 1972 and 1973 was no greater than previously, either for major hypotensive drugs or for the major diuretics.

Because most people newly on treatment in 1973 were not cases that were notified in 1971, factors besides notification itself must have increased awareness of blood pressure among local doctors and in the community generally. Table 2 shows that our interventions in Albury were quite numerous, although the ones following screening were mostly unplanned. At the preliminary meeting with local doctors, we aimed for acceptance of the screening idea without altering current therapeutic practice, because this was one of the things we wanted to find out. Publicity was designed to inform the community, to reassure about financial costs and to emphasize a continuing normal relationship between individuals and their doctors whatever the findings on screening might be. Contact between individuals and the screening team occurred only through the initial census, the filling in of a questionnaire, the BP

TABLE 2. List of Interventions in the Community in Albury in
Relation to Screening for Blood Pressure in September 1971

Oct. 1970	Preliminary meeting with local doctors. Census (completed April 1971)
Sept. 1971	Publicity Questionnaires and screening invitations sent Blood pressure measurements 2 weeks later
Oct. 1971	Notification of DBP $\geqslant$ 110 mm Hg to subjects and their local doctors
Jan. 1972	Follow-up inquiry to doctors
April 1972	Report on findings to local doctors
Aug. 1972	Talk to local doctors on investigation and treatment of hypertension
Feb. 1973	Talk to local doctors on renal aspects of hypertension
April 1973	Follow-up inquiry to local doctors
July 1973	Follow-up inquiry to subjects screened
Sept. 1973	Supplementary follow-up inquiry to subjects

measurement and, for those with DBP $\geqslant$ 110 mm Hg, the letter
of notification.

In retrospect, the striking feature of this list (Table 2) is the
number of contacts we made with local doctors — six in the 18
months following screening. Some 90% of the doctors attended
the postscreening talks which were arranged through the local
medical society by Dr. W. B. Stephens, the specialist physician
in Albury and a member of the investigating team. It would
have been tempting to emphasize the importance of the close
relationship that developed with the local doctors as an
important determinant of the increased treatment rate. However, we can make some tentative comparison with sequels to a
similar screening exercise which we undertook in an inner
suburb of Melbourne in 1972,[9, 10] in which personal contacts
between the screening team and the far more numerous local
doctors were minimal. In Melbourne, only 60% of notified
people had attended their doctors at three months postscreening, compared with 90% in Albury. However, responses to
a first follow-up letter, received so far from about 70% of those
screened, indicate that at 18 months postscreening the treatment rate has also risen sharply. As in Albury, about 11% of

those who, when screened, said they had never been told they had high blood pressure now say they are on treatment and, once again, the majority were not subjects notified as having DBP $\geqslant$ 110 mm Hg.

Comparison of experience in other studies will help to identify which of the many factors associated with screening are the main determinants of sequels such as these. The increased treatment rates presumably result either from doctors taking blood pressures more often, taking action more frequently as a result of their findings, or both. Evidently, in Australia, such sequels can and do occur in the context of the normal health care system.

Summary

If widespread community screening for hypertension were initiated, subjects needing to be checked and possibly treated might be dealt with within the local health care system. Since little is known of what happens to subjects handled in this way, the status of 1,515 people aged 50-59 screened in 1971 in a prevalence study in Albury, Australia, was examined 21 months later. The treatment rate in the screened sample had nearly doubled, from 12% to 21%. Two thirds of those newly on treatment in 1973 were not among those notified on the basis of the finding of a DBP $\geqslant$ 110 mm Hg in 1971. Factors related to this screening episode which may have contributed to the increased treatment rate, which occurred within the context of the normal health care system, were discussed.

References

1. Stamler, J., Stamler, S. and Pullman, T. N. (eds.): *The Epidemiology of Hypertension.* New York:Grune and Stratton, 1967.
2. Cutler, J. L., Ramcharan, S. F., Feldman, R. et al: Multiphasic checkup evaluation study. 1. Methods and population. *Prev. Med.,* 2:197, 1973.
3. Wilber, J. A. and Barrow, J. G.: Reducing elevated blood pressure. Experience found in a community. *Minnesota Med.,* 52:97, 1969.
4. Wilber, J. A., Millward, D., Baldwin, A. et al: The Atlanta Community High Blood Pressure Program. Methods of community hypertension screening. *Circ. Res.,* 31 (suppl. 2): 101, 1972.
5. Schoenberger, J. A., Stamler, J., Shekelle, R. B. et al: Current status of hypertension control in an industrial population. *JAMA,* 222:559, 1972.

6. Prineas, R. J., Stephens, W. B. and Lovell, R. R. H.: Blood pressure and its treatment in a community. The Albury Blood Pressure Study. *Med. J. Aust.*, 1:5, 1973.

7. Prineas, R. J., Stephens, W. B. and Lovell, R. R. H.: Early consequences of screening for hypertension in a community. *Clin. Sci. Molec. Med.*, 45:475, 1973.

8. Lovell, R. R. H., Stephens, W. B., Prineas, R. J. et al: Some sequels to screening an Australian community for hypertension: A follow-up in Albury. *Med. J. Aust.*, 1974, in preparation.

9. Lovell, R. R. H. and Prineas, R. J.: The identification and treatment of hypertensives in two Australian urban communities. *Int. J. Epidem.*, 3:25, 1974.

10. Lovell, R. R. H. and Prineas, R. J.: Differences in blood pressure measurements and prevalence of hypertension between Australian-born and Italian-born middle-aged men and women in Melbourne. *Med. J. Aust.*, 2:893, 1974.

Discussion

Dr. Tyroler: I would like to echo and support your concern, Dr. Lovell, for the effect on the medical organizational structure and, equally, the effect on the social structure and the response of patients and the need for caution and controlled trials. However, I would also like to point out that we have been talking about community control from a very narrow perspective. I don't mean to belittle it. It is extraordinarily important. But, if we were completely successful at present in screening, referring, diagnosing, treating and achieving follow-up, at best we would be engaged in secondary prevention. We might achieve our goals of reduction of morbidity and mortality as we have laid them out. But we are all aware of the fact that this is just the beginning of the exercise. I would like to suggest that when we speak about control, we should keep in mind the challenge that Dr. Stamler put to us to speak about primary prevention. At our next ten years' meeting, based upon some of the ground-breaking work that has been reported at this symposium, hopefully we will have primary prevention tools. We have heard much here about poverty and social disorganization. I would like to try to reconcile the apparent disparity between Dr. Schoenberger's findings of no effect of poverty and the findings that Dr. Borhani and Dr. Stamler reported for mortality statistics. Those who have been fortunate enough or perhaps unfortunate enough to live and work in the rural South recognize that the phenomenon of poverty, particularly in the black population, is so widespread and the variation is so small, that there is little or no opportunity to test this variable and its effects upon blood pressure. You can't really test for the effects of poverty in that particular setting. The hope for the future, of course, is that poverty will not remain forever and there might be variation to be observed.

You have mentioned the fact that you have looked into a poverty area. Did you simultaneously look at blood pressure levels or just treatment levels? Did you observe the effect of poverty? If so, was it in the similar direction?

Dr. Lovell: We only looked at treatment level. In the poorer area we found the same phenomenon as in Albury — the treatment rate had gone up and in the preliminary replies, it had gone up to the same extent. May I echo your and Dr. Stamler's point about the lesson that I hope perhaps might be the main lesson for our proceedings and that is this question of primary prevention. I just find it terribly hard to contemplate the possibility that one out of five people in my age group should be taking pills for the rest of his life.

Dr. Hatano: Since I am from the World Health Organization, you may wonder what, under the circumstances, World Health Organization is doing. Actually, after consultation with experts including Doctors Lovell, Holland and Dollery, we have embarked upon a pilot study on hypertension control in the community using the hypertension register as a tool.

Participating centers are from all over the world, for example, Mongolia, Japan, Nigeria, Jamaica and in several European countries. We prepared general guidelines about the level of blood pressure and at what age treatment should be given, but the decision is left to the treating physician. We put emphasis on the education of general practitioners and populations. This is done in various ways in different countries. Evaluation of the program will be made in five years.

Dr. Dollery: Dr. Freis' data are the best, but are based upon pressures after six to eight weeks on placebo medication. We know from other studies that if we translate that into single casual readings, we will probably have to add 10 mm Hg to 12 mm Hg. So, when you say treat at 105 mm Hg diastolic, you are saying, "treat at somewhere around 115 mm Hg to 117 mm Hg

diastolic on single casual readings." Those who are going into
hypertension control programs must bear this level in mind.
They must also remember what was said about Dr. Freis' paper,
that a great many of the complications were in those who had
already suffered complications. So, one cannot take the VA
data and translate it directly to unselected hypertensive
individuals in the community. That is why at the meeting held
at the World Health Organization a little while ago, Dr. Holland
and I argued strenuously that there is a range of pressures,
perhaps in this range of casual diastolic readings of 90 mm Hg
to 115 mm Hg, where we really don't know what the impact of
a community control program would be. Obviously, there is a
level of diastolic pressure, perhaps on a casual reading it is 115
mm Hg on up, where we can say from the VA data that we need
to treat. I am interested that among the epidemiologists here,
who I have always felt were some of the most scientific
physicians in the community, that this wave of enthusiasm for
treatment in that middle range is running somewhat ahead of
the evidence. The reason why it is important is that every time
you shift your criteria 5 or 10 mm Hg down, you are talking
about treating millions of additional people.

Dr. Lovell: I not only agree entirely with Dr. Dollery, but
what causes me great disquiet is whether this enthusiasm, this
attempt to put marking points, isn't rubbing off on members of
the profession generally, causing them to react by treating
people as suggested in one of the slides I showed.

Dr. Stamler: I am sorry, but I am afraid that I cannot let Dr.
Dollery "off the hook" with that argument, because we have
another responsibility and this is what we are really discussing —
the responsibility all physicians always have (including researchers) to arrive at a best judgment from the presently available
data. A few years ago, before the VA published their trial data,
we had the same debates. I can recall very vividly disagreeing
with colleagues who argued against treatment for practically all
but malignant hypertension. Clearly we were then giving best
judgment in the absence of any data from good randomized
controlled trials. Some of us were then emphasizing that the
insurance companies had been giving us data for decades about
the risks of hypertension, data fully confirmed by the Framingham, Gas Company, Western Electric, Albany, Minnesota, Los

Angeles, etc., prospective epidemiologic studies. Considerable information was by then available — ie, ten years ago — on the side and toxic effects of the antihypertensive medications, so that one could weigh risks of high blood pressure versus risks of the pharmacologic agents for lowering blood pressure. Based on such assessments, many of us arrived at the best judgment that for a wide range of persons with "benign" (what a misnomer!) hypertension — markedly at risk of premature sickness, disability and death — the best judgment was to treat, and the judgment to follow the path of therapeutic nihilism (a la Goldring and Chasis), of "judicious" neglect was really injudicious, *not* best judgment. I agree with Dr. Dollery that you need to add up to 10 mm Hg to the VA average levels to get comparative casual levels. In any case, we as leaders in population care have to offer best medical judgments today about nutritional, hygienic and pharmacologic treatment for *all* at greater risk due to hypertension.

Finally, I cannot agree that the problems of compliance are so huge and mysterious that they justify doing nothing about screening and detection. If that position had been taken 50 or 75 years ago, we would not have TB under control. Of course, if you use inadequate health delivery operations — "classically" oriented on acute care for sick people, and overworked to boot — as referral centers for hypertensives detected in mass screening, it's easy to "prove" how big the compliance problem is, how "apathetic" hypertensive patients are, etc. Our experience in the Hypertension Detection and Follow-up Program, and the Coronary Prevention Evaluation Program in Chicago is that satisfactory compliance can be achieved in a *majority* of hypertensives with modern methods of long-term care.

Now, the second big issue is a little different. Once you make a judgment, do you have to wait for years for control trials before you begin community programming on the notion that until we check everything out, community programming with continuing evaluation is impossible? That, I think, is the essence of Dr. Sackett's position. I don't agree with that, for a variety of reasons, including, by the way, the initial year of experience in the Hypertension Detection and Follow-Up Program, on the ability to go into communities with good effective care and to treat well.

Dr. Holland: As an epidemiologist, perhaps I could make just a very brief comment and that is to quote Sir Austin Bradford Hill. He stated that there is only one opportunity to determine whether any form of treatment is effective and that is at the start. If we don't do it now, we will never be able to find out because it will not be ethically possible to do the trials that Doctors Sackett, Lovell, Dollery and I have been talking about here. As Dr. Dollery has stated, we do not have the evidence in the "middle ground" — if we don't get it now, we never will.

Dr. Simpson, New Zealand: One of the problems here is the level of cutoff point for treatment. There is no doubt that with these community surveys, two things are being done: certain people with relatively low blood pressures are being picked up and, often, are now being treated. However, in addition, there are those with the high figures, who have previously been going undetected, and who are referred for treatment. In agreement with Dr. Stamler, I think this is the important point at the moment. If one is looking at pure cost-effectiveness, one would be picking out those people who have very high blood pressures and treating them. Anyone who works in a hospital knows that patients come along quite frequently with severe complications which could have been avoided if the severe hypertension had been detected sooner. I don't believe that the problem of community surveys for those with very high pressures need necessarily be mixed up with the problem of knowing what to do with people with relatively low pressures. If only we could do wider screening to pick out the very high blood pressures, I suspect that more benefit would ensue.

Community Studies of Hypertension in Glasgow

V. M. Hawthorne, M.D., D. A. Greaves, M.B., B.S.
and D. G. Beevers, M.B., B.S.

The estimated total population of Scotland in 1972 was 5,235,300. Of these, 1,698,200 lived in the Central Clydeside Conurbation[1] where the City of Glasgow with its population of 861,898[2] is the major center of an area with a soft water supply and an excess mortality from cardiovascular and other diseases compared with the rest of Scotland, England and Wales.[3] Diseases of the circulatory system[4] (pp. 390-458) are the leading cause of death in Scotland. In 1972 they accounted for 54.6% of a total mortality, comprising 17,399 men and 18,095 women to which ischemic heart disease[4] (pp. 410-414) contributed 10,763 male and 8,238 female deaths representing 32.4% and 25.9%, respectively, of the national mortality. In recent years, the annual increase in ischemic heart disease in the United Kingdom has been greater than in the United States, but not as marked as in Northern Europe.[5,6] A comparison of age-specific death rates in 1969 showed these to be about the same in men and women as in the United States and Finland, but higher than in Czechoslovakia, Singapore, Sweden and Japan.[7] As in many other centers with comparable problems, considerable epidemiological interest attaches to hypertension and to the possibilities of early detection and treatment in the primary prevention of ischemic heart disease and of cerebrovascular disease[4] (pp. 430-438) which is responsible for about 10,000 deaths in Scotland annually.

During the last nine years, a small cardiorespiratory screening unit, based jointly on the Department of Community

V. M. Hawthorne, M.D., F.R.C.P. (Glas.), F.F.C.M.; D. A. Greaves, M.B., B.S., and D. G. Beevers, M.B., B.S., *Department of Community Medicine, University of Glasgow, Ruchill Hospital, Glasgow, Scotland.*

Medicine at Glasgow University and on the Glasgow Mass Miniature Radiography Service and using the facilities of that service to secure access to defined groups of the Scottish population, has developed techniques for the assessment of cardiorespiratory parameters in the general population and in specific occupational groups in the West of Scotland. Prospective studies now in progress include one involving 10,000 subjects in occupational and general population groups. This particular study has contributed to a collaborative random controlled trial of stopping smoking in the prevention of cardiorespiratory disease[9] and the occupational component has provided the data for a study of the prevalence of hyperlipoproteinemia.[10] In addition, the general population sample drawn from the Burgh of Renfrew[11,12] has acted as a pilot for the general population study of tuberculosis, hypertension and cardiorespiratory disease of 20,000 subjects which is now in progress in the Burgh of Paisley.[13] Some of the problems of estimating prevalence and incidence, making diagnoses and arranging for the disposal and follow-up of patients suspected of having hypertension are outlined here.

Material and Methods

Renfrew, with a population of 19,000 and Paisley, the adjacent town and the largest burgh in Scotland with a population of 95,000 people, are urban burghs situated about seven miles from Glasgow. Door-to-door censuses of 6,534 (99.1% response) households appearing on the burgh assessor's rating list in Renfrew and of 9,515 (96.9% response) households canvassed so far in the first three sectors of Paisley have identified 3,810 men and women between the ages of 45 and 64 years in Renfrew and 5,337 in Paisley who were eligible and capable of attending for screening examination.

Response

In Renfrew, 3,000 (78.7%) − 1,407 (78.7%) males and 1,593 (78.8%) females − attended for examination in 1972; and 1,062 (79.6%) males and 1,201 (79.6%) females eligible and capable of attending for reexamination in 1973 − about 60% of those originally eligible in 1972 − returned for examination in

1973. In Paisley, 4,018 (70.8% — range 78.0%-68.4%) men and women from 5,337 persons eligible and capable of attending for examination have attended from the first three of ten sectors which are to be examined in that town between February 1974 and June 1976.

All were offered a timed appointment to attend a temporary examination center (Fig. 1) situated as close as possible to the middle of the district under study. Before attending, each patient was asked to complete a standard questionnaire* which included symptoms of cardiovascular and respiratory disease. At the temporary examination center ten subjects arrived every ten minutes during each afternoon and evening session. Individual questionnaires were checked and standard investigations lasting approximately 20 minutes were undertaken by a staff of about

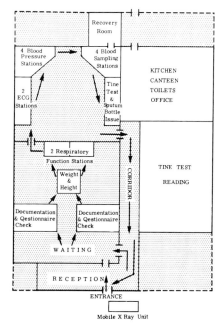

Fig. 1. Layout of a temporary examination center.[1][2]

---

*Available from VMH.

Figures 1-3 from *British Medical Journal.*[1][2]

40 permanent, part-time and voluntary Red Cross workers as follows:

Measurement was made of height and weight; forced expiratory volume in one second was observed using a Garthur Vitalograph with the subject standing, the best of two expirations being recorded. A six-lead electrocardiogram (leads I, II, III, aVR, aVL and aVF) was taken in the sitting position. Blood pressure was estimated while seated by observers trained on standardized tapes[14] using the London School of Hygiene and Tropical Medicine sphygmomanometer[15] with a cuff of 12 × 22 cm.

A 10 ml nonfasting blood sample was taken for plasma cholesterol in both Renfrew and Paisley and for electrolytes, urea, blood sugar and plasma potassium concentration (centrifuged within two hours) in Renfrew only. In both burghs, a tuberculin Tine test (Lederle) and a 70 mm miniature chest x-ray were made and sputa collected for direct examination and culture as part of the study of tuberculosis.[13]

The cost of the whole examination was estimated at £4.31 per person.

All subjects with abnormalities requiring immediate attention were referred directly to their general practitioner. This group included patients with a diastolic blood pressure of 115 mm Hg or more confirmed by two observers. Subjects with diastolic blood pressures between 100 and 114 mm Hg in Renfrew and between 95 and 114 mm Hg in Paisley were recalled for secondary screening examination within 12 weeks. All subjects with blood pressure sustained within these ranges were referred to special clinics established in cooperation with the general practitioners in their health center in Renfrew under the direction of Dr. Gareth Beevers of the Glasgow MRC Blood Pressure Unit and in the outpatient department of the Royal Alexandra Infirmary in Paisley under the consultant supervision of Dr. Hugh Conway. Risk scores were calculated on a scale derived from the Framingham study[16] and high-risk smokers outside the range of blood pressure abnormality described above, randomly allocated to a controlled trial of the effects of discontinuance of smoking.

The Renfrew examinees were offered reexamination on the anniversary of their original examination in 1972. For both study populations, mortality is reported monthly by the Registrar General in Scotland and morbidity annually by the Research and Intelligence Unit of the Scottish Home and Health Department through medical record linkage with the Scottish Hospital Inpatient Statistics (SHIP). Additional linkage has been established with the West of Scotland Oncological Organisation and the local tuberculosis department. The written permission to consult NHS records is obtained from all examinees.

The outpatient clinics for those with blood pressure sustained above the limits defined above at the general practitioner health center at Renfrew and in the outpatient department of the Royal Alexandra Infirmary in Paisley were staffed by a registrar from the Western Infirmary in Glasgow and from the local hospital together with a nurse/secretary. At Paisley the clinic was staffed by a group of general practitioners from that area under the supervision of two consultant physicians. Ten new patients and an appropriate number of "return" patients are seen on three evenings each week as part of the MRC trial of "mild to moderate" hypertension.

Results

Figure 2 shows that in Renfrew there was no evidence of a bimodal distribution of subjects with and without hypertension.[17]

In both Renfrew and Paisley, after 12 weeks, reexamination of those with elevation of blood pressure above the limits described above reduced these numbers substantially. In Renfrew 476 (15.8%) of those initially screened had blood pressure > 100 mm Hg but ultimately only 165 (5.5%) of the whole sample were referred to the clinic after secondary screening. Table 1 shows the corresponding reduction in numbers identified at primary screening, effected by secondary screening following an interval of 8 to 12 weeks in the first three sectors in Paisley.

Examination of the general practitioners' records in the Renfrew Health Center showed that, in addition to 468 (15.6%) patients detected as having an elevated blood pressure by the screening unit, a further 168 hypertensives whose blood pressure was within normal limits at the time of the survey were identified from the general practitioners' records, thus making a

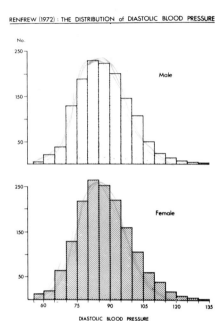

Figure 2.

total of 636 (21.1%) of the whole sample as having had elevated blood pressure at one time or another or being on treatment at the time of the survey examination (Table 2). Two hundred and fifty-five of those identified as hypertensive initially by screening, representing 8.5% of the whole sample or 54.5% of all detected by screening, had no record of high blood pressure in the general practitioners' records.

TABLE 1. The Census and Screening Response and Yields at Primary and Secondary Screening in the First Three Sectors of Paisley 1974

| | Response | | Yield | |
	Household census	Primary screening	Primary screening 95 mm Hg	Secondary screening 90 to 109 mm Hg
Glenburn	96.8%	1,880 (76.0%)	533 (28.3%)	313 (17.2%)
Foxbar	96.5%	1,457 (78.0%)	319 (21.9%)	180 (12.4%)
Mossvale	97.6%	681 (68.4%)	154 (22.6%)	75 (11.0%)

TABLE 2. Prevalence of Hypertension Related to
General Practitioners' National Health Service Records
(Renfrew Burgh Survey 1972 n = 3000 45-64 yrs)

Identified by screening as having diastolic blood pressure ≥ 100 mm Hg		
No entry in NHS record	255 (54.5%)	
Details of treatment in NHS record	73 (15.6%)	
Not yet traced	140 (29.9%)	
	468 (100.0%)	468 (15.6%)
Identified by general practitioners' NHS records and with diastolic blood pressure < 100 mm Hg		
Entry regarding raised blood pressure in GPNHS records	113 (67.3%)	
Entry regarding treatment of raised blood pressure in GPNHS records	55 (32.7%)	
	168 (100.0%)	636 (21.1%)

In Renfrew blood pressure observations were repeated on the anniversary of the initial examination (Fig. 3). In 93 (3.0%) persons, blood pressure had risen above 100 mm Hg diastolic. Mean blood pressure and standard deviations for the whole of the study population remained constant over the year (Table 3) and, as will be seen, rises and falls in blood pressure in the whole group were evenly distributed.[1] [2]

Medical Record Linkage

To date, 307 male and 72 female deaths have been notified by the Registrar General from 15,000 registered examinees. The crude mortality two years after the initial survey of Renfrew was 37 (2.63%) males and 17 (1.07%) females, 19 (1.4%) of the male and 4 (0.25%) of the female deaths being attributed to rheumatic, hypertensive, ischemic and other types of heart disease.[4] [pp. 343-429] Ischemic heart disease[4] [pp. 410-414] rates were 17 (1.2%) and two (0.1%) in men and women, respectively.

Two hundred and sixty-four possible admissions of subjects in the Renfrew sample to hospitals throughout Scotland were notified by the Scottish Home and Health Department to the screening unit from scrutiny of the Scottish Hospital In-patients' Statistics data file in March 1973. Excluding repeated

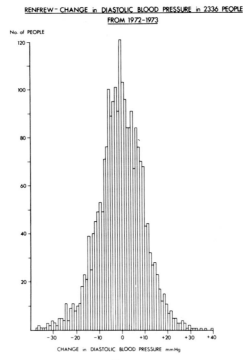

RENFREW – CHANGE in DIASTOLIC BLOOD PRESSURE in 2336 PEOPLE
FROM 1972–1973

Figure 3.

admissions of the same subject, 147 (55.7%) were correctly notified, the proportion of correctly linked cases diminishing from 69 (93.2%) for admissions to hospitals in the Renfrew and Paisley area to 73 (62.9%) for admissions to hospitals in Glasgow. Only five (6.7%) notifications for the rest of the country were confirmed. Morbidity rates from all causes were 63 (4.6%) in men and 82 (5.1%) in women. The incidence of rheumatic, hypertensive, ischemic and other types of heart disease[4] (pp. 393-429) was nine (0.6%) for men and six (0.37%) for women. There were six (0.4%) male and four (0.3%) female admissions for ischemic heart disease.[4] (pp. 410-414)

Discussion

The report of the Joint Working Party of the Scottish Home and Health Department on the integrated health service[18]

TABLE 3. The Mean and S.D. of Systolic and Diastolic Blood Pressure in Males and Females Examined in the Renfrew Burgh Survey in 1972 and 1973[12]

		Males								Females							
		45-49 yrs		50-54 yrs		55-59 yrs		60-64 yrs		45-49 yrs		50-54 yrs		55-59 yrs		60-64 yrs	
		1972	1973	1972	1973	1972	1973	1972	1973	1972	1973	1972	1973	1972	1973	1972	1973
Systolic Blood Pressure	No.	403	230	377	257	340	218	289	204	449	229	415	301	377	256	351	254
	Mean	142.8	140.9	147.3	144.9	153.5	151.7	156.9	153.3	145.2	142.6	149.7	150.1	158.3	158.1	163.7	164.9
	S.D.	20.4	18.8	22.9	22.2	24.1	24.9	25.1	24.3	21.9	21.8	23.2	23.0	24.7	24.8	23.9	25.8
Diastolic Blood Pressure	No.	403	230	377	257	340	218	289	204	449	229	415	301	377	256	351	254
	Mean	86.5	87.0	87.3	86.7	88.0	88.2	87.6	86.5	84.0	84.3	85.8	88.9	88.7	88.8	90.9	91.3
	S.D.	12.4	11.9	11.4	10.8	13.2	13.1	13.7	12.2	11.9	10.9	11.9	10.8	12.6	11.8	13.3	12.7

which came into being on April 1, 1974, commenting on the fact that Scotland had the worst mortality rates for both sexes at most ages compared with other Western countries and on the unfavorable position of Scotland in regard to diseases of the cardiovascular and respiratory systems, emphasized the heavy burden of diagnosis and care that falls in consequence on the health services and the need for the medical profession to carry its advice and expertise, not only to the individual patient, but further than that to families and the general population. To assist hospital doctors and general practitioners in the integrated health service to meet this need, a specialist in community medicine, combining the duties of both medical administrator and the public health doctor of the old 1948 health service, was created. The new specialist is charged with the responsibility of investigating and assessing the health needs of whole populations, the healthy as well as the sick, in order to determine priorities for the delivery of medical care, the prevention of disease and the promotion of health. In many ways, the joint approach to the whole community by the three types of doctor in Renfrew and Paisley, the location of the Renfrew hypertension clinic in the general practitioner health center and the staffing of both clinics in Renfrew and Paisley by hospital doctors and general practitioners working together in the treatment and surveillance of patients identified by the community medicine team, exemplifies one aspect of a disease-orientated approach to health problems which should become much easier in the integrated service.

There are, of course, many problems in detecting occult disease in whole populations. Response in Renfrew was 78%, a rate identical with that in the general population of Tiree and with the mean rate in surveys of occupational groups examined at that time.[19] It was a little higher than in Paisley in 1974. Health visitor follow-up of defaulters contributes about 5% to the general population response rates which vary inversely in both general populations and occupational groups by social class.

Apart from reconciling the need to gain access to everyone in a defined population with the need to respect the rights of those who expressly do not wish to participate in epidemiologic surveys, there are problems in estimating the true prevalence and incidence of high blood pressure in respondents. At times and particularly in the ranges of "mild" to "moderately" raised blood pressure (90-109 mm Hg diastolic), hypertension seems like a will-o'-the-wisp. In Renfrew, for example, at a cutting point of 100 mm Hg diastolic, a yield of 476 (15.8%) "hypertensives" after primary screening is reduced to 243 (8.0%) at secondary screening after an interval between 8 and 12 weeks. In Paisley, initial numbers seem to be similarly reduced in the same interval to attendance at the hypertension clinic; and reduction can continue again if there is delay in the start of treatment. There are also early indications that mean levels of blood pressure continue to fall even in placebo groups in trials. That this should occur despite the use of approved techniques of standardization, teaching tapes and quality control suggests that the phenomenon, which would not diminish the prognostic significance of a casual elevation of blood pressure, may be a real one in studies of apparently healthy populations.

The problem is further compounded by the Renfrew reexamination survey after one year. An annual incidence of 3% at a cutting point of 100 mm Hg diastolic is useful information, but what of the observation that the proportions with raised and lowered blood pressures are evenly distributed around the modal value; and that age- and sex-specific group means and standard deviations are virtually unchanged from one year to the next? Is there some sort of perennial cycle of variation in individuals? Again, there was no evidence of a bimodal distribution into subjects with and without hypertension in the Renfrew population.[17] If this is so, who then have the "casual" elevations of blood pressure which ultimately prove significant?

The medical record linkage facilities which exist in Scotland are reported here for the first time in relation to an epidemiologic survey of a whole community. In the trial "run" of the linkage system here reported, nearly half of the identifications were wrong, but an accuracy of 75% was available without further corroboration by excluding all notifications outside the Glasgow and Paisley areas. The exclusion of notifications from outside the Glasgow area might be acceptable as numbers build up. The inclusion of patients' addresses in the linkage notification system would not only increase accuracy, but reduce considerably the clerical work of checking notifications.

The use and value of mortality record linkage in assessing predictions of risk and the relative risks of different risk factors have already been demonstrated,[21] but morbidity record linkage has much to offer the epidemiologist beyond the provision of earlier if "softer" end points than death. Large-scale prospective studies can be free of the need for reexamination and the inevitable 20% loss in response over a one- to two-year interval. If the ethical and medicolegal problems of confidentiality of medical information could be resolved, prevalence and incidence morbidity rates of census-identified nonrespondents not attending surveys at any time could be ascertained to the benefit of accuracy and completeness in survey data.

Although the urgent need for natural history data, derived from epidemiologic studies of whole populations, fully justifies mass health examinations,[22] their use as practical procedures in preventive medicine has yet to be evaluated. In the primary prevention of coronary artery disease, a multiphasic procedure including risk factors other than hypertension and indeed other disease entities like stroke, as joint objectives for primary prevention, is an important requirement for the economic use of an expensive medical resource. In Scotland, the ideal locus for these activities is the general practitioner health center where the records system obviates the need for a census to provide the sampling frame and offers, at the same time, an additional direct source of medical record linkage data. Ultimately, the value of primary prevention and the place of nonepisodic care of disease in the apparently healthy population must depend upon the effectiveness of the procedure in reducing demand on the whole of the health resources available to the health service. Above all, in noninfectious disease, effectiveness will depend upon the individual patient's recognition of his own need and his willingness, often as an asymptomatic patient, to comply with advice and accept treatments which may radically change his life style and personal perception of well-being.

Summary

An account is given of the method and some of the findings in three major prospective epidemiologic surveys[9-13,19,21] using multiphasic screening procedures, including standardized blood pressure observations[14,15] in mass health examinations,[22] presently in progress for some 34,000 subjects identified by occupational group from the wages roll or by census from three general populations in the Island of Tiree and in the Burghs of Renfrew and Paisley in the West of Scotland.

Some aspects of the problems of estimating the true prevalence and incidence of hypertension and determining who should be treated and the early use of medical record linkage to derive morbidity data are discussed in the context of the new integrated national health service in Scotland.[18]

Acknowledgments

The work described in this report is supported by grants administered by the Finance Officer of the University of Glasgow, from the Medical Research Council, the Renfrewshire King Edward Memorial Trust and the Scottish Home and Health Department.

The various studies mentioned have been made in cooperation with the Glasgow University Departments of Pathological Biochemistry and Medical Cardiology, the Glasgow University Computing Service; the MRC Blood Pressure and the MRC Epidemiology and Medical Care Units; the Department of Epidemiology and Medical Statistics of the London School of Hygiene and Tropical Medicine; the National Health Service Register; the Research and Intelligence Unit of the Scottish Home and Health Department; the Royal Alexandra Hospital, the general practitioners of Renfrew, Paisley and the West of Scotland, and the occupational health and public health (now community medicine) departments of the organizations and areas in which the surveys took place.

References

1. Registrar General Scotland Annual Report Part 1, Mortality Statistics, No. 118, H.M.S.O., Edinburgh, 1972.
2. M.O.H. Annual Report, Corporation of the City of Glasgow, 1972.
3. Howe, G. M.: *National Atlas of Disease Mortality in the United Kingdom*, revised edition, The Royal Geographic Society. London: Thomas Nelson and Sons, 1970.
4. *International Statistical Classification of Diseases, Injuries and Causes of Death*, eighth revision, W.H.O., Geneva, 1965.

5. *W.H.O. Epidem. Vit. Stat. Rep.*, 20:535, 1967.
6. *W.H.O. Chronicle*, 23:351, 1969.
7. *World Health Stat. Annual* (1969), Vol. 1, W.H.O. Geneva, 1972.
8. Peart, W. S.: *Clin. Sci. Molec. Med.*, 45:675, 1973.
9. Report of the Working Group on Epidemiological Studies of Ischaemic Heart Disease, W.H.O. Regional Office for Europe, 1969.
10. Lorimer, A. R., Cox, F. C., Greaves, D. A. et al: Prevalence of hyperlipoproteinaemia in apparently healthy men. *Brit. Heart J.*, 36:192, 1974.
11. Hawthorne, V. M.: Prevalence of cardio-respiratory disease in a Scottish Burgh, B.T.T.H. Review. *Tubercle*, 3:34, 1973.
12. Hawthorne, V. M., Greaves, D. A. and Beevers, D. G.: Blood pressure in a Scottish town. *Brit. Med. J.*, 3:600, 1974.
13. Hawthorne, V. M.: An epidemiological method to improve tuberculosis control. *Scot. Med. J.*, 14:22, 1969.
14. Rose, G. A.: *Lancet*, 1:673, 1965.
15. Rose, G. A., Holland, W. W. and Crawley, E. A.: *Lancet*, 1:296, 1964.
16. Truett, J., Cornfield, J. and Kannel, W.: *J. Chronic Dis.*: 20:511, 1967.
17. Pickering, G. W.: *High Blood Pressure*, ed. 2. London:Churchill, 1968, p. 229.
18. Report of the Joint Working Party, Scottish Home and Health Department, Doctors in an integrated service, H.M.S.O., Edinburgh, 1971.
19. Hawthorne, V. M., Gillis, C. R., Lorimer, A. R. et al: Blood pressure in a Scottish island community. *Brit. Med. J.*, 2:651, 1969.
20. Metropolitan Life Insurance Company, Blood pressure Insurance Experience and its Implications, New York, 1961.
21. Hawthorne, V. M., Gillis, C. R. and Maclean, D. S.: Monitoring health in Scotland. *Int. J. Epidem.*, 1:387, 1972.
22. W.H.O., Report of Technical Discussions at 24th World Health Assembly, 424, 5, 3, 1971.

Discussion

Dr. Hawthorne: May I comment. Your own paper showed that the U.K. emigrants had lower blood pressures than the indigenous Australian population.

Dr. Lovell: The Australians and the Scots are equally bad.

Dr. Borhani: I enjoyed your presentation as everybody else did. Did I hear you correctly that 54.5% of those discovered with diastolic blood pressure equal or over 100 were not known to their general practitioners?

Dr. Hawthorne: Yes, these are new identifications, completely new detection in a screening program.

Dr. Borhani: Of those who were known to general practitioners only 29% were under treatment?

Dr. Hawthorne: Only 15.6%. No information was available in 29.9%. But the question is whether they were under effective treatment or not. I would gather that a substantial number were not under effective treatment.

Dr. Borhani: The picture in Scotland is not different from the picture in the United States.

Dr. Hawthorne: This is our feeling but I would also, in fairness to general practitioners, say that the other side of the coin was the false negatives. If you remember, they had a reasonable number of people under good treatment and who were in the group without hypertension on examination.

Dr. Borhani: It is very important for us to emphasize that two major problems keep coming up regardless of where the data are from. One is that at least 50% of people in any community with diastolic blood pressure of 90-95 and over, at any given time, are not known to the practitioners of medicine or themselves. Second, that physicians by and large, apparently all over the world, are not treating their patients to push for an optimal diastolic blood pressure.

Hypertension in Framingham

W. B. Kannel, M.D. and P. Sorlie

Over the past decade, findings from prospective epidemiologic investigations of the evolution of cardiovascular disease at Framingham and elsewhere have served to confirm and emphasize the importance of hypertension as a precursor of cardiovascular morbidity and mortality.[1] At Framingham, the role of blood pressure in the development of clinical manifestations of coronary heart disease, atherothrombotic brain infarction, congestive failure and occlusive peripheral arterial disease has been explored in detail.[2-5] The impact of each component of the blood pressure has been examined as well as its role as an ingredient of a cardiovascular risk profile.[6] Most important, factors affecting morbidity and mortality in hypertension before organ damage have been delineated. Efforts to learn the determinants of essential hypertension in the general population have been less fruitful, although some clues have been provided.[7]

Methods

The basic method of analysis employed is to examine prospectively the rate of development of major cardiovascular events in two years in relation to characterization of each subject according to age, sex, personal attributes and living habits at the beginning of each biennium.[8,9] It records all the cardiovascular events that have evolved in the population sample, including those not hospitalized or under medical care. Follow-up surveillance for cardiovascular mortality has been virtually complete; only 2% have been completely lost after 18 years. Almost 85% have received every possible biennial examination and the rest have been seen at less frequent intervals.

W. B. Kannel, M.D., M.P.H., F.A.C.P., F.A.C.C., *Director, Framingham Study, NHLI; Lecturer, Harvard Medical School, Research Associate, Boston University and* P. Sorlie, *Biometrics Section, NHLI, NIH, Bethesda, Md.*

Each subject was examined every two years, at which time personal attributes including blood chemistries, blood pressure, relative weight, ECG, cigarette history and a variety of other observations were made.[8,9] A complete cardiovascular examination was obtained on each subject using standardized forms for uniformity of assessment. Diagnostic criteria employed have been published elsewhere.[8,9] All suspect cases were reviewed by a panel of investigators to determine if they met minimum criteria. Suspect cerebrovascular accidents were seen in the hospital by a neurologist assigned to the study to help establish the specific type of stroke with greater precision. Only half the cases suspected of a major cardiovascular event were accepted after the review process.

To determine the net and joint contribution of blood pressure to risk of each cardiovascular event, taking into account other major contributors to their incidence, multivariate analysis employing the methods of Truett-Cornfield and Duncan-Walker were applied.[10,11] In order to examine the relation of various factors to trends in blood pressure over time, a bivariate regression was performed ($y = a + b_1 x_1 + b_2 x_2$) where the dependent variable (y) was the trend in blood pressure (slope of systolic blood pressure from exam 3 to last known), x_1 is the *baseline* value of the specified characteristic and x_2 the *change* from exam 3 to the last exam taken, divided by the number of exams. From this analysis, it is possible to determine whether the baseline of the characteristic or its *change* is associated with the trend in systolic blood pressure.

Mortality

It is difficult to judge mortality attributable to hypertension from death certificate information alone because of incomplete information on the certificate, as well as changing fashions in death certification practices. It is particularly difficult to arrive at a true assessment of the contribution of hypertension to mortality from vital statistics because only those listing hypertension as the direct underlying cause are included. The atherosclerotic diseases to which hypertension is a major contributor are often excluded. Hypertension not only kills directly, but it also accounts for about a third of the 800,000 deaths each year from coronary attacks and strokes. Paul, in a survey of the epidemiology of hypertension, points out the

striking downward trend in mortality attributed to hypertension in the United States and elsewhere, beginning in 1940
and extending through 1972.[1] He discounts changes in fashions
in death certification as the explanation, but finds that it
cannot be attributed to better treatment (the trend downward
preceded effective antihypertensive agents and hypertension is
still undertreated) or to less inflammatory renal disease.

A more realistic appraisal of the impact of hypertension on
mortality can be obtained from a prospective examination of
mortality in general and from cardiovascular disease in particular, in relation to antecedent blood pressure status. This reveals
that the total mortality of hypertensives, as well as cardiovascular mortality in particular, is at least double that of
"normotensive" persons (Fig. 1). Also, even borderline eleva-

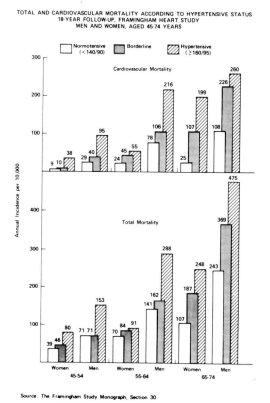

Figure 1.

556 W. B. KANNEL AND P. SORLIE

tions carry an excess mortality. As expected, the proportion of deaths due to cardiovascular disease increases with the blood pressure (Table 1). About 37% of men and 51% of women who

TABLE 1. Proportion of Deaths Due to Cardiovascular Disease*
Men and Women 45-74
Framingham Study: 18 Year Follow-Up

Men	45-54	55-64	65-74	Women	45-54	55-64	65-74
Normotensive	40	55	44	Normotensive	24	34	23
Borderline	57	65	61	Borderline	22	54	58
Hypertensive	62	75	55	Hypertensive	48	60	80
Total	51	65	55	Total	29	50	64

*C-V disease: coronary disease, brain infarction, congestive heart failure.

died of cardiovascular disease had antecedent hypertension ($\geq$ 160/95 mm Hg). If borderline elevations are included ($\geq$ 140/90 mm Hg), then 73% of men and 81% of women had some degree of antecedent hypertension.

Evidently, it is blood pressure per se that kills, for risk of cardiovascular mortality mounts in proportion to the antecedent blood pressure, even within the "nonhypertensive" range

TABLE 2. Regression of Cardiovascular Mortality
on Specified Risk Factors
Men and Women 45-74
Framingham Study: 18 Year Follow-Up

	Standardized Regression Coefficient*		T-Value	
	Men	Women	Men	Women
Systolic Blood Pressure	.388	.458	7.3	6.6
Diastolic Blood Pressure	.240	.282	4.1	3.7
Glucose	.210	.283	5.3	7.2
Cigarettes	.212	.144	3.5	1.8
Metropolitan Relative Weight	-.105	.095	-1.6	1.2
Cholesterol	.064	.161	1.1	2.4
Cardiac Enlargement x-ray	.535	.687	11.0	8.9
ECG-LVH	.443	.407	14.8	11.5
ECG-I-V Block	.260	.177	8.1	4.0
ECG-NSA	.201	.250	4.2	4.3
Vital Capacity/Height	-.379	-.637	-6.2	-8.3
Heart Rate	.330	.226	5.9	3.0

*Standardized — average over age groups.

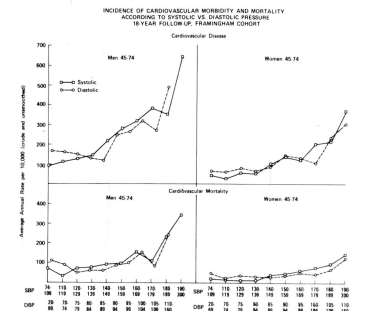

INCIDENCE OF CARDIOVASCULAR MORBIDITY AND MORTALITY
ACCORDING TO SYSTOLIC VS. DIASTOLIC PRESSURE
18-YEAR FOLLOW-UP, FRAMINGHAM COHORT

Scales for systolic and diastolic blood pressure adjusted for differences in their distributions.

Figure 2.

(Fig. 2). Comparing the regression coefficients for the various contributors to cardiovascular mortality (suitably standardized for the different units of measurement), it is clear that blood pressure — discounting factors such as ECG-LVH, x-ray cardiac enlargement or a low vital capacity which signify preclinical disease itself — is the most powerful risk factor (Table 2).

Morbidity

Compared to "normotensives," "hypertensive" persons develop a marked excess of the major cardiovascular diseases. In the age group 45-74, they develop at least twice as much occlusive peripheral arterial disease, about three times as much coronary disease, more than four times as much congestive failure and over seven times the incidence of brain infarction as do "normotensives" (Fig. 3). Even borderline hypertension carries a substantial risk of cardiovascular events. The risk is proportional to the height of the blood pressure (Fig. 2).

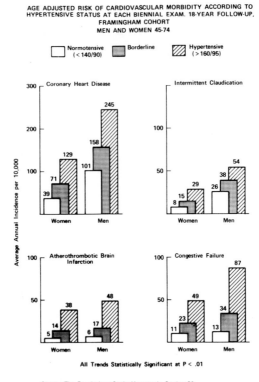

AGE ADJUSTED RISK OF CARDIOVASCULAR MORBIDITY ACCORDING TO
HYPERTENSIVE STATUS AT EACH BIENNIAL EXAM. 18-YEAR FOLLOW-UP.
FRAMINGHAM COHORT
MEN AND WOMEN 45-74

Source: The Framingham Study Monograph, Section 30

Figure 3.

Although the relative impact of hypertension is greater for stroke and congestive failure, the absolute risk is greatest for coronary heart disease. The incidence of coronary disease in hypertensives exceeds that of all the other cardiovascular sequelae combined (Fig. 3).

Factors Influencing Prognosis

In addition to the height and character of the blood pressure elevation, a number of factors have been identified which influence the prognosis associated with hypertension. It is widely recognized that those with presymptomatic evidence of organ involvement such as retinal changes,[1][2] proteinuria (Table 3), and x-ray cardiac enlargement and ECG changes (Table 4) will fare far worse than those without such findings. It

TABLE 3. Risk of Death from Cardiovascular Disease According to
Albuminuria at Biennial Exam
Men and Women 45-74
Framingham Study: 18 Year Follow-Up

Men	Albuminuria	Annual Incidence Per 10,000				T-Value**
		45-54	*55-64*	*65-74*	*45-74**	
	Absent	41	112	176	87	
						4.55
	Present	227	270	421	235	
Women						
	Absent	13	38	117	37	
						3.68
	Present	36	127	301	114	

*Age-Adjusted
**Bivariate: Age and Albuminuria

TABLE 4. Risk of Cardiovascular Death According to Evidence
of Cardiac Impairment on ECG and X-Ray
Men and Women 45-74
Framingham Study: 18 Year Follow-Up

Average Annual incidence rate per 10,000 (Age-Adjusted 45-74)

	ECG-LVH	
	Men	Women
Absent	72	32
Present-possible	221	105
Present-definite	637	329

Non-Specific S-T and T		
Absent	85	37
Present	166	84

I-V Block		
Absent	85	38
Present	314	137

X-Ray Cardiac Enlargement		
Absent	61	21
Present-possible	126	47
Present-definite	253	107

All association of incidence and impairment significant at .01 level.

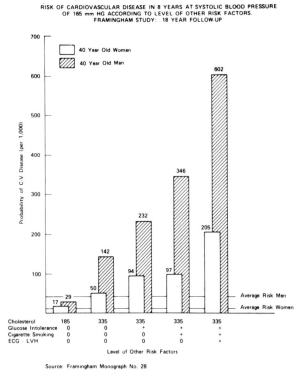

Figure 4.

is not as well appreciated that persons with a "hypertensive" blood pressure (eg, 165 mm Hg systolic) will vary widely in their risk, depending upon other risk factors present (Fig. 4), allowing risk assessment and prophylactic treatment before organ damage has occurred.

Age and Sex

One of the misconceptions about hypertension is the notion that elevated blood pressure is an "essential" feature of growing old which compensates for the stenotic vessels in order that blood flow to vital organs can be maintained. It is also believed that women tolerate hypertension better than men. There is little evidence to support either of these contentions.

While pressures tend to rise with age, an examination of cardiovascular morbidity and mortality according to age reveals, in each sex, no indication that hypertension is better tolerated in the old than in the young (Table 5, Fig. 1). Also, while at any

TABLE 5. Risk of Cardiovascular Events
According to Blood Pressure Status
Men and Women 45-74
Framingham Study: 18 Year Follow-Up

	Men			Women		
	Average Annual Incidence Per 1000 Population					
Age	*Normal*	*BHBP*	*HBP*	*Normal*	*BHBP*	*HBP*
45-54	8.3	14.6	23.4	2.4	5.0	8.9
55-64	15.5	29.3	44.4	6.2	14.2	22.7
65-74	16.4	31.9	52.3	8.3	24.9	33.2
45-74*	12.4	21.1	35.3	5.7	10.4	18.8

*Age-Adjusted Rates

	Regression Coefficients		T-Value	
	Men	Women	Men	Women
45-54	0.534	0.662	5.52	4.47
55-64	0.554	0.639	6.62	6.23
65-74	0.613	0.579	4.20	4.02

age the incidence of cardiovascular morbidity and mortality at any blood pressure level is greater in men than women, the gradients of risk according to blood pressure within each sex (as indicated by the regression coefficients) are almost identical at all ages (Table 5). For each of the major cardiovascular events, in the multivariate as well as the univariate case, coefficients for the regression of incidence on blood pressure are as large for women as for men (Table 6). Thus, hypertension is a threat to life at any age in either sex.

In addition to age and sex, the character, height and persistence of the blood pressure elevation are usually taken into account in assessing the clinical significance of hypertension.

Casual Blood Pressure

Clinical teaching dictates that since blood pressure is a normally variable phenomenon, it is essential to obtain basal levels of pressure with the subject in a relaxed and rested state and the need for treatment judged on these findings. Casual pressures are regarded as misleading and treatment based on them ill-advised. There is some merit in this clinical impression, but it has resulted in too wanton a disregard of casual pressure elevations.

TABLE 6. Regression of Major Cardiovascular Events on
Systolic Blood Pressure in the Two Sexes
Men and Women 45-74
Framingham Study: 18 Year Follow-Up

Regression Coefficient	Coronary Disease		Brain Infarction		Intermittent Claudication	
	Women	Men	Women	Men	Women	Men
Univariate	.022	.017	.029	.032	.023	.014
Bivariate	.018	.015	.026	.029	.019	.010
Multivariate	.016	.012	.019	.027	.013	.007

Regression Coefficient	Congestive Heart Failure		Total C-V Disease	
	Women	Men	Women	Men
Univariate	.026	.028	.022	.021
Bivariate	.023	.025	.018	.018
Multivariate	.016	.016	.014	.015

Bivariate = Age and SBP
Multivariate = Age and SBP and Cholesterol, Glucose, Cigarettes, ECG-LVH
All coefficients are statistically significant at p < .01 level with exception of I.C. in men.

It has been ascertained from 24-hour monitoring of blood pressure that pressure is an extremely variable phenomenon with an average range of variation of 50 mm Hg.[13,14] Even though blood pressure shows this great variability, casual blood pressures are reasonably characteristic of persons from one examination to the next. In fact, they correlate surprisingly well (r=0.5 - 0.8) even 18 years apart (Table 7).

More to the point, prospective epidemiologic data at Framingham have consistently revealed that risk of cardio-vascular events is strikingly related to casually determined pressures (Fig. 3). This excess risk is not confined to those whose basal as well as casual pressures are elevated, for it can be demonstrated even when those in whom the two pressures are similar are excluded (Table 8).

Truly basal blood pressures are not available at Framing-ham, but it was possible to examine the risk of cardiovascular events in relation to the minimum versus the maximum pressure obtained by the physician in the course of a one-hour cardiovascular examination. Since the lower of the two is closer to the basal pressure, a comparison may perhaps throw some light on the value of basal pressures. Because this comparison has meaning only if the two readings differ substantially,

TABLE 7. Correlation of Systolic Blood Pressure
Between Biennial Examinations
Men and Women
Framingham Study

Exams	Men	Women
1,2	.750	.802
1,3	.695	.767
1,4	.677	.742
1,5	.602	.704
1,6	.583	.684
1,7	.568	.643
1,8	.521	.609
1,9	.482	.588
1,10	.466	.554

TABLE 8. Risk Function Coefficients for Regression
of Cardiovascular Disease Incidence on
Minimum (Most Basal) vs. Maximum
Systolic Pressure*   Men and Women 35-74
Framingham Study: 18 Year Follow-Up

		No. of Cases	Pop. at Risk	Standardized Coefficients	T-Value
Maximum Systolic Blood Pressure					
	Men	42	1040	.363	2.70
	Women	46	1727	.516	4.01
Minimum Systolic Blood Pressure					
	Men	42	1040	.293	2.08
	Women	46	1727	.478	3.64

*Restrictions: Includes only those with greater than 20 mm Hg difference in the two examiner's blood pressures.

analysis of their relation to subsequent cardiovascular disease was confined to those who showed at least a 20 mm Hg difference in systolic pressures.

An examination of the coefficients for the regression of incidence of cardiovascular disease on the minimum versus maximum systolic pressure obtained at time of examination reveals that each is strongly related to sequelae of hypertension with no evidence that more basal pressures predict any better than casual ones (Table 8). On the basis of the foregoing, it would seem most unwise to disregard casual blood pressure elevations since even those whose basal pressures are substantially lower (more than 20 mm Hg) are at increased risk.

Borderline Hypertension

"Hypertension" is said to exist when pressures exceed some arbitrary value (eg, 160/95 mm Hg designated by the World Health Organization). While this has pragmatic utility and will identify persons who are generally at increased risk, such categorical assessments are inefficient. With regard to the risk of cardiovascular sequelae, blood pressure is best treated as a continuous variable, since the risk is related to the blood pressure level with no critical value where "normotension" leaves off and "hypertension" begins (Fig. 2). It has been pointed out by Paul,[1] based on pooled data from epidemiologic studies in the United States and also demonstrated at Framingham, that "borderline" blood pressure elevations carry a substantial cardiovascular risk.[2-6] Nevertheless, most clinicians have continued to await the appearance of "definite hypertension" before treatment in the belief that few cardiovascular events occur before the borderline pressure progresses to "true hypertension."

Evidence from Framingham, based on biennial reclassification of subjects according to "hypertensive status" and age, reveals that *while in the borderline range* persons are subject to about a doubled risk of cardiovascular morbidity and mortality (Table 9).

Blood Pressure versus Hypertension

Among "hypertensives" the risk of a cardiovascular event rises with the height of the blood pressure. This is also true for those with borderline elevations and even within the "normal" range of pressures (Fig. 5). Thus, it is *blood pressure* that kills and produces cardiovascular sequelae. If the rate of development of cardiovascular disease is plotted on a logarithmic scale in relation to systolic blood pressure, it is readily apparent, from either the actually observed or logistically fitted rates, that a specified increment in systolic pressure at the low end of the systolic pressure range results in the same percent change in risk as when it occurs at the upper end of the systolic pressure range. For each 10 mm rise in pressure there is approximately a

TABLE 9. Risk of Cardiovascular Events According
to Blood Pressure Status (Significance of Borderline Elevations)
Men and Women 45-74
Framingham Study: 18 Year Follow-Up

	C-V Mortality			C-V Events		
	Average Annual Mortality Per 1000 Persons					
	Normal	BHBP	HBP	Normal	BHBP	HBP
Men						
45-54	2.9	4.0	9.5	8.3	14.6	23.4
55-64	7.8	10.6	21.6	15.5	29.3	44.4
65-74	10.8	22.6	26.0	16.4	31.9	52.3
45-74*	5.8	9.7	16.0	12.4	21.1	35.3
Women						
45-54	0.9	1.0	3.8	2.4	5.0	8.9
55-64	2.4	4.5	5.5	6.2	14.2	22.7
65-74	2.5	10.7	19.9	8.3	24.9	33.2
45-74*	2.2	4.0	7.2	5.7	10.4	18.8

*Age-adjusted rates.
All trends significant at $p < .001$ level.

30% increase in the rate of development of cardiovascular disease. Although at any level of pressure the rates are lower in women than men, the risk *gradients* are essentially parallel (Fig. 5).

Systolic Blood Pressure

It is customary to judge the need for treatment of hypertension from the diastolic pressure, more or less ignoring the systolic pressure. This concept of hypertension control derives from the contention that diastolic pressure more than systolic reflects the increase in peripheral resistance; the belief that the cardiovascular sequelae of hypertension are more closely related to diastolic pressure; and the notion that antihypertensive pharmaceuticals are less effective in reducing systolic pressure and owe their efficacy to lowering diastolic pressure. There is little evidence to support any of these contentions.

Increased total peripheral resistance does not preferentially increase diastolic pressure so it is illogical to regard the concomitant rise in systolic pressure as only a secondary phenomenon.[15] Almost all hypertensives have a decreased

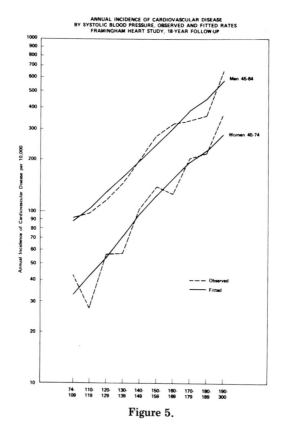

Figure 5.

arterial capacitance and a widened pulse pressure and any increase in their peripheral resistance actually causes more systolic than diastolic hypertension.

More to the point, there is little evidence to support the contention that the cardiovascular consequences of hypertension are best predicted from the diastolic component of blood pressure. Direct assessment of this hypothesis at Framingham comparing subsequent cardiovascular disease incidence in persons classified by their systolic versus their diastolic pressure reveals nothing to suggest superiority of the diastolic pressure (Fig. 2). Using regression analysis suitably standardized for the different range of values for systolic and diastolic pressure (and even taking age and other contributors to cardiovascular incidence into account by multivariate analysis), nothing emerges to suggest a greater impact of diastolic pressure for any

TABLE 10. Standardized Coefficients for Regression of
Systolic vs. Diastolic Pressure on Incidence of Specified C-V Events
Men and Women 45-74
Framingham Study: 18 Year Follow-Up

| | Men | | Women | |
	Systolic	Diastolic	Systolic	Diastolic
Coronary Heart Disease	.352	.300	.478	.364
Cerebrovascular Accident	.576	.546	.589	.544
Intermittent Claudication	.250	-.021	.536	.388
Congestive Heart Failure	.606	.423	.596	.451
Any Cardiovascular Disease	.419	.342	.470	.378
Cardiovascular Death	.388	.240	.458	.282

Source: Monograph # 30.

TABLE 11. Incidence of Cardiovascular Disease According to
Systolic Pressure at Diastolic Pressures Below 90 mm Hg
Men and Women 55-74   Framingham Study

| Systolic Blood | Age-Adjusted Annual Incidence per 10,000 | |
Pressure (mm Hg)*	Men	Women
140-159	277	176
160-179	296	191

*Too few cases of C-V disease occurred in too small a population risk to allow
estimates outside this range of systolic pressure.

major cardiovascular event in either sex (Table 10). In fact, for
each specified cardiovascular disease in each sex, the coefficients are uniformly larger for systolic pressure.

Furthermore, an examination of incidence rates of cardiovascular disease in relation to systolic blood pressure in persons
with diastolic pressures less than 90 mm Hg suggests that even
isolated elevation of systolic pressure is important (Table 11).
More extensive data are available elsewhere which would
substantiate this claim.[16,17] In fact, gradients of risk on
systolic pressure in the low diastolic segment of the population
do not seem different from those of the general population.

Evidence of Cardiac Impairment

The most prominent precursor of congestive failure in the
general population is hypertension, which is found in the
background of 75% of persons who develop this end stage of

cardiovascular disease.[4] Once overt congestive failure ensues in the hypertensive, half will be dead within five years despite the usual medical management.[4] "Hypertensives" have a four- to sixfold risk of congestive failure compared to "normotensives," and even borderline elevations carry more than a twofold increased risk (Fig. 3).

Even more subtle evidences of cardiac impairment including ECG abnormalities and x-ray cardiac enlargement in persons free of overt congestive failure carry a substantially increased risk of cardiovascular mortality (Table 4). These ECG findings and x-ray enlargement are especially common in hypertensives compared to the general population.

ECG-LVH, in particular, is strikingly related to blood pressure. The higher the pressure (systolic as well as diastolic) the more likely is this finding to appear (Fig. 6). Once hypertensives develop this finding they are in great jeopardy of a lethal cardiovascular outcome. Within five years, 32% of men with definite ECG-LVH will die of a cardiovascular catastrophe (Table 12). Over 21% of all cardiovascular mortality in Framingham was preceded by this finding. In persons who develop the ECG abnormality congestive failure will occur at ten times the rate of the general population. Awaiting the appearance of this finding before treatment would seem imprudent and failure to treat vigorously when it appears, downright negligent. The ECG finding evidently reflects more than simple hypertensive hypertrophy (when accompanied by S-T and T-wave changes as well as increased voltage). At any level of pressure, and whether or not otherwise at high or low risk, those with ECG-LVH are at distinctly greater risk (Table 13).

Cardiovascular Risk Profile

Although the risk of cardiovascular disease in hypertensives is in general high, it is not uniformly so. Because risk can vary so widely, depending upon the actual size of the blood pressure elevation, whether or not evidence of organ damage is already present, and depending upon the level of other cardiovascular risk factors (Fig. 4), it seems most logical to conceptualize blood pressure as an ingredient in a cardiovascular risk profile.

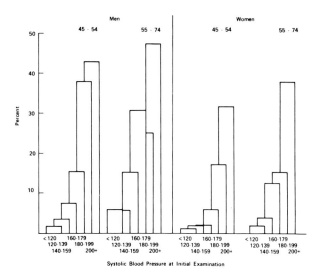

PERIOD PREVALENCE* OF LEFT VENTRICULAR HYPERTROPHY
ACCORDING TO SYSTOLIC BLOOD PRESSURE AT INITIAL EXAM.
MEN AND WOMEN 45 - 74

* Proportion of Persons Manifesting Definite (i.e. with S-T and T changes) ECG-LVH
on any of First Seven Exams.

Figure 6.

TABLE 12. Incidence of Cardiovascular Morbidity and Mortality
According to ECG-LVH
Men and Women 45-74
Framingham Study: 18 Year Follow-Up

Mortality	5 Year Age-Adjusted Incidence (Per 100)							
	Cardiovascular Mortality		Coronary Mortality		Sudden Death		Overall Mortality	
LVH-ECG	M	F	M	F	M	F	M	F
None	3.6	1.6	1.4	0.5	0.8	0.2	6.7	3.6
Possible	11.1	5.2	3.7	1.0	2.1	0.4	16.4	8.6
Definite	31.8	16.4	9.5	1.8	5.5	0.7	37.6	19.6

Morbidity	C-V Disease		Coronary Disease Other than AP		Brain Infarction		Congestive Failure	
LVH-ECG	M	F	M	F	M	F	M	F
None	9.1	4.7	4.6	1.5	0.8	0.6	1.4	1.0
Possible	18.5	11.7	9.0	2.2	1.7	2.1	4.2	3.2
Definite	35.9	27.9	17.3	3.3	3.5	6.9	12.5	10.2

TABLE 13. Risk of Developing Cardiovascular Disease According to
ECG-LVH Status, Blood Pressure and Other Risk Factors
35 Year Old Man
Framingham Study: 18 Year Follow-Up

Risk in 8 Years (Per 1000)								
ECG-LVH SBP:	105	120	135	150	165	180	195	
Absent	6	7	9	11	14	18	23	Non-Smoker
							Low Risk:	Chol. 185
Present	16	20	25	32	40	50	62	No Glucose Intol.
Absent	114	140	171	207	248	295	346	Smokes
							High Risk:	Chol. 335
Present	269	318	371	428	486	545	602	Glucose Intol.

Monograph #28

By means of ordinary office procedures and simple laboratory tests it is now possible to select persons — while still
asymptomatic and before organ damage has occurred — for
management of hypertension. Synthesizing information which
includes systolic blood pressure level, serum cholesterol concentration, blood glucose, cigarette habit and ECG-LVH into a
composite risk estimate, it can be more logically determined,
than by pressure alone, if the patient needs treatment.[18] It can
be seen from handbooks computed for this purpose[8] that the
risk of a 40-year-old male with a 165 mm Hg pressure (systolic)
having a cardiovascular event in eight years is as high as 60% if
all factors are unfavorable or as low as 3% if all else is optimal
(Table 14). Because of this 20-fold difference in the range of
risk in persons who would qualify for a diagnosis of "hypertension" it is necessary to ascertain the risk profile if over- or
undertreatment is to be avoided.

Atherosclerosis

In the past, the cardiovascular sequelae most closely linked
to hypertension have been intracerebral hemorrhage, dissecting
aneurysm, hypertension with renal failure and hypertensive
encephalopathy. The atherosclerotic complications were somehow accorded a lesser place as direct sequelae of hypertension.
On the contrary, the hypertension in such persons was regarded
as a compensatory response to atherosclerosis in order to
maintain blood flow to vital organs through narrowed vessels.[19]

Specified Characteristics: The Framingham Study, 18 Year Follow-up. 40-Year-Old Man

LVH-ECG Negative — Does Not Smoke Cigarettes

	SBP	105	120	135	150	165	180	195
Glucose Intolerance Absent	CHOL							
	185	12	15	19	23	29	37	46
	210	15	19	24	31	39	48	60
	235	20	26	32	40	51	63	79
	260	27	34	42	53	66	82	102
	285	35	44	55	69	86	106	131
	310	46	58	72	90	111	136	167
	335	61	76	94	116	142	173	210
Glucose Intolerance Present	CHOL							
	185	21	27	33	42	52	65	81
	210	28	35	44	55	68	85	105
	235	37	46	57	71	89	110	135
	260	48	60	75	93	115	141	172
	285	63	78	97	119	147	178	216
	310	82	101	125	153	186	224	267
	335	106	130	159	193	232	277	326

LVH-ECG Negative — Smokes Cigarettes

	SBP	105	120	135	150	165	180	195
Glucose Intolerance Absent	CHOL							
	185	20	25	32	40	50	63	78
	210	27	33	42	53	66	82	101
	235	35	44	55	69	85	106	130
	260	46	58	72	89	110	135	165
	285	60	75	93	115	141	172	208
	310	78	97	120	147	179	216	259
	335	101	125	153	186	225	268	317
Glucose Intolerance Present	CHOL							
	185	36	45	57	71	88	109	134
	210	48	60	74	92	114	140	170
	235	62	77	96	119	145	177	214
	260	81	100	124	152	184	222	266
	285	105	129	158	192	231	275	325
	310	134	164	199	239	285	335	389
	335	171	207	248	295	346	401	459

LVH-ECG Positive — Does Not Smoke Cigarettes

	SBP	105	120	135	150	165	180	195
Glucose Intolerance Absent	CHOL							
	185	33	41	51	64	80	99	122
	210	43	54	67	83	103	127	156
	235	56	70	87	108	133	162	197
	260	73	91	113	138	169	204	245
	285	95	117	144	176	212	254	301
	310	122	150	183	220	264	312	364
	335	156	190	229	273	322	375	432
Glucose Intolerance Present	CHOL							
	185	58	73	90	111	137	167	202
	210	76	94	116	143	174	210	252
	235	98	121	148	181	218	261	309
	260	126	155	188	227	270	319	372
	285	161	195	235	280	330	384	441
	310	203	244	290	340	395	453	511
	335	253	300	351	407	464	523	581

LVH-ECG Positive — Smokes Cigarettes

	SBP	105	120	135	150	165	180	195
Glucose Intolerance Absent	CHOL							
	185	56	70	86	107	132	161	195
	210	73	90	112	137	168	203	244
	235	94	117	143	174	211	253	300
	260	122	149	181	219	262	310	362
	285	155	189	227	271	320	373	430
	310	196	236	281	331	385	442	500
	335	245	291	341	396	454	512	571
Glucose Intolerance Present	CHOL							
	185	97	120	147	180	217	259	307
	210	125	154	187	225	269	317	371
	235	160	194	234	278	328	382	439
	260	202	242	288	339	393	450	509
	285	251	298	349	405	462	521	579
	310	308	360	416	474	533	591	646
	335	371	428	486	545	602	657	708

Framingham men aged 40 yrs have an average SBP of 129 mm Hg and an average serum cholesterol of 228 mg%. Seventy percent smoke cigarettes, 0.3 percent have definite IVH by ECG and 3.3 percent have glucose intolerance. At these average values the probability of developing cardiovascular disease in eight years is 41/1000.

Recent evidence from clinical trials that the benefits of controlling hypertension are confined to those effects (judged *direct* hypertensive manifestations) other than atherosclerosis, has served to reinforce this notion.[19]

However, the evidence linking hypertension to atherosclerotic disease is massive[20] and based upon animal experiments,[21-23] necropsy studies, angiographic observations and clinical comparisons. Despite this and acknowledging a close association between hypertension and clinical manifestations of coronary heart disease, some conclude that it is not clear that hypertension per se, in the absence of other atherogenic factors, can cause atherosclerosis.[24] The fact that vein grafts placed in the high pressure circulation to bypass arterial obstructions develop atherosclerosis while failing to do so in their usual low pressure situation suggests that blood pressure per se may induce atherosclerosis, or is at least one factor.

Whether directly causal or only a contributor, systolic or diastolic hypertension is powerfully related to the rate of clinical atherosclerotic events (Fig. 3) and this relationship holds even when the impact of other major contributors is accounted for (Table 6). This is true even when blood pressure status was evaluated a decade or more before the appearance of the clinical atherosclerotic events[2,3] so it is unlikely that the atherosclerosis was demanding an increased pressure in order to sustain flow. In addition to atherothrombotic brain infarction and intermittent claudication (Fig. 3), risk of every clinical manifestation of coronary heart disease was strikingly related to blood pressure status (Fig. 7).

Persuasive evidence that hypertension induces accelerated atherogenesis comes not only from epidemiologic data and animal experiments, but also from observations on the distribution of atheromata in the circulation in man. These suggest that blood pressure may in fact play a crucial role. Atheromata are more numerous and appear earlier in segments of the circulation with the greatest pressure and turbulence of flow.[25,26] Although bathed by the same lipid-laden blood, atherosclerosis is seldom encountered in low pressure segments of the circulation unless pathology produces hypertension. There are evidently some pressures below which atheromata seldom develop.

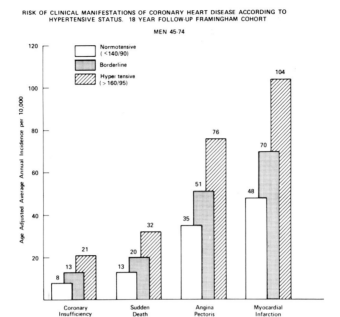

RISK OF CLINICAL MANIFESTATIONS OF CORONARY HEART DISEASE ACCORDING TO
HYPERTENSIVE STATUS. 18 YEAR FOLLOW-UP FRAMINGHAM COHORT

MEN 45-74

Source: The Framingham Study Monograph, Section 30

Figure 7.

Determinants of Hypertension

While the cardiovascular consequences of hypertension and now even the pathologic physiology are well understood, the determinants of blood pressure level in the general population are not. If we knew the cause of essential hypertension we could explore the possibility for prevention of hypertension itself. Until that becomes possible we can attack the problem only by controlling already elevated pressures.

An examination of possible environmental precursors of hypertension provides few solid clues. Salt intake has been incriminated, but convincing proof is lacking.[27,28] Psychological factors are believed to play a role, but convincing evidence to support this contention is lacking. The sloth and gluttony leading to obesity which has been promoted by modern affluent societies has, on the other hand, been convincingly incriminated.

More so than environmental factors, genetic predisposition has been accorded a major role.[29,30] Hypertension is indeed a family affair but this does not necessarily reflect only genetic influences for families share more than genes.

Genetic Susceptibility

There seems little doubt that an increased susceptibility to hypertension in man is inherited.[29,31-35] Genetically induced hypertension can be reliably produced in rats.[30,36,37] Some have been bred to be supersensitive to salt so that they develop accelerated hypertension when fed salt early in life.[30,37] The hemodynamic characteristics of the hypertension in these susceptible rats closely resemble those in essential hypertension. Genetic susceptibility to hypertension in humans is not as conclusively demonstrated. Families share an environment and even spouses tend to share a propensity to hypertension.[7] Correlation of spouses' pressures did not increase with the duration of marriage, so assortative mating may be a factor.

Factors Affecting Trends in Blood Pressure

Aside from familial vulnerability, changes in a number of personal attributes of participants in the Framingham Study were found to be associated with corresponding changes in systolic pressure and associated with steeper trends in pressure over time. The strongest of these were relative weight and serum cholesterol which changes were mirrored by changes in systolic pressure in both sexes (Table 15). An increase in relative weight of five units corresponds to an increase in systolic blood pressure of 3.3 mm Hg (Fig. 8). There is a relationship of weight gain to serum cholesterol value which might explain the association between cholesterol and blood pressure noted. However, even though there is a 0.18-0.40 correlation between cholesterol change and change in relative weight, the relation between cholesterol change and change in blood pressure persists in multivariate analysis which takes weight into account.

Hematocrit changes were significantly associated with changes in blood pressure in women but not in men. A rising

TABLE 15. Factors Associated with Trends in Systolic Pressure
Men and Women 35-64
Framingham Study: 14 Year Follow-Up

		T-Values for Significance of Multivariate Regression Coefficients – Average Over Age Groups	
		Baseline Value	Change in Characteristic
Relative Weight	Men	-1.26	5.91
	Women	0.73	9.60
Serum Cholesterol	Men	0.29	3.46
	Women	0.58	5.72
Pulse Rate	Men	-0.57	4.68
	Women	-2.01	1.84
Blood Glucose	Men	0.31	2.76
	Women	0.31	0.01
Hematocrit	Men	-0.14	-0.49
	Women	-0.92	2.49
Vital Capacity	Men	-1.61	-1.89
	Women	-2.53	1.65

CHANGE IN SYSTOLIC BLOOD PRESSURE ACCORDING TO
CHANGE IN RELATIVE WEIGHT BETWEEN BIENNIAL EXAMS

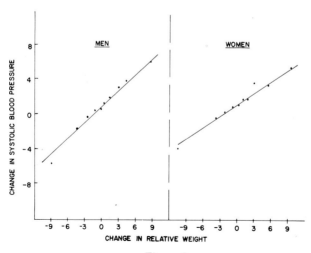

Figure 8.

pulse rate was associated with an increasing blood pressure, more prominently in men (Table 15). Low vital capacities at baseline were associated with higher pressures. The reasons for these correlations with blood pressure are unclear, but they do provide clues to pathogenesis. Hematocrit might be a reflection of blood volume or erythropoietic elaboration from an ischemic kidney. Pulse rate could reflect anxiety, sympathetic autonomic imbalance or a poor myocardium.

Menopause

It is tempting to attribute the steeper rise in systolic pressure with advancing age in women than men to the menopause. It has also been suspected that the narrowing gap in incidence of cardiovascular disease between the sexes with advancing age is due to loss of immunity of women as they undergo the menopause. This might, in part, be a product of the age trend in blood pressure in the sexes. An examination of the blood pressure change in women who have undergone the menopause (natural or surgical) in comparison to women the same age who have not (comparing premenopausal, in-menopause and postmenopausal pressures) reveals only trivial differences which are not statistically significant (Table 16).

Diabetes

An association between diabetes and hypertension has been noted, and hypertensive heart disease[1] and congestive heart failure have been observed to occur more frequently in diabetics. Although renal involvement such as intercapillary glomerulosclerosis is associated with hypertension, the explanation for most hypertension in diabetics is still obscure.

In the Framingham cohort only in men was a significant relationship of change in glucose under observation related to observed trends in blood pressure. In neither sex was the baseline value related (Table 15).

Environmental Determinants

There are some indications that powerful environmental influences may be at work in determining the high prevalence of hypertension. The downward trend in deaths attributed to

TABLE 16. Systolic Blood Pressure According to Menopausal Status
Women 40-51
Framingham Study: 18 Year Follow-Up

Type of Menopause		Mean Systolic Blood Pressure (mm Hg)		
		Menopausal	Control*	T-Value
Natural (817 women)				
SBP Measured:	Exam prior to menopause	130.6	128.6	1.66
	Exam of menopause	131.8	130.2	1.23
	Exam following menopause	132.4	131.3	0.89
Surgical				
Hysterectomy Only or				
Unilateral Oophorectomy (114 women)				
SBP Measured:	Exam prior to menopause	127.2	125.9	0.53
	Exam of menopause	125.5	127.0	-0.81
	Exam following menopause	130.5	129.5	0.42
Bilateral Oophorectomy (183 women)				
SBP Measured:	Exam prior to menopause	129.1	127.4	1.19
	Exam of menopause	131.0	128.5	1.48
	Exam following menopause	131.2	129.5	0.93

*Control Group: Women, matched by age, who remained premenopausal through the exam following matched menopausal exam.

hypertension, if not an artifact of reporting, would suggest this.[38] Also, higher pressures have been correlated with the degree of acculturation of primitive tribes in the South Pacific and higher mortality has been reported in blacks and among whites with rudimentary educations.[38] Local and regional differences in the prevalence of hypertension have been reported[1]; a lower prevalence of hypertensive cardiovascular disease has been found in hard water areas[39] and altitude seems to play a role in Peru.[40]

Obesity

Of the various factors examined for an association with trends in blood pressure in the Framingham cohort, changes in relative weight and cholesterol were the strongest, as judged from the size of their standardized regression coefficients (Table 17). Regression analysis shows a highly significant relationship of weight change to change in blood pressure, but not to basal weight level per se (Table 15). For men 55-64 the standardized coefficient for change in relative weight is 1.287, indicating that

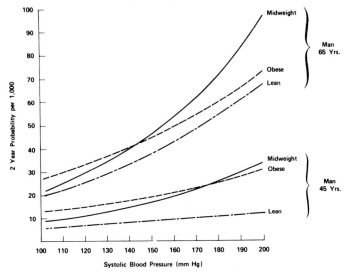

FITTED PROBABILITY OF DEVELOPING CORONARY HEART DISEASE
IN A MAN 45 YRS. AND 65 YRS., BY WEIGHT GROUP AND BLOOD PRESSURE
FRAMINGHAM STUDY: 18-YEAR FOLLOW-UP

Figure 9.

TABLE 17. Significant Standardized Coefficients for Regression
of Trend in Blood Pressure on Change in Specified Attributes:
Men and Women 45-54

| | Standardized Regression Coefficients | |
	Men	Women
Framingham Relative Weight	1.046	0.871
Serum Cholesterol	1.037	0.846
Heart Rate	0.395	0.660
Vital Capacity	*1	0.490
Hematocrit	*1	0.489

*1Coefficient not significantly different from zero.

one standard deviation in weight change will result in a 1.3 mm
Hg change in blood pressure in two years, or 6.5 mm Hg in ten
years.

Some question the importance of elevated pressures in the
obese as either resulting from a fat arm artifact or a less virulent
type of hypertension. Since the relationship of hypertension
and obesity can be demonstrated using forearm blood pressures,

the fat arm artifact seems an unlikely explanation.[41] An examination of the incidence of cardiovascular disease in relation to blood pressure in different weight classes reveals nothing to suggest that blood pressure is innocuous in the obese (Fig. 9).

Psychosocial Factors

A few psychosocial indices are available and these may be examined for their relation to hypertension. For example, those reporting the use of tranquilizers may have more emotional problems than the rest of the population, or at least think they do. Framingham data suggest that pressures of those taking tranquilizers are little different from those who do not (Table 18).

TABLE 18. Systolic Blood Pressure According
to Tranquilizer Use (Exams 9+10)
Framingham Study

		Mean Systolic Pressure Tranquilizers		Mean Change In Systolic Pressure Tranquilizers				Population Tranquilizers	
		0	+	0/0	0/+	+/+	+/0	0	+
Men									
	Under 60	134.5	137.7	1.3	1.4	5.8	10.1	865	50
	60 and Over	142.2	143.7	-0.7	4.2	-0.9	3.6	666	43
Women									
	Under 60	131.8	134.6	0.6	0.2	2.2	3.3	1050	117
	60 and Over	151.6	151.8	0.1	-2.5	1.2	-2.7	911	69

	Standard Deviation			
	Men		Women	
	0	+	0	+
Under 60	20.1	23.7	20.1	23.0
60 and Over	21.6	26.2	25.0	23.7

Loss of a spouse is an emotionally and socially disruptive event. A comparison of blood pressures in married and widowed persons in the Framingham cohort reveals higher pressures in the widowed than in the married in each sex (Table 19). The difference is more pronounced under age 60. While the differences are significant in those under 60, there is still an intervening age difference in the broad comparison age groups

TABLE 19. Systolic Blood Pressures in Widowed vs. Married
Subjects (Exam 9). Men and Women 45-78
Framingham Study: 16 Year Follow-Up

| | | Mean Systolic Pressure | | Standard Deviation | | Number | |
		Married	Widowed	Married	Widowed	Married	Widowed
Men							
	Under 60	134.3	144.1	20.2	21.0	858	20
	60 and Over	142.3	146.5	21.8	23.2	637	50
Women							
	Under 60	131.5	136.0	20.4	23.4	912	85
	60 and Over	151.3	152.4	26.4	23.1	524	342

TABLE 20. Regression of Systolic Blood Pressure on Alcohol
Consumed (Exam 4) Men and Women 35-64
Framingham Study

| | Regression Coefficient – Bivariate (SBP × Relative Weight) | | | | | |
| | Men | | | | Women | |
Age	Mean Alcohol Intake*	B	T-Value	Mean Alcohol Intake*	B	T-Value
All Subjects						
35-44	25.0	.049	3.43	8.8	.060	2.13
45-54	24.1	.063	2.90	6.4	-.009	-0.15
55-64	22.4	.079	2.48	5.1	.130	1.72
Alcohol Drinkers Only						
35-44	29.5	.054	3.73	13.0	.081	2.86
45-54	30.2	.070	3.03	11.5	.042	0.66
55-64	30.1	.068	1.97	11.0	.189	2.34

*Oz./Mo.

used and when the greater age of the widowed is taken into
account, the differences are somewhat reduced.

Although it may reflect other things, such as physical
fitness, the *pulse rate* during a routine medical examination
with the subject at rest usually reflects apprehension in a
medical environment. At initial exam, there was a modest
association of blood pressure and heart rate (r=.24).

Coffee, alcohol and *cigarettes* are common social practices
which might affect blood pressure. There is a small but positive
correlation (0.13) of systolic pressure and alcohol intake in the
Framingham cohort. Regression analysis reveals a modest but
significant relationship of systolic pressure to alcohol intake

PERCENT PREVALENCE OF HYPERTENSION
BY ALCOHOL CONSUMPTION AT EXAM. 4; FRAMINGHAM STUDY

MEN

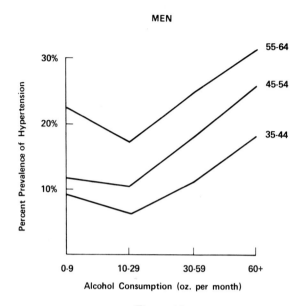

Figure 10.

(Table 20) independent of associated weight. This translates into sizable differences in the prevalence of "hypertension" (> 160/95 mm Hg) in relation to alcohol intake (Fig. 10). There is a doubled prevalence in those who drink more than 60 oz/month, compared to light drinkers, who seem to fare slightly better than those who do not drink at all.

Excessive *coffee intake*, because of the pharmacologic effect of caffeine, might be expected to influence blood pressure more than transiently. There is no association between coffee intake and blood pressure in men, but a slight negative relationship is seen in women (Table 21).

Persons who smoke *cigarettes* in general have slightly *lower* blood pressures than those who do not, probably because they weigh less. Also, those who quit smoking generally experience a rise in blood pressures, presumably because of a slight weight gain. However, the changes noted are trivial and not statistically significant (Table 22).

TABLE 21. Systolic Blood Pressure According to Daily Coffee Intake:
6th Biennial Exam   Men and Women 35-65
Framingham Study

Cups of Coffee Per Day	Age:	Average Systolic Blood Pressure Men					
		35-39	40-44	45-49	50-54	55-59	60+
0		131.2	131.1	132.9	126.2	134.4	141.8
1		124.8	124.8	129.7	137.7	134.1	151.5
2		125.0	127.7	132.2	134.1	134.3	141.9
3		125.4	127.3	133.0	135.5	139.2	137.0
4		125.7	131.7	130.7	129.3	141.0	137.5
5		125.9	127.6	135.9	129.6	136.3	136.6
6		134.8	131.4	132.4	133.0	146.6	129.2
7		134.7	129.8	129.4	131.6	140.5	130.1
				Women			
0		116.6	127.9	129.1	143.2	143.8	150.0
1		118.0	123.4	134.1	139.8	146.4	156.2
2		116.6	128.1	128.5	137.3	148.0	149.4
3		115.3	124.4	129.9	140.7	144.4	154.3
4		119.2	122.1	126.9	133.7	138.2	159.5
5		120.3	120.3	122.6	134.3	135.6	147.7
6		117.9	119.9	131.2	132.1	148.6	146.5
7		117.7	120.7	127.2	133.7	137.9	136.0

TABLE 22. Change in Systolic Blood Pressure
with Change in Cigarette Habit.
Men < 65 Years
Framingham Study

	No.*	Average Change in Systolic Blood Pressure (mm Hg)
Quit Smoking	544	1.6
Continued Smoking	4078	0.7
Took up Smoking	246	0.6
Continued Non-Smoking	3120	0.7

*Number of changes; not number of persons.

Impact of Antihypertensive Therapy

With hypertension so highly prevalent, the introduction of
effective antihypertensive agents into the community might be
expected to have altered blood pressures recently as compared
to the past. Prior to the fifth biennial examination at

TABLE 23. Percent First on Anti-Hypertensives at Exams 4-10

| SYS BP* | Men Percent | | | |
	35-44	45-54	55-64	65-74
LT 120	0.40	0.43	0.58	2.90
120-129	0.45	0.76	0.73	1.46
130-139	0.56	0.96	1.23	2.05
140-149	2.26	2.23	2.49	1.66
150-159	7.75	5.74	7.12	7.02
160-169	10.42	8.25	8.55	7.02
170-179	12.50	18.89	15.44	14.81
180-189	23.08	27.27	23.75	14.29
190-199	25.00	26.92	30.61	17.39
200+	40.00	27.78	36.73	20.83
TOTAL	1.63	2.49	4.21	4.46

| SYS BP* | Women Percent | | | |
	35-44	45-54	55-64	65-74
LT 120	0.88	1.91	1.23	1.47
120-129	1.31	2.25	1.58	4.58
130-139	2.82	2.70	2.93	3.60
140-149	3.45	5.30	5.86	5.95
150-159	10.53	10.84	6.35	7.97
160-169	10.71	14.76	11.60	9.47
170-179	22.22	20.77	16.28	16.13
180-189	22.22	31.43	17.45	20.25
190-199	40.00	33.33	40.85	26.92
200+	42.86	53.33	39.58	32.26
TOTAL	2.20	5.04	6.69	8.96

*On exam preceding the first use of antihypertensive drugs.

Framingham there was little available for the treatment of hypertension except hexamethonium, sympathectomy, veratrum alkaloids and phenobarbitol. No potent oral anti-hypertensive agents with acceptable side effects suitable for asymptomatic ambulatory hypertensives were available.

An examination of the use of these agents in the Framingham cohort reveals that at almost any level of pressure and every age women are put on the drugs more often than men. Of course, there is an increase in the percent on drugs with increasing blood pressure, and a pronounced increase comes after 150 mm Hg (Table 23). The small percentage under treatment for pressures below 140 mm Hg probably represents diuretics prescribed for edema. By exam seven about 12% of the cohort were receiving antihypertensive drugs including diuretics. It is of interest, however, that even at 200 mm Hg in the Framingham cohort there are still less than 50% on antihypertensive drugs! This in a community where the cohort is routinely examined every two years, blood pressure findings are reported to the physician and the patient advised to see his physician.

Examination of age trends in blood pressure in those on antihypertensive drugs versus those who never received them reveals, of course, higher pressures in those on drugs. However, the rate of rise is measurably greater after exam five (when antihypertensive drugs came into more common use) in those who have never received antihypertensive drugs, especially in women (Fig. 11). This suggests some impact of antihypertensive therapy in those who claimed that they had taken the medicine as shown in Table 24. This table gives the mean systolic pressure at the last examination for those on antihypertensive drugs compared to the systolic pressure predicted for them from that terminal examination assuming that they did not take antihypertensive drugs. This reveals that pressures are slightly lowered by antihypertensive drugs and that the greater reduction occurs at higher blood pressure.

Although the difference in pressures between those on treatment and the general population has been narrowing over

TABLE 24. Mean Systolic Blood Pressure at Last Examination Among Those on Antihypertensive Drugs at Least One Examination (Exams 4-10) Comparing Actual and Predicted Values Men and Women 36-68   Framingham Study

Systolic Blood Pressure at Exam Prior to Therapy	No.	Mean Systolic Blood Pressure		
		Actual Value Observed on Treatment	Predicted Value*	Difference (Estimated Effort of Rx)
<140	(161)	136	139	- 3
140-159	(223)	151	154	- 3
160-179	(228)	162	166	- 4
180+	(219)	171	182	-11

*Prediction is based on linear regression of systolic blood pressure on initial level in those free of antihypertensive therapy.

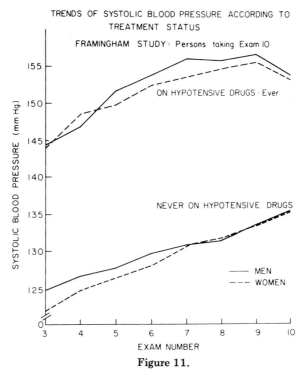

TRENDS OF SYSTOLIC BLOOD PRESSURE ACCORDING TO
TREATMENT STATUS

FRAMINGHAM STUDY : Persons taking Exam IO

Figure 11.

the years, it is clear that the introduction of antihypertensive therapy into the Framingham cohort has had a disappointing impact on blood pressure. This is very likely a consequence of the failure of physicians to perceive the hazard of asymptomatic hypertension and of their patients to understand that they are in jeopardy, as well as difficulty in obtaining long-term adherence to antihypertensive regimens.

Clinical and Preventive Implications

Cardiovascular disease is a disastrous medical entity which really doesn't begin with crushing chest pain, hemiplegia, a bout of pulmonary edema or claudication in an extremity, but with subtle signs like asymptomatic hypertension. Despite truly spectacular progress in cardiology over the past quarter century, cardiovascular mortality continues to take a huge annual toll. This is because the bulk of the mortality is from coronary heart disease and sudden unexpected death is the characteristic mode of exitus. Also, once infarcted, neither the brain nor the myocardium can be restored by any means, nor can a myocardium or kidney which has used up all its reserve and compensatory mechanisms be resurrected. The nature of cardiovascular disease is such that treatment directed only at already symptomatic disease, no matter how ingenious or successful, can not achieve a substantial reduction in cardiovascular morbidity and mortality. Only a preventive approach, correcting precursors which lead to organ damage, can have a substantial impact. Chief among these contributors requiring attention is hypertension.

The high prevalence of risk factors, including hypertension, justifies a *public health approach* to hypertensive cardiovascular disease. One in ten adults has a level of cardiovascular risk factors which more than doubles the already too high general risk. However, in hypertension, we do not know which elements of the ecology need to be modified in the community although salt intake and living habits which promote obesity are suspect.

In the present state of knowledge, there is less resistance to a preventive medical approach which focuses attention on highly vulnerable persons for specific prophylactic medical management of hypertension. Problems exist here, too, because of the asymptomatic state of the candidate for antihypertensive management. Unfortunately, many physicians appear to consider management of presymptomatic hypertensives meddlesome and have trouble perceiving such hypertension as "disease" requiring treatment. Furthermore, most physicians lack skill in achieving sustained lowering of blood pressure in asymptomatic ambulatory patients, and patients seem unable to cooperate for long periods.

We are evidently doing a poor job in informing the general population about the nature and significance of hypertension to themselves and their families so that they can be motivated to act in their own behalf. While many know that cigarettes, overeating, lack of exercise, cholesterol, diabetes and hypertension are bad for their health, they seem powerless to do anything about it. They appear to be victims of an affluent society which promotes the faulty habits they must avoid.

It is clear that both the physician and the prime candidate for cardiovascular disease are going to need considerable assistance in their joint endeavor to avoid the sequelae of hypertension. To be successful this must be accomplished with as little disruption of life style as possible. Acceptable alternatives must be provided for all restrictions imposed. Antihypertensive regimens that are too complex and too restrictive are not likely to succeed.

There is surprising resistance to recommendations to treat hypertension which will have to be overcome. We should have come a long way from the days when "essential" hypertension was considered essential to ensure flow to vital organs with a compromised circulation and a "benign" condition. There is nothing benign or essential about asymptomatic hypertension at any age in either sex, whether labile or fixed, systolic or diastolic.

Summary

The Framingham Heart Study, a prospective cardiovascular study of 5,209 men and women, has identified systolic blood pressure as the major factor in a set of measurable attributes which can identify those persons who are at high risk of developing cardiovascular disease. There is a continuous exponential increase in risk as blood pressure increases. The fact that the blood pressure measurement is a casual reading does not reduce its ability to predict those at high risk.

Factors found to be associated with systolic pressure on a cross-sectional basis were weight, alcohol intake and hemoglobin. Factors associated with trend in systolic blood pressure were weight change, serum cholesterol change, pulse rate change, blood glucose change in men, hematocrit change in women and baseline vital capacity.

Antihypertensive drug therapy was used more by women than men but even in those with high systolic pressure (200 mm Hg or more), less than 50% were put on antihypertensive drugs. These drugs as used in the community had some effect in reducing the mean systolic pressure (reduction of 6%), particularly in those whose systolic pressure was over 180 mm Hg.

References

1. Paul, O.: A survey of the epidemiology of hypertension. 1964-1974. *Mod. Conc. Cardiov. Dis.*, 43:99-102, 1974.
2. Kannel, W. B., Gordon, T. and Schwartz, M. J.: Systolic vs. diastolic

blood pressure and risk of coronary heart disease: The Framingham Study. *Amer. J. Cardiol.*, 27:335-346, 1971.

3. Kannel, W. B., Wolf, P. A., Verter, J. et al: Epidemiologic assessment of the role of blood pressure in stroke: The Framingham Study. *JAMA*, 214:301-310, 1970.

4. Kannel, W. B., Castelli, W. P., McNamara, P. M. et al: Role of blood pressure in the development of congestive heart failure: The Framingham Study. *New Eng. J. Med.*, 287:781-787, 1972.

5. Kannel, W. B. and Shurtleff, D.: The natural history of arteriosclerosis obliterans. *Cardiov. Clin.*, 3:37-52, 1971.

6. Kannel, W. B. and Dawber, T. R.: Hypertension as an ingredient of a cardiovascular risk profile. *Brit. J. Hosp. Medicine*, 2:508-524, 1974.

7. Kannel, W. B. and Dawber, T. R.: Hypertensive cardiovascular disease: The Framingham Study. In Onesti, G., Kim, K. E. and Moyer, J. H. (eds.): *Hypertension: Mechanisms and Management*. New York:Grune & Stratton, 1973, pp. 93-110.

8. McGee, D.: The probability of developing certain cardiovascular diseases in 8 years at specified values of some characteristics. *DHEW*, Public. No. (NIH), 74-618, 1973.

9. Gordon, T., Sorlie, P. and Kannel, W. B.: Coronary heart disease, atherothrombotic brain infarction, intermittent claudication — A multivariate analysis of some factors related to their incidence. Framingham Study, 16-year follow-up. DHEW, Public. NHLI, NIH, 1971.

10. Truett, J., Cornfield, J. and Kannel, W. B.: A multivariate analysis of the risk of coronary heart disease in Framingham. *J. Chronic Dis.*, 20:511-524, 1967.

11. Walker, S. H. and Duncan, D. B.: Estimation of the probability of an event as a function of several independent variables. *Biometrika*, 54:167-179, 1967.

12. Breslin, D. J., Gifford, R. W., Jr. and Fairbairn, J. F. 2d: Essential hypertension. A twenty-year follow-up study. *Circulation*, 33:87-97, 1966.

13. Bevan, A. T., Hanour, A. J. and Stott, F. H.: Direct arterial pressure recordings in unrestricted man. *Clin. Sci.*, 36:329-344, 1969.

14. Richardson, D. W., Vetrovic, G. W. and Williamson, W. C.: Effect of sleep on blood pressure in patients with hypertension. In *Hypertension*. Third Hacknanmann Symposium. Lea & Febiger, 1973.

15. Koch-Weser, J.: The therapeutic challenge of systolic hypertension. *New Eng. J. Med.*, 289:481-483, 1973.

16. Colandrea, M. A., Friedman, G. D., Nichaman, M. Z. et al: Systolic hypertension in the elderly. An epidemiologic assessment. *Circulation*, 41:239-245, 1970.

17. Gubner, R. S.: Systolic hypertension: A pathogenetic entity. Significance and therapeutic considerations. *Amer. J. Cardiol.*, 9:773-776, 1962.

18. Gordon, T. and Kannel, W. B.: Multiple contributors to coronary risk. Implications for screening and prevention. *J. Chron. Dis.*, 25:561-565, 1972.

19. Chasis, H.: Appraisal of antihypertensive drug therapy. *Circulation*, 50:4-8, 1974.
20. Freis, E. D.: Rebuttal: Appraisal of antihypertensive drug therapy. *Circulation*, 50:9-10, 1974.
21. Deming, Q. B., Mosbach, E. H., Bevans, M. et al: Blood pressure, cholesterol content of serum and tissues and atherogenesis in the rat. *J. Exp. Med.*, 107:581-598, 1958.
22. Moses, C.: Development of atherosclerosis in dogs with hypercholesterolemia and chronic hypertension. *Circ. Res.*, 2:243-247, 1954.
23. Bronte-Stewart, B. and Heptinstall, R. H.: The relationship between experimental hypertension and cholesterol-induced atheroma in rabbits. *J. Path. Bact.*, 68:407-417, 1954.
24. Hollander, W.: Hypertension, antihypertensive drugs and atherosclerosis. *Circulation*, 48:1112-1127, 1973.
25. Sako, Y.: Effects of turbulent blood flow and hypertension on experimental atherosclerosis. *JAMA*, 179:36-40, 1962.
26. Duncan, L. E., Jr.: Mechanical factors in the localization of atheromata. In John, R. D. (ed.): *Evolution of the Atherosclerotic Plaque*. Chicago:University Press, 1963.
27. Dahl, L. K. and Love, R. A.: Etiological role of sodium chloride in essential hypertension in humans. *JAMA*, 164:397-400, 1957.
28. Grollman, A.: The relationship of salt and diet to diastolic hypertension. *Amer. J. Cardiol.*, 9:700-703, 1962.
29. McKusick, V. A.: Genetic factors in cardiovascular diseases. I. The four major types of cardiovascular disease. *Mod. Conc. Cardiov. Dis.*, 28:535-542, 1959.
30. Dahl, L. K., Heine, M. and Tassinari, L.: Effects of chronic excess salt ingestion. Evidence that genetic factors play an important role in susceptibility to experimental hypertension. *J. Exp. Med.*, 115:1173-1190, 1962.
31. Thomas, C. B.: Heritage of hypertension. *Amer. J. Med. Sci.*, 224:367-376, 1952.
32. Miall, W. E. and Oldham, P. D.: The hereditary factor in arterial blood pressure. *Brit. Med. J.*, 5323:75-80, 1963.
33. Thomas, C. B.: Familial patterns in hypertension and coronary heart disease. *Circulation*, 20:25-29, 1959.
34. Platt, R.: Heredity in hypertension. *Lancet*, 1:899-904, 1963.
35. Pickering, G. W.: *High Blood Pressure*. New York:Grune and Stratton, 1955.
36. Smirk, F. H. and Hall, W. H.: Inherited hypertension in rats. *Nature, (London)*, 182:727-728, 1959.
37. Okamoto, K. and Poki, K.: Development of a strain of spontaneously hypertensive rats. *Jap. Circ. J.*, 12:943-952, 1964.
38. Moriyama, I. M., Krueger, D. E. and Stamler, J.: *Cardiovascular Disease in the U. S.* Harvard University Press, 1971, pp. 157, 141, 155, 156.
39. Fodor, J. G., Abbott, E. C. and Rusted, I. E.: An epidemiologic study of hypertension in Newfoundland. *Canad. Med. Ass. J.*, 108:1365-1368, 1973.

40. Marticorena, E., Ruiz, L., Severino, J. et al: Systemic blood pressure in white men born at sea level: Changes after long residence at high altitudes. *Amer. J. Cardiol.*, 23:364-368, 1969.
41. Kannel, W. B., Brand, N., Skinner, J. J. et al: The relation of adiposity to blood pressure and development of hypertension. The Framingham Study. *Ann. Intern. Med.*, 67:48-59, 1967.

Discussion

Dr. Winkelstein: As always, when you tell us about Framingham there is something new to be learned. In view of the fact that the risk, which we have all known, is continuous, ie, the increase in risk of developing a complication of high blood pressure is continuous over the whole range, how would you recommend deciding when to start treating? At what level?

Dr. Kannel: I tried to indicate that by suggesting that hypertension is best looked upon or conceptualized as an ingredient of a cardiovascular risk profile in which one uses the actual blood pressure level in conjunction with other powerful contributors to cardiovascular risk. By synthesizing this information, one can obtain a composite risk estimate. This, on the one hand, prevents overtreating those whose risk is quite modest and undertreating, on the other hand, those whose risk is quite substantial. I think one should use the actual blood pressure value in conjunction with other factors.

Dr. Kass: Along these lines, there was one aside that you threw in that was of particular interest and this was the matter of whether some evidence of end organ damage was or was not necessary before the risks began to accumulate. Is there a great deal of indication, from your data, that people may have a significant mortality without having developed some evidence of preceding end organ damage? The alternative would be to wait until that showed up and then institute treatment.

Dr. Kannel: As I indicated, cardiovascular events occur quite regularly in people who do not progress to the stage where they have identifiable end organ damage. Even at borderline levels of pressure, in certain persons one finds a very substantial increased risk. This usually occurs most prominently in people whose cholesterol values tend to be high and/or who smoke cigarettes. But they do not invariably occur in persons who show ECG evidence of cardiovascular involvement or heart enlargement on x-ray. There is a substantial morbidity and mortality in those who do not reach that stage.

Dr. Kass: Have you had a chance to take a look at whether in the absence of end organ damage such events occur in the absence of high cholesterol or high smoking?

Dr. Kannel: I was trying to indicate that even a 165 mm pressure carries a very low risk if everything else is optimal. So the blood pressure alone does not seem to be enough.

Dr. Labarthe, Minnesota: There has been a question for some time of the possibility of an excess in mortality in the very lowest blood pressure group, and this does appear in the data you showed for systolic pressure for females in the Framingham Study. If this is real, it may have important implications for our usual assumption, "the lower the pressure the better," in control programs. Is there an explanation for that aspect of your data?

Dr. Kannel: It is always hard to tell if you are dealing with a U-shaped distribution, as you well know. I suspect that that is not real, but I do not know how you can really test it because the population at risk is rather small. I think the safest assumption would be that the lower the pressure the better off you are. Nobody I know of has a large enough sample of people with these really low pressures to describe these people and to really get stable rates to compare with the average for people their age. I had hoped the Pooling Project might do that but they did not seem interested.

Dr. Stamler: First, on systolic versus diastolic as a predictor: This is in many ways a sterile argument, since the correlation coefficient between the two is about 0.7, hence they are bound to be very similar in predicting risk. It is not surprising, therefore, that the evidence indicates systolic is as good a predictor as diastolic. But I think we have a peculiar methodological problem which needs to be teased out of these data, ie, the problem of pure systolic hypertension, a sign of already existent disease, usually atherosclerotic disease. Second, you made a remark in your summary about the average rise in blood pressure. I think it is important to note, and I would assume in Framingham you have been working on this, that this average rise in blood pressure with age is a composite including a segment of the population that starts low and stays low.

Finally, do you have a slide on the relationship of blood pressure in men and women, younger or older, to noncardiovascular mortality including mortality from malignancy?

Dr. Kannel: With respect to the issue of isolated systolic hypertension, there is no question that there is a disproportionate rise in systolic blood pressure with age and that this is attributable to an inelastic vasculature. Roy Dawber has demonstrated that if one measures elasticity from pulse wave recordings using the dicrotic notch as a measure of elastic recoil that one will find that those with inelastic vessels do have and develop more atherosclerotic disease. Furthermore, they do this at any level of pressure. So there is no question that rigid vessels seem to be more susceptible to atherosclerotic events or measure the atherosclerotic process. But I think the converse is also true, namely, that in any rigidity of the vessel, the pressure contributes to risk. I do not know any way to answer this question except by a clinical trial which addresses itself to the issue — is it beneficial to reduce isolated, systolic hypertension? This seems more feasible in young people where the pressure is modifiable and still variable and labile. It does not seem as likely to be acceptable in very old people where attempts to lower this type of pressure are often associated with intolerable symptoms. However, I would point out from our work in the geriatric hospital in Framingham that about half of these isolated systolic hypertensions in the elderly are quite labile and that we have seen many of these put on treatment and they are able to tolerate it. These old people do fall down and a lot of people attribute this to postural problems associated with treatment. It is our impression that the number of falls is just as great in those not on treatment. Old people just fall down a lot. So it is hard to know what is going on.

The Georgia Experience in Hypertension Control

J. Gordon Barrow, M.D.

The prevalence of hypertension in Georgia studies is similar to that in other areas of the country. Two predominantly rural counties and one urban area have been well studied.

Wilber[1] reported a true random sample of rural Baldwin County, Georgia, including all persons over 15 years of age in every fourth household in the county. Racial distribution in the county was 40% black and 60% white. Three thousand eighty-four persons (96.8% of the sample) were examined; 17.5% of the sample had hypertension ($\geq$ 160/95) and 3% had normal blood pressure but were on current therapy for hypertension.

Mean BP, by age and race, is shown in Figure 1. The distribution of diastolic pressure in each sex and race is shown in Figures 2 and 3.

McDonough et al[2] have studied another rural county, Evans County, Georgia. The study population included all persons 40 through 74 years of age and a 50% random sample of all persons 15 through 39 years of age. Racial make-up was 38% black and 62% white. Mean BP was higher than Baldwin County at all ages for both races in this group (Fig. 4). Although the method of dividing the group into normotensive vs hypertensive persons differs in the Baldwin County and Evans County studies, a comparison of the two studies utilizing either mean BP or only diastolic pressure confirms this impression. Whereas only 13.4% of the Baldwin County population had a diastolic pressure of 95 mm or greater, 28.4% of the Evans County population had a diastolic of 100 or greater. No valid explanation for this difference has been determined. It is interesting to note that

J. Gordon Barrow, M.D., *Coordinator, Georgia Regional Medical Program, Atlanta, Ga.*

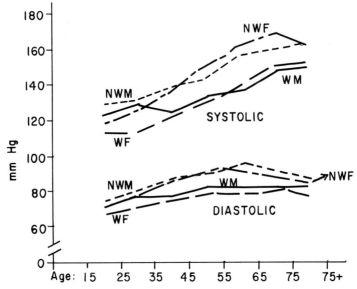

Fig. 1. Baldwin County Hypertension Study: Mean systolic and diastolic blood pressure, by race, sex and age.

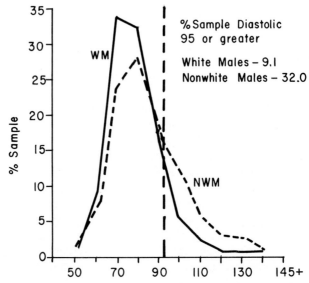

Fig. 2. Baldwin County Hypertension Study: Percentage distribution of diastolic blood pressure for males, by race.

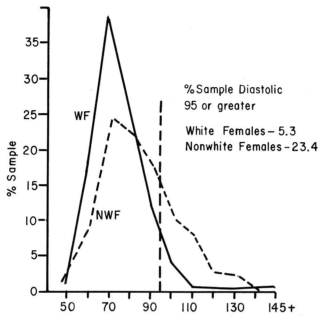

Fig. 3. Baldwin County Hypertension Study: Percentage distribution of diastolic blood pressures for females, by race.

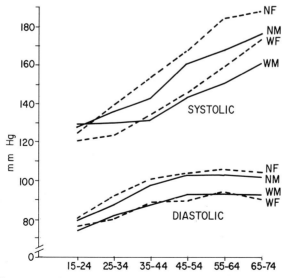

Fig. 4. Systolic and diastolic blood pressure by age group, sex and race.

Evans County lies in the coastal plain area which has the highest prevalence of stroke in the country.

The third study[3] was made in six urban census tracts of metropolitan Atlanta, Georgia, containing 23,000 persons 15 years or older, about 95% black. Only about 6,000 persons were examined and these were not randomly selected. Comparison with the census data showed that more females, especially in the older age groups, participated voluntarily.

Prevalence of hypertension was similar to that in Baldwin County although again it must be kept in mind that the method of classification differed and that the purpose of the study was not to study the epidemiology of hypertension, but to learn the best methods of conducting community screening for the control of the condition.

We have learned from the Georgia studies that hypertension in the community is largely asymptomatic and many are unrecognized. Forty-one percent of the Baldwin County hypertensives and 19% of the Atlanta hypertensives had never been told their blood pressure was elevated. At the time of screening, prior awareness of their disease (Table 1) was highest in white females and lowest in black males, probably relating to the relative frequency with which these groups visit doctors.

Our studies have also shown that many who have hypertension are currently on no treatment. Seventy percent of the hypertensives in Baldwin County and 43% of those in Atlanta were not on any treatment, partly as a result of not being aware of the disease, but also because it was asymptomatic and not considered important by the patient.

Untreated hypertension is widely known by the medical profession to be an important risk factor for the premature development of coronary disease, stroke or renal disease. Not as well known is the importance of hypertension of even mild degree in the teenage population. The group in Evans County, Georgia,[4] found that 11% of a group of young people (15-25 years old) had a BP of 140/90 or greater. Seven years later they reexamined the group and 11 out of 30 patients had developed sustained hypertension. Two of these had died from cerebral hemorrhage while four others had cardiomegaly, proteinuria and/or an abnormal electrocardiogram. Five had sustained hypertension without evidence of complication; 7 still had borderline hypertension and 12 had become normotensive. This

TABLE 1. Baldwin County Hypertension Survey, 1962:
Percent with No Prior Knowledge of Hypertension
among Combined Hypertensives, by Race and Sex

Combined Hypertensives (Systolic 160 or >, Diastolic 95 or >)	Percent with No Prior Knowledge
All	41
White male	42
White female	19
Nonwhite male	57
Nonwhite female	37

unexpectedly high incidence of sustained hypertension with early complications certainly implies that hypertension in the young must be recognized and treated early.

Long-term control of hypertension with appropriate drug therapy is now possible in at least 95% of most populations and since drug control has been shown to reduce significantly complications of the disease, at least in moderate or severe hypertension, we felt it was urgent to learn quickly how best to control this disease in the general population.

As a result of these epidemiologic findings, the Atlanta study was designed to study various methods of screening and follow-up in the community to compare their relative cost effectiveness. The Baldwin County Study[1] had shown that a door-to-door survey, utilizing public health nurses, was highly effective; however since most homes had to be revisited several times — often at night and on the weekend — and since highly skilled public health nurses are in short supply and are relatively costly, other methods were tried in Atlanta.

Screening Methods

Three approaches were used. First, a mass media campaign followed by a letter to each target household inviting everyone to come to a nearby community center for screening resulted in only 10% participation by the target population.

Next, a door-to-door survey, utilizing specially trained nonprofessionals from within the community, working during daylight hours, was tried. Only 50% of the households visited had anyone at home and in 13% of the households in which someone was found at home, screening was refused. Those screened tended to be older females when compared to census data.

The most efficient of the three approaches tried was late afternoon and evening shopping center screening utilizing a mobile van staffed by specially trained nonprofessionals. Those screened were much more representative of the population and the number screened per unit of time was greater than with the other two methods. It is realized, however, that only a representative sample of the population was reached by this method. If it is desirable and economically feasible to reach an entire population, the door-to-door method, utilizing repeated visits at night and on weekends as was done in the Baldwin County Study, is most effective.

Referral and Follow-up

Even after the hypertension is recognized and the patient referred for treatment, results are far from encouraging. The Atlanta study showed that making the patient aware he has hypertension and referring him to his physician resulted in only 50% of the patients actually seeing a physician during the next 12 months. About 74% of those who saw the physician were actually treated and about 73% of these maintained treatment for at least a year.

In Baldwin County, the number of hypertensives in the community under treatment was doubled (from 25% to 50% of the hypertensives) by the total community screening program and referral to a physician, but by the end of four years this had fallen to about 35% with no special program of follow-up. In only 20% of the hypertensives was the hypertension under good control (average diastolic pressure less than 95 mm Hg).

Use of the public health nurse in a program of continued home follow-up after the initial screening increased the hypertensives under treatment by a physician from 25% at the initial screening to 86% two years later, and in 80% of the total group the blood pressure was under good control.

We were interested to learn why treatment for hypertension was discontinued. Table 2 shows a breakdown of the reasons given by a group in Baldwin County who had discontinued treatment. In the Atlanta group, findings were similar except

TABLE 2. Baldwin County Hypertension Survey, 1962:
Reasons Why Treatment for Hypertension
Was Discontinued

Number giving reasons	104
Total*	110%
Financial considerations	16
Didn't realize should continue	12
Felt better	30
Take when needed	16
Miscellaneous	36

*Totals more than 100 because some gave more than one reason.

that financial considerations were given as a reason in only 4.8% of the patients.

We have learned from this that simple referral of hypertensives in the community to their physicians for treatment without follow-up is an unsatisfactory way to control hypertension in the community.

Use of Nonphysicians in Treatment

The very large number of hypertensives who need treatment in the community has led us to study the use of specially trained nurses or physician assistants to supervise both treatment and follow-up of a group of patients.

A group of registered nurses with no previous special training or experience in hypertension was given two weeks of intensive training in the management of this disease. The pathophysiology of hypertension was discussed, but the major emphasis was on the evaluation of the patient and on the pharmacology of the drugs used in treating hypertension and their side effects. They were then taught to use a written stepwise protocol approach to the diagnosis and long-term management of the hypertensive patient.

They were given the responsibility for a group of hypertensives identified in the screening program. The patients were unselected except that they had no private physician and were not eligible for the municipal charity hospital. It was explained to each patient that specially trained nurses would manage their high blood pressure under the close supervision of a physician who would always be available and would review their progress periodically.

A standard history, physical and laboratory examination were carried out. A stepwise treatment protocol was followed after diagnosis. In general, patients were given a thorough review of their problem after the work-up was completed and the severity of their problem was explained to them in detail. The need for lifetime treatment as well as the importance of regular daily medication was explained to them.

Appointments were made at two week intervals until the blood pressure was controlled. Drugs were added in stepwise fashion at standard dosages until the diastolic blood pressure averaged lower than 90 mm Hg. When this level was reached, the patient was maintained on this step. There was also emphasis on a potassium-rich low-salt diet and on weight control. Regular follow-up was stressed.

A preliminary analysis of our results to date indicates the following:

1. Nurses are excellent therapists for asymptomatic hypertensive patients and are very effective in their patient education.
2. Patients accept them almost universally.
3. Only 10%-15% of patients discontinue treatment within a year.
4. Forty percent of patients (some with diastolic blood pressure as high as 120) can be controlled on diuretics alone.
5. Seventy-five percent of patients can be controlled on a diuretic plus reserpine.
6. Ninety-five percent can be controlled on a diuretic, reserpine and hydralazine.
7. The physician must assume moral and legal responsibility. He must check the history, physical and laboratory work with the patient personally. He must review and sign all orders on each patient visit, and he must be available to see the patient whenever the nurse or the patient may request.

We see no reason why primary physicians could not institute a similar plan in their own offices. Whereas follow-up and patient education is very poorly done or not done at all in most physicians' offices, the use of these specially trained nurses could assure good patient education and management and more adequate follow-up with a much more economical use of the physician's time and less cost to the patient.

Where community outpatient services exist, either in indigent patient facilities or in heart association sponsored clinics, similar arrangements can be used.

Discussion

With a public health problem as serious and as widespread as hypertension, it is urgent that an organized control program be devised. There is no evidence that the public education program currently underway will significantly change the number of hypertensive patients under treatment. Scattered screening programs with voluntary participation will not solve the problem. We need an organized screening program involving all persons from 15 to 65 years of age at least once every five years with a yearly reappraisal of all those in the borderline or mild hypertension groups. I personally do not see any way of accomplishing this without some mandatory element. Perhaps, if national health insurance becomes a reality, screening for hypertension (and certain other diseases) should be required at the time an eligibility card is granted or renewed.

In my opinion, we do not yet have sufficient evidence to warrant treatment of borderline or mild hypertension, but close follow-up of these cases is essential. In the younger age groups particularly, treatment should be instituted if it is felt to be justified by the individual's physician.

Moderate to severe hypertension should clearly be treated and use of nurses and other allied health professionals using step-care protocols as described in this paper will enable this large number of cases to be absorbed into the medical care system with maximum efficiency.

Follow-up and extensive patient education is essential to proper management and must be assured in any system of care. Use of these principles in a nationwide program of hypertension recognition and care should enable us to control this disease in our lifetime.

602 J. G. BARROW

References

1. Wilber, J. A.: Detection and control of hypertensive disease in Georgia, U.S.A. In Stamler, J., Stamler, R. and Pullman, T. J. (eds.): *The Epidemiology of Hypertension.* New York:Grune and Stratton, 1967, pp. 439-448.
2. McDonough, J. R., Garrison, G. E. and Hames, C. G.: Blood pressure and hypertensive disease among Negroes and whites. *Ann. Intern. Med.,* 61:208, 1964.
3. Wilber, J. A. and Barrow, J. G.: Hypertension — a community problem. *Amer. J. Med.,* 52:653, 1972.
4. Heyden, S., Bartel, A. G. and McDonough, J. R.: Elevated blood pressure levels in adolescents, Evans County, Georgia. *JAMA,* 209:1683, 1969.

Discussion

Dr. Holland: What was the actual cost to a patient, in your study, who was referred to a doctor? If he went to a doctor what would he have had to pay?

Dr. Barrow: We did a cost study on that and it ranged from $30 a year to over $300 a year. The doctor charged whatever his normal charge was, and the cost varied with how extensive his work-up was and how often he saw the patient in the follow-up.

Dr. Finnerty: I was delighted to hear Dr. Barrow because he knows we share the same enthusiasm for nurses. I think really the time has come to put this concept into the private office. It must be accepted by repeated pilot demonstrations in the doctor's office that yes, the nurse can do it as well or better than the physician, and that his office will make as much if not more money. There is the secret, you are everybody's friend until you are in the pocketbook. We have a study going in which we are putting a private nurse into a doctor's office in two settings, out in the country and downtown Washington. The nurse is going to take over, just as you are saying here. The Blue Shield people are going to pay the patient's bill as if the patient saw the doctor. This is the first time the Blue Shield is endorsing preventive medicine. They do not want this advertised yet. If it is successful, if there is better control of pressure and the doctor makes more money, we are in. It is not enough for us all to talk to each other who are in city hospitals and in the university; we have to get out where the average patient is.

Dr. Barrow: I agree that the payment is very critical and I think we have gotten Medicare to pay in our area but not Medicaid and it is run by the same department.

Dr. Miller, Maryland: I like to have nurses too but from where are we going to get them?

Dr. Barrow: I think we have only just begun to explore just how far we can go with the use of nonprofessional personnel. As you know, there is information that high school students can be used to follow these step protocols. We have to do a good bit more work before we know just how far down in the subprofessional level we can go.

Dr. Milller: That was really my point. Let us not put all our emphasis on nurses. There are other people who do this kind of thing.

Dr. Haynes, Canada: One of the things which you did not mention is whether once the nurse stops going to those patients, in the subsequent follow-up they had not really dropped their adherence to treatment. I do not know of any method of improving adherence to treatment that is self-sustaining.

Dr. Barrow: It follows that if there is not a good follow-up program that is continuous, the treatment begins to taper off substantially.

Dr. Sackett: Concerning the economics of the situation from a Canadian perspective, it is a cause for concern that nurse-practitioners are being put into a fee-for-service system; this has grave implications in terms of costs. Ontario has adopted a somewhat different approach based in part on a randomized clinical trial showing similar clinical outcomes for patients randomly allocated to be treated by nurses and by physicians.* It has adopted a salaried nurse-practitioner program which will give a greater amount of care at a lower incremental cost. As you described your program, you are giving a greater amount of care but you are going to have a substantial increment in cost. I think this is going to be financially self-defeating.

Dr. Holland: Can I comment also on one aspect just mentioned. May I urge that these trials of physician's assistants,

---

*Spitzer, W. O., Sackett, D. L., Sibley, J. C. et al: The Burlington randomized trial of the nurse practitioner. *New Eng. J. Med.*, 290:251-256, 1974.

nurses, what have you, be done as proper experiments in which one measures other things than purely the clinical outcome. There are not only the costs. There are also the attitudes and the reactions of the patients, the families and the providers of the service. I hope we do not enter into the same mistakes as we have done with cytology and other procedures which have been introduced without proper evaluation.

Dr. Barrow: We have actually measured patient satisfaction and family satisfaction and other things as well as the success in treating blood pressure.

Dr. Holland: But you do not have a control group, so you cannot say which is better.

Dr. Meneely, Louisiana: Have there been any readings on the purely medicolegal aspect of this approach to the problem?

Dr. Barrow: We have an opinion from the Attorney General of Georgia received before we went into this, which says that as long as the nurse has been delegated this responsibility by a physician and is working under his supervision that what she does is legal.

Dr. Meneely: How does his insurance carrier feel about that?

Dr. Barrow: The insurance rates have not gone up. As a matter of fact, the malpractice rates in Georgia are substantially lower than in most parts of the country.

Urban Programs in Hypertension

Frank A. Finnerty, Jr., M.D.

Any community program, urban or suburban, designed to detect and follow up patients with hypertension must consist of four rather integrated activities: (1) screening, (2) referral, (3) diagnosis and (4) treatment.

Screening

Who Should Screen?

It is not only essential to gain the cooperation of key members of the community, eg, ministers, civic leaders, youth leaders, but it is also very helpful to have them on the team. When screening in our high schools, for example, we have found it particularly advantageous to have several intelligent and motivated students whom we have previously taught the technique of blood pressure recording actually work with us. Similarly, when screening in supermarkets or churches, or wherever any screening activity is going on, having a well-known member of the community identify with us greatly enhances the cooperation of the subjects and the efficiency of the operation.

In addition to community participation, screening programs are ideally manned by paramedics, retired nurses, nursing, dental, medical and pharmacy students and police and fire fighting personnel. The physician truly does not need to be involved in this phase, although his presence may certainly lend sophistication, enhance compliance and is, of course, always good public relations.

Frank A. Finnerty, Jr., M.D., *Professor of Medicine, Georgetown University and Georgetown University Medical Division, District of Columbia General Hospital, Washington.*

Where to Screen?

From a practical standpoint, screening should be carried out "where the action is." Several years ago, we had a great deal of success screening in supermarkets, particularly at the beginning of the month, when welfare and social security checks were being cashed.[1] With civic leaders encouraging the subjects to come over to our blood pressure tables, which were manned by medical students, 500 subjects were screened during one summer weekend; 210 of those were found to be hypertensive. Although screening in such areas does not identify the entire community (necessary for an epidemiologic study), 61% of the subjects in three census tracts were screened simply and efficiently in a three-month period. We also had good success in carrying out our screening activities at the voting polls where a large number of residents were gathered at one time.

It must be emphasized that house-to-house canvassing in previously laid out census tracts is the only way to determine the true incidence of disease in a community. Since such data are currently being obtained in the Hypertension Detection and Follow-up Program study supported by the National Heart and Lung Institute, and since the goal of a community program should be the finding and treating of hypertensive subjects wherever they live, this expensive and timeconsuming method of screening need not be repeated. Screening should be carried out, therefore, where groups of people are gathered at times convenient to them.

Screening activities must be dovetailed with treatment and follow-up facilities. Screening by itself will produce little benefit unless the medical facilities of the community are willing to be organized and willing to accept reponsibility for appropriate evaluation and treatment. The medical society particularly must be made aware of the screening activities since many physicians feel very protective of their patients. Thus, a patient found to be hypertensive at the supermarket may indeed be normotensive when he goes to his physician. If the physician then conveys to the patient the idea that both of them have wasted time, both may become antagonistic toward the program.

Before setting up any community screening program, it would be well to make sure that patients who are already under medical care, whether in the doctor's office, hospital, or clinic, are actually having their blood pressure taken and treated if elevated. That many physicians do not routinely record blood pressure is obvious when one visits the offices of dermatologists, ophthalmologists, surgeons, and so on. Some of these clinics or offices do not even own a blood pressure cuff.

A great many hypertensives would surely be discovered if every patient who went to any medical facility for any reason would have his blood pressure recorded. Our group recently trained high school students to record blood pressure and then placed them in clinics where blood pressure recording was not a routine — for example, orthopedics, urology and dermatology. The incidence of undiagnosed, untreated hypertension was 43% in the city hospital, 39% in the University hospital and 38% in a community hospital.[2] The lack of routine recording of blood pressure is not peculiar to office or clinic practice. A nurse working with our group recently recorded blood pressures on hospitalized patients in a city hospital who were not on the medical or obstetrical services. Of the 13,000 blood pressures recorded, 400 were over 150/100 mm Hg, 285 did not know they were hypertensive, and only 8 were under therapy.[3] It would seem, in this regard, that we should clean our own house before going out into the community.

Referral

The importance of making a verification appointment shortly after the patient has been initially screened and found to be hypertensive was brought out in the pilot phase of our Hypertension Detection and Follow-up Study. When there was more than one week's duration between the verification appointment and the time the patient was initially screened, there was a 50% no-show rate. Subsequent experience demonstrated that when a verification visit was scheduled 24-48 hours after the initial screening, the incidence of no-shows fell to below 5%. It would also seem important, particularly in a private practice setting, to verify an elevated blood pressure at least once before referring the patient to a private doctor. Verifying the elevated pressure on the scene is obviously more practical than sending the patient elsewhere. The waste of time and lack of accomplishment from screening alone was brought

up by the nationally advertised screening activities recently
conducted in New Orleans. Despite the fact that over 30,000
subjects were screened in a single weekend and 38% were found
to be hypertensive, there has been follow-up on actually less
than 5%.

Diagnosis

Gifford[3] has found that less than 6% of 5,000 consecutive
hypertensive patients first seen at the Cleveland Clinic (where
emphasis is on diagnosis of secondary types of hypertension)
have secondary hypertension. We thoroughly agree with his
conclusions that these findings would hardly warrant an
exhaustive search for secondary hypertension in every patient.
Indeed, one of the major drawbacks of the practicing physician
accepting the responsibility of caring for any hypertensive
patient is the fear of criticism from his peers that he did not
"work up the patient completely or promptly." He is also
reluctant to spend the patient's money for undergoing the costs
of sophisticated, expensive, routine laboratory procedures.

Since 85%-90% of the hypertensive population has the
essential variety, since at least 75% of these patients have mild
forms of the disease which can readily be treated with effective
simple therapy and since 70% of hypertensive patients are over
40 years of age, we recommend the following work-up for the
asymptomatic patient over 40 years of age.

1. Documentation of a diastolic pressure over 95 mm Hg
    on at least three independent visits.
2. A careful history with emphasis on the cardiovascular
    and renal systems and a complete physical examination.
3. Blood glucose (preferably two hours postprandial),
    serum creatinine, serum potassium, and serum choles-
    terol. (Although not directly related to hypertension, an
    elevated cholesterol represents an important risk factor
    for coronary disease.)
4. Urinalysis.
5. ECG.
6. Chest x-ray.

These examinations are readily available, easy to perform
and relatively inexpensive, can be performed by the nurse
(except for an x-ray) and conform in general to the recom-

mendations of the hypertensive study group of the Inter-Society Commission for Heart Disease Research. The history and physical examination are the most important. They not only establish the degree of vascular disease and the presence or absence of major target organ involvement, but frequently provide telltale clues of the presence of secondary types of hypertension. Most types of secondary hypertension can at least be suspected from a careful history, physical examination and simple laboratory data. Any patient suspected of having secondary hypertension should obviously be referred to a physician for appropriate verification.

It should also be emphasized that patients *at any age* with accelerated hypertension, patients who do not respond satisfactorily to treatment, or patients who cannot or will not tolerate effective doses of antihypertensive drugs need to be referred to their physician for an exhaustive work-up for secondary hypertension.

Let us be honest with ourselves! The long-term routine care of the hypertensive patient offers no challenge. Just as we rely on specially trained nurses in the coronary intensive care unit, we must become aware of their value in the follow-up of hypertensive patients. Once the hypertensive patient has been initially evaluated and placed on a therapeutic regimen by a physician and has reached a status quo situation, the patient can ideally be followed by a nurse or health assistant working under the nurse. The nurse, challenged by this assignment, establishes a meaningful relationship with the patient, which then allows her to motivate the patient to take medication and remain under care for the rest of his or her life.

Wherever such projects have been carried out, they have been successful. The Amos Project at Ft. Belvoir, the Ambulatory Care Project at the Beth-Israel Hospital in Boston and the Hypertension Detection and Follow-up Program in inner city Washington are a few examples. Utilization of the specially trained nurse and paramedical personnel goes a long way toward eliminating the overcrowded clinics and teaches patients and doctors that it is not necessary for the doctor to examine the patient on every visit. Utilizing paramedical personnel in this way allows taking advantage of already existing facilities and bypasses the need for construction of new buildings.

Specific examples would include placing the health assistant with supporting personnel (when necessary) in the private practitioner's (or private group) office, in VD clinics, in birth control clinics, in general medical clinics in hospitals where the back-up facilities would be immediately available, in neighborhood health clinics, in multiphasic screening clinics and, finally, in rheumatic fever clinics (as planned by the Georgia Heart Association) where the emphasis could easily be changed (and/or extended) to following hypertensive subjects.

In our clinic at District of Columbia General Hospital, with a trained nurse effectively directing the clinic in consultation with a physician and assisted by two paramedics, 30-40 patients can easily be seen each day. Doubling the paramedical personnel (ours are recruited from the community and trained by the clinic staff) can usually double the number of patients such a clinic can handle. Considering the roughly 8:1 cost ratio of physicians to paramedical personnel, this arrangement leads to substantial economic savings and frees the doctor to carry out other duties.

Treatment

The key to the success of this approach lies in the basic assumption that the vast proportion of hypertensive patients have mild or moderately severe disease which can be easily treated, often on a regimen of one pill a day. The major obstacle to effective treatment is patient noncompliance. Patients either stop appearing for "regular check-ups" or stop taking their medication. To counteract this noncompliance, the medical profession (doctors, nurses or paramedics) must use the leverage of personal identification with the patient to stimulate motivation to the long course of therapy. In our inner city clinic, a well-trained, understanding paramedic has substituted for the doctor in this personal relationship with the patient. Once this relationship has been established, time can then be spent in motivating and educating the patient rather than merely reassuring him. Indeed, this personal relationship (each patient has his own paramedic) has been instrumental not only in controlling the blood pressure but also in decreasing the drop-out rate from 42% to 4%.

Many studies[5,6] have demonstrated that the simpler the treatment, the more likely the patient will remain on therapy. The greatest compliance obviously follows a regimen of one pill a day. In this regard, the good effect of a combination of thiazides plus reserpine in the Veterans Administration Study[7] should be emphasized. The addition of a third drug, hydralazine, resulted in only a 4 mm average further reduction in diastolic pressure. If those patients whose diastolic pressure was between 114 and 129 mm Hg could be controlled by these medications — two of which can be combined in a single tablet — surely good control of the blood pressure can be obtained with these medications in the vast majority of the hypertensive population who have only mild disease. A recent study in our inner city population has also demonstrated that in 70% of newly discovered hypertensive patients, the diastolic blood pressure was brought to 90 mm Hg or below by either a thiazide alone or a thiazide plus reserpine, eg, a pill a day.[1]

Conclusion

It is not our intent to advocate that the treatment of all patients with hypertension be relegated to the specially trained nurse or paramedical person. Certainly those patients with moderately severe or severe disease must be under the constant attention of the physician, since they frequently require complicated therapeutic regimens, careful dosage adjustments, monitoring of electrolytes and kidney function and, at times, hospitalization. This small group of patients should be under the direct care of the physician until blood pressure has returned to normal and a stable therapeutic regimen has been established.

It is hoped, however, that these pilot studies will stimulate other physicians, both in hospitals and in private practice, to identify and treat more hypertensive patients and to use specially trained nurses and paramedical personnel in their long-term management.

References

1. Finnerty, F. A., Jr., Shaw, L. W. and Himmelsbach, C.: Hypertension in the inner city: II. Detection and follow-up. *Circulation*, 47:76-78, 1973.

2. Wilson, M., Mroczek, W. J. and Finnerty, F. A., Jr.: Early detection of hypertension: The role of out-patient clinics and their nurses. *JAMA* (In press.)
3. Finnerty, F. A., Jr.: The hypertension problem: What we can do about it. *Circulation*, 48:681-683, 1973.
4. Finnerty, F. A., Jr.: Hypertension: New techniques for improving patient compliance. *Hypertension Handbook.* West Point, Pa.:Merck Sharp & Dohme, pp. 117-124, 1974.
5. Francis, V., Korsch, B. M. and Morris, M. J.: Gaps in doctor-patient communication. Patients' response to medical advice. *New Eng. J. Med.*, 280:535, 1969.
6. Marston, M. V.: Compliance with medical regimens: A review of the literature. *Nurs. Res.*, 19:312, 1970.
7. Veterans Administration Cooperative Study Group on Antihypertensive Agents; Effect of Treatment on Morbidity: Results in Patients with Diastolic Pressures Averaging 115 through 129 mm Hg. *JAMA*, 202: 1028, 1967.

Discussion

Dr. Stamler: I think Dr. Finnerty would agree on the following points: (1) baseline work-up should include a serum uric acid and a blood count , (2) simple therapy with one pill a day can accomplish control of blood pressure in a sizable proportion of cases and (3) when there is concomitant cigarette smoking and/or hypercholesterolemia and/or gross obesity and/or hyperglycemia, and consequently risks are markedly compounded, our health counselor, nurse practitioner, etc., can play a very important role in the nutritional and hygienic management also.

Mr. Eckenfels, Illinois: My comment has to do with screening. From my experience in both the Mile Square community, an inner city ghetto on the west side of Chicago and Holmes County, a poor, black, rural community in Mississippi, we found that prior to any screening a good demographic base is essential for evaluation and epidemiological purposes. In other words, you need a good denominator that accounts for the total population you hope to reach. Relying on U.S. Census figures can be a problem. For example, in Holmes County we uncovered underenumeration because some households were difficult to locate, and in Mile Square we found overenumeration due to rapid housing deterioration and urban-renewal. A reliable population census is absolutely essential to assure accurate coverage of the population to be screened. It is also helpful in making systematic assignments.

Dr. Finnerty: I have no objection to what you are saying. My point would be that if you want to go out and get everybody and identify your population, then you really have to do a house-to-house canvass. That is currently being done I hope in such a way that this will not have to be done again. This is the expensive way to do it. Once it has been done then let us get on with it, let us go out and treat people. In order to find them you must go where they are.

Dr. Holland: Before everybody accepts the value of screening, may I comment that a randomized controlled trial of screening in Britain has not demonstrated any change in mortality at the end of five years and we found no difference in levels of blood pressures between those people who were screened regularly and those who received their normal medical care. Obviously, our situation is different from that of the black population of Washington, but I would urge you to do a proper randomized control trial because otherwise you will be finding yourself in the same difficulties that everybody has landed in when introducing new methods of medical care of not really knowing whether you were achieving anything useful.

Dr. Finnerty: My only comment would be that the people in Britain must be significantly different from our inner city blacks because wherever we screen or wherever I hear screening is done in black populations, 50% of the people do not know they have hypertension. How are you going to treat if they do not know they have hypertension and if you cannot find them?

Mrs. Stamler: One big feature of the Hypertension Detection and Follow-up Program (HDFP) is placing a very large share of patient management in the hands of nonphysicians, under the general leadership of physicians, using a very carefully worked out protocol with very careful monitoring. I believe that in the course of examining long-term adherence rates in this program, compared to those randomly referred to usual care, we will get an answer to some of these questions. I also believe HDFP will help very much to answer the question of whether a screening program followed by a very careful referral, treatment and follow-up effort will influence mortality. A plain screening program with no follow-up or treatment is very likely not to influence mortality.

Dr. Simpson, New Zealand: We also make a lot of use of paramedical personnel and I am sure they do an excellent job. I just wonder whether it is wise to have the same person both take the blood pressure and be responsible for keeping it down. Does Dr. Finnerty feel that there is any problem of bias?

Dr. Finnerty: I think there is bias but it does not override the other advantages. In my private office my nurse takes the pressure, I take the pressure, and they are always violently different, but I go by mine.

Dr. Schoenberger: I would like to make two points. In Chicago we carried out a mass screening project in industry over a number of years and we have rescreened almost 5,000 of these individuals. The prevalence of hypertension has actually gone up, indicating that our screening and referral process was entirely ineffective. We used the most effective referral methods we could under the terms of the study. Much of this might have been a reflection of the incidence of new cases, but nevertheless one could conclude that there had been no impact on the problem from the screening effort. The second point I would like to make is that the Harris poll which was done for the National Heart and Lung Institute showed that 77% of a random sample of the public indicated that their blood pressures had been taken within the preceding year. Our data confirm what everybody else has pointed out, namely that the majority of people are unaware that they are hypertensive. This would clearly indicate that doctors not only are failing to do anything about hypertension when they find it, but they are not even informing the patients. So I think, again, that the emphasis should not be on screening. The first emphasis, in my judgment, should be on educating the practicing physician of the value of treatment.

Dr. Finnerty: I would surely agree and would make one more comment that the worst thing as far as putting a fence around finding hypertension has been the specialization of medicine. Often there is not a blood pressure cuff in a surgeon's office, or in an ophthalmologist's, or dermatologist's office. Before talking about community programs, we should clean up our own house. We should make it mandatory, as the AMA says, that every patient who goes to any medical or dental facility should have his blood pressure checked.

Comment: It seems that it might be useful to remember to be honest with ourselves. We have heard all stages of the problem elucidated yet we do not know whether the treatment is effective (as evidenced by the carrying forward of clinical trials) and we do not know very much about the various methods of application of our knowledge to the community. We have evidence that screening and case finding may be no more effective than self-presentation and self-selection of patients. So I would like to second Dr. Holland's plea that most of these activities, at the present time, should be carefully controlled. I think it should be placed on record that we are not yet in a position simply to go forward with service programs without building in careful, controlled and scientific evaluation.

Dr. Finnerty: My answer to that is that there has been more than enough proof that patients whose diastolic pressure is more than 105 have a much greater mortality if they are not treated and that the complications — stroke, heart failure, kidney failure — are the direct result of blood pressure.

Dr. Tuomilehto, Finland: We have in Finland a very high incidence of cardiovascular diseases. Two years ago we started with a community control program in North Karelia County to prevent them. One part of that community program is the community control of hypertension. We found that when we get people who are hypertensive on treatment, we also learn that most of those patients also have high cholesterol levels and many of them smoke. We found that the best way to help such hypertensive population groups is to build up the system with hypertensive patients coming to the office and at that time have them discuss with the nurse the nature of cardiovascular diseases, diet habits and smoking habits. It may be useful when we are building up the system of high-risk cardiovascular persons to start with hypertensive patients who have high cholesterol values and who smoke to get the risk level for complications lower more effectively than in traditional anti-hypertensive drug treatment.

Dr. Labarthe, Minnesota: I would just like to add to the record the possibility that there may be wide differences among populations in the level of compliance in screening programs. Dr. Hunt has initiated studies of screening, referral and long-term management in rural communities surrounding

Rochester. We have been quite surprised to note that within a two-week period, after 195 persons were identified as hypertensive in a central screening program, 193 had appeared voluntarily as recommended for their appointments with no special effort to contact them. The two delinquents were telephoned and one came in and the other went to her physician. In the four months since that initial screening, only 3% of those who were confirmed as hypertensive have not continued their regular scheduled appointments. I hope this is not a unique experience.

The Australian National Blood Pressure Study

John Abernethy, B. Med. Sc., M.B., Ch. B.

Introduction

A full description of the Australian National Blood Pressure Study has been published elsewhere.[1] In brief, it is a single blind therapeutic trial designed to test the hypothesis that compared to placebos active antihypertensive therapy is effective in reducing the morbidity and mortality from strokes, hypertensive and ischemic heart disease and renal disease and by a margin of 30% in a population of subjects aged 30-69 with uncomplicated mild hypertension. For purposes of this study mild hypertension is defined arbitrarily as a mean diastolic pressure between 95 and 109 mm Hg and a mean systolic pressure less than 200 mm Hg, the mean pressures being based on pairs of casual readings taken on two separate occasions approximately one week apart.

Recruitment of suitable subjects for the therapeutic trial is a three-stage process, two preliminary screening stages conducted by trained nonmedical personnel followed by a full-scale medical examination including ancillary investigations (ECG, biochemistry). In order to obtain sufficient numbers and a significant outcome, the study is dispersed in space and time, ie, it is a multicentric study and will continue for five years. Screening commenced in three centers, two in Melbourne and one in Perth, in mid-1973 and is now complete. Screening at a fourth center in Sydney started in April 1974 and is still in progress. The screening of 57,000 subjects has yielded 2,212

John Abernethy, B.Med.Sc., M.B., Ch. B., *Study Director, National Blood Pressure Study, National Heart Foundation of Australia, Canberra City, Australia.*

subjects for the trial, a yield of 3.9%. Current predictions are that a total of 80,000 screened is necessary to achieve a total yield of 3,200, the number required to achieve significance; these numbers are, however, subject to review.

The purposes of this paper are to present some interim results on the three-stage screening procedure and to discuss some of the problems faced in attempting to achieve a satisfactory outcome to the therapeutic trial.

Primary Screening Stage (S1)

Subjects from particular suburban areas or occupational groups are invited to attend a conveniently located screening center, usually a specially equipped bus. After details of age, sex and country of birth, previous history of knowledge of or treatment of hypertension have been recorded, two consecutive readings are taken with a random zero sphygmomanometer. All subjects with a mean $DBP > 95$ or mean $SBP > 200$ and no history of antihypertensive treatment in the past three months are invited to return on a second occasion about one week later. In the following presentation of data from the three centers with completed screening programs, it is to be noted that the sample is nonrandom by virtue of the selection of particular suburban and occupational groups and because of the element of self-selection involved.

Prevalence of hypertension based on one pair of readings at the primary stage is of the order of 23%. This figure is made up of the proportion of subjects admitting to antihypertensive

TABLE 1. Blood Pressure (mm Hg) of 37,899 Untreated Subjects Attending Primary Screening

	Systolic *Mean ± S.D.*	*Diastolic* *Mean ± S.D.*
First reading	137.92 ± 23.09	82.01 ± 13.42
Second reading	135.71 ± 22.03	82.29 ± 13.05
Mean	136.82 ± 22.07	82.15 ± 12.84
Difference (1-2)	2.21 ± 9.39	-0.28 ± 6.43

treatment (7%) plus those untreated subjects found to be hypertensive.

Comparison of First and Second Readings
in Untreated Subjects (Table 1)

On the average, the systolic pressure is 2 mm lower on the second reading but the diastolic readings are virtually identical. The mean of two readings has a standard deviation of the same order as that of the individual readings because the population variance is relatively large compared to the within-subject variance.

In the following figures curves have been drawn by eye through mean values; the data are to be further analyzed by polynomial regression so that variance can be reliably assigned to the various factors.

Blood Pressure, Age and Sex in Untreated Subjects (Fig. 1)

The population was analyzed by five-year age groups. Diastolic pressure reaches a maximum in the 55-59 age group.

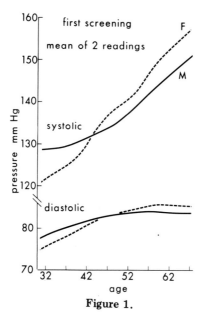

Figure 1.

The higher pressure of males in the lower age groups is the converse of the situation in the higher age groups.

Blood Pressure, Age and Country of Birth
in Untreated Subjects (Fig. 2)

U.K. migrants have significantly lower pressures than their Australian counterparts and a similar pattern is seen in Italian migrants.[2] A number of lines of evidence point to the fact that there are factors operating other than those of self-selection or medical selection of migrants.[3]

Secondary Screening Stage (S2)

Fourteen percent of the total screened attend S2, these subjects having been classed as untreated hypertensives at S1. After two further readings the mean of the four readings becomes the major determinant in final selection for the trial. On these more stringent criteria 9% of the total are now found to be hypertensive but 1.5% of the total screened are excluded because the pressures are above the critical upper limits set for defining mild hypertensives. A further 2.5% are excluded

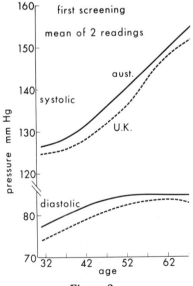

Figure 2.

because of a history of angina or stroke or some complicating illness such as diabetes, gout, asthma or in females because of pregnancy or use of contraceptive pills. Particular note is taken of hypertensives in the moderate-to-severe range. They are advised to attend the family doctor and their response to this advice is followed up. Using the two-stage screening as a criterion and including those attending S1 on treatment prevalence would now be defined as being of the order of 16%.

Comparison of Mean Pressures at Primary
and Secondary Screening (Untreated Hypertensives)
(Table 2 and Fig. 3)

Both systolic and diastolic pressures are lower at S2 by mean values of 6.5 and 7.7 mm Hg, respectively. This relationship varies somewhat with age, the differences being slightly greater at either end of the age range.

Third Stage

The clinical examination and induction into the trial comprise the third stage. Five percent of all screened subjects enter the third stage and are subjected to history taking and physical examination and ancillary investigations (ECG, serum potassium, uric acid, cholesterol and creatinine). One sixth of these are excluded because of ischemic heart disease, use of antidepressant drugs or defined illness or social situations likely to interfere with clinic attendance in the long-term trial. Only a

TABLE 2. Blood Pressure (mm Hg) of 5,391 Untreated Hypertensives at Primary (S1) and Secondary (S2) Screenings

	Systolic Mean ± S.D.	Diastolic Mean ± S.D.
S1 (mean of 2 readings)	163.43 ± 20.36	102.37 ± 7.45
S2 (mean of 2 readings)	156.89 ± 21.92	94.71 ± 11.65
Mean (S1 + S2)/2	160.16 ± 19.41	98.53 ± 8.22
Difference (S1 - S2)	6.54 ± 16.82	7.66 ± 10.59

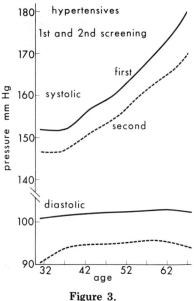

Figure 3.

small fraction (3%) of those eligible actually decline to enter the trial. Each subject is then randomly assigned either to an active treatment regime or to a regime of matching placebos. However, if the mean diastolic pressure on the day of the clinic is below the critical level of 95 mm Hg, issue of tablets to the subject is deferred. These subjects, initially about 15% of the total randomized, are asked to return at four-month intervals and are not issued tablets until this is indicated.

Difficulties Encountered in Conducting the Therapeutic Trial

One difficulty has been that the yield from screening into the trial is low (about half that predicted). A more pressing problem is that the current estimate of numbers required to achieve a significant outcome (3,200 randomized in a five-year trial) may be an underestimate because of certain unpredictable factors:

    1. The current rate of occurrence of trial end points is lower than expected possibly by as much as half. This

may have arisen because of the active selection of what amounts to a low-risk group.

2. The age structure of the present trial population is lower than previous estimates based on a smaller sample.

3. The attenuation of the trial population by defaulting was previously estimated at 25% over five years. Currently, it is about 10% over one year which might indicate a five-year rate of up to 50%.

4. The estimates of numbers required are based on a margin of benefit of treatment of 30% over five years. There are a number of factors operating to attenuate this margin:

   (a) Reduction of the effective difference between the active and placebo groups by the 15% who receive no tablets in the first instance.

   (b) Fall in diastolic pressure in the subjects on placebos. In one center analyzed at four months, the mean fall in diastolic pressure in the actively treated group was 8 mm Hg, but the placebo group also showed a fall of 4 mm Hg.

   (c) If (as is possible) no benefit accrues from treatment with respect to the incidence of ischemic heart disease, then the effective margin will again be considerably reduced particularly because ischemic heart disease end points may account for 75% of the total end points.

5. Attenuation of the control group by withdrawal of subjects whose pressures rise above the critical limits. This is necessitated by ethical considerations. The selective removal of high-risk subjects from the control group is therefore unavoidable even though it may prejudice the outcome of the trial. There are a number of compromise solutions to this problem but none are entirely satisfactory. For example, minimal antihypertensive therapy could be instigated in order to keep the pressure within the mild hypertension range. We have chosen an alternative solution which to some extent duplicates the dilemma facing doctors in the management of mild hypertension. Once it has been established that the critical limits are being consistently exceeded,

the subject is given full antihypertensive treatment. This subgroup may be used in conjunction with the remainder of the control group to answer a subsidiary question as to whether to initiate treatment as soon as mild hypertension is recognized or to delay treatment until the moderate-to-severe range is encountered. Currently, some 2.6% of the control group have entered this category after having been on placebos for up to one year.

Factors Which May Reduce the Numbers Required

Since risk (and therefore the trial end point rate) increases with age, extending the length of the trial by, say, one year would be an advantage. Furthermore, if the treatment effect is a cumulative one (rather than constant in time), then the effective margin would also increase with time, an additional advantage.

The rate of defaulting may decrease with time according to experience in other therapeutic trials.

The proportion of subjects not on tablets will probably decrease progressively.

As the trial progresses the diastolic pressures of the control group may tend to rise and thus increase the therapeutic margin.

The possibility of pooling results with those from a similar trial being conducted by the Medical Research Council of the United Kingdom has influenced the planning of both trials and is therefore an available option.

References

1. Abernethy, J. D.: The Australian National Blood Pressure Study. *Med. J. Aust.*, 1:821-824, 1974.
2. Ulman, R. and Abernethy, J. D.: The blood pressure of Australian and Italian immigrants in the Australian National Blood Pressure Study. (Submitted for publication.)
3. Stenhouse, N. S. and McCall, M. G.: Differential mortality from cardiovascular disease in migrants from England and Wales, Scotland and Italy, and native-born Australians. *J. Chronic Dis.*, 23:423-431, 1970.

Appendix

The Australian National Blood Pressure Study

Management Committee: Dr. S. R. Reader (Chairman), Dr. G. E. Bauer, Professor A. E. Doyle, Dr. K. Edmondson, Dr. T. H. Hurley, Professor P. I. Korner, Dr. P. Leighton, Professor R. R. H. Lovell, Professor M. G. McCall, Dr. J. M. McPhie, Mr. D. Oldfield, Professor M. J. Rand and Professor H. M. Whyte.

Directors of Study Centers: Dr. M. Bullen (Royal Melbourne Hospital), Dr. W. F. Heale (Austin Hospital), Dr. M. Lamb (Perth), Dr. J. Baker (Sydney).

Sponsors: The sponsors are the National Heart Foundation, National Health and Medical Research Council, Life Insurance Medical Research Fund of Australia and New Zealand, The Ramaciotti Foundations for Medical Research and Raine Bequest Medical Research Fund.

Discussion

Dr. Lovell: Dr. Abernethy has been very creditable in spending his whole time telling us about the difficulties. This is a very important area of activity and we shall gain nothing by glossing over the difficulties.

Dr. Winkelstein: It is interesting to note that your results indicate the systolic blood pressure to be in a sense a more stable measurement than the diastolic and this might have a bearing on the initial screening for trials where it is necessary to screen literally tens to hundreds of thousands of people in order to identify study groups. In the Hypertension Detection and Follow-up Program we use the diastolic blood pressure which might turn out to be considerably more costly than if we used the more stable systolic measurement for initial identification.

Dr. Abernethy: I just have one comment about that. You have decided it is more stable and you take that from the fact the change from the first to second screening was 6% for diastolic and 4% for the systolic.

Dr. Hoobler, Michigan: I had hoped you would comment on the incidence of those individuals who went up to 109 and particularly when they get to 109, do they stay there or do they drop back? Is this a spontaneous variation or a real advance of disease?

Dr. Abernethy: Our criteria for exit from trial are more stringent than for entry into it. We require that three successive blood pressures on three separate clinic visits each be above 109 mm. Using these criteria, so far, we have eliminated 2.3% from the control group in approximately a year.

Dr. Freis: You certainly did not get much reduction of blood pressure in your treatment group compared to that with the placebo. I want to comment that in mild hypertension it is more difficult to reduce the blood pressure than it is when the blood pressure is very high. The decrement is always much smaller in any kinds of trials that have been carried out in this regard. It may be necessary in some individuals to use combination therapy if you want to get a sizable decrement in blood pressure.

Dr. Stamler: First, a word of encouragement about one of your problems. In many trials, the dropout rate is not linear but it is higher in the first year. I offer you the hope that that might be the case on your 50% over five years. It may be nearer 25%. I would like to enter into the record my own conclusion that I do not believe any of the data we saw here really permit a conclusion that systolic pressure is more stable than diastolic. Further, I would like to comment that the observation that there is greater difficulty in lowering pressure in "mild hypertension" really has nothing to do with the inherent ability of blood pressure to be treated, but with the approach of doctors to pushing the medication and their insecurity about doing so in the face of their uncertainty of the benefit-risk ratio.

Dr. Prineas, Minnesota: Dr. Abernethy, since this is a single-blind trial and you have such small differences between the treated and control groups, could you tell us who takes the blood pressures?

Dr. Abernethy: The protocol lays down that if possible, and it is not always possible, a trained, nonmedical person, in fact one of the screeners, takes the blood pressure.

Implementation and Evaluation of Community Hypertension Programs

Nemat O. Borhani, M.D.

Introduction

Although the death rate attributed to hypertension and hypertensive heart disease has been declining steadily during the past decades,[1] high blood pressure remains a serious health problem in the United States. The toll of death and disability inflicted by uncontrolled hypertension and hypertensive heart disease is indeed a challenge to the health profession and the society as a whole — a challenge that demands an immediate and nationally coordinated response. Diseases caused by, or resulting from, high blood pressure cast a much larger shadow than is outlined by their attendant rates of mortality and morbidity. The very possibility of these diseases insults the achievement of growing older and, to this extent, it afflicts us all.

To the extent that mortality and morbidity associated with uncontrolled high blood pressure increases with age,[1-3] growing older remains a social and an economic liability rather than a valued confirmation of human potential. On the one hand, by judicious application of the results of our research in the control of infectious diseases, we have succeeded in extending the life expectancy of our fellow man. On the other hand, and perhaps ironically, men and women who have deferred immediate or fragmented pleasures in favor of a lifetime sense of purpose are too often denied both because of the diseases

Nemat O. Borhani, M.D., *Professor and Chairman, Department of Community Health, School of Medicine, University of California, Davis.*

associated with high blood pressure. In short, too many people are dying of hypertension and hypertensive heart disease (a total of 24,712 deaths in 1969) just when they are needed most and when they should be celebrating the rewards of seniority in human affairs.

It may be argued that since the needs for community hypertension control programs are immediate, a categorical approach will serve the community best. Although there seems to be little doubt of the benefits of judicious medical treatment in control of high blood pressure and its complications,[4-7] certain practical problems still exist, however, that may diminish this potential benefit. For example, drugs used to lower the blood pressure are not without toxicity and other pharmacologic side effects. We do not know under what conditions the problems in administering treatment will overcome the benefits of treatment. Further, we do not know the level of blood pressure that is optimal for good health and longevity. If we accept the level that is derived from the actuarial data[8] (ie, diastolic blood pressure of 70 mm Hg), many questions arise concerning the problems involved, not only in assuring a therapeutic regimen that will achieve such a goal (ie, reducing the diastolic blood pressure to 70 mm Hg), but also in inducing participants to comply with the regimen. These and many related questions of substantial importance must be answered before the value of community hypertension control programs is universally accepted. For this reason, the issue of the need for community hypertension control programs and the implementation of such programs must be viewed in total context of the epidemiology of hypertension, the potential impact of its control and the cost benefit of such control programs.

This paper briefly reviews (1) the epidemiology of hypertension; (2) the rationale and evidence supporting the need for initiating community hypertension control programs; and (3) the issues that must be carefully considered in planning and implementing such programs. Also presented is a simple mathematical model that my colleagues and I have developed for evaluation of the potential impact of community hypertension control programs.[9]

A Brief Review of the Epidemiology of Hypertension

Prevalence

Epidemiologic surveys[10-12] in the United States indicate a diastolic blood pressure of 90 mm Hg and above in 15% of the whites and 30% of the blacks. Frequency distributions of systolic and diastolic blood pressure in the adult population of the United States are depicted in Figures 1 and 2. As can be

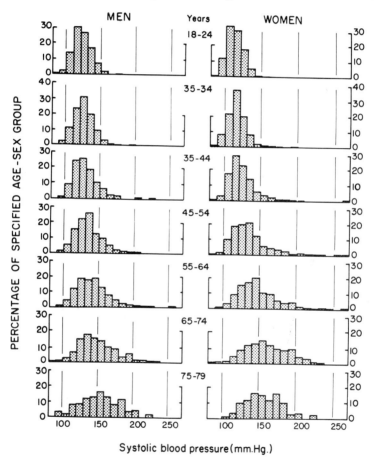

Fig. 1. Frequency distribution of systolic blood pressure by age and sex. United States adult population, National Health Survey 1960-1962.

630 N. O. BORHANI

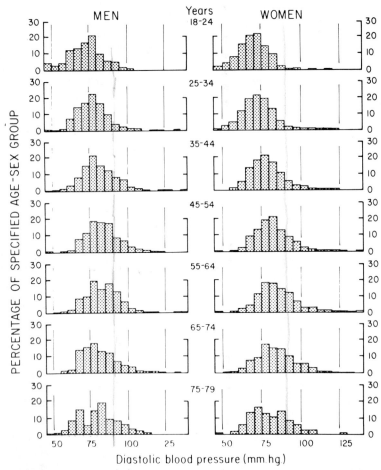

Fig. 2. Frequency distribution of diastolic blood pressure by age and sex.
United States adult population, National Health Survey 1960-1962.

seen, both systolic and diastolic blood pressures rise with age.
The frequency distributions of both assume a unimodal curve,
skewed to the right, and without any evidence of a clear
distinction between "normal" and "abnormal" levels. In other
words, there is no dividing line to separate low blood pressure
from high blood pressure. It should be emphasized that, as
pointed out by Sir George Pickering,[3,13] any consideration of
the course and natural history of elevated blood pressure in
terms of a dividing line is "fallacious." Arterial blood pressure is
a "biologic quantity" and "its adverse effects are related

numerically to it."[1][3] This well-known epidemiologic observation has a tremendous implication in planning and implementing community hypertension control programs. For, as demonstrated by actuarial data, mortality and morbidity increase proportionally with blood pressure even in the range not generally considered extreme by accepted clinical criteria.[2][8] Also, since blood pressure increases with age, any community hypertension control program should be designed according to the age composition of the target population; the yield in screening and the number of individuals eligible for referral, treatment and follow-up would depend upon the age composition of the target population.

In addition to age, the frequency distribution of blood pressure varies by sex and race. Table 1 shows that the percent

TABLE 1. Frequency Distribution at Various Critical Levels of Diastolic Blood Pressure, Adult Population of United States Aged 18-79 Years (National Health and Examination Survey 1960-62)

Whites						
Levels of Diastolic Blood Pressure mm Hg	Males		Females		Total	
	Number	Percent	Number	Percent	Number	Percent
115 and more	339	0.7	497	1.0	836	0.9
110 and more	582	1.2	688	1.3	1270	1.3
105 and more	1245	2.7	1304	2.5	2549	2.6
100 and more	2235	4.8	2436	4.8	4671	4.8
95 and more	4258	9.1	4255	8.3	8513	8.7
90 and over	7778	16.7	7505	14.7	15283	15.6
Less than 90	38782	83.3	43678	85.3	82460	84.4

Negroes						
Levels of Diastolic Blood Pressure mm Hg	Males		Females		Total	
	Number	Percent	Number	Percent	Number	Percent
115 and more	116	2.2	318	5.1	434	3.8
110 and more	248	4.8	417	6.7	665	5.8
105 and more	356	6.9	638	10.3	994	8.7
100 and more	538	10.4	881	14.2	1419	12.4
95 and more	1176	22.6	1338	21.5	2514	22.0
90 and over	1683	32.4	1779	28.6	3462	30.3
Less than 90	3513	67.6	4438	71.4	7951	69.7

distribution in any given level of blood pressure differs considerably between the two sexes and by race. For example, a diastolic blood pressure of 90 mm Hg and above is found in 14.7% of white females and 16.7% of white males. Corresponding percentages for blacks are 28.6 and 32.4.

The particular problem of blood pressure of blacks assumes added significance in planning and implementing community hypertension control programs. In addition to the National Health Survey, numerous clinical and epidemiologic studies have consistently shown an excess of elevated blood pressure in the black. Figure 3, including data from four such studies,

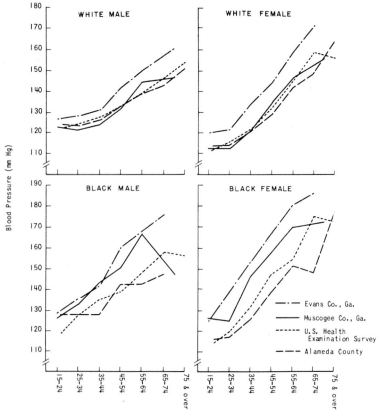

Fig. 3. Mean systolic blood pressure of four selected surveys by race, sex and age.

shows that for each age group the mean systolic blood pressure is higher for blacks than for whites. Prevalence data also indicate that complications of elevated blood pressure, such as hypertensive heart disease, have a higher frequency in blacks than in whites. Figure 4 presents data on the distribution of hypertensive heart disease by age, sex and race in the United States as reported by the National Health Survey. Again,

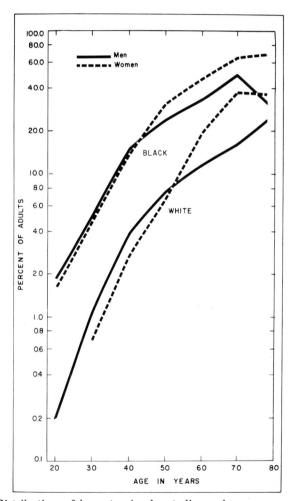

Fig. 4. Distribution of hypertensive heart disease by age, race and sex. United States adult population, National Health Survey 1960-1962.

hypertensive heart disease is more frequent in blacks, both males and females, than in whites. These data suggest that the course and natural history of diseases resulting from elevated blood pressure are perhaps different in blacks from those in whites. This particular inference from the available epidemiologic data should be considered seriously in planning and implementing community hypertension control programs.

Thus, the prevalence of hypertension depends upon age, sex and race. But the distribution of blood pressure is also known to be influenced by other socioeconomic, cultural, educational and occupational factors.[14] All of these factors must be considered in planning a community hypertension control program. Finally, the words "prevalence of hypertension" carry with them the implicit understanding that an arbitrary cutoff point (or dividing line) has been used in calculating this "prevalence." It should be emphasized, however, that for planning and implementing community hypertension control programs, such dividing lines do not mean that an artificial definition of hypertension will be used clinically. Rather, they reflect the implicit answer provided by administrators of community hypertension control programs to the crucial question of the pressure level at which one should begin treatment. As pointed out by Sir George Pickering, "The answer to this most important question can be a sterile exercise of great danger to the well-being of the patient, or it may be used constructively to further the patient's own interest. The latter should be the objective of every physician."[3] We feel it should also be the objective of every community hypertension control program.

Community hypertension control programs can use as a general guide the World Health Organization criteria of systolic blood pressure of 160 mm Hg or above and/or diastolic blood pressure of 95 mm Hg or above. On the basis of these criteria, the prevalence of hypertension among the adult population of the United States is estimated at 10%-15%. This would amount to more than 20 million American adults. More alarming than the sheer number is the fact that the elevated blood pressures in the majority of these people are either undetected, untreated or inadequately treated. Table 2 shows the estimated reservoir of people with elevated blood pressure that is undetected or untreated. These data, derived from three different studies, all

TABLE 2. Estimated Reservoir of Undetected and Untreated Individuals
With Elevated Blood Pressure

Characteristics of Populations Surveyed	Baldwin County Georgia - 1962 N = 3084	National Health Survey 1960 - 1962 N = 6672	Alameda County Calif. - 1966 N = 2495
% c̄ elev. BP ≥160 sys. ≥ 95 dia.	17.5%	15.2%	13.0%
% pop. on med. for hyp.	6.0%	6.5%	5.9%
% c̄ elev. BP on med. for hyp.	18.3%	23.2%	16.9%**
Total hyp. pop.* % unknown	630 (41.0%)	1214 (42.8%)	420** –
% of total hyp. pop. on med.	29.7%	35.7%	35.7%**
% of total hyp. "under control"	14.0%	16.3%	22.6%
% of those on med. "under control"	47.0%	45.6%	63.3%

* Total hyp. pop. = those with BP ≥160 systolic and/or 95 diastolic at time of survey plus those on medication for hypertension with survey pressures below those levels.

**In determining proportions on medication, etc., systolic level of 165 instead of 160 was used.

demonstrate the same phenomenon: not more than 23% of people with elevated blood pressure are on treatment, and of these, only about one half are considered to be under control. Here lies the challenge in planning and implementing community hypertension control programs.[14,15]

Hypertension as a Risk of Mortality

Approximately 70% of middle-aged deaths in the United States are from diseases associated with elevated blood pressure, such as hypertensive heart disease, congestive heart failure, renal failure, stroke and coronary artery disease.

Studies by life insurance companies provide some of the best data relating blood pressure and deaths. By far, the largest and most widely quoted body of data on mortality and elevated blood pressure levels is that published by the Build and Blood Pressure Study,[2] which covered the experience of 26 large life insurance companies under some 4 million policies issued to men and women from 1935 to 1953.[8] Among the most significant findings of the Build and Blood Pressure Study of the Society of Actuaries was that the rate of mortality increased proportionally with blood pressure level, even in the range not generally considered extreme by clinical criteria, and that mortality was lowest among persons with blood pressures distinctly below average. In other words, insofar as longevity is concerned ". . . average blood pressures are significantly higher than optimal blood pressures . . ."[8] In addition, data on mortality are consistent with the concept that arterial blood pressure is a biologic quantity and that ". . . its adverse effects are related numerically to it,"[13] and that within specified ranges of either systolic or diastolic blood pressure, there is a rise in mortality as the other pressure increases. Each of the measured blood pressure components (systolic or diastolic) appears to contribute to the risk of death, and both components interact positively with each other; thus, a given diastolic blood pressure at higher level of systolic blood pressure carries a greater risk of mortality than the same diastolic blood pressure at a lower level of systolic blood pressure.[2,8,16]

In addition to the information from actuarial studies, data accumulated in recent years from different prospective epidemiologic studies indicate a marked and consistent rise in death rate with increasing levels of systolic and/or diastolic blood pressure.[17-23] None of those reports, however, suggest a critical cutoff point, or threshold, or dividing line value of blood pressure that can be used as a predictor of mortality. They all confirm the concept that the level of blood pressure is indeed a continuous variable when it is considered as a risk of mortality. In other words, the higher the level of blood pressure, the greater the risk of death. The relationship is nonlinear, however, although the association between blood pressure and risk of mortality is a continuum. That is, the risk of death is much greater in the higher ranges of blood pressure than in the lower ranges. This epidemiologic observation is of significant importance in planning and implementing community hypertension control programs because, even though blood pressure influences the risk of mortality at all levels, priority for treatment should obviously be directed toward individuals with blood pressures in the higher range of the distribution. Such priorities will be dictated by limitations in financial and other resources of the community.

Hypertension as a Risk of Morbidity

In addition to its positive influence on the risk of mortality, the elevated blood pressure is known to be an important risk factor in the incidence of coronary heart disease, congestive heart failure, cerebrovascular and related diseases.[22-30] Figure 5 presents, based on the Framingham Study, the association between blood pressure and risk of an acute episode of coronary heart disease, in a 45-year-old man. All other prospective studies show a regular and marked increase in coronary heart disease with blood pressure, either systolic or diastolic. As with data on mortality, there is no apparent cutoff point or dividing line in any level of blood pressure above which people are at risk of developing coronary heart disease and below which they are free from it. It should be noted that according to the available evidence, the risk of developing coronary heart disease as associated with blood pressure is a relative risk, not absolute. That also has significant implications for hypertension control programs. In other words, this important finding will affect the size of the population considered to be at risk and the expected efficacy of treatment.

A relationship similar to that for coronary heart disease exists between the levels of blood pressure and incidence of cerebrovascular disease (ie, stroke). Although the positive association between high blood pressure and incidence of stroke is more dramatic than that of coronary heart disease and has been recognized clinically for many years, only a few population studies have been conducted to provide quantitative estimates of risk.[24,25,29] By and large, the risk of brain infarction and/or hemorrhage rises sharply with the corresponding increase in the level of blood pressure. In the Framingham Study Population,[24] for example, the risk of stroke was approximately five times as high in hypertensives (ie, systolic blood pressure of 160 mm Hg and over and/or diastolic blood pressure of 95 mm Hg and over) as in normotensives. In

PROBABILITY OF DEVELOPING CORONARY HEART DISEASE IN SIX YEARS
BY SYSTOLIC BLOOD PRESSURE, CHOLESTEROL, LEFT VENTRICULAR HYPERTROPHY
BY ECG, CIGARETTE SMOKING AND GLUCOSE INTOLERANCE
(THE FRAMINGHAM STUDY)

45 YEAR OLD MAN

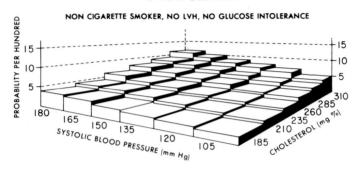

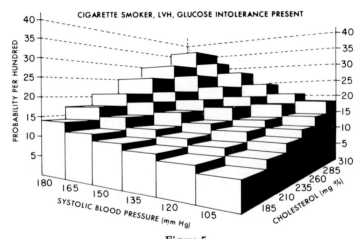

Figure 5.

terms of relative risk, the gradient of association between levels of blood pressure and incidence of stroke is much steeper for stroke than it is for myocardial infarction.

Evidence for Effectiveness of Antihypertensive Therapy

Thus far, we have briefly considered the magnitude of the problem of high blood pressure and the increased risk of mortality and morbidity associated with it. The available data reviewed to this point are based on nonexperimental observational surveys and cannot by themselves justify therapeutic regimens or community hypertension control programs. Therefore, we must now consider, from an epidemiologic point of view, the available evidence from controlled clinical trials regarding the effectiveness of antihypertensive therapy. Originally, three randomized trials of treatment of essential hypertension were reported, each demonstrating a significantly lower incidence of morbidity and mortality in the treated than in the untreated group.[4-7] One of these, the Veterans Administration Cooperative Study Group on Antihypertensive Agents,[4,5] was a prospective randomized double-blind therapeutic trial conducted among male veterans. The 523 patients selected for the study were randomized into placebo and active treatment groups. Active treatment consisted of a combination of hydrochlorothiazide, reserpine and hydrolazine. The risk of morbid events was substantially reduced in the actively treated group, indicating that judicious medical treatment of high blood pressure not only reduces the level of blood pressure but decreases the risk of morbidity and mortality associated with it. As might be expected, benefits of treatment were more dramatic and immediate at higher blood pressures than at moderate or mild pressures. As noted earlier it is an important epidemiologic observation that the risk of morbid events (and death) increases much more sharply in the higher ranges of blood pressure than in the lower ranges. The dramatic findings of the VA Cooperative Study Group, demonstrating a significant and immediate response to treatment among those whose diastolic blood pressures were in the range of 115-129 mm Hg, coupled with our epidemiologic knowledge of an increased risk in the higher ranges of blood pressure, emphasize the need for instituting appropriate measures and procedures so that all individuals with diastolic blood pressure of 115 mm Hg and over can be brought under treatment without delay. These observations also point up the importance of recognizing the time required for beneficial effect of antihypertensive therapy to become apparent in community programs. Generally, this time element depends upon the chosen level of blood pressure for entry into the program.

It should be pointed out that our epidemiologic estimates of risk in relation to blood pressure are based on *casual* readings of blood pressures obtained from observational surveys in *general* population groups. In contrast, our present knowledge of the effectiveness of the antihypertensive therapy is limited to data obtained from clinical trials among *selected* hypertensive individuals with *sustained* elevations in blood pressure. As important and as dramatic as the findings of the VA Study are, the question of their *general* applicability to the population at large in the community remains unanswered at present. Furthermore, we do not know the feasibility and the effectiveness of mass antihypertensive therapy directed toward those with moderate or mild elevations of blood pressure. Fortunately, several population-based epidemiologic studies are underway in the United States and Europe (eg, the U. S. National Heart and Lung Institute's Hypertension Detection and Follow-Up Program) that may, in a few years, shed some light on these important issues. We must await the completion of these studies and review their findings before making any definitive statements about most of the debatable and controversial questions that surround the issue of advocating mass community hypertension control programs.

Notwithstanding the controversial questions and uncertainties about the feasibility of mass antihypertensive therapy, community hypertension control programs are being developed throughout the United States. It is essential, therefore, that present knowledge of the epidemiology of high blood pressure be used in the orderly planning and implementation of these programs. The most important criterion to consider is to plan and implement a program that permits *accurate* assessment of intervention.

Epidemiologic Considerations in Planning Community Hypertension Control Programs

Considering the magnitude of the problem of high blood pressure, the need for feasible and effective community hypertension control programs is apparent. Since we do not have answers to all questions that surround the issue of the need for community hypertension control programs, we must recognize that planning and implementation of these programs represent a great challenge to the medical profession as a whole. We are dealing with a massive community health problem affecting 15%-20% of the adult population; a large number of those affected are not aware of their malady and have no symptoms to guide them in seeking medical care; they must be sought among the general and presumably healthy population. Yet, we do not have adequate scientific information to guide us in our efforts. We do not know what the level of blood pressure is above which the people in the community must be brought into the program and treated; we do not know what methods in behavioral sciences might best keep the general public motivated to join the program and stay with it; we do not know the reasons for compliance and noncompliance with a life-long therapeutic regimen. These and a host of many related questions need answers. Yet we must proceed without them in planning and implementing community programs to reduce the tragic toll of high blood pressure. This is, indeed, a challenge. Not only do we have to seek out asymptomatic hypertensives, but we must be prepared to provide them with adequate diagnostic and therapeutic facilities and, above all, to maintain among them a high level of motivation so that they will participate in the program and adhere to the therapeutic regimen. All these, in the absence of any clinical symptoms, are difficult to achieve. As indicated in the report of the Inter-Society Commission for Heart Disease Resources, " . . . solution to the problems of detection and maintenance of effective treatment for populations of hypertensives will require long-term planning and the allocation of sufficient funds . . . "[30] Further, high blood pressure as a *community* rather than an *individual* health problem is a relatively new concept that needs public acceptance. It is, therefore, necessary to articulate and define, in precise terms, the basic elements and requirements of a community hypertension control program in the very early stages of planning. Also, it is essential to establish, and adhere to, a rigorous design that permits accurate assessment of the effectiveness of these programs. As a minimum, the following steps must be taken in the design of a community hypertension control program: (1) definition of the population to be served, and identification of the high-risk groups in it; (2) definition of method and criteria for blood pressure measurements, referral mechanism, diagnostic procedures and the therapeutic regimen that will follow; these criteria must include provisions that guarantee completion of the referral to a final medical decision on disposition of the patient. Too often, referral procedures fall short of guaranteeing that the patient is seen by a qualified physician and his case is disposed of in the most appropriate manner; such a practice is a disservice to the patient and to the community; (3) definition of method and criteria for monitoring participants' compliance and surveillance for morbid events as well as adverse effects of the therapy; and (4) definition of criteria and method that will be used for the assessment of the effectiveness of the program; these criteria should be in terms of the program's cost-benefit and the indices of community health.

Whatever the design and the administrative structure, the role of practicing physicians in planning and implementing community hypertension control programs is crucial. Practicing physicians must be convinced, on scientific ground, of the need for the program and must be willing to participate. Other members of the health profession should also be approached and convinced of the need. They must all become familiar with the objectives, methods of implementation and means of evaluation of the program. Otherwise, they will not feel themselves part of the program and will not support it. Without such support, the program will fail. A program that fails in midstream is worse than no program at all; it will cause needless waste of community resources and will create credibility gaps by unfulfilled promises.

It should be noted that the role of practicing physician is singled out here because he, by tradition, has assumed the role of primary screener for hidden diseases in his patient. Every time a physician examines a patient, he is (or should be) screening for diseases other than those for which the patient has sought his counsel. Further, after successful completion of the original screening, the burden of diagnostic work-up, classification of the patient, treatment and follow-up falls, ordinarily, on the practicing physician. For all these reasons, the practicing physician's understanding of the program and his full cooperation are essential ingredients of a community hypertension control program. Practicing physicians' opinions must be sought before any effort to detect, diagnose and treat hypertensive individuals in a community has begun. This particular aspect of planning the program (securing of practicing physicians' full cooperation) may be easy or very difficult, depending upon the size and character of the community. But it is vital to the program.

Since the need for community hypertension control programs is acute and immediate, a strong argument can be mounted as to the necessity for establishing a categorical approach to the control of high blood pressure, separate from the current sources of medical care in the community. One of the most attractive arguments in favor of such a categorical approach is to cite the situation of the already overworked and overcommitted private practitioner. Should an already overburdened private physician now undertake to educate himself, in his scanty free time, in the vagaries of measurement of blood pressure, in newer details of diagnosis and in the complexities of the wide array of drugs, each with its own toxicity, pharmacological side effects and cost? Proponents of categorical approach answer this question in the negative and advocate planning and implementing a community program completely (or sometimes partially) outside the mainstream of American medicine. In doing so, the most important element of planning a community hypertension program could be bypassed. That is, the planners may feel no need to secure complete cooperation of practicing physicians for implementation of the program. This practice, although it may be administratively convenient, is detrimental to the community and should be avoided. All efforts instead should be directed toward the education of practicing physicians so that they can appreciate the need for the program, participate freely in its planning and cooperate fully in its implementation. Under the present system of medical care in the United States, and in terms of available resources and manpower, the establishment of an isolated categorical program for control of high blood pressure is unwise. It will not succeed and it will thus be detrimental to the community. Further, categorical programs do have definite problems that diminish their effectiveness despite their seeming utility. Not the least of these problems is the fact that any categorical program, regardless of how effectively it is administered, will tend to compartmentalize the patient and isolate him from the truly comprehensive health care system he needs most. Hence, we cannot yet determine precisely which administrative mechanism is most appropriate for a community hypertension control program, and the answer will not be easy to obtain. In the meantime, community hypertension programs should be incorporated into the available source(s) of medical care in the community, and the contribution of practicing physicians should be considered essential to successful implementation of the program. Therefore, either all of the physicians in the community, or an appropriately representative group of them, should participate in the original planning and in the discussion of questions important to the development of the program. Some of the most important items that should be considered at the very early phase of planning are the following questions:

Who Should Be Treated?

As mentioned earlier, the criteria for choosing crucial levels of blood pressure must be established early and adhered to throughout the program. At present, the World Health Organization criteria seem to be most feasible for early detection, treatment and follow-up programs in hypertension. These criteria are systolic blood pressure of 160 mm Hg or above and/or diastolic blood pressure of 95 mm Hg or above. Ideally, all patients who meet these criteria during the original screening should be rescreened at least on one (or perhaps two) subsequent occasions, to determine the lability of blood pressure and confirm the sustained elevation. The ideal goal for reduction in blood pressure of these individuals should be to bring their diastolic blood pressure down at least 10 mm Hg below the baseline (to 85 mm Hg or below). Obviously, if the baseline pressure chosen is around 100 mm Hg or above, and achievement of the original goal of bringing it down by 10 mm Hg to a level of 90 mm Hg (or above, as the case may be) has not produced untoward side effects, it would be desirable to push the therapeutic regimen further to an ultimate goal of 85 mm Hg. Since the relationship between blood pressure and risk of mortality and morbidity is a continuous one (ie, no cutoff point or threshold), it seems logical to lower the diastolic blood pressure as much as the patient can tolerate. It should be emphasized that there is no magic in the goal blood pressure level cited above (ie, diastolic blood pressure of 85 mm Hg). Actuarial data indicate very clearly that ". . . the blood pressures optimal for longevity are those below 110 mm Hg systolic and 70 mm Hg diastolic. . . ."[8] The crucial issues, therefore, are as follows: What is the level of blood pressure that requires treatment? What is the optimal goal blood pressure to be achieved for an individual patient in community hypertension control programs? Answers to those questions must await the completion of currently ongoing epidemiologic studies such as the NHLI's Hypertension Detection and Follow-up Program. In the meantime, medical judgment and judicious and careful observation and surveillance of the patient are essential for achieving an optimal goal blood pressure that does not harm the patient. That is the reason we believe that full participation of an informed practicing physician is essential to the success of community hypertension control programs.

Referral

Physicians practicing in the community should agree with the criteria and method adopted by the program for the disposition of newly discovered hypertensive patients who need care. Ordinarily, they may accept these patients into their private practice. If that is the arrangement, they must know in advance that they are required to follow these patients according to the terms of the protocol of the program. This point cannot be overemphasized. In some instances, physicians may participate in programs with other arrangements for delivery of needed care to patients who are discovered during screening (eg, a categorical antihypertension control program). Even in that situation, all elements of the program, including referral and follow-up mechanisms, should be discussed with private physicians, and their cooperation must be sought. It should be emphasized that screening for hypertension without prior development of a workable system for adequate comprehensive care is a *disservice* to the community and should be avoided.

Diagnostic Procedures

The big question always is, "How much of a work-up will be necessary for a hypertensive patient?" The acceptable level of "compromise" between an "ideal" work-up and a "minimum" work-up must be decided upon very early in planning the program. Physicians in the community who participate in the preliminary planning discussions must agree and adhere to the accepted level of work-up. In addition, the level of work-up should be flexible enough that the welfare and safety of the patient are not jeopardized by sheer economic efficiency. The welfare of the patient should always remain the guiding light for any administrative decision in planning community hypertension control programs. Obviously, the cost of the work-up — to the patient, to the program and to the community — must be considered seriously. Program staff and those who ultimately make these decisions must be familiar with current epidemiologic, clinical and pharmacologic data on hypertension, so that their decisions will be based on current scientific evidence rather than personal subjective experiences and feelings. By and large, a complete physical examination, including urinalysis, routine blood chemistries, chest x-ray and a 12-lead electrocardiogram will suffice in the preliminary work-up of a hypertensive patient. Tests such as hormone assays, rapid-sequence IVP and angiographic studies should be reserved for defined and specific purposes. Rigid and specific criteria for administering these tests must be established before the program begins and adhered to during the life of the program. Laboratory data that are "nice to have" should be sought only when there are specific clinical reasons for having them available for the welfare of the patient.

Reporting

There must be an effective mechanism for feedback of information to and from practicing physicians and leaders of the community. Physicians, in particular, should find it easy to report their observations on the program participants (most of whom are their patients) to the program administrators. Likewise, program staff must have at their disposal an agreed upon and accepted method of communicating their daily observation to practicing physicians. Both physicians and program staff can have a choice of completing, periodically, predesignated forms or questionnaires for transmission of needed information. Whatever the method, it should be discussed candidly with private physicians and others *before* the program gets underway. The procedure agreed upon should be faithfully followed.

Community Involvement

As recommended by the Inter-Society Commission for Heart Disease Resources,[30] any community program for control of high blood pressure must begin with an intensive and specific professional and public education aimed at securing the support of an informed community. All aspects of the program, benefits as well as potential adverse effects, must be explained to the public in specific terms, without creating fear or anxiety. It has been our experience that people appreciate being informed about the elements of a community health program that will require their participation. The whole process of public education, if it is done effectively, can pay handsome dividends in motivating the people to participate in the program and stay with it. Leaders in the medical profession (Medical Society and the specialty associations) should be consulted first and reminded of serious health hazards of uncontrolled hypertension. They should be reminded also of the uncertainties that exist at present about the "wisdom" of treating those with mild or moderate hypertension. At the same time, the medical profession should be consulted in earnest and be made aware of the recent evidence demanding systematic identification and treatment of those with severe hypertension. The medical profession should also be reminded that there are no cutoff points in the relationship between the level of blood pressure and risk of mortality and morbidity. Theoretically, at least, lowering any level of blood pressure should be beneficial to health. Nevertheless, the lack of scientific evidence for early detection and treatment of mild to moderate hypertensives should be stressed. These points are important to emphasize because our experience, and that of others, has shown that the success of a community hypertension control program depends, most of all, upon a candid, detached and objective appraisal of the scientific evidence available when the program is planned, not on what could (or should) prove true later on.

The public should be reminded that hypertension is not curable (except for proven cases of secondary hypertension) and requires continuous evaluation. Once the diagnosis of hypertension is established, the patient must be under medical surveillance for the rest of his life. The public must be made aware of the extreme importance of faithful adherence to the program and compliance with its medical regimen. The possible

N. O. BORHANI

and potential side effects of antihypertensive therapy should be explained to the public in its proper context; the reasons for these side effects and the methods of preventing and/or tolerating them should be explained fully before an "informed consent" for participation in the program is obtained. Since people fear the unknown most, the entire spectrum of expectations under a continuous antihypertensive regimen should be explained in precise terms to alleviate their fear. They should be assured that professional help will be available and accessible when needed.

Our experience has been that the leaders of the community and, in fact, all citizens are eager and enthusiastic about learning of and participating in the program. These people will contribute many good ideas for its implementation. Community leaders should be urged to learn as much as possible about the program and requested to explain its features to others in the community. In other words, the public education aspect of the program should aim at increasing the number of informed influential advocates of the program in the community. Our experience has shown the great importance of the knowledge and skill of informed civic leaders in reaching other people in the community, explaining the program's objectives to them and encouraging their participation. They should be used to the maximum. Their support is needed in the extremely difficult problem of persuading the asymptomatic individuals who feel well and believe themselves "healthy" that they must give life-long adherence to antihypertensive therapy.

Another important aspect of reaching community leaders and securing their support early in the planning stage is to guarantee orderly administration of the program and the highest possible rate of participation. For example, the leaders in industry and business can be asked to give "time off" to their employees to participate in the program. If these leaders are convinced of the value of the program, there would be little difficulty in their agreeing to such an arrangement. This will encourage participation in the program and will reduce non-compliance. Obviously, since every community has different organizations, groups and leaders, the method of planning must be tailored to the specific characteristics of each community. The basic principle of educating the public and facilitating participation in the program remains the same for all communities.

Other Activities

Implementation of a successful community hypertension control program involves, besides the items mentioned above, a series of important ancillary activities:

Training of personnel. Training programs must be concerned, most of all, with techniques of taking and recording blood pressure and the methods of interview. The administrators of community hypertension control programs should anticipate that, by and large, the majority of staff they recruit into the program will be inexperienced in the techniques of blood pressure measurement, interview and patient education, referral procedures and follow-up methods. Therefore, a wholesome and effective training program must be developed before the staff is recruited. The entire staff must go through all phases of the training program. Every member of the staff should be tested and certified, upon completion of the training program. This process of in-service training and certification should be repeated from time to time, perhaps at least once every year. An important point is that all staff members must be tested for eyesight and hearing. Staff who will be engaged in taking and recording blood pressure should be retested for hearing periodically, perhaps twice every year.

Well-trained interviewers are vital to the success of any community hypertension control program. Involvement of patients from the community depends very heavily upon the skill of the interviewers, who contact them first. Of course, the interviewers should understand and believe in the importance of the job they are performing. They must be convinced that they are helping the community maintain its health. The attitude of interviewers toward their job, and toward the program as a whole, will have a significant effect on the success of the program. A positive and cheerful attitude, coupled with training in techniques of interviewing and dealing with people, will enhance smooth and effective operation of the program.

In addition, the training curriculum should include items on the epidemiology of hypertension, in terms of its magnitude, hazards to health and the value and benefits of early detection and treatment. Obviously, the extent of such a training program depends upon the local situation and sophistication of the staff and cannot be generalized. In-service training of a staff for a community hypertension control program must be tailored to the needs of the staff and the special characteristics of the community.

Forms. Like other programs in community health a hypertension control program will require a series of forms designed to suit the *specific needs* of the program. They should be simple to administer and easy to interpret. Any program will be damaged by forms that are too complicated, too lengthy and too diffuse. All items to be incorporated into these forms must be scrutinized against the specific needs and objectives of the program. Exclude the merely "nice to have" and items designed for a "fishing expedition." Each form must have the sole purpose of serving orderly administration of the program in terms of intake, referral, follow-up and data retrieval for analysis and evaluation of the effectiveness of the program. As a minimum, each program should develop the following forms:

1. *Informed consent:* This form should very clearly and specifically make the nature of the program clear to the participant. Participants should be requested to sign it *only* after there is evidence they are fully informed of all aspects of the program.

2. *Baseline data:* These forms should include a minimum of sociodemographic information and relevant medical characteristics of participants in terms of blood pressure, height, weight, pulse rate and a brief history of the cardiovascular system.

3. *Screening data:* These forms should include the results of screening. The nature of the program will dictate the number and nature of these forms. They should be simple and short. It is advantageous to precode these forms so that the data can be processed immediately after intake.

4. *Referral data:* The referral form should be capable of identifying the disposition of those screened; it should be simple and specific.

5. *Diagnostic and therapeutic data:* These data should be recorded, as appropriate, in special forms and coded for processing immediately after intake. The form should be easy to manage by the physician and should be developed in consultation with those physicians who will have to complete it. Too

often, complicated forms are developed that will not be used by physicians in the clinic. This practice is too costly and detrimental to the program and should be avoided.

6. *Follow-up data:* Like the referral data form, this should be specific and to the point. Its main purpose is to identify the follow-up status of the participant, any end point (ie, death), side effects and other information relevant to the evaluation of the program.

7. *Miscellaneous data:* Depending upon the size of the program and other local characteristics, other forms such as laboratory form, notification of death form and release of information form may be developed. The important point to emphasize is that regardless of the number of forms, simplicity and utility must be the overriding principle in designing each form.

Evaluation

Although the evidence is now convincing that early detection and control of high blood pressure reduce mortality and morbidity, the effectiveness of such programs must be evaluated continuously and objectively. The concept of evaluation of effectiveness is fundamental to the control of high blood pressure itself. For example, in the United States with its large pool of undiagnosed and untreated hypertensives, the yield from screening would be large, possibly as high as 10%-15% of the adult population. Assuming that diagnostic work-up and treatment would follow these screening programs, a large burden would be placed on existing manpower, facilities and resources. Hence, before widespread community screening programs are initiated, it is necessary to determine whether community hypertension control programs would be beneficial in fostering community health and thus justify their cost.

There are, of course, different methods of evaluating any community health program and a hypertension control program is no exception. These programs could be, for example, evaluated on the basis of how many persons in the community were screened, how many were found to be hypertensive, how many were referred for further diagnostic work-up and/or treatment and many similar indices. It should be pointed out, however, that none of the above-mentioned indices is sufficient to evaluate objectively the true benefit, and cost effectiveness, of a community hypertension control program. In the final analysis, the most important objective of a community hypertension control program should be to achieve "a significant reduction in mortality and morbidity" that could be attributed to the program. For this reason, any evaluation program must, by necessity, be designed on epidemiologic principles and should be capable of following the cohort of population under observation over time and accurately assessing the effectiveness of the program. The end points that will be used for this assessment should be defined before the program begins. Also, the evaluation program should take into account the migration pattern of the cohort under observation, the compliance to the program and the rate of withdrawal.

Based on available epidemiologic data and by making some assumptions, we have developed a mathematical model[9] believed to be capable of evaluating the potential impact of a community hypertension control program. This model incorporates the parameters of status of hypertension in the community (eg, normotensives, new hypertensives and old hypertensives), the characteristics of the cohort under observation (eg, withdrawal from the program or death), specific end points (eg, death due to hypertension or any other cause), intervention and nonintervention stages and different patterns of migration. In constructing this mathematical model, we calculated the expected incidence of a specific end point (eg, mortality from all causes) among a cohort of white normotensive men aged 30-69 (with diastolic blood pressure of 87 mm Hg or less). With this rate used as a standard, we then compared the mortality experience of two hypothetical cohorts of hypertensive men, aged 30-69: one group left with uncontrolled hypertension, and the other with their elevated blood pressure brought under control. We then measured the effectiveness (impact) of the intervention program by comparing the mortality experience of the two cohorts. The methodology for, and the parameters used in, development of this model are reported elsewhere.[9] It should be noted, however, that we recognize two levels of impact of a hypertension control program, each of which can be calculated in mathematical terms. We define these two as follows: (1) *clinical impact*, to represent the percentage ratio of the difference between expected and observed cases of end points to the number of observed cases in the group with elevated blood pressure, as determined at the original screening program; (2) *community impact*, to represent the percentage ratio of the same difference to the total number of observed cases in the total population of the cohort under observation, irrespective of the level of their blood pressure at the time of original screening. A detailed description of these terms and their application to assessment of the effectiveness of a community hypertension control program is reported elsewhere.[16]

Conclusion

Community impact of a hypertension control program can be measured in terms of either the impact of the program on total mortality (ie, mortality from all causes) or the impact upon mortality related specifically to high blood pressure. Figures 6 and 7 represent the results of the application of our model to a hypothetical community (10,000 white men aged 30-69 undergoing a hypertension control program). Figure 6 demonstrates the community impact of a successful hypertension control program in terms of the effect of the program on total mortality in the community. Figure 7 presents community impact in terms of deaths due to hypertension-related causes. Both figures consider different rates of migration and adherence to the program. It can be seen that if the assumptions underlying the construction of this model are valid, the potential community impact of a successful hypertension control program would be a reduction of at least 30% in total mortality and a reduction of approximately 50% in deaths related to hypertension over a ten-year period. Obviously, at this time, we can only speculate on the utility of this model, since it has not as yet been tested in an actual community program. Nevertheless, these data indicate that a community hypertension control program can be evaluated objectively in terms of its potential impact on the health of the community. Evaluation is possible and the idea should be pursued.

Clinical impact of a successful community hypertension control program denotes reduction in mortality (from all causes

Annual Percentage Reduction In Death Rates Due to All Causes
As a Result of Hypertension Intervention (Community Impact) Under
Two Assumptions of Follow-Up and Two Migration Patterns

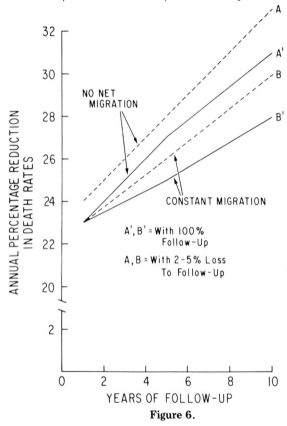

Figure 6.

Annual Percentage Reduction in Death Rates Due to
Hypertension-Related Causes as a Result of
Hypertension Intervention (Community Impact) Under
Two Assumptions of Follow-Up and Two Migration Patterns

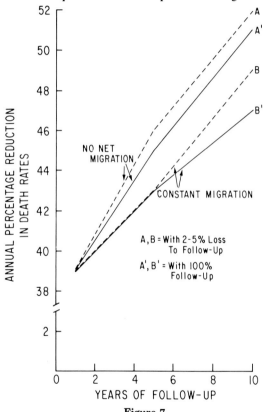

Figure 7.

or hypertension-related causes) only among hypertensive individuals discovered at the time of the original screening. The results obtained in the application of our model to the same hypothetical population, in terms of determining the clinical impact of the program, demonstrate that at the end of a ten-year period the clinical impact of a successful program is about 50% reduction in total mortality among hypertensive individuals.

Obviously, if community hypertension control programs have a success anywhere near what we found by application of our model to a hypothetical community of 10,000 white men, justification of such community health programs in terms of impact on community health versus costs would be less difficult than hitherto anticipated.

Finally, we believe one of the most important aspects of our findings in applying our model to a hypothetical community of 10,000 men is that the migration pattern of people apparently has only a minor effect on the evaluation of the impact. This finding, if it proves to be true, has a very important and significant implication in planning and implementing community hypertension control programs. It is very difficult, if not impossible, to monitor people's movement in a free society, not to mention the extreme cost of such monitoring. Our data thus far indicate that the impact of a hypertension control program is affected very little by the pattern of migration, as can be seen from Figures 6 and 7. If that proves to be true, there could be a significant reduction in the cost of community hypertension control programs and a significant increase in their acceptability by the people whose cooperation and participation we seek.

References

1. *Mortality Trends for Leading Causes of Death.* United States, 1950-69. Vital and Health Statistics, Series 20, No. 16. U. S. Dept. of Health, Education, and Welfare.
2. *Society of Actuaries Data on Build and Blood Pressures Study, Vol. 1.* Chicago:Society of Actuaries, 1959.
3. Pickering, G.: Hypertension: Definition, natural histories, and consequences. In Laragh, J. E. (ed.): *Hypertension Manual.* New York:York Medical Books, 1973.
4. Effects of treatment on morbidity in hypertension: Results in patients with diastolic blood pressure averaging 115 mm Hg. V-A Cooperative Study. *JAMA* 262:1028, 1967.

5. Effects of treatment on morbidity in hypertension: Results in patients with diastolic blood pressure averaging 90-114 mm Hg. V-A Cooperative Study. *JAMA*, 213:1143, 1970.

6. Hamilton, M.: *Selection of Patients for Antihypertensive Therapy, Principles and Practice*. Gross, F. (ed.). New York:Springer-Verlag, Inc., 1966, pp. 196-211.

7. Wolff, W. and Linderman, R. D.: Effects of treatment in hypertension. Results of a controlled study. *J. Chronic Dis.*, 19:227-240, 1966.

8. Lew, E. A.: High blood pressure, other risk factors and longevity, the insurance view point. In Laragh, J. H. (ed.): *Hypertension Manual*. New York:York Medical Books, 1973.

9. Borhani, N. O., Franti, C. E. and Kraus, J. F.: An epidemiological model for evaluating community and clinical impact of hypertension intervention programs. Submitted for publication.

10. *Blood Pressure of Adults, by Race and Area*. United States 1960-62: Report of the National Center for Health Statistics, Series 11, No. 5, 1964.

11. *Blood Pressure of Adults by Age and Sex*. United States 1960-62: Report of the National Center for Health Statistics. Series 11, No. 4, 1964.

12. *Hypertension and Hypertensive Heart Disease in Adults*. United States 1960-1962. Report of the National Center for Health Statistics, Series 11, No. 13, 1966.

13. Pickering, G.: *High Blood Pressure*. New York:Grune and Stratton, Inc., 1968.

14. Borhani, N. O.: *The Alameda County Blood Pressure Study*. A Monograph. Berkeley, California:U.C. Press, 1968.

15. Wilber, J. A. and Barrow, J. G.: Hypertension. A community problem. In Laragh, J. H. (ed.): *Hypertension Manual*. New York:York Medical Books, 1973.

16. Borhani, N. O., Labarthe, D., Remington, R. et al: The control of elevated blood pressure in the community — An epidemiologic perspective. *Heart and Lung*, 3:477-488, 1974.

17. Borhani, N. O. (ed.): *Medical Basis for Comprehensive Community Hypertension Control Programs*. DHEW Publication No. (HRA) 74-3800, Government Printing Office, 1974.

18. Kannel, W.: Some factors affecting morbidity and mortality in hypertension. *Milbank Mem. Fund Quart.*, 74:116, 1969.

19. Stamler, J., Stamler, R. and Pullman, T. (eds.): *The Epidemiology of Hypertension*. New York:Grune and Stratton, Inc., 1967.

20. Stamler, J.: *On the Natural History and Epidemiology of Hypertension*. Proceedings of the Prague Symposium. Prague:State Medical Publishing House, 1969.

21. Borhani, N. O.: Prevention at the community level of mortality and morbidity associated with hypertension. *Heart and Lung*, 1:384-393, 1972.

22. Borhani, N. O., Hechter, H H. and Breslow, L.: Report of a ten-year follow-up study of the San Francisco longshoremen. *J. Chronic Dis.*,

16:1251, 1963.
23. Borhani, N. O.: Magnitude of the problem of cardiovascular-renal diseases. In Lilienfeld, A. (ed.): *Chronic Disease and Public Health.* Baltimore, Md.:The Johns Hopkins Press, 1966.
24. Kannel, W.: Epidemiologic assessment of the role of blood pressure in stroke. *JAMA,* 214:301, 1970.
25. Chapman, J.: Epidemiology of vascular lesions affecting the central nervous system. *Amer. J. Pub. Health,* 56:191, 1966.
26. Cassel, J. C.: Evans County cardiovascular and cerebrovascular epidemiologic study. *Arch. Intern. Med.,* 128:887-889, 1971.
27. Stamler, J.: *Lectures in Preventive Cardiology.* New York:Grune and Stratton, Inc., 1967.
28. Primary prevention of the atherosclerotic diseases. Report of Inter-Society Commission for Heart Disease Resources. *Circulation,* 42:A-55, 1970.
29. Kannel, W. and Dawber, T.: Vascular disease of the brain — epidemiologic aspects. *Amer. J. Public Health,* 55:1355-1366, 1965.
30. Guidelines for the detection, diagnosis, and management of hypertensive populations. Report of Inter-Society Commission for Heart Disease Resources. *Circulation,* 44:A-263, 1971.

Discussion

Dr. Stamler: I would like to open the discussion with a reminder to everyone of the very fine address that Dr. Oglesby Paul gave at the Tenth Anniversary of the Council on Epidemiology of the American Heart Association, in which he urged all of us in epidemiology to be a little bolder. I would also like to open my remarks by pointing out what Dr. Theodore Cooper said here in the first session about the need to emphasize five areas including (1) the prevention of disease, (2) systems reform for improvement in the financing of health care and (3) assurance of quality. I make these points to emphasize that data are available from the VA controlled field trials unequivocally demonstrating the efficacy of therapy in men with average diastolic blood pressures 105 and above. There must be conservatively 2 million such people in the United States. Whatever the judgmental aspects on beginning antihypertensive drug treatment for those in the 90-104 range in relation to such factors as age, sex, presence of other risk factors and target organ damage, the group with diastolic pressures of 105 and above itself presents a huge, immediate and unequivocal health challenge not requiring further trials, but rather requiring getting on with the job of care and learning how to do it properly through the proper evaluation of ongoing care programs, as distinct from further trials. The urgency of this is not only in regard to quality performance, it is also in terms of the priorities in our country, in which we professionals should assume big responsibilities, priorities which are a little out of order, when $1 billion is available for dialysis, but only $2 or $4 million is available for hypertension education, not to mention comparative priorities between health and other budget categories (space, highways, defense, for example). As far as I can determine, next to nothing is available for hypertension programming of the type we are talking about at this symposium.

Dr. Sackett: At this morning's session we were considering medical versus surgical therapy for hypertension. We were unanimous in condemning any attempt to justify surgery because of the absence of proper randomized clinical trials. We were impressed by the contrast between the effort, enthusiasm and dedication of the surgical workers (which were certainly great and certainly admirable) and the evidence which they were able to present (which was inadequate). I think that we now have been asked to accept similarly unproven maneuvers for making physicians treat hypertension and for making patients take their medication. The issue here is not efficacy; it is delivery. It is even more surprising to be urged to go ahead now when we recognize that randomized clinical trials to answer some of these questions, albeit not all of them, are already underway and are not yet completed. I think that these randomized clinical trials are going to be as surprising to us as were the trials for coronary care units and for aorto-coronary bypass grafting. For example, we are currently completing Phase I of a randomized clinical trial of clinical strategies for attempting to improve compliance with antihypertensive therapy. Our work, as well as the work of others who have looked very carefully at teaching patients about their disease and its treatment, suggests that it has no effect upon improving compliance with antihypertensive therapy. I think that we should be cautioning against going into community-wide screen-

ing programs, until we have these answers, because I think that
we otherwise will have a substantial price to pay in terms of
credibility and ultimate success.*

Dr. Borhani: I agree with that. I was talking specifically in
terms of mild and moderate hypertension and not the categories
that Dr. Freis' data showed unequivocally that you must treat
and if you don't treat them they will die of stroke. As
epidemiologists, we have an obligation to our society, to our
own colleagues, to ourselves, to do something to see to it that
this most important major public health problem of our time is
approached properly, so that 10 or 20 years from now, we will
not regret it.

Dr. Kannel: I just want to comment with respect to what
Dr. Stamler said. I would like to reinforce the notion that we
have a very serious deficiency in dealing effectively with
hypertension, particularly in regard to the physician's role in
this problem. Surely, we need controlled trials in order to see
how best to implement effective programs in the community.
But it has been shown, it seems to me, unequivocally, that
severe hypertensive patients live longer and develop fewer
cardiovascular sequelae when treated. It is a great pity to find in
a city, such as Framingham, Massachusetts, that only 50% of
people with systolic pressures over 200 mm Hg are receiving
medicine. Also, Dr. Schoenberger has pointed out that while
one half of the hypertensive patient population is "undetected"
in the community, 75% of these people have had their blood
pressures taken. Therefore, the problem isn't undetected blood
pressure elevations but rather it is the fact that the physician is
unwilling to perceive these elevated blood pressures as life-
threatening conditions. I think that this is a very serious
problem that deserves our attention. We can forget about the
mild hypertension, in which the skeptical may question the
need for treatment, but how about the severe hypertensive
patients? A recent survey found about 80% of people entering
teaching hospitals with hypertension leave the hospital with the
hypertension, without the diagnosis being made and with no
treatment given. I think that this is a shame.

---

*Sackett, D.L.: Screening for disease: Cardiovascular diseases. *Lancet*,
2:1189-1191, 1974.

Dr. Borhani: The main issue is that we are getting involved with medical care delivery; we are getting into new public health programs, which have no precedents in our society in terms of disease control. We don't know anything about the ways and methods that will best serve the patient population. This is the problem which I think that we, as epidemiologists, have to be concerned with. This does not mean that we should relax our efforts in terms of seeing to it that physicians do indeed treat people who have diastolic blood pressures of 115 mm Hg and over.

The Hypertension Detection and Follow-up Program

The Steering Committee*

The National Institutes of Health have recently initiated a major study on the ability of antihypertensive agents to reduce morbidity and mortality in the general population. The purpose of this report is to review the developments which led up to this program, to outline its purpose and scope and to report some early findings of this community effort, known as the Hypertension Detection and Follow-up Program.

During the 1950s and 1960s prospective studies of entire populations, subpopulations or probability samples from such populations were instituted at Framingham,[1] Albany,[2] Los Angeles,[3] Tecumseh,[4] Chicago[5] and Minneapolis.[6] These studies identified elevated arterial blood pressure as a prominent risk factor for morbidity and mortality from cardiovascular disease. However, they were not designed to determine whether reduction of blood pressure was accompanied by reduction of disease and death.

In 1967 and 1970, two important papers appeared summarizing the studies done with the U. S. Veterans Administration by a cooperative group led by Dr. Edward Freis. These papers reported a carefully controlled randomized clinical trial of antihypertensive agents. The initial paper, appearing in 1967, summarized the results for patients with mean outpatient diastolic pressures at entry between 115 and 129 mm Hg. The beneficial effect of therapy was so marked that the study originally designed to continue for five years was concluded for these patients after an average of only 20.7 months of therapy

---

*Prepared on behalf of the Steering Committee by H. G. Langford, M.D., J. Payne, M.D., R. D. Remington, Ph.D. and J. Stamler, M.D.

for the active drug group and 15.7 months for the placebo patients (who had a briefer period of follow-up because of the larger number of terminating events).[7] In 1970, the results were reported for the remainder of the patients, with initial diastolic blood pressures averaging 90 through 114 mm Hg. Again, a highly significant reduction in morbid events occurred in the treated group.[8]

It is necessary to emphasize several aspects of the design of the VA trial, for the need for another program springs from what was and what was not answered by that study.

The VA study determined the effect of therapy on selected patients, ie, people who had presented themselves to the VA for some reason. Patients not likely to continue therapy were ruled out as far as possible. Patients had to maintain a blood pressure of 90 mm Hg diastolic or above from the fourth through the sixth day of hospitalization and also have a pressure of 90 mm Hg diastolic or above when they appeared at the clinic at the time therapy was initiated. Women were not represented, and young adults were not well represented in the study. This indicates that the trial involved patients of more than average reliability and those who were probably sicker than comparable individuals selected by casual blood pressure alone.

Two aspects of the results deserve further attention. First, although there was a significant reduction of terminating events in the subgroup with initial diastolic pressures of 105 to 114 and in the total group of treated patients, the relative reduction was somewhat less and not statistically significant in those with pressures of 90-104. Second, there was not a significant reduction in the rate of occurrence of myocardial infarction. The trend was toward improvement, at least in regard to sudden death and fatal myocardial infarction. A larger sample or a longer period of observation might have provided a definite answer. Therefore, the approaches described above left unanswered several questions:

1. Can hypertensives in an entire community be identified, brought under modern pharmacological management and kept under such management?
2. Will intervention on hypertension identified in the population of the community at large reduce the occurrence of associated disease and death?

3. Does therapeutic efficacy exceed toxicity in the mild hypertensive and justify long-term treatment?
4. Is pharmacologic control of elevated blood pressure effective in the young adult? In the female?
5. Will the occurrence of myocardial infarction and coronary death be decreased by antihypertensive therapy?

In October 1970, the National Heart and Lung Institute of the National Institutes of Health appointed a special panel to consider the implications for public health of the epidemiologic and therapeutic studies discussed above and to consider whether any additional clinical trials were needed in hypertension. It recommended that "the first priority need is to determine the effectiveness of antihypertensive therapy in reducing morbidity and mortality from hypertension in the general population. Such studies should include both sexes, all races in a community, and preferably younger as well as the middle-age ranges. Such a study would not have a placebo group, but could allow randomization of subjects for comparison of optimum drug regimens versus the customary medical care in the community."

A new investigative approach was needed to implement these guidelines. This approach would attempt to study hypertensive disease in the community and to alter its course and consequences, while providing for simultaneous comparison observations for continuous program evaluation. This approach has several implications for study design:

1. There must be nearly complete case finding in the community.
2. There can be few, if any, exclusions.
3. Though randomization is essential, the use of placebos and therefore blind technique is not possible.
4. Participants on whom the study is not systematically intervening long term must be observed, but as unobtrusively as possible. Their status must be known, but not altered except as dictated by ethical concern for the welfare of the severe hypertensive.
5. The lack of blindness requires reliance on "harder" end points, such as mortality from all causes — in any case a key, or *the* key, end point.

    6. Large numbers of patients are required.

    7. A multiclinic design is essential to obtain the large numbers which must be followed.

The Hypertension Detection and Follow-up Program (HDFP) is the first example of the implementation of this approach. In 1971 and 1972, financial awards were made by the NHLI to 14 clinical centers, a coordinating center, a central biochemistry laboratory, and an electrocardiogram interpretation center (see Appendix).

The populations in the 30-69 age range screened in the 14 clinical centers were either all residents in a few census tracts, probability samples of entire cities or of groups of census tracts, or all employees in selected industries.

The primary hypothesis to be tested in this program is whether total mortality over five years of follow-up among a Stepped Care group (intensively treated by the 14 research centers) could be significantly reduced over that of a Regular Care group. To determine the sample size necessary to test this primary hypothesis several estimates had to be made.

First, the age and sex composition of the population to be screened was estimated using U. S. Census data. The race composition was estimated using demographic data from the nine initial clinical centers. Next, using results of the National Health Examination Survey, the expected number and age-sex-race composition of the hypertensive group to be identified from the population to be screened was estimated. Mortality results from the national cooperative Pooling Project, stratified by five-year age groups and initial diastolic blood pressure, were then applied to the expected hypertensive population in the HDFP. The data from the Pooling Project were for white males only. Assumptions had to be made concerning expected mortality for the hypertensives of the other sex-race groups in the HDFP. From these results it was further estimated, based on Pooling Project and Framingham data, that mortality among the Stepped Care group could perhaps be reduced by 40% over the Regular Care group if the diastolic blood pressure of the Stepped Care group could be reduced long term to 90 mm Hg or less, or at least 10 mm Hg, whichever was lower.

It was determined that the null hypothesis of no difference in mortality between the two groups should be tested against an alternative hypothesis of a 40% reduction in mortality among the Stepped Care group compared with the Regular Care group.

Sample size was determined using the result above together with a Type I error of 0.05 and a Type II error of 0.10 (ie, a power of 90% of detecting a difference in mortality of 40% or greater), considering that the follow-up of the Stepped and Regular Care groups would be five years in duration. Furthermore, it was estimated that over the five years of follow-up, no more than 50% of the Stepped Care group would drop out of the program in the following pattern: 25% dropout in the first year, 10% in the second year and 5% in each of the last three years.

These assumptions and estimations yielded a sample size of 10,500 hypertensives, age 30-69 — 5,250 randomized to Stepped Care and 5,250 randomized to Regular Care. One hundred and seventy thousand individuals were screened in order to enroll this required number. A two-stage screening process was used. An interviewer personally contacted the individual household and constructed a census roster of everyone residing in the household. (In Chicago, where industries were used, the contact was made at the place of employment.) Following completion of the household enumeration form, individuals within the target age range who were at home at that time were screened for blood pressure elevation. Three readings were taken in the sitting position with a conventional mercury manometer. If the average fifth phase (disappearance of sound) diastolic pressure on the second and third readings was 95 mm Hg or over, the individual was invited to attend, within 48 hours if possible, a special clinical center for a secondary blood pressure screening. For individuals within the age range but not at home at the time of initial contact, appointments for screening were made before the interviewer left. A major effort was made to screen everyone in the enumerated age-eligible target group, and a 95% success rate overall was obtained. At the second stage screen in the clinic, four blood pressure readings were taken, again in the sitting position. This time the first and third readings were made with the conventional sphygmomanometer, and the second and fourth were made with the Hawksley random zero device, which concealed the true zero point on the scale until after the reading. It was believed essential to have some mechanism to avoid the biases inherent in standard blood pressure determination. All persons taking blood pressures were carefully trained and had to pass an examination. However, it was felt that even careful training would not completely eliminate bias, especially at the decision points.

When the pressure with the random zero device averaged 90 mm Hg or above for the two readings, the individual was considered hypertensive for the purpose of the program. As anticipated, this two-stage screen reduced the yield of hypertension below that produced by one single blood pressure determination.

For individuals considered hypertensive, further health history information was taken, blood and urine specimens collected, and ECGs and chest x-rays completed. An unopened randomization envelope was drawn and attached to the data recording form. This sealed envelope contained instructions for assignment of the participant either to his usual sources of care or to our Program Stepped Care group. A second clinic visit was scheduled within a week, repeat blood and urine specimens were collected, further baseline blood pressures were measured, a physical examination was administered and the randomization envelope was opened. Randomization was stratified by the clinical center and by the level of diastolic blood pressure at the first clinic visit into three strata: 90-104, 105-114 and 115 or over. Individuals assigned to regular care were referred to their personal physician for management; if no such physician was identified, assistance was provided in finding a source of care. For those referred to their usual source of care who showed target organ damage or severe elevation of blood pressure (115 mm Hg diastolic or higher), substantial efforts were made to insure that an initial contact for care was made. In very severe cases, treatment was begun at the special care center while the permanent source of care was being sought for those assigned to the Regular Care group.

A trial of the therapeutic effect of antihypertensive drugs may be designed in two ways. Either a fixed dose may be used or the blood pressure may be reduced to a predetermined level. The HDFP has chosen the second approach. Those who enter with a diastolic pressure of 100 mm Hg or above have a goal blood pressure of 90 mm Hg. Our concept of the goal blood pressure is that we must attempt to get the pressure at least that low. If it can be held lower without distressing side effects, we feel that we should gratefully accept this greater lowering, for the prospective studies show that the effect of blood pressure on mortality is graded and continuous from well below 80 mm Hg.

If the participant enters with pressure between 90 and 100, a 10 mm Hg drop is the goal.

Individuals participating in the active treatment program given by our special facilities are called Stepped Care participants, for the mode of blood pressure control is to adjust therapy progressively in stepwise fashion until goal blood pressure is obtained. Those therapy steps are as follows:

1. Chlorthalidone in the dosage range 50 mg on alternate days to 100 mg daily.
2. Chlorthalidone 50-100 mg, reserpine 0.25 mg, once daily.
3. Add hydralazine (10 mg three times a day to 50 mg four times a day).
4. Chlorthalidone plus hydralazine plus guanethidine. Chlorthalidone (50 mg three times daily to 50 mg four times daily). Guanethidine (10 mg daily to 200 mg daily).

Stepped Care participants proceed through these steps in accordance with their blood pressure response. The aim is to bring each participant's pressure to goal as rapidly and safely as feasible and with as little drug as possible. At each step except the last, a maximum period of time a participant can remain at that step without reaching goal is specified. Exceptions to the basic plan are provided for because of history (eg, of depression), toxicity or specific side reactions. All Stepped Care participants are seen at a frequency determined by their clinical status, but mandatory visits are scheduled every four months.

All the Stepped Care and Regular Care participants are to be seen at annual intervals. The present plans call for follow-up visits after one and three years, consisting of a home interview. The two, four and five year contacts will include a clinical examination.

The goal of enrolling 10,500 participants was attained in 15 months. The majority of the active Stepped Care participants have been brought to goal blood pressure by the first or second steps of therapy. Many of the patients are still proceeding through the steps, ie, have not had their medicines increased to the full permissible amount. Nevertheless, from 50% to 80% of the Stepped Care patients attending the Program facilities are at goal blood pressure within four months of therapy. From 80% to 94% of individuals randomized to Stepped Care are keeping appointments faithfully.

Therefore, at this stage it seems reasonable to conclude that the HDFP has an excellent chance of determining if an all-out community attack on hypertension can significantly improve cardiovascular and all-cause morbidity and mortality in persons with hypertension in the United States.

This has an important impact on decisions concerning the level of blood pressure for which pharmacologic treatment is likely to be beneficial as well as the best means of carrying out a community attack on hypertension.

References

1. The Framingham Study. Section 3, Kannel, W. B. and Gorden, T. (eds.). DHEW Publications NO (NIH) 74-599, 1974, U. S. Government Printing Office, Washington, D. C.
2. Doyle, J. T.: Risk factors in coronary heart disease. *New York J. Med.*, 63:1317, 1963.
3. Chapman, J. M. and Massey, F. J.: The interrelationship of serum cholesterol, hypertension, body weight, and risk of coronary disease: Results of the first ten years follow-up in the Los Angeles Heart Study. *J. Chronic Dis.*, 17:933, 1964.
4. Epstein, F. H., Ostrander, L. D., Jr., Johnson, B. C. et al: Epidemiological studies of cardiovascular disease in a total community — Tecumseh, Michigan. *Ann. Intern. Med.*, 62:1170, 1965.
5. Stamler, J., Lindberg, H. A., Berkson, D. M. et al: Prevalence and incidence of coronary heart disease in strata of the labor force of a Chicago industrial corporation. *J. Chronic Dis.*, 11:405-420, 1960.
6. Keys, A., Taylor, H. L., Blackburn, H. et al: Coronary heart disease among Minnesota business and professional men followed fifteen years. *Circulation*, 28:381, 1963.
7. Effects of treatment on morbidity in hypertension: Results in patients with diastolic blood pressures averaging 115 through 129 mm Hg. Veterans Administration Cooperative Study Group on Antihypertensive Agents. *JAMA*, 202:1028-1034, 1967.
8. Effects of treatment on morbidity in hypertension: Results in patients with diastolic pressures averaging 90 through 114 mm Hg. *JAMA*, 213:1143-1152, 1970.

Appendix

Policy Advisory Board
Hypertension Detection and Follow-Up Program

Alvin P. Shapiro, M.D. (Chairman)
Professor of Medicine
University of Pittsburgh
School of Medicine
M-252 Scaife Hall
Pittsburgh, Pennsylvania 15213
(412) 624-2486

Glenn E. Bartsch, Ph.D.
Biometry Division
School of Public Health
1325 Mayo Memorial Building
Minneapolis, Minnesota 55455
(612) 373-8038

Kenneth G. Berge, M.D.
Consultant in Medicine
Mayo Clinic, East 8
200 First Street, S.W.
Rochester, Minnesota 55901
(507) 282-2511

Edward D. Frohlich, M.D.
Professor of Medicine
Health Sciences Center
University of Oklahoma
800 N.E. 13th Street
Oklahoma City, Oklahoma 73104
(405) 271-4736

Richard H. Gadsden, Ph.D.
Professor of Biochemistry and
    Clinical Pathology
Medical University of South Carolina
80 Barre Street
Charleston, South Carolina 29401
(803) 792-3237

Edward W. Hawthorne, M.D.
Department of Physiology and Biophysics
Howard University College of Medicine
520 W Street, N.W., Room 2414
Washington, D. C. 20001
(202) 636-6330

David L. Sackett, M.D.
Department of Clinical Epidemiology
    and Biostatistics
McMaster University Medical Center
1400 Main Street West, Room 2-738
Hamilton 16, Ontario, Canada
(416) 525-9140 x2420

Joseph A. Wilber, M.D.
Director, Adult Health Section
Georgia Department of Public Health
618 Ponce de Leon, N.E.
Atlanta, Georgia 30334
(404) 894-5122

The Hypertension Detection Follow-Up Program is a collaborative study supported by contracts from the National Heart and Lung Institute. Key centers and selected senior staff members of the program include the following:

Clinical Centers
    Atlanta, Ga.
        E. Tuttle, M.D., N. Shulman, M.D., S. Heymsfield, M.D.
    Baltimore, Md.
        G. Entwisle, M.D., A. Apostolides, Ph.D.
    Birmingham, Ala.
        A. Oberman, M.D., H. W. Schnaper, M.D.

Boston, Mass.
   E. H. Kass, M.D., Ph.D., J. O. Taylor, M.D., B. F. Polk, M.D.
Chicago, Ill.
   J. Stamler, M.D., R. Stamler, M. H., F. C. Gosch, M.D.
Davis, Calif.
   N. O. Borhani, M.D., D. T. Mason, M.D.
East Lansing, Mich.
   S. A. Daugherty, M.D., Ph.D., R. M. Daugherty, M.D., Ph.D.
Evans County, Ga.
   C. G. Hames, M.D., I. Krishan, M.D.
Georgetown, Washington, D. C.
   F. A. Finnerty, M.D.
Los Angeles, Calif.
   M. H. Maxwell, M.D., R. Detels, M.D.
Minneapolis, Minn.
   R. Berman, M.D., S. Fetcher, Ph.D.
New York, N. Y.
   M. D. Blaufox, M.D., S. Wasserthiel, Ph.D.
Salt Lake City, Utah
   C. H. Castle, M.D.

Coordinating Center

Houston, Tex.
   M. Hawkins, Ph.D., D. Curb, M.D., G. Cutler, Ph.D.

ECG Center

Minneapolis, Minn.
   R. Prineas, M.D.

Laboratory Center
Chicago, Ill.
   K. Schneider, M.D.

National Heart and Lung Institute staff

Bethesda, Md.
   W. Zukel, M.D., G. Payne, M.D., M. Halperin, Ph.D.

Subject Index